# ESSENTIALS OF
# *Athletic Injury Management*

## *Eighth Edition*

**William E. Prentice, Ph.D., A.T.C., P.T., F.N.A.T.A.**
Professor, Coordinator of the Sports Medicine Specialization,
Department of Exercise and Sports Science
The University of North Carolina at Chapel Hill
Chapel Hill, North Carolina

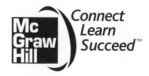

Connect
Learn
Succeed™

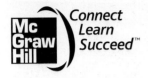
Published by McGraw-Hill, an imprint of The McGraw-Hill Companies, Inc., 1221 Avenue of the Americas, New York, NY 10020. Copyright © 2010, 2008, 2005, 2002, 1999, 1995, 1991, 1987. All rights reserved. No part of this publication may be reproduced or distributed in any form or by any means, or stored in a database or retrieval system, without the prior written consent of The McGraw-Hill Companies, Inc., including, but not limited to, in any network or other electronic storage or transmission, or broadcast for distance learning.

This book is printed on acid-free paper.

1 2 3 4 5 6 7 8 9 0 DOC/DOC 0 9

ISBN: 978-0-07-337657-8
MHID: 0-07-337657-4

Vice President Editorial: *Michael Ryan*
Editorial Director: *William Glass*
Executive Editor: *Christopher Johnson*
Director of Development: *Kathleen Engelberg*
Developmental Editor: *Gary O'Brien, Van Brien & Associates*
Editorial Coordinator: *Lydia Kim*
Marketing Manager: *William Minick*
Media Project Manager: *Tom Brierly*
Production Editor: *Alison Meier*
Design Coordinator: *Ashley Bedell*
Photo Research: *Brian J. Pecko*
Production Supervisor: *Tandra Jorgensen*
Production Service: *Jill Eccher*
Composition: *10/12 Meridien by Macmillan Publishing Solutions*
Printing: *45# New Era Matte Plus, R. R. Donnelley & Sons*

Credits: A credits section for this book begins on page 640 and is considered an extension of the copyright page.

### Library of Congress Cataloging-in-Publication Data

Prentice, William E.
  Essentials of athletic injury management / William E. Prentice.—8th ed.
      p. cm.
  Includes bibliographical references and index.
  ISBN-13: 978-0-07-337657-8 (alk. paper)
  ISBN-10: 0-07-337657-4 (alk. paper)
  1.  Sports medicine. 2.  Sports injuries—Prevention. 3.  Physical education and training.  I. Title.
  RC1210.A749 2010
  617.1'027—dc22
                                                          2009030562

The Internet addresses listed in the text were accurate at the time of publication. The inclusion of a Web site does not indicate an endorsement by the authors or McGraw-Hill, and McGraw-Hill does not guarantee the accuracy of the information presented at these sites.

**www.mhhe.com**

# Contents in Brief

# Contents

# Preface

## WHO SHOULD USE THIS TEXT?

The majority of students who take courses about the prevention and management of injuries that typically occur in an athletic population have little or no intention of pursuing athletic training as a career. However, it is also true that a large percentage of those students who are taking these courses are doing so because they intend to pursue careers in coaching, fitness, physical education, or other areas related to exercise and sport science. For these individuals, some knowledge and understanding of the many aspects of health care for both recreational and competitive athletes is essential for them to effectively perform the associated responsibilities of their job. The eighth edition of *Essentials of Athletic Injury Management* is written for those students interested in coaching, physical education, and the fitness profession.

Other students who are personally involved in fitness, or training and conditioning, may be interested in taking a course that will provide them with guidelines and recommendations for preventing injuries, recognizing injuries, and learning how to correctly manage a specific injury. Thus, *Essentials of Athletic Injury Management* has been designed to provide basic information on a variety of topics, all of which relate in one way or another to health care for the athlete.

*Essentials of Athletic Injury Management* was created from the foundations established by another well-recognized textbook, *Arnheim's Principles of Athletic Training,* currently in its fourteenth edition. Whereas *Arnheim's Principles of Athletic Training* serves as a major text for professional athletic trainers and those individuals interested in sports medicine, **Essentials of Athletic Injury Management is written at a level more appropriate for the coach, fitness professional, and physical educator.** It provides guidance, suggestions, and recommendations for handling athletic health care situations when an athletic trainer or physician is not available.

## ORGANIZATION AND COVERAGE

The eighth edition of *Essentials of Athletic Injury Management* provides the reader with the most current information possible on the subject of prevention and basic care of sports injuries. The general philosophy of the text is that adverse effects of physical activity arising from participation in sport should be prevented to the greatest extent possible. However, the nature of participation in physical activity dictates that sooner or later injury may occur. In these situations, providing immediate and correct care can minimize the seriousness of an injury.

Overall, this text is designed to take the beginning student from general to more specific concepts. Each chapter focuses on promoting an understanding of the prevention and care of athletic injuries.

*Essentials of Athletic Injury Management* is divided into three parts: *Organizing and Establishing an Effective Athletic Health Care System, Techniques for Preventing or Minimizing Sport-Related Injuries,* and *Recognition and Management of Specific Injuries and Conditions.*

Part One, *Organizing and Establishing an Effective Athletic Health Care System,* begins in Chapter 1 with a discussion of the roles and responsibilities of all the individuals on the "sports medicine team" who in some way affect the delivery of health care to the athlete. Chapter 2 provides guidelines and recommendations for setting up a system for providing athletic health care in situations where an athletic trainer is not available to oversee that process. In today's society, and in particular for anyone who is remotely involved with providing athletic heath care, the issue of legal responsibility and, perhaps more importantly, legal liability is of utmost concern. Chapter 3 discusses ways to minimize the chances of litigation and also to make certain that both the athlete and anyone who is in any way involved in providing athletic health care are protected by appropriate insurance coverage.

Part Two, *Techniques for Preventing or Minimizing Sport-Related Injuries,* discusses a variety of topics that both individually and collectively can reduce the chances for injury to occur. Chapter 4 emphasizes the importance of making certain that the athlete is fit to prevent injuries. Chapter 5 discusses the importance of a healthy diet, giving attention to sound nutritional practices and providing sound advice on the use of dietary supplements. Chapter 6 provides guidelines for selecting and using protective equipment. Chapter 7 details how to assess the severity of an injury and then provides specific steps that should be taken to handle emergency situations. Chapter 8 provides guidelines that can help reduce the chances of spreading infectious diseases by taking universal precautions dealing with bloodborne pathogens. Chapter 9 looks at ways to minimize the potentially negative threats of various environmental conditions on the health of the athlete. Chapter 10 discusses the more common taping techniques that can be used to prevent new injuries from occurring and old ones from becoming worse. Chapter 11 includes a brief discussion of the general techniques that may be used in rehabilitation following injury. Chapter 12 discusses the psychology of preparing to compete and proposes recommendations for how a coach should manage an injury.

Part Three, *Recognition and Management of Specific Injuries and Conditions,* begins with Chapter 13, which defines and classifies the various types of injuries that are most commonly seen in the physically active population.

Chapters 14 through 22 discuss injuries that occur in specific regions of the body, including the foot; the ankle and lower leg; the knee; the hip, thigh, groin, and pelvis; the shoulder; the elbow, wrist, forearm, and hand; the spine; the thorax and abdomen; and the head, face, eyes, ears, nose, and throat. Injuries are discussed individually in terms of their most common causes, the signs of injury you would expect to see, and a basic plan of care for that injury. Chapter 23 provides guidelines and suggestions for managing various illnesses and other health conditions that may affect athletes and their ability to play and compete. Chapter 24 focuses specifically on issues related to substance abuse and the potential effects on the athlete. Chapter 25 provides special considerations for injuries that may occur in young athletes.

## NEW TO THIS EDITION

Based on reviewer comments, a substantial effort has been made to improve the quality of the illustrations throughout this text. Most of the outdated line drawings have been replaced with photographs that more clearly demonstrate and emphasize the points made in the text. Approximately 190 new photos have been included as replacement for outdated photos.

In addition, numerous changes and clarification have been made in content throughout the entire text.

### Chapter 1

- Clarification on CPR/AED certifications for certain members of the sport medicine team.
- Two new photos illustrating fitness professionals' roles in the sports medicine team.

### Chapter 2

- Updated terminology throughout to reflect current health care facilities.
- Updated list of recommended basic athletic training room and field kit supplies.

### Chapter 3

- Clarified purpose and audience for the chapter.
- Reorganized insurance section.

### Chapter 4

- Revised coverage of dynamic and static stretching.
- Several new photos illustrating proper techniques for stretches and exercises.

### Chapter 5

- Clarification on the use of herbal supplements.

- New discussion of the effectiveness of organic foods.
- New coverage of anorexia athletica.

## Chapter 6

- Updated to include the latest information on safety equipment.
- Many new photos showing new safety and rehabilitative equipment.

## Chapter 7

- Updated and expanded information on AEDs and CPR.
- Information on "Hands-only CPR."
- New Focus Box on consent forms for minors.
- New flowcharts on appropriate emergency procedures and flowchart for adult and child CPR.
- New photos for CPR and other emergency techniques.

## Chapter 8

- Added brief discussion of using appropriate gloves.
- Included new photos that better show wounds that frequently occur in sports.

## Chapter 9

- New illustration that shows the correlation between temperature and relative humidity in heat index.
- Updated terminology throughout to reflect current trends.
- New recommendations for preventing heat illness.

## Chapter 10

- Clarification on who should apply tape.
- Clarification on the steps of several taping techniques.
- Several new and updated photos and illustrations.

## Chapter 11

- New discussion of therapeutic versus conditioning exercise.
- New content and photos on reestablishing core stability.

## Chapter 12

- Added brief introduction and focus box discussing the role of the coach and other fitness professionals in helping athletes deal with injury.

## Chapter 13

- New introduction discussing injury causes and prevention.
- New and enhanced photos and illustrations of muscle strains, osteoarthritis, and tissue healing.

## Chapter 14

- New introduction on assessments that states recommendations on referrals to medical staff.
- New, updated, and enhanced photos that show a variety of conditions, injuries, protection, and rehabilitation options.

## Chapter 15

- New introduction on assessments that states recommendations on referrals to medical staff.
- New, updated, and enhanced photos that show a variety of conditions, injuries, protection, and rehabilitation options.

## Chapter 16

- New introduction on assessments that states recommendations on referrals to medical staff.
- New, updated, and enhanced photos that show a variety of conditions, injuries, protection, and rehabilitation options.
- New information on knee plica.

## Chapter 17

- New introduction on assessments that states recommendations on referrals to medical staff.
- New, updated, and enhanced photos that show a variety of conditions, injuries, protection, and rehabilitation options.
- New information on femoral stress fractures.
- New information on hip labral tear.

## Chapter 18

- New introduction on assessments that states recommendations on referrals to medical staff.
- New, updated, and enhanced photos that show a variety of conditions, injuries, protection, and rehabilitation options.

## Chapter 19

- New introduction on assessments that states recommendations on referrals to medical staff.
- New, updated, and enhanced photos that show a variety of conditions, injuries, protection, and rehabilitation options.

## Chapter 20

- New introduction on assessments that states recommendations on referrals to medical staff.
- New introduction to special tests clarifies the role of non-medical personnel in recognizing potential red flags associated with injuries.
- New, updated, and enhanced photos that show a variety of conditions, injuries, protection, and rehabilitation options.

## Chapter 21

- New introduction on assessments that states recommendations on referrals to medical staff.
- New, updated, and enhanced photos that show a variety of conditions, injuries, protection, and rehabilitation options.

## Chapter 22

- Expanded information on cerebral concussion.
- New, updated, and enhanced photos that show a variety of conditions, injuries, protection, and rehabilitation options.

## Chapter 23

- New recommendations on referrals to medical staff.
- New information on testicular and breast cancer.
- New photos on common skin infections and MRSA.

## Chapter 24

- New information on crystal methamphetamine, ecstasy, and other recreational drugs.
- Updated coverage of Androstenedione.

## Chapter 25

- New coverage of where injuries occur and proven interactions.
- Updated information on coaching qualifications.

## Appendix A

- Expanded and updated the discussion of employment settings and opportunities for athletic trainers.

## PEDAGOGICAL FEATURES

- *Chapter objectives.* Objectives are presented at the beginning of each chapter to reinforce learning goals.
- *Focus Boxes.* Important information is highlighted to provide additional content that supplements the main text.
- *Margin information.* Key concepts, selected definitions and pronunciation guides, helpful training tips, and illustrations are placed in margins throughout the text for added emphasis and ease of reading and studying.
- *Illustrations and photographs.* The illustrations have been significantly upgraded with many line drawings replaced by photographs. Approximately 190 new photos have been included.
- *Critical thinking exercises.* Included in every chapter, these brief case studies correspond with the accompanying text and help students apply the content just learned. Solutions for each exercise are located at the end of the chapters.

- *Athletic Injury Management Checklists.* New checklists prepared specifically to help organize the details of a specific procedure when managing athletic health care.
- *Chapter summaries.* Chapter content is summarized and bulleted to reinforce key concepts and aid in test preparation.
- *Review questions and class activities.* A list of questions and suggested class activities follows each chapter for review and application of the concepts learned.
- *References.* All chapters have a bibliography of pertinent references that includes the most complete and up-to-date resources available.
- *Annotated bibliography.* To further aid in learning, relevant and timely articles, books, and topics from the current literature have been annotated to provide additional resources.
- *Websites.* A list of useful websites is included to direct the student to additional relevant information that can be found on the Internet.
- *Color throughout the text.* A second color appears throughout the text to enhance overall appearance and accentuate and clarify illustrations.
- *Glossary.* A comprehensive list of key terms with their definitions is presented at the end of the text.
- *Appendixes.* For those students interested in learning more about athletic training, Appendixes A and B provide information about employment settings for the athletic trainer and the requirements for certification as an athletic trainer.
- *Back cover.* Helpful charts for metric and celsius conversions are found inside the back cover.

## INSTRUCTOR'S RESOURCE MATERIALS

### Computerized Test Bank

McGraw-Hill's Computerized Testing is the most flexible and easy-to-use electronic testing program available in higher education. The program allows instructors to create tests from book-specific test banks. It accommodates a wide range of question types, and instructors may add their own questions. Multiple versions of the test can be created. The program is available for Windows, Macintosh, and Linux environments. It is located in the Online Learning Center.

### PowerPoint Presentation

Developed for the eighth edition by Jason S. Scibek, Ph.D., ATC, from Duquesne University, a comprehensive and extensively illustrated PowerPoint presentation accompanies this text for use in classroom discussion. The PowerPoint presentation may also be converted to outlines and given to students as a handout. You can easily download the PowerPoint presentation from the McGraw-Hill website at www.mhhe.com/prentice/8e. Adopters of the text can obtain the login and password to access this presentation by contacting your local McGraw-Hill sales representative.

## INTERNET RESOURCES

### Online Learning Center

**www.mhhe.com/prentice8e** This website offers resources to students and instructors. It includes downloadable ancillaries, Web links, student quizzes, additional information on topics of interest, and more. Resources for the instructor include:

- Instructor's Manual
- Downloadable PowerPoint presentations
- Links to professional resources

Resources for the student include:

- Flashcards
- Review materials
- Interactive quizzes

### eSims

**www.mhhe.com/esims** eSims is an online assessment tool that provides students with computerized simulation tests with instant feedback that emulate the actual Athletic Training certification exam. It is available with each new purchase of *Essentials of Athletic Injury Management.* (It is also available for purchase online too!) Check out eSims at the address above.

## ACKNOWLEDGMENTS

Special thanks are extended to Gary O'Brien, my Development Editor on this and several additional projects. As always he has provided invaluable guidance in the preparation of the eighth edition of *Essentials of Athletic Injury Management.*

Jill Eccher, who has been the Senior Project Manager on several of my recent texts, has become someone that I rely on quite heavily to make sure all of the countless details are taken care of. She makes the process a lot less stressful and I know that I can always count on her diligence.

Amanda Andrews, PhD, ATC, from Troy University and Linda Stark Bobo, PhD, ATC, from Stephen F. Austin University have been responsible for preparing the Instructor's Manual and Test Bank that accompany this text. Jason Scibek from Duquesne University has prepared the PowerPoint presentation. Their efforts have provided a much needed educational resource for individuals teaching a course in athletic injury management, and I certainly appreciate the manner in which they have completed their parts of this project.

I would also like to thank the following individuals who served as reviewers for their input into the revision of this text:

*Gary Ward*
**Missouri State University**

*Vanessa Rettinger*
**Anderson University**

*Doris Flores*
**California State University**

*Thomas Cappaert*
**Central Michigan University**

*Mike Goforoth*
**Virginia Tech**

*Connie DeVries*
**Community College of Rhode Island**

*Brian Hatzel*
**Grand Valley State University**

*Jason Pachter*
**SUNY—Plattsburgh**

Finally, I would like to thank my family, Tena, Brian, and Zach, for always being an important part of everything I do.

**William E. Prentice**

# Applications at a Glance

# PART 1

## Organizing and Establishing an Effective Athletic Health Care System

# Fitness Professionals, Coaches, and the Sports Medicine Team: Defining Roles

## CHAPTER 1

*When you finish this chapter you will be able to:*

- Define the umbrella term *sports medicine*.
- Identify various sports medicine organizations.
- Contrast athletic health care in organized versus recreational sport activities.
- Discuss how fitness professionals, including personal fitness trainers and strength and conditioning coaches, relate to the sports medicine team.
- Describe the role of an individual supervising a recreational program in athletic injury management.
- Analyze the role of the athletic administrator in the athletic health care system.
- Describe the role of the coach in injury prevention, emergency care, and injury management.
- Identify the responsibilities of the athletic trainer in dealing with the injured athlete.
- Describe the role of the team physician and his or her interaction with the athletic trainer.
- Explain how the sports medicine team should interact with the athlete.
- Identify other members of the sports medicine team and describe their roles.

Millions of individuals in our American society participate on a regular basis in both organized and recreational sports or physical activities. There is great demand for well-educated, professionally trained personnel to supervise and oversee these activities. Among those professionals are coaches, fitness professionals such as strength and conditioning specialists and personal fitness trainers, recreation specialists, athletic administrators, and others interested in some aspect of exercise and sport science.

Ironically, participation in any type of physical activity places the "athlete" in situations in which injury is likely to occur. Athletes who engage in organized sports and/or recreational activities have every right to expect that their health and safety will be a high priority for those who supervise or organize those activities. Thus it is essential to have some knowledge about how injuries can best be prevented or at least minimized. Should injury occur, it is critical to be able to recognize that a problem exists, to learn how to correctly provide first-aid care, and to then refer the athlete to the appropriate medical or health care personnel for optimal treatment. However, it must be emphasized that these well-trained professionals are NOT health care professionals. In fact, attempting to provide health care to an injured or ill athlete is in most states illegal and likely violates the practice acts of several different professional health care provider groups licensed by the state to give medical care to an injured athlete.

**The intent throughout this text is to provide students who intend to become coaches, fitness professionals, recreation specialists, athletic administrators, physical education teachers, exercise physiologists, biomechanists, sport psychologists, or sport nutritionists with an introduction or exposure to a variety of topics that in some way or another relate to athletic injury management.** The purpose of this chapter is to introduce the members of the sports medicine team with whom these professionals are likely to interact throughout their careers. Specific roles and responsibilities of each member of the sports medicine team in managing the health care of the athlete will be discussed in detail.

## WHAT IS SPORTS MEDICINE?

The term *sports medicine* refers generically to a broad field of medical practice related to physical activity and sport. The American College of Sports Medicine (ACSM) has defined sports medicine as multidisciplinary, including the physiological, biomechanical, psychological, and pathological phenomena associated with exercise and sports. The clinical application of the work of these disciplines is performed to improve and maintain an individual's functional capacities for physical labor, exercise, and sports. It also includes the prevention and treatment of diseases and injuries related to exercise and sports. The field of sports medicine encompasses under its umbrella a number of more specialized aspects of dealing with the physically active or athletic populations that may be classified as relating either to performance enhancement or to injury care and management (Figure 1-1). Those areas of specialization that are primarily concerned with performance enhancement include exercise physiology, biomechanics, sport psychology, sports nutrition, strength and conditioning, personal fitness training, coaching, and physical education. Areas of specialization that focus more on health care and injury/illness management specific to the athlete are the practice of medicine (physicians and physician assistants), athletic training, sports physical therapy, massage therapy, dentistry, osteopathic medicine, orthotists/prosthetists, sports chiropractic, and sports podiatry. Certainly, some of the specializations listed under this umbrella could be concerned with both performance enhancement and injury care and management (for example, sports nutrition).

### Sports Medicine Organizations

A number of professional organizations are dedicated to sports medicine. Professional organizations have many goals: (1) to upgrade the field by

Many professional organizations are dedicated to achieving health and safety in sports.

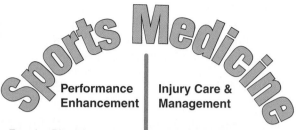

**Figure 1-1**

Areas of specialization under
the sports medicine
"umbrella"

**Sports Medicine**

| Performance Enhancement | Injury Care & Management |
|---|---|
| Exercise Physiology | Practice of Medicine |
| Biomechanics | (Physicians, Physicians Assistants) |
| Sport Psychology | Athletic Training |
| Sports Nutrition | Sports Physical Therapy |
| Strength & Conditioning | Sports Massage Therapy |
| Personal Fitness Training | Sports Dentistry |
| Coaching | Osteopathic Medicine |
| Physical Education | Orthotists/Prosthetists |
| | Sports Chiropractic |
| | Sport Podiatry |

devising and maintaining a set of professional standards, including a code of ethics; (2) to bring together professionally competent individuals to exchange ideas, stimulate research, and promote critical thinking; and (3) to give individuals an opportunity to work as a group with a singleness of purpose, thereby making it possible for them to achieve objectives that, separately, they could not accomplish. Addresses and websites for these organizations are listed in Focus Box 1-1.

**1-1**    *Focus Box*

**List of Professional Sports Medicine Organizations**

- American Academy of Pediatrics, Sports Committee, 1801 Hinman Ave., Evanston, IL 60204 www.aap.org
- American Board of Physical Therapy Specialists, American Physical Therapy Association, 1111 North Fairfax St., Alexandria, VA 22314 apta.edoc.com
- American College of Sports Medicine, 401 W. Michigan St., Indianapolis, IN 46202-3233 www.acsm.org
- American Orthopaedic Society for Sports Medicine, Suite 202, 70 West Hubbard, Chicago, IL 60610 www.sportsmed.org
- National Athletic Trainers' Association, 2952 Stemmons Freeway, Dallas, TX 75247 www.nata.org
- National Collegiate Athletic Association, Competitive Safeguards and Medical Aspects of Sports Committee, 700 W. Washington St., P.O. Box 622, Indianapolis, IN 46206-6222 www.ncaa.org
- The National Federation of State High School Athletic Associations, 11724 Plaza Circle, P.O. Box 20626, Kansas City, MO 64195 www.nfsha.org
- National Strength and Conditioning Association, P.O. Box 38909, Colorado Springs, CO 80937-8909 www.nsca-lift.org
- American Osteopathic Academy of Sports Medicine, 7600 Terrace Ave., Middleton, WI 53562 www.aoasm.org

Many of the national organizations interested in athletic health and safety have state and local associations that are extensions of the larger bodies. National, state, and local sports organizations have all provided extensive support to the reduction of illness and injury risk to the athlete.

## ATHLETIC HEALTH CARE IN ORGANIZED VERSUS RECREATIONAL SPORTS ACTIVITIES

The system or methods by which athletic health care is delivered by members of the sports medicine team to a large extent depend on whether the activity is organized or recreational. An organized activity refers to a situation that is generally competitive in which there is some type of team or league involvement, as would be the case with secondary school, collegiate, and professional athletic teams. With organized sport activities, the primary players on the sports medicine team are employed on either a full-time or part-time basis by a school or organization and include the coach, the athletic trainer, and a physician who is designated as a "team" physician. At the collegiate and professional levels, a strength and conditioning coach, a sports nutritionist, a sports massage therapist, and a sport psychologist are also usually involved. In organized sport activities, the athletic health care system is generally well organized and comprehensive and in many instances the sports medicine coverage would be considered highly sophisticated.

Certainly a recreational sport activity can be competitive. However a recreational activity is one that is done more for leisure and free time enjoyment and involves a much less formal structure with many of the organizers being primarily volunteers. These include city- or community-based recreational leagues and teams. Many individuals choose to engage in fitness-oriented exercise activities such as running or weight training as a recreational activity. These "recreational athletes" may decide to hire personal fitness trainers to help them with their fitness programs. Should injury occur, they are likely to consult their family physician, an athletic trainer, a sports chiropractor, or a sports physical therapist. Athletic health care for recreational athletes is generally provided on a fee-for-care basis.

## THE PLAYERS ON THE SPORTS MEDICINE TEAM

Providing health care to the athlete requires a group effort to be most effective.[26] The sports medicine team involves a number of individuals, each of whom must perform specific functions relative to caring for the injured athlete.[3,8]

### How Does the Fitness Professional Relate to the Sports Medicine Team?

Earlier in this chapter, the term *fitness professional* was used to refer to personal fitness trainers, strength and conditioning coaches, and others interested in exercise and sport sciences. In this group we may also include physical education teachers, exercise physiologists, biomechanists, sport psychologists, and sport nutritionists. If we consider the "sports medicine umbrella" model, the focus of this group is on improving performance. Certainly there is an argument to be made that if athletes achieve a high level of fitness through training and conditioning, they are not only more likely to perform athletically at a higher level but they are also less likely to sustain some type of activity-related injury. Therefore, there is a relationship between those areas that specialize in performance enhancement and those that focus on health care in that both groups are concerned with injury prevention.

### Personal Fitness Trainers

A personal fitness trainer is responsible for designing comprehensive exercise or fitness programs for an individual client based on that person's health history, capabilities, and objectives for fitness.[11] Once thought of as a service for the rich and famous, people from all income levels are using personal fitness trainers to increase their fitness levels and to get advice about living a healthy lifestyle.

Personal fitness trainers first began to appear in the late 1970s. The intensive growth in the number of personal fitness trainers began in the late 1980s. The personal fitness training industry has grown in acceptance, to some extent in credibility, and definitely in the number of personal fitness trainers in the last 10 years. It is estimated that there are currently over 65,000 personal trainers in North America, who offer their services to a variety of people and businesses. While associations and certification agencies can count the number of personal fitness trainers in their organization, many personal fitness trainers have one or more certifications and belong to more than one professional organization, making it almost impossible to accurately assess the number of certified personal fitness trainers in the United States.

Unfortunately, no single standard qualification is required before a person can practice as a personal fitness trainer. About 400 organizations in the United States offer certification to personal fitness trainers. Of that number, only a few are considered legitimate by most professionals. Among the most respected are the American College of Sports Medicine (ACSM), the National Academy of Sports Medicine (NASM), the National Strength and Conditioning Association (NSCA), and the American Council on Exercise (ACE).[13] These organizations have specific requirements based on tested and practical knowledge, mandatory retesting at renewal periods, and continuing education. A recent trend by some of these organizations is to require that its certified personal fitness trainers have a formal educational degree in exercise science or a related field.[15] However, the requirements for other organizations are not so strict. Some award certification after taking a correspondence course over the Internet, or after attending as little as a weekend or single day training session. Individuals who hire personal fitness trainers should check qualifications and certifications.

**All personal fitness trainers should be certified in CPR/AED (cardiopulmonary resuscitation/automated external defibrillator) by either the American Red Cross, the American Heart Association, or the National Safety Council. They should also be certified in first aid by the American Red Cross or the National Safety Council.**

Personal fitness training is without question the strongest growth segment of the fitness industry, and this trend is expected to continue as personal fitness trainers are beginning to offer a variety of services that go beyond a general exercise program.[11] Personal fitness trainers are increasingly providing services in postrehabilitation training, sports conditioning, special medical needs, and weight management to a variety of specific client populations including prenatal women, adolescents, and older persons.

### Strength and Conditioning Coaches

The responsibility for making certain that an athlete is fit for competition depends on the personnel available to oversee this aspect of an athletic program. At the professional level and at most colleges and universities, a full-time strength and conditioning coach is employed to conduct both team and individual training sessions. Many, but not all, strength coaches are certified by the National Strength and Conditioning Association (NSCA). This association has more than 30,000 members. It is the responsibility of the strength and conditioning coach to communicate freely and work in close cooperation with both the athletic trainers and the team coaches to ensure that the athletes achieve an optimal level of fitness.[30] **All strength and conditioning coaches should be certified in CPR/AED by either the American Red Cross, the American Heart Association, or the National Safety Council. They should also be certified in first aid by the American Red Cross or the National Safety Council.**

If an athlete is injured and is undergoing a rehabilitation program, it should be the strength and conditioning coach's responsibility to communicate with the athletic trainer as to how the conditioning program should be limited and/or modified.[16] The athletic trainer must respect the role of the strength and conditioning coach in getting the athlete fit. However, the responsibility for rehabilitating an injured athlete clearly belongs to the athletic trainer. The athletic trainer should be allowed to critically review the training and conditioning program designed by the strength and conditioning coach and to be very familiar with what is expected of the athletes on a daily basis. The athletic trainer should dictate what an injured athlete can or cannot do when engaging in a strength and conditioning program.

In the majority of high school settings, a strength and conditioning coach is not available. In this situation either the athletic trainer or team coach often assumes the role of a strength and conditioning coach in addition to his or her athletic training or coaching responsibilities. The athletic trainer or coach frequently finds it necessary not only to design training and conditioning programs but also to oversee the weight room and to educate young, inexperienced athletes about getting themselves fit to compete. The athletic trainer must cooperate with team coaches in supervising the training and conditioning program.

## How Does a Recreation Specialist Relate to the Sports Medicine Team?

Recreation specialists organize, plan, and oversee leisure activities and athletic programs in local recreation, camp, and park areas; in playgrounds; in health clubs and fitness centers; in the workplace; and in theme parks and tourist attractions. An essential responsibility for any individual overseeing a recreational program is to ensure that the recreational environment is as safe as possible to minimize the risk of injury. Should injury occur to a participant the recreation specialist should be able to provide immediate and correct first aid and then refer the injured person to appropriate medical personnel. **All recreation specialists should be certified in CPR/AED by either the American Red Cross, the American Heart Association, or the National Safety Council. They should also be certified in first aid by the American Red Cross or the National Safety Council.**

*Recreation and parks directors* serve as advisors to local and state recreation and park commissions and manage comprehensive recreation programs in a variety of settings. They are responsible for developing budgets for recreation programs. *Recreation supervisors* serve as liaisons between the director of the park or recreation center and the recreation leaders. They plan, organize, and manage recreational activities to meet the needs of a variety of populations and oversee recreation leaders. Recreation supervisors with more specialized training may also direct special activities or events or oversee a major activity such as aquatics, gymnastics, or performing arts. *Recreation leaders* are primarily responsible for the daily operation of a recreation program. They organize and direct participants; schedule use of facilities; lead and give instruction in dance, drama, crafts, games, and sports; maintain equipment; and ensure appropriate use of recreation facilities. *Activity specialists* provide instruction and coach groups in specialties such as swimming or tennis. *Camp counselors* lead and instruct campers in outdoor-oriented forms of recreation, such as swimming, hiking, horseback riding, and camping.

A *recreational therapist* may be considered a health care provider. Recreational therapists work in acute health care settings, such as hospitals and rehabilitation centers or in long-term and residential care facilities. Their job is to treat and rehabilitate individuals with specific health conditions, usually in conjunction or collaboration with physicians, nurses, psychologists, social workers, and physical and occupational therapists. Recreational therapists use leisure activities—especially structured group programs—to improve and maintain their clients' general health and well-being. They also provide interventions that help prevent the client from suffering further medical problems and complications related to illnesses and disabilities.

## The Role of the Athletic Administrator in the Sports Medicine Team

Without question, an athletic administrator, overseeing both collegiate and secondary school athletic programs, has a significant impact on the sports medicine team. The athletic administrator is responsible for hiring personnel who will make up the sports medicine team including the coaches, the strength and conditioning coach, the athletic trainer, the team physician, a sports nutritionist, and a sport psychologist. It is essential for the athletic administrator to make certain that each individual hired has the appropriate credentials and that they are willing and able to work in close cooperation with the other members of the sports medicine team. The athletic administrator should make certain that policies and procedures, a risk management plan, and emergency action plans are developed for the athletic health care system. The administrator is also responsible for establishing a budget for funding all aspects of an athletic health care program including salaries, supplies and equipment, and purchasing necessary insurance (see Chapter 3). The consistent support and commitment to an athletic health care program on the part of an athletic administrator can have a tremendous impact on the success of the athletic program.

## The Role of a Coach in the Sports Medicine Team

It is critical for the coach to understand the specific roles and responsibilities of each individual who could potentially be involved in the sports medicine team. This becomes even more critical if there is no athletic trainer to oversee the health care and the coach is forced to assume this responsibility. It must be stressed that individual states differ significantly in the laws that govern what nonmedical personnel can and cannot do when providing health care. **Coaches have the responsibility to clearly understand the limits of their ability to function as a health care provider in the state where they are employed.**

The coach is directly responsible for preventing injuries by seeing that athletes have undergone a preventive injury conditioning program. The coach must ensure that sports equipment, especially protective equipment, is of the highest quality and is properly fitted. The coach must also make sure that protective equipment is properly maintained.[26] A coach must be keenly aware of what produces injuries in his or her particular sport and what measures must be taken to avoid them (Figure 1-2). A coach should be able, when called on to do so, to apply proper first aid. This knowledge is especially important in serious head and spinal injuries. **All coaches (both head and assistants) should be certified in CPR/AED by either the American Red Cross, the American Heart Association, or the National Safety Council. Coaches should also be certified in first aid by the American Red Cross or the National Safety Council.**[27] For the

All head and assistant coaches should be certified in CPR/AED and first aid.

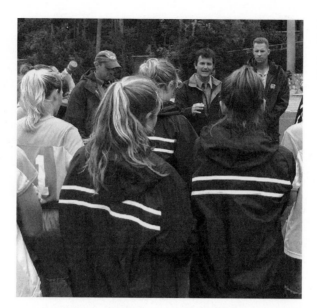

**Figure 1-2**

The coach is directly responsible for preventing injuries in his or her sport.

coach, obtaining these certifications is important in being able to provide correct and appropriate health care for the injured athlete. But it is also true that not having these certifications can potentially have some negative legal implications for the coach and his or her employer.

It is essential that a coach have a thorough understanding of the skill techniques and environmental factors that may adversely affect the athlete. Poor biomechanics in skill areas such as throwing and running can lead to overuse injuries of the arms and legs, whereas overexposure to heat and humidity may cause death. Just because a coach is experienced in coaching does not mean that he or she knows proper skill techniques. Coaches must engage in a continual process of education to further their knowledge in their particular sport through organizations such as the American Sport Education Program (ASEP) or the National Council for Accreditation of Coaching Education (NCACE). When a sports program or specific sport is without an athletic trainer, the coach very often takes over this role.

Coaches work closely with athletic trainers; therefore both must develop an awareness and an insight into each other's problems so that they can function effectively. The athletic trainer must develop patience and must earn the respect of the coaches so that his or her judgment in all medical matters is fully accepted. In turn, the athletic trainer must avoid questioning the abilities of the coaches in their particular fields and must restrict opinions to athletic training matters. To avoid frustration and hard feelings, the coach must coach, and the athletic trainer must conduct athletic training matters. In terms of the health and well-being of the athlete, the physician and the athletic trainer have the last word. The athletic director must back this position at all times.

**Figure 1-3**

Coaches should work closely with athletic trainers and physicians to provide health care for the injured athlete.

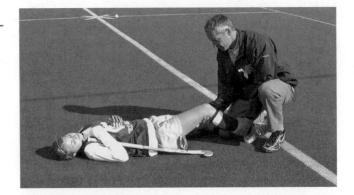

## The Roles and Responsibilities of the Athletic Trainer

It is essential for a coach or an other fitness professional who is working with an athletic trainer to gain an appreciation of the roles and responsibilities that an athletic trainer assumes in caring for the athletes (Figure 1-3). If the coach does not have an athletic trainer, many of those responsibilities may fall on the coach.

Of all the professionals charged with injury prevention and health care provision for the athlete, perhaps none is more intimately involved with the athlete than the athletic trainer.[26] The athletic trainer is the one individual who deals with the athlete from the time of the initial injury, throughout the period of rehabilitation, until the athlete's complete, unrestricted return to practice or competition.[26] The athletic trainer is most directly responsible for all phases of health care in an athletic environment, including preventing injuries from occurring, providing initial first aid and injury management, evaluating and diagnosing injuries, and designing and supervising a timely and effective program of rehabilitation that can facilitate the safe and expeditious return of the athlete to activity.[20,21] Athletic trainers are employed by schools and school systems, colleges and universities, professional athletic teams, sports medicine clinics, corporations in industry, and less "traditional" organizations such as the performing arts, NASCAR, NASA, the military, medical equipment sales/support, and the like[12,19,32] (see Appendix A).

Employment settings for athletic trainers:

- schools
- school systems
- colleges and universities
- professional teams
- clinics/hospitals
- corporations
- NASCAR, NASA, military, etc.
- performing arts

The athletic trainer must be knowledgeable and competent in a variety of sports medicine specialties if he or she is to be effective in preventing and treating injuries to the athlete.[1,21] The Board of Certification has established specific requirements that must be met for an individual to become certified as an athletic trainer.[21] These requirements include a combination of both academic coursework and clinical experience in athletic training settings (see Appendix B). Once these requirements for certification have been met and the individual passes a certification exam, that person earns the credential **ATC.** *(In this text all references to athletic trainers imply that this individual has met the requirements for certification set forth by the Board of Certification.)* Focus Box 1-2 further

**ATC**
Credential of an individual who is certified as an athletic trainer.

### Clarifying Roles

The terms *training* and *athletic training* are often confused. Historically, training implies the act of coaching or teaching. In comparison, athletic training has traditionally been known as a field within the allied health care professions that is concerned with prevention, management, evaluation, and rehabilitation of injuries related to physical activity.[24]

Recently, there has been confusion in the general public between the terms *trainers, certified athletic trainers, personal fitness trainers,* and *strength and conditioning coaches.* A *trainer* refers to someone who trains dogs or horses. A *certified athletic trainer* (certified by the Board of Certification) is a highly educated allied health care professional who is a credentialed specialist in athletic training. These individuals hold the credential ATC. Certified athletic trainers play a major role in the health care of the physically active in general and the athlete in particular.[23] *Personal fitness trainers* may also have some level of certification from any one of at least 400 existing certifying organizations. They are primarily concerned with developing fitness and wellness and improving levels of physical conditioning in a healthy population. Strength and conditioning coaches (certified by the National Strength and Conditioning Association) work primarily with athletes at the professional or collegiate levels to enhance their levels of physical conditioning and optimize performance.

clarifies the differences between an athletic trainer and a personal fitness trainer. The specific roles and responsibilities of the athletic trainer will differ and, to a certain extent, will be defined by the situation in which he or she works.[10,21] Different states have different requirements as to who can call themselves an athletic trainer. It should be reemphasized that trainers working with athletes should be certified athletic trainers (ATC).

### Injury Prevention

A major responsibility of the athletic trainer is to make the competitive environment as safe as possible to reduce the likelihood of injury. The athletic trainer is responsible for conducting physical examinations and preparticipation screenings to identify conditions that predispose an athlete to injury (see Chapter 2), and educating parents, coaches, and athletes about the risks inherent to sport participation. Injury prevention includes (1) ensuring appropriate training and conditioning of the athlete (see Chapter 4); (2) monitoring environmental conditions to ensure safe participation (see Chapter 10); (3) selecting, properly fitting, and maintaining protective equipment (see Chapter 6); (4) explaining the importance of proper nutrition (see Chapter 5); and (5) using medications appropriately.

Roles and responsibilities of the athletic trainer:
- prevention of athletic injuries
- clinical evaluation and diagnosis
- immediate care
- treatment, rehabilitation, and reconditioning
- organization and administration
- professional responsibilities

### Clinical Evaluation and Diagnosis

The athletic trainer must be skilled in recognizing the nature and extent of an injury through competency in injury evaluation. The athletic trainer must be able to efficiently and accurately evaluate an injury (see Chapter 7). The athletic trainer is responsible for referring the athlete to appropriate medical care or support services.

## Immediate Care

Once the initial on-the-field assessment is done the athletic trainer then must assume responsibility for administering appropriate first aid to the injured athlete and for making correct decisions in the management of acute injury (see Chapter 7).[25] Thus the athletic trainer must possess sound skills not only in the initial recognition and evaluation of potentially serious or life-threatening injuries but also in emergency care.

The athletic trainer is required to be certified in CPR/AED and should be certified in first aid by the American Red Cross or the National Safety Council.

## Treatment, Rehabilitation, and Reconditioning

An athletic trainer must be proficient in designing and supervising rehabilitation and reconditioning protocols that make use of appropriate rehabilitative equipment, manual (hands on) therapy techniques, or therapeutic modalities (see Chapter 12). In certain settings the athletic trainer may work closely with physical therapists and/or strength and conditioning specialists in designing functional return to play activities.

## Organization and Administration

The athletic trainer is responsible for the organization and administration of the athletic training program, including maintaining health and injury records for each athlete, developing emergency action plans, requisitioning and maintaining an inventory of necessary supplies and equipment, submitting insurance information to insurance companies, supervising assistants, athletic training students and establishing policies and procedures for day-to-day operation of the athletic training program (see Chapter 2).

## Professional Responsibilities

The athletic trainer must educate the general public, in addition to a large segment of the various allied medical health care professions, as to exactly what athletic trainers are and what their roles and responsibilities are. This education is perhaps best accomplished by holding professional seminars, publishing research in scholarly journals, meeting with local and community organizations, and, most important, doing a good and professional job of providing health care to the injured athlete.[22]

## Responsibilities of the Team Physician

The team physician assumes a number of roles and responsibilities with regard to injury prevention and the health care of the athlete.[2,18,28]

### Compiling Medical Histories

The team physician should be responsible for compiling medical histories and conducting physical examinations for each athlete, both of which can provide critical information that may reduce the possibility of injury.[29] Preparticipation screening by both the athletic trainer and

**◀◀ 1-1 Critical Thinking**
Exercise

A basketball player suffers a grade 2 ankle sprain during midseason of the competitive schedule. After a 3-week course of rehabilitation, most of the athlete's pain and swelling have been eliminated. The athlete is anxious to get back into practice and competitive games as soon as possible and subsequent injuries to other players have put pressure on the coach to force this player's return. Unfortunately the athlete is still unable to perform functional tasks (cutting and jumping) essential in basketball.

? Who is responsible for making the decision regarding when the athlete can fully return to practice and game situations?

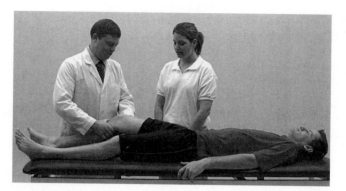

**Figure 1-4**

In treating the athlete, the physician supervises the athletic trainers.

physician is important in establishing baseline information to be used for comparison should injury occur during the season.

### Diagnosing Injury

The team physician should assume responsibility for diagnosing an injury and should be keenly aware of the program of rehabilitation as designed by the athletic trainer following the diagnosis[31] (Figure 1-4).

### Deciding on Disqualification

The physician should determine when an athlete should be disqualified from competition on medical grounds and must have the final say in when an injured athlete may return to activity. The physician's judgment must be based not only on medical knowledge but also on knowledge of the psychophysiological demands of a particular sport.[1]

### Attending Practices and Games

A team physician should make an effort to attend as many practices, scrimmages, and competitions as possible. This attendance obviously becomes very difficult at an institution with twenty or more athletic teams.[9]

It is essential that the team physician promote and maintain consistently high quality care for the athlete in all phases of the sports medicine program.[6,17]

## The Relationship Between the Sports Medicine Team and Athlete

If a coach has an athletic trainer and/or a physician who work together in providing health care, the relationships that exist can significantly affect the success of that team or athletic program.[5] The major concern of everyone on the sports medicine team should always be the athlete. If not for the athlete, the coach, athletic trainer, and team physician would have nothing to do in sports. All decisions made by the physician, coach, and athletic trainer ultimately affect the athlete. It should be clear that the physician working in cooperation with the athletic trainer assumes the responsibility of making the final decisions about medical care for the

Team physicians must have absolute authority in determining the health status of an athlete who wishes to participate in the sports program.

**1-2 Critical Thinking**
Exercise

What are some things that a
coach working in cooperation
with an athletic trainer can do
to help minimize the chances of
injury?

athlete from the time of injury until full return to activity.[7] The coach
must defer and should always support the decisions of the medical staff
in any matter regarding health care for the athlete.

This is not to say, however, that the coach should not be involved
with the decision-making process. For example, during the time the athlete is rehabilitating an injury, there may be drills or technical instruction sessions that the athlete can participate in that will not exacerbate
the existing problem. Thus the coach, the athletic trainer, and the team
physician should be able to negotiate what the athlete can and cannot
do safely in the course of a practice.

Athletes are frequently caught in the middle between coaches who
tell them to do one thing and medical staff who tell them something
else. Close communication between the coach and athletic trainer is
essential so that everyone is on the same page.

Any personal relationship takes some time to grow and develop. The
relationship between the coach and the athletic trainer is no different.
The athletic trainer must demonstrate to the coach his or her capability to correctly manage an injury and guide the course of a rehabilitation program. It will take some time for the coach to develop trust and
confidence in the athletic trainer. The coach must understand that what
the athletic trainer wants for the athlete is exactly the same as what the
coach wants—to get an athlete healthy and back to practice as quickly
and safely as possible.

The injured athlete must always be informed and made aware of
the why, how, and when factors that collectively dictate the course of
an injury rehabilitation program. Both the coach and the athletic trainer
should make it a priority to educate student-athletes about injury prevention and management. Athletes should learn about techniques of
training and conditioning that may reduce the likelihood of injury. They
should be well informed about their injuries and about listening to what
their bodies are telling them to prevent reinjury.

## The Importance of the Family in the Sports Medicine Team

In a high school or junior high school setting, the coach, the athletic
trainer, and the physician must also take the time to explain to and
inform the parents about injury management and prevention.[3] With an
athlete of secondary school age, the parents' decisions regarding health
care must be of primary consideration.

In certain situations, particularly at the high school and middle school
levels, many parents will insist that their child be seen by their family
physician rather than by the individual who may be designated as the
team physician. It is also likely that the choice of a physician will be
dictated by the parents' insurance plan (e.g., HMO, PPO). This creates
a situation in which the athletic trainer must work and communicate
with many different "team physicians." The opinion of the family physician must be respected even if the individual has little or no experience
with injuries related to sports.

The coach, athletic trainer, and team physician should make certain that the athlete and their family are familiar with the Health Insurance Portability and Accountability Act (HIPAA), which regulates how individuals who have health information about an athlete can share that information with others and not be in violation of the privacy rule. HIPAA was created to protect a patient's privacy and limit the number of people who could gain access to the athlete's medical records. HIPAA regulations will be discussed in more detail in Chapter 2.

## Other Members of the Sports Medicine Team

A sports program may use a number of support health services. Those people may include a nurse; physicians in specialties such as orthopedics, dentist, and podiatrist; physician's assistants; strength and conditioning coaches; nutritionist; sport psychologists; exercise physiologists; biomechanists; physical therapists; equipment personnel; and referees.

### Nurse

As a rule, the nurse is not usually responsible for the recognition of sports injuries. Education and background, however, render the nurse quite capable in the recognition of skin disease, infections, and minor irritations. The nurse works under the direction of the physician and in liaison with the athletic trainer and the school health services.

### Physicians

A number of physicians with a variety of specializations can aid the sports medicine team in treating the athlete.

**Dermatologist**   A dermatologist should be consulted for problems and lesions occurring on the skin.

**Gynecologist**   A gynecologist is consulted in cases where health issues in the female athlete are of primary concern.

**Family medicine physician**   A physician who specializes in family medicine is concerned with supervising or providing medical care to all members of a family. Many team physicians in colleges and universities and particularly at the high school level are engaged in family practice.

**Internist**   An internist is a physician who specializes in the practice of internal medicine. An internist treats diseases of the internal organs by using measures other than surgery.

**Neurologist**   A neurologist specializes in treating disorders of and injuries to the nervous system. Consultation with a neurologist is warranted in certain common situations in athletics, such as cases of head injury or peripheral nerve injury.

**Ophthalmologist**   Physicians who manage and treat injuries to the eye are ophthalmologists. An optometrist is an individual who evaluates and fits patients with glasses or contact lenses.

**Orthopedist**   The orthopedist is responsible for treating injuries and disorders of the musculoskeletal system. Many colleges and universities have a team orthopedist on their staff.

Support personnel concerned with athletes' health and safety:
- nurse
- school health services
- physicians
- dentist
- podiatrist
- sports chiropractors
- orthotist/prosthetist
- physician's assistant
- strength and conditioning coach
- sport psychologist
- sports physical therapist
- exercise physiologist
- biomechanist
- nutritionist
- massage therapists
- emergency medical specialist
- equipment personnel
- referees

**Osteopath**   An osteopath is a trained medical doctor who uses manual therapy and manipulation of joints extensively in his or her practice.

**Pediatrician**   A pediatrician is concerned with the practice of caring for or treating injuries and illnesses that occur in young physically active children and adolescents.

**Psychiatrist**   Psychiatry is a medical practice that deals with the diagnosis, treatment, and prevention of mental illness.

### Dentist

The role of team dentist is somewhat analogous to that of team physician. He or she serves as a dental consultant for the team and should be available for first aid and emergency care. Good communication between the dentist and the coach or athletic trainer should ensure a good dental program. The team dentist has three areas of responsibility:

1. Organizing and performing the preseason dental examination.
2. Being available to provide emergency care when needed.
3. Fitting mouth protectors.

### Podiatrist

Podiatry, the specialized field dealing with the study and care of the foot, has become an integral part of sports health care. Many podiatrists are trained in surgical procedures, foot biomechanics, and the fitting and construction of orthotic devices for the shoe. Like the team dentist, a podiatrist should be available on a consulting basis.

### Physician's Assistants

Physician's assistants (PAs) are trained to assume some of the responsibilities for patient care traditionally done by the physician. They assist the physician by conducting preliminary patient evaluations, arranging for various hospital-based diagnostic tests, and dispensing appropriate medications. A number of athletic trainers have also become PAs in recent years.

### Strength and Conditioning Coach

Many colleges and universities and some high schools employ full-time strength coaches to advise athletes on training and conditioning programs. Athletic trainers should routinely consult with these individuals to advise them about injuries to a particular athlete and exercises that should be avoided or modified relative to a specific injury.

### Sports Psychologists

The sports psychologist can advise the athlete on matters related to the psychological aspects of the rehabilitation process. The way the athlete feels about his or her injury and how it affects his or her social, emotional, intellectual, and physical dimensions can have a substantial effect on the course of a treatment program and how quickly the athlete may

**1-3 Critical Thinking**
Exercise

A new high school has hired a coach to establish and develop the football program. Unfortunately, the school does not have enough funds to also hire an athletic trainer. Thus the coach must assume the responsibility of creating a safe playing environment for the athletes.

? What considerations should the coach make to ensure that his athletes will be competing under the safest possible conditions?

return to competition. The sports psychologist uses different intervention strategies to help the athlete cope with injury.

### Sports Physical Therapists

Some athletic trainers use sports physical therapists to supervise the rehabilitation programs for injured athletes while the athletic trainer concentrates primarily on getting a player ready to practice or compete. A number of athletic trainers are also physical therapists.

The individual who achieves both certification as an athletic trainer and licensure as a physical therapist is extremely well qualified to function in various sports medicine settings, including both the private clinic and the colleges and universities.

### Sports Chiropractors

Chiropractors make use of spinal and extremity manipulation techniques to treat most musculoskeletal conditions.

### Orthotist/Prosthetist

These individuals custom fit, design, and construct braces, orthotics, and support devices based on physician prescriptions.

### Exercise Physiologists

The exercise physiologist can significantly influence athletic performance by giving input regarding training and conditioning techniques, body composition analysis, and nutritional considerations.

### Biomechanist

A biomechanist is a scientist who studies and investigates how athletes move. The biomechanist analyzes movement techniques using mathematical models and makes corrections and adjustments that can potentially increase efficiency of movement, thus improving performance.

### Nutritionists

Increasingly, individuals in the field of nutrition are becoming interested in athletics. Some large sports programs engage a nutritionist as a consultant who plans eating programs that are geared to the needs of a particular sport. He or she also assists individual athletes who need special nutritional counseling.

### Sports Massage Therapists

A qualified massage therapist has training and experience in all areas of massage. They may use their skills primarily in the precompetition and postcompetition phases of an athletic event.

### Emergency Medical Specialist (EMS)

These individuals are indispensable in providing transport to the injured athlete to a medical care facility.[4]

### Equipment Personnel

Sports equipment personnel are becoming specialists in the purchase and proper fitting of protective equipment. They work closely with the coach and the athletic trainer.

### Referees

Referees must be highly knowledgeable regarding rules and regulations, especially those that relate to the health and welfare of the athlete. They work cooperatively with the coach and the athletic trainer. They must be capable of checking the playing facility for dangerous situations and equipment that may predispose the athlete to injury. They must routinely check athletes to ensure that they are wearing adequate protective pads.

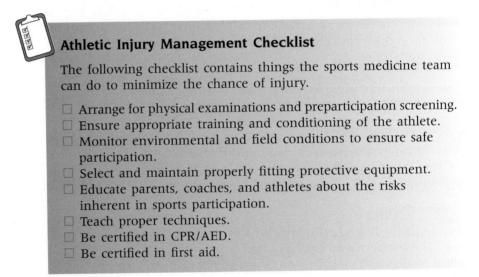

**Athletic Injury Management Checklist**

The following checklist contains things the sports medicine team can do to minimize the chance of injury.

☐ Arrange for physical examinations and preparticipation screening.
☐ Ensure appropriate training and conditioning of the athlete.
☐ Monitor environmental and field conditions to ensure safe participation.
☐ Select and maintain properly fitting protective equipment.
☐ Educate parents, coaches, and athletes about the risks inherent in sports participation.
☐ Teach proper techniques.
☐ Be certified in CPR/AED.
☐ Be certified in first aid.

## SUMMARY

- The term *sports medicine* has many connotations, depending on which group is using it. The term encompasses many different areas of sports related to both performance enhancement and injury care and management.
- Athletic health care is delivered differently in organized and recreational sport activities.
- Both personnel who concentrate on performance enhancement (such as fitness professionals and coaches) and personnel who focus on health care are concerned with injury prevention.
- Providing health care to the athlete requires a group effort to be most effective.
- The coach must ensure that the environment and the equipment that is worn are the safest possible, that all injuries and illnesses

are properly cared for, that skills are properly taught, and that conditioning is at the highest level.

- The athletic trainer is responsible for preventing injuries from occurring, for providing initial first aid and injury management, for evaluating injuries, and for designing and supervising a program of rehabilitation that can facilitate the safe return to activity.

- The team physician is responsible for preparticipation health examinations; for diagnosing and treating illnesses and injuries; for advising and teaching athletic trainers; for attending games, scrimmages, and practices; and for counseling the athlete about health matters.

- Other members of the sports medicine team may include nurses, physicians in specializations such as orthopedics, dentists, podiatrists, physician's assistants, strength and conditioning coaches, nutritionists, sport psychologists, exercise physiologists, biomechanists, physical therapists, chiropractors, equipment personnel, and referees.

---

*Solutions to Critical Thinking* Exercises

**1-1** Ultimately the team physician is responsible for making that decision. However, that decision must be based on collective input from the coach, the athletic trainer, and the athlete. Remember that everyone in the sports medicine team has the same ultimate goal—returning the athlete to full competitive levels as quickly and safely as possible.

**1-2** To help prevent injury the athletic trainer should (1) arrange for physical examinations and preparticipation screenings to identify conditions that predispose an athlete to injury; (2) ensure appropriate training and conditioning of the athlete; (3) monitor environmental conditions to ensure safe participation; (4) select and maintain properly fitting protective equipment; and (5) educate parents, coaches, and athletes about the risks inherent to sports participation.

**1-3** The coach should be responsible for designing an effective conditioning program; be responsible for ensuring that protective equipment is of the highest quality, properly fitted, and properly maintained; be able to apply proper first aid; be certified in CPR and first aid; and be aware of the environmental factors that may adversely affect the athlete.

## REVIEW QUESTIONS AND CLASS ACTIVITIES

1. What areas of specialization are encompassed under the general heading of sports medicine?
2. List some of the professional sports medicine organizations.
3. How should the sports medicine team work together to provide optimal health care for the athlete?
4. What are the responsibilities of a coach or fitness professional who must assume the role of a health care provider when an athletic trainer is not available?

5. What are the specific roles of the athletic trainer in overseeing the total health care of the athlete?
6. Discuss the role of the team physician as an important member of the sports medicine team.
7. What special impact can other members of the sports medicine team have in providing health care for the athlete?

## REFERENCES

1. Arnold B, Gansneder B, VanLunen B: 1998. Importance of selected athletic trainer employment characteristics in collegiate, sports medicine clinic and high school settings, *J Ath Train* 33(3):254.
2. Boyd, J: 2007. Understanding the politics of being a team physician. *Clinics in sports medicine* 26(2):161.
3. Brukner, P, Khan, K: 2002. Sports medicine: the team approach. In Brukner, P. (ed.), *Clinical sports medicine*. 2nd rev. ed., Sydney, McGraw-Hill.
4. Courson, R, Henry, G: 2005. Communication: the critical element in emergency preparation. *Athletic therapy today* 10(2):16.
5. Durgin, G: 2002. Advice: athletic directors sharing thoughts and actions. Utilizing athletic trainers within your program. *Interscholastic athletic administration* 28(4):20.
6. Editorial, 2001. The ethics of selecting a team physician. "Show me the money" shouldn't be part of the process, *Sports medicine digest* 23(4):37–38.
7. Finkam, S: 2002. The athletic trainer or athletic therapist as physician extender, *Athletic therapy today* 7(3):50–51.
8. Fu, F, Tjoumakaris, F, Buoncristiani, A: 2007. Building a sports medicine team. *Clinics in sports medicine* 26(2):173.
9. Herring, SA, Bergfeld, J, Boyd, J, et al. 2001. Sideline preparedness for the team physician: a consensus statement, *Medicine and science in sports and exercise* 33(5):846–849.
10. Kahanov, L, Andrews, L: 2001. A survey of athletic training employers' hiring criteria, *Journal of athletic training* 36(4):408–412.
11. Keller, J: 2004. "Fitness professional" among the fastest-growing jobs, *IDEA fitness journal* 1(5):13.
12. Kirkland, M: 2005. Increasing diversity of practice settings for athletic trainers. *Athletic therapy today* 10:5:1.
13. Lofshult, D: 2004. Personal fitness trainer certification. *IDEA health & fitness source* 22(3):15.
14. Lyznicki J, Riggs J, Champion H: 1999. Certified athletic trainers in secondary schools: report of the council on scientific affairs, American Medical Association, *J Ath Train* 34(3):272.
15. Malek, M.H.; Nalbone, D.P.; Berger, D.E.; Coburn, J.W.: 2002. Importance of health science education for personal fitness trainers, *Journal of strength and conditioning research* 16(1):19–24.
16. Massey, C.D.; Maneval, M.W.; Phillips, J.; Vincent, J.; White, G.; Zoeller, B.: 2003. An analysis of teaching and coaching behaviors of elite strength and conditioning coaches, *Journal of strength and conditioning research* 16(3):456–460.
17. Matheson, G: 2005. Advocating injury prevention: the team physician's role. *Physician and sportsmedicine* 33(8):1.
18. Mellion MB, Walsh WM: 2002. The team physician. In Mellion MB, editor: *Sports medicine secrets*, Philadelphia, Elsevier Health Sciences.

19. Mensch, J, Mitchell, M: 2008. Choosing a career in athletic training: exploring the perceptions of potential recruits. *Journal of Athletic Training* 43(1):70.

20. National Athletic Trainers Association Education Council: 2006. Athletic training educational competencies. 5th ed. Dallas, NATA.

21. National Athletic Trainers Association: 2004. *Role Delineation Study*. 5th ed. Dallas, NATA.

22. Peer, K: 2007. Ethics education: the cornerstone of foundational behaviors of professional practice. *Athletic therapy today* 12(1):2.

23. Perkins, SA, Judd, MR: 2001. Certified athletic trainers: providing better health care for sport participants, *Strategies* 15(2):27–28.

24. Popke, M: 2001. Vision quest: certified athletic trainers have spent years seeking respect in the high school ranks. Are they finally getting it? Maybe, *Athletic business* 25(12):69–70; 72; 74–77.

25. Potter, B: 2006. Developing professional relationships with emergency medical services providers, *Athletic therapy today* 11(3):18.

26. Prentice W: 1991. The athletic trainer. In Mueller F, Ryan A, editors: *Prevention of athletic injuries: the role of the sports medicine team*, Philadelphia, Davis.

27. Ransone J, Dunn-Bennett L: 1999. Assessment of first-aid knowledge and decision making of high school athletic coaches, *J Ath Train* 34(3): 267.

28. Rich BS: 1993. All physicians are not created equal; understanding the educational background of the sports medicine physician, *J Ath Train* 28(2):177.

29. Ruskin, BI, Goldsmith, LM: 2002. The role of the team physician, *Sports law administration & practice* 9(2):9–10.

30. Steinbach, P.: 2003. Training ways: strength and conditioning coaches weigh their options amid an abundance of diverse techniques designed to enhance the performance of today's elite athletes; *Athletic* 27(7):66–74.

31. Team Physician Consensus Statement: 2002. *Medicine and science in sports and exercise* 32(4):877–878.

32. Xerogeanes, J: 2007. The athletic trainer as orthopedic physician extender. *Athletic therapy today* 12(1):1.

## ANNOTATED BIBLIOGRAPHY

Cartwright L, Pittney W: 2000. *Athletic training for student assistants*, Champaign, IL, Human Kinetics.

*A practical guide for student athletic training assistants including their roles and responsibilities within the sports medicine team.*

Hannum S: 2000. *Professional behaviors in athletic training*, Thorofare, NJ, Slack.

*Focuses on essentials of effective career development. Addresses many skills students will require to build their image as health care professionals, such as communication, critical thinking, networking, interpersonal skills, and recognition of cultural differences.*

Mueller F, Ryan A: 1991. *Prevention of athletic injuries: the role of the sports medicine team*, Philadelphia, Davis.

*Provides an in-depth discussion of the various members of the sports medicine team.*

Prentice W: 2011. *Arnheim's principles of athletic training*, 14th ed. New York, McGraw-Hill.

*Discusses the sports medicine team approach paying particular attention to the role of the athletic trainer in providing health care to the athlete.*

Earle, R., Baechle, T: 2004. *NSCA's essentials of personal training*, Champaign, IL, Human Kinetics.

NSCA's Essentials of Personal Training *is the ideal authoritative resource for personal trainers, health and fitness instructors, exercise scientists, and other fitness professionals.*

ACSM's resources for the personal trainer, 2004. Philadelphia, Lippincott, Williams and Wilkins.
*A guide for working and becoming certified as a personal fitness trainer.*

Van Ost L, Manfre K: 2003. *Athletic training student guide to success*, Thorofare, NJ, Slack.
*This text emphasizes the roles and responsibilities of the student athletic trainer necessary to make them successful as health care professionals.*

## WEB SITES

American Academy of Orthopaedic Surgeons: www.aaos.org
*Presents general public information and information to its members. The public information is in the form of patient education brochures and a description of the organization and a definition of orthopedics.*

American College of Sports Medicine: www.acsm.org
*The mission of the American College of Sports Medicine is to advance and integrate scientific research to provide educational and practical applications of exercise science and sports.*

American Orthopaedic Society for Sports Medicine: www.sportsmed.org
*Dedicated to educating health care professionals and the general public about sports medicine; access is provided to the American Journal of Sports Medicine and a wide variety of links to related sites.*

American Sports Medicine Institute: www.asmi.org
*The American Sports Medicine Institute's mission is to improve the understanding, prevention, and treatment of sports-related injuries through research and education. In addition to stating this mission, the site provides access to current research and journal articles.*

Athletic Trainer.com: athletictrainer.com
*Specifically designed to give information to athletic trainers, including students and those interested in athletic training; provides access to interesting journal articles and links to several additional informative Web sites.*

National Athletic Trainers Association: www.nata.org
*Presents a description of the athletic training profession, the role of an athletic trainer, and how to become involved in athletic training.*

NCAA: www.ncaa.org
*Provides general information about the NCAA and the publications that the NCAA circulates; is useful for those working in the collegiate setting.*

# Organizing and Administering
# an Athletic Health Care Program

*When you finish this chapter you will be able to:*

- Identify the rules of operation that should be enforced in an athletic health care program.
- Explain budgetary concerns for ordering supplies and equipment.
- Explain the importance of the preparticipation physical examination.
- Identify the records that an athletic health care program must maintain.
- Describe a well-designed athletic health care facility.

Operating an effective athletic health care program requires careful organization and administration regardless of whether the setting is a high school, college, or university, or at the professional level.[15] **This chapter is directed toward coaches and other fitness professionals who do not have a certified athletic trainer to supervise or oversee an athletic health care program and who, by default, must develop and/or administer such a program.** It looks at the administrative tasks required for successful operation of an athletic health care program, including facility design, policies and procedures, budget considerations, organizing preparticipation physical examinations, and record keeping.

## ESTABLISHING RULES OF OPERATION FOR AN ATHLETIC HEALTH CARE PROGRAM

Every athletic health care program must develop policies and procedures that carefully delineate the daily routine of the program.[3] This is imperative for handling health problems and injuries.[1,12,22]

It is first necessary to decide exactly who will be taken care of in the athletic health care facility. The athletic administrator or school principal must decide the extent to which the athlete will be served. For example, will prevention and care activities be extended to athletes for the entire year, including summer and other vacations, or only during the competitive season? A policy should clarify whether students other than athletes, athletes from other schools, faculty, and staff are to receive care.[23] Often legal concerns and the school liability insurance dictate who, other than the athlete, is to be served.

### Providing Coverage

A concern of any athletic program is to try to provide the most qualified health care possible to the athlete. Unfortunately, as indicated in

*Every athletic health care program must develop policies and procedures that carefully delineate the daily routine of the program.*

## CHAPTER 2

Organizing and Establishing
an Effective Athletic Health
Care System

The members of the school
board at All-American High
School voted to allocate
$25,000 to renovate a 25 foot by
40 foot storage space and to
purchase new equipment for an
athletic training health care
facility. The athletic administrator has been asked to provide
the school principal with a wish
list of what should be included
in this facility. It has been
estimated that the physical
renovation will cost
approximately $17,000.

? How may this space be best
used, and what type of equipment should be purchased to
maximize the effectiveness of
this new facility?

Chapter 1, budgetary limitations often dictate who is responsible for overseeing the health care program for the athletes. Ideally an institution hires a certified athletic trainer who is primarily responsible. In some cases, schools rely on a nurse to provide care. And in other situations in which there are no athletic trainers or nurses, health care responsibility usually falls on the coach. Regardless of who is in charge of the health care program, policies must be established concerning how to best provide coverage to various athletic teams.[16] High schools with limited available supervision may only be able to provide athletic training facility coverage in the afternoons and during vacation periods. Ideally, high-risk sports should have a certified athletic trainer and physician present at all practices and contests.

## Athletic Health Care Facility Policies

The athletic health care facility should be used only for the prevention and care of sports injuries.[4] Too often the athletic health care facility becomes a meeting or club room for teams and athletes. Unless definite rules are established and practiced, room cleanliness and sanitation become an impossible chore. Focus Box 2-1 lists some important athletic health care facility policies. Specific policies regarding emergency protocols (Chapter 7), lightning (Chapter 10), heat stress (Chapter 10), and fluid replacement (Chapter 10) will be discussed later in the text.

**2-1** *Focus Box*

**Rules and Policies of the Athletic Health Care Facility**

- *Cleated shoes are not allowed.* Dirt and debris tend to cling to cleated shoes; therefore cleated shoes should be removed before athletes enter the athletic training facility.

- *Game equipment must remain outside.* Because game equipment such as balls and bats add to the sanitation problem, it should be kept out of the athletic health care facility. Athletes must be continually reminded that the athletic health care facility is not a storage room for sports equipment.

- *Shoes must be kept off treatment tables.* Because shoes tend to contaminate treatment tables, they must be removed before any care is given to the athlete.

- *Athletes should shower before receiving treatment.* The athlete should make it a habit to shower before being treated if the treatment is not an emergency. This procedure helps keep tables and therapeutic modalities sanitary.

- *Roughhousing and profanity are not allowed.* Athletes must be continually reminded that the athletic health care facility is for injury care and prevention. Horseplay and foul language lower the basic purpose of the athletic health care facility.

- *No food or smokeless tobacco is allowed.*

---

( 2-2 )　*Focus Box*

---

**Suggestions for Maintaining a Sanitary Environment**

- Sweep the gymnasium floors daily.
- Clean and disinfect drinking fountains, showers, sinks, urinals, and toilets daily.
- Air out and sanitize lockers frequently.
- Clean wrestling mats and wall mats daily.
- Urge the use of clean dry towels each day for each individual athlete.
- Issue individual equipment and clothing to each athlete to avoid skin irritations.
- Do not allow swapping of equipment and clothing.
- Launder and change clothing frequently.
- Allow wet clothing to dry thoroughly before the athlete wears it again.

---

## Keeping Facilities Clean

The practice of good hygiene and sanitation is of the utmost importance in an athletic health care program. Preventing infectious diseases is a direct responsibility of the coach, whose duty it is to see that all athletes are surrounded by as hygienic an environment as is possible and that each individual is practicing sound health habits. Chapter 8 discusses the management of bloodborne pathogens. The coach must be aware of and adhere to guidelines for the operation of an athletic care facility as dictated by the Occupational Safety and Health Administration (OSHA).

Focus Box 2-2 lists guidelines to help maintain a sanitary environment.

Cleaning responsibilities in most schools are divided between the athletic training or coaching staff and the maintenance crew. Care of permanent building structures and trash disposal are usually the responsibilities of maintenance, whereas upkeep of specialized equipment falls within the province of the coaches or athletic trainers. Division of routine cleaning responsibilities may be organized as suggested in Focus Box 2-3.

*Good hygiene and sanitation are essential for an athletic training program.*

## Establishing Health Habits for the Athlete

To promote good health among the athletes, the coach and/or the athletic trainer should encourage sound health habits. Focus Box 2-4 provides a checklist that may be a useful guide for coaches, athletic trainers, and athletes.

## Providing Emergency Phones

The installation or availability of an emergency telephone adjacent to all major activity areas or the availability of a mobile phone is a must. It should be possible to use this phone to call outside for emergency aid or to contact the athletic health care facilities when additional assistance is required. Walkie-talkies are also useful when practices or games occur at several different facilities simultaneously. These devices can greatly enhance communication without incurring a tremendous expense.

## Emergency Action Plan

In cooperation with existing community-based emergency health care delivery systems, the individual developing an athletic health care program should develop a systematic plan for accessing the emergency medical system and subsequent transportation of the injured athlete to an emergency care facility.[1,8,13] Meetings should be scheduled periodically with EMTs or paramedics who work in the community to make certain that they understand their role as a provider of emergency health care.

It is important to communicate the special considerations for dealing with athletic equipment issues before an emergency arises.[5] Focus Box 2-5 provides a sample for the emergency action plan. Chapter 7 discusses the emergency management plan in detail.

---

**2-5** *Focus Box*

---

### Sample Emergency Action Plan

*Emergency action plan for women's ice hockey*

**Emergency Personnel**

Certified athletic trainer and athletic training students on site for practice and competition: additional sports medicine staff accessible from main athletic health care facility (across street from arena)

**Emergency Communication**

Fixed telephone line in ice hockey satellite athletic health care facility (_____-_____)

**Emergency Equipment**

Supplies (AED, trauma kit, splint kit, spine board) maintained in ice hockey satellite athletic health care facility; additional emergency equipment accessible from athletic health care facility across street from arena (_____-_____)

**Roles of First Responders**

Immediate care of the injured or ill student athlete
Emergency equipment retrieval

**Activation of emergency medical system (EMS)**

**911 call (provide name, address, telephone number; number of individuals injured; condition of injured; first aid treatment; specific directions; other information as requested)**

Direct EMS to scene
  Open appropriate doors
  Designate individual to "flag down" EMS and direct to scene
Scene control: Limit scene to first aid providers and move bystanders away from area

**Venue Directions**

Ice hockey arena is located on corner of _____ Street and _____ Street adjacent to _____. Two gates provide access to the arena: _____ Street; drive leads to arena as well as rear door of complex (locker room, athletic training room)

**Sports Medicine Staff and Phone Numbers**

| | |
|---|---|
| Athletic Trainer in Charge | 929-0000 |
| Head Athletic Trainer | 929-0001 |
| Team Physician | 929-0002 |

---

From *NCAA Sports Medicine Handbook 2000–2001.*

Organizing and Establishing
an Effective Athletic Health
Care System

Keeping adequate records is
of major importance in the
athletic health care program.

Preparticipation health
examination:
• medical history
• physical examination
• maturity assessment
• orthopedic screening

All-American High School offers
eighteen sports, which are divided into six fall, six winter, and
six spring sports. The school has
a total of approximately 500
athletes, and approximately 200
of them are involved in the fall
sports. A preparticipation exam
must be arranged and administered so that each athlete can
be cleared for competition.

? How can the preparticipation
exams be set up to most efficiently clear 200 athletes for
competition in the fall sports?

# RECORD KEEPING

Record keeping is a major responsibility in an athletic health care program.
**There is no choice when it comes to keeping records!** Keeping
records and filling out forms is time consuming and to some extent annoying. Nevertheless, in a time in which lawsuits are the rule rather than the
exception, accurate and up-to-date records are an absolute necessity. In
addition to keeping medical records, injury reports, treatment logs, personal information cards, injury evaluations and progress notes, supply and
equipment inventories, and annual reports must be maintained.

## Administering Preparticipation Health Examinations

The primary purpose of the preseason health examination is to identify
whether an athlete is at risk before he or she participates in a specific
sport.[17,18] The preparticipation examination should consist of a medical
history, a physical examination, and a brief orthopedic screening. Information obtained during this examination will establish a baseline to which
comparisons may be made following injury.[2] The examination may reveal
conditions that could warrant disqualification from certain sports. The
examination will also satisfy insurance and liability issues (see Chapter 3).

The preparticipation physical may be administered on an individual
basis by a personal physician, or it may be done using a station examination system with a team of examiners.[20] Examination by a personal
physician has the advantage of yielding an in-depth history and an ideal
physician-patient relationship. A disadvantage of this type of examination is that it may not be directed to detection of factors that predispose
the athlete to a sports injury.[33]

The most thorough and sport-specific type of preparticipation examination is the station examination.[20] This method can provide the
athlete with a detailed examination in a short time. A team of nine
people is needed to examine thirty or more athletes. The team should
include two physicians, two medically trained nonphysicians (nurse,
athletic trainer, physical therapist, or physician's assistant), and five
managers, athletic training students, or assistant coaches who are
assigned specific tasks during the preparticipation exam based on their
level of expertise.

A preparticipation exam should include all of the following items.

### Medical History

A medical history form should be completed before the physical examination and orthopedic screening; its purpose is to identify any past or
existing medical problems. This form should be updated for each athlete every year. Medical histories should be closely reviewed by the
physician, the coach, and the athletic trainer so that they will be prepared should some medical emergency arise. Necessary participation
release forms and insurance information should be collected along with
the medical history (Figure 2-1).

**MEDICAL HISTORY FORM**

DATE OF EXAM_____

Name_____ Sex _____ Age _____ Date of birth _____

Grade _____ School _____ Sport(s) _____

Address _____ Phone _____

Personal physician _____

*In case of emergency, contact*

Name_____ Relationship_____ Phone (H) _____ (W) _____

**Explain "Yes" answers below.**
**Circle questions you don't know the answers to.**

| | Yes | No |
|---|---|---|
| 1. Has a doctor ever denied or restricted your participation in sports for any reason? | ☐ | ☐ |
| 2. Do you have an ongoing medical condition (like diabetes or asthma)? | ☐ | ☐ |
| 3. Are you currently taking any prescription or nonprescription (over-the-counter) medicine or pills? | ☐ | ☐ |
| 4. Do you have allergies to medicines, pollens, foods, or stinging insects? | ☐ | ☐ |
| 5. Have you ever passed out or nearly passed out DURING exercise? | ☐ | ☐ |
| 6. Have you ever passed out or nearly passed out AFTER exercise? | ☐ | ☐ |
| 7. Have you ever had discomfort, pain, or pressure in your chest during exercise? | ☐ | ☐ |
| 8. Does your heart race or skip beats during exercise? | ☐ | ☐ |

9. Has a doctor ever told you that you have (check all that apply):

☐ High blood pressure ☐ A heart murmur
☐ High cholesterol ☐ A heart infection

| | Yes | No |
|---|---|---|
| 10. Has a doctor ever ordered a test for your heart? (for example, ECG, echocardiogram) | ☐ | ☐ |
| 11. Has anyone in your family died for no apparent reason? | ☐ | ☐ |
| 12. Does anyone in your family have a heart problem? | ☐ | ☐ |
| 13. Has any family member or relative died of heart problems or of sudden death before age 50? | ☐ | ☐ |
| 14. Does anyone in your family have Marfan syndrome? | ☐ | ☐ |
| 15. Have you ever spent the night in a hospital? | ☐ | ☐ |
| 16. Have you ever had surgery? | ☐ | ☐ |
| 17. Have you ever had an injury, like a sprain, muscle or ligament tear, or tendonitis, that caused you to miss a practice or game? If yes, circle affected area below: | ☐ | ☐ |
| 18. Have you had any broken or fractured bones or dislocated joints? If yes, circle below: | ☐ | ☐ |
| 19. Have you had a bone or joint injury that required x-rays, MRI, CT, surgery, injections, rehabilitation, physical therapy, a brace, a cast, or crutches? If yes, circle below: | ☐ | ☐ |

| Head | Neck | Shoulder | Upper arm | Elbow | Forearm | Hand/ fingers | Chest |
|---|---|---|---|---|---|---|---|
| Upper back | Lower back | Hip | Thigh | Knee | Calf/shin | Ankle | Foot/toes |

| | Yes | No |
|---|---|---|
| 20. Have you ever had a stress fracture? | ☐ | ☐ |
| 21. Have you been told that you have or have you had an x-ray for atlantoaxial (neck) instability? | ☐ | ☐ |
| 22. Do you regularly use a brace or assistive device? | ☐ | ☐ |
| 23. Has a doctor ever told you that you have asthma or allergies? | ☐ | ☐ |

| | Yes | No |
|---|---|---|
| 24. Do you cough, wheeze, or have difficulty breathing during or after exercise? | ☐ | ☐ |
| 25. Is there anyone in your family who has asthma? | ☐ | ☐ |
| 26. Have you ever used an inhaler or taken asthma medicine? | ☐ | ☐ |
| 27. Were you born without or are you missing a kidney, an eye, a testicle, or any other organ? | ☐ | ☐ |
| 28. Have you had infectious mononucleosis (mono) within the last month? | ☐ | ☐ |
| 29. Do you have any rashes, pressure sores, or other skin problems? | ☐ | ☐ |
| 30. Have you had a herpes skin infection? | ☐ | ☐ |
| 31. Have you ever had a head injury or concussion? | ☐ | ☐ |
| 32. Have you been hit in the head and been confused or lost your memory? | ☐ | ☐ |
| 33. Have you ever had a seizure? | ☐ | ☐ |
| 34. Do you have headaches with exercise? | ☐ | ☐ |
| 35. Have you ever had numbness, tingling, or weakness in your arms or legs after being hit or falling? | ☐ | ☐ |
| 36. Have you ever been unable to move your arms or legs after being hit or falling? | ☐ | ☐ |
| 37. When exercising in the heat, do you have severe muscle cramps or become ill? | ☐ | ☐ |
| 38. Has a doctor told you that you or someone in your family has sickle cell trait or sickle cell disease? | ☐ | ☐ |
| 39. Have you had any problems with your eyes or vision? | ☐ | ☐ |
| 40. Do you wear glasses or contact lenses? | ☐ | ☐ |
| 41. Do you wear protective eyewear, such as goggles or a face shield? | ☐ | ☐ |
| 42. Are you happy with your weight? | ☐ | ☐ |
| 43. Are you trying to gain or lose weight? | ☐ | ☐ |
| 44. Has anyone recommended you change your weight or eating habits? | ☐ | ☐ |
| 45. Do you limit or carefully control what you eat? | ☐ | ☐ |
| 46. Do you have any concerns that you would like to discuss with a doctor? | ☐ | ☐ |

**FEMALES ONLY**

| | Yes | No |
|---|---|---|
| 47. Have you ever had a menstrual period? | ☐ | ☐ |

48. How old were you when you had your first menstrual period?_____

49. How many periods have you had in the last 12 months? _____

Explain "Yes" answers here: _____
_____
_____
_____
_____
_____
_____

**I hereby state that, to the best of my knowledge, my answers to the above questions are complete and correct.**

Signature of athlete_____ Signature of parent/guardian_____ Date_____

**Source: Used with Permission from the Physician and Sports Medicine.**

**Figure 2-1**

Sample medical history form

### Physical Examination

The physical examination should include assessment of height, weight, body composition, blood pressure, pulse, vision, skin, teeth, ears, nose, throat, heart and lung function, abdomen, lymphatics, genitalia, maturation index, and—if funds allow—urinalysis and blood work (Figure 2-2).

### Maturity Assessment

Maturity assessment should be part of the physical examination as a means of protecting the young athlete. Most commonly used methods are the circumpubertal (sexual maturity), skeletal, and dental assessments. Of the three, Tanner's five stages of assessment, indicating maturity of secondary sexual characteristics, is the most expedient for use in the station method of examination (see Chapter 25 for detailed discussion).[36]

### Orthopedic Screening

Orthopedic screening may be done as part of the physical examination or separately by the athletic trainer. An example of a very quick orthopedic screening examination appears in Table 2-1; it usually takes about 90 seconds. A more detailed orthopedic examination may be conducted to assess strength, range of motion, and stability at various joints.

**TABLE 2-1** Orthopedic Screening Examination

| Activity and Instruction | To Determine |
|---|---|
| Stand facing examiner | Acromioclavicular joints; general symmetry |
| Look at ceiling, floor, over both shoulders; touch ears to shoulders | Cervical spine motion |
| Shrug shoulders (examiner resists) | Trapezius strength |
| Abduct shoulders 90 degrees (examiner resists at 90 degrees) | Deltoid strength |
| Full external rotation of arms | Shoulder motion |
| Flex and extend elbows | Elbow motion |
| Arms at sides, elbows 90 degrees flexed; pronate and supinate wrists | Elbow and wrist motion |
| Spread fingers; make fist | Hand or finger motion and deformities |
| Tighten (contract) quadriceps; relax quadriceps | Symmetry and knee effusion; ankle effusion |
| Perform a lunge with each leg | Hip, knee, and ankle motion |
| Stand with back to examiner | Shoulder symmetry; scoliosis |
| Knees straight, touch toes | Scoliosis, hip motion, hamstring tightness |
| Raise up on toes, raise heels | Calf symmetry, leg strength |

## PHYSICAL EXAMINATION FORM

Name_____ Date of birth_____

Grade_____Weight _____% Body fat (optional)_____Pulse_____BP___/_____ (___/____,___/____)

Vision  R 20 /_____  L 20 /_____     Corrected: Y  N     Pupils: Equal _____  Unequal _____

| Follow-Up Questions on More Sensitive Issues | Yes | No |
|---|---|---|
| 1. Do you feel stressed out or under a lot of pressure? | ☐ | ☐ |
| 2. Do you ever feel so sad or hopeless that you stop doing some of your usual activities for more than a few days? | ☐ | ☐ |
| 3. Do you feel safe? | ☐ | ☐ |
| 4. have you ever tried cigarette smoking, even 1 or 2 puffs? Do you currently smoke? | ☐ | ☐ |
| 5. During the past 30 days, did you use chewing tobacco, snuff, or dip? | ☐ | ☐ |
| 6. During the past 30 days, have you had at least 1 drink of alcohol? | ☐ | ☐ |
| 7. Have you ever taken steroid pills or shots without a doctor's prescription? | ☐ | ☐ |
| 8. Have you ever taken any supplements to help you gain or lose weight or improve your performance? | ☐ | ☐ |
| 9. Questions from the Youth Risk Behavior Survey (http://www.cdc.gov/HealthyYouth/yrbs/index.htm) on guns, seatbelts, unprotected sex, domestic violence, drugs, etc. | ☐ | ☐ |

Notes:_____

| | NORMAL | ABNORMAL FINDINGS | INITIALS* |
|---|---|---|---|
| **MEDICAL** | | | |
| Appearance | | | |
| Eyes/ears/nose/throat | | | |
| Hearing | | | |
| Lymph nodes | | | |
| Heart | | | |
| Murmurs | | | |
| Pulses | | | |
| Lungs | | | |
| Abdomen | | | |
| Genitourinary (males only)† | | | |
| Skin | | | |
| **MUSCULOSKELETAL** | | | |
| Neck | | | |
| Back | | | |
| Shoulder/arm | | | |
| Elbow/forearm | | | |
| Wrist/hand/fingers | | | |
| Hip/thigh | | | |
| Knee | | | |
| Leg/ankle | | | |
| Foot/toes | | | |

*Multiple-examiner set-up only.
†Having a third party present is recommended for the genitourinary examination.

Notes:_____

Name of physician (print/type)_____ Date _____

Address _____ Phone _____

Signature of physician _____, MD or DO

*Used with permission from ©2004 American Academy of Family Physicians, American Academy of Pediatrics, American College of Sports Medicine, American Medical Society for Sports Medicine, American Orthopedic Society for Sports Medicine, and American Osteopathic Academy of Sports Medicine.*

**Source: Used with Permission from the Physician and Sports Medicine.**

**Figure 2-2**

Sample physical examination form

### Sport Disqualification

As discussed previously, sports participation involves risks. Most conditions that warrant a recommendation for disqualification can be identified during a preparticipation health evaluation and should be noted in the medical history.[26] Because of the Americans with Disabilities Act, a physician cannot legally disqualify athletes from competing because of an existing medical problem. They can only recommend that the athlete voluntarily choose not to participate. In general, the athlete who has lost one of two paired organs such as eyes or kidneys is cautioned against playing a collision or contact sport.[33] Such an athlete should be counseled into participating in a noncontact sport. The athlete with one testicle, or one or both that are undescended, must be apprised that there is a small risk, which is substantially minimized with the use of an athletic supporter and a protective device.

## Release of Medical Records

The coach, athletic trainer, or other members of the sports medicine team may not release an athlete's medical records to anyone either in writing or verbally without written consent. If the athlete wishes to have medical records released to colleges or universities, professional sports organizations, insurance companies, the news media, or any other group or individual, he, she, the parent, or the guardian must sign a waiver that specifies which information is to be released.

### HIPAA Regulations

The Health Insurance Portability and Accountability Act (HIPAA) regulates how any member of the sports medicine team who has health information about an athlete can share that information with others.[9] The regulation guarantees that athletes have access to their medical records, gives them more control over how their protected health information is used and disclosed, and provides a clear avenue of recourse if their medical privacy is compromised. Authorization by an athlete to release medical information is not necessary on a per-injury basis. A blanket authorization signed by the athlete at the beginning of the year will suffice for all injuries and treatment done during the course of participation for that year. These one-time, blanket authorizations must indicate clearly what information may be released, to whom, and for what length of time.[19]

### FERPA Regulations

The Family Educational Rights and Privacy Act (FERPA) is a law that protects the privacy of student educational records. It has been suggested that in some instances medical records should be kept along with a student's educational records and thus the right to privacy of medical records would be protected under FERPA instead of HIPAA. FERPA gives parents certain rights with respect to their children's educational records. These rights transfer to the student when he or she reaches the age of 18 or attends a school beyond the high school level. Students to whom the rights have been transferred are "eligible students." Parents or eligible students have the right to inspect and review the student's educational records maintained by the school. Parents or eligible students have the right to request that a school correct records that they believe to be inaccurate or misleading. Schools must have written permission from the parent or eligible student to release any information from a student's educational records.

### Injury Reports

An injury report serves as a record for future reference (Figure 2-3). If the emergency procedures followed are questioned at a later date, a person's memory of the details may be somewhat hazy, but a report completed on the spot provides specific information. In a litigation situation, questions may be asked about an injury that occurred 3 years in the past. All injury reports should be filed in an administrator's office. The reports should be made out in triplicate, with one copy sent to the school health office, one to the physician, and one retained.

### Treatment Log

Each athletic health care facility should have a sign-in log available for the athlete who receives any service. Emphasis is placed on recording treatments for the athlete who is receiving daily therapy for an injury. As with injury records, treatment logs often have the status of legal documents and are used to establish certain facts in a civil litigation, an insurance action, or a criminal action following injury. These are subject to HIPAA and FERPA regulation and must be kept private.

### Personal Information Card

An athlete's personal information should be maintained in a file card or database. This card is completed by the athlete at the time of the health examination and serves as a means of contacting the family, personal physician, and insurance company in case of emergency. This information is efficiently stored on a PDA if available.

### Injury Evaluation and Progress Notes

The injured athlete should be evaluated by an athletic trainer, physical therapist, or physician who must record this information in some consistent format. If no athletic trainer or physician is available, the coach should either recommend to the parents or make arrangements for the athlete to be seen by a local physician, who must document the diagnosis in a medical record.

### Supply and Equipment Inventory

A major responsibility of anyone who oversees athletic health care is to manage a budget, most of which is spent on equipment and supplies. Every year an inventory must be conducted and recorded on such items as new equipment that is needed, equipment that needs to be replaced or repaired, and expendable supplies that need replenishing.

**2-3 Critical Thinking**
Exercise

One of the responsibilities of overseeing an athletic health care program is maintaining accurate records for every athlete.

? What kinds of records or types of information should be included in these records?

A major problem often facing athletic administrators is obtaining an adequate budget.

Name _____ Sport _____ Date: ___ / ___ / ___ Time: _____ Injury number: _____
Player I.D. _____ Age: _____ Location: _____ Intercollegiate-nonintercollegiate
Initial injury    Recheck    Reinjury        Preseason—Practice—Game        Incurred while participating in sport: yes ___ no ___
Description:  How did it happen? _____
_____
Initial impression: _____
_____
_____

| SITE OF INJURY | BODY PART | | STRUCTURE | Treatment _____ |
|---|---|---|---|---|
| 1 Right | 1 Head | 25 MP joint | 1 Skin | _____ |
| 2 Left | 2 Face | 26 PIP joint | 2 Muscle | _____ |
| 3 Proximal | 3 Eye | 27 Abdomen | 3 Fascia | _____ |
| 4 Distal | 4 Nose | 28 Hip | 4 Bone | _____ |
| 5 Anterior | 5 Ear | 29 Thigh | 5 Nerve | _____ |
| 6 Posterior | 6 Mouth | 30 Knee | 6 Fat pad | _____ |
| 7 Medial | 7 Neck | 31 Patella | 7 Tendon | _____ |
| 8 Lateral | 8 Thorax | 32 Lower leg | 8 Ligament | _____ |
| 9 Other | 9 Ribs | 33 Ankle | 9 Cartilage | _____ |
| | 10 Sternum | 34 Achilles tendon | 10 Capsule | _____ |
| | 11 Upper back | 35 Foot | 11 Compartment | _____ |
| **SITE OF EVALUATION** | 12 Lower back | 36 Toes | 12 Dental | _____ |
| 1 SHS | 13 Shoulder | 37 Other | 13 _____ | _____ |
| 2 Athletic Trn Rm. | 14 Rotator cuff | | | Medication _____ |
| 3 Site-Competition | 15 AC joint | _____ | _____ | _____ |
| 4 _____ | 16 Glenohumeral | | | _____ |
| | 17 Sternoclavicular | **NONTRAUMATIC** | **NATURE OF INJURY** | _____ |
| **PROCEDURES** | 18 Upper arm | 1 Dermatological | 1 Contusion | _____ |
| 1 Physical exam | 19 Elbow | 2 Allergy | 2 Strain | _____ |
| 2 X-ray | 20 Forearm | 3 Influenza | 3 Sprain | _____ |
| 3 Splint | 21 Wrist | 4 URI | 4 Fracture | _____ |
| 4 Wrap | 22 Hand | 5 GU | 5 Rupture | _____ |
| 5 Cast | 23 Thumb | 6 Systemic infect. | 6 Tendonitis | _____ |
| 6 Aspiration | 24 Finger | 7 Local infect. | 7 Bursitis | _____ |
| 7 Other | | 8 Other | 8 Myositis | Prescription dispensed |
| | | | 9 Laceration | 1 Antibiotics    5 Muscle relaxant |
| _____ | | | 10 Concussion | 2 Antiinflammatory  6 Enzyme |
| | | | 11 Avulsion | 3 Decongestant   7 _____ |
| | | | 12 Abrasion | 4 Analgesic |
| | | | 13 _____ | **INJECTIONS** |
| **DISPOSITION** | **REFERRAL** | **DISPOSITION OF INJURY** | | |
| 1 SHS | 1 Arthrogram | 1 No part. | | 1 Steroids |
| 2 Trainer | 2 Neurological | 2 Part part. | Degree | 2 Antibiotics |
| 3 Hospital | 3 Int. Med. | 3 Full part. | 1°  2°  3° | 3 Steroids-xylo |
| 4 H.D. | 4 Orthopedic | | | 4 _____ |
| 5 Other | 5 EENT | | | |
| | 6 Dentist | | | |
| | 7 Other | Previous injury _____ | | |

**Figure 2-3**        Source: Courtesy D. Bailey, California State University at Long Beach.

Athletic injury record form

## Annual Reports

Most athletic administrators require an annual report on the functions of the athletic health care program. This report serves as a means for making program changes and improvements. It commonly includes the number of athletes served, a survey of the number and types of injuries, an analysis of the program, and recommendations for future improvements.

## DEVELOPING A BUDGET

One of the major problems administrators face is to obtain a budget of sufficient size to permit the institution to perform a creditable job of providing health care to the athlete.[34] Many high schools fail to make any budgetary provisions for athletic health care except for the purchase of tape, bandages, and a medical bag that contains a minimum amount of equipment.[27] Many schools fail to provide a room and any of the special facilities that are needed to establish an effective athletic health care program. Some school boards and administrators fail to recognize that the functions performed in the athletic health care facility are an essential component of the athletic program and that even if no specialist is used, the facilities are nonetheless necessary.[26] Colleges and universities do not usually face this problem to the extent that high schools do. By and large, athletic health care is recognized as an important aspect of the college athletic program.

Budgetary needs vary considerably within programs; some require only a few thousand dollars, whereas others spend hundreds of thousands of dollars. The amount spent on building and equipping an athletic health care facility, of course, is entirely a matter of local option. In purchasing equipment, immediate needs as well as availability of personnel to operate specialized equipment should be kept in mind.[29]

Budget records should be kept on file so that they are available for use in projecting the following year's budgetary needs. They present a picture of the distribution of current funds and serve to substantiate future budgetary requests. Expenditures for individual items vary in accordance with different administrative philosophies. An annual inventory must be conducted at the end of the year or before replenishing supplies and equipment. Accurate records must be kept to justify future requests.[28]

## Ordering Supplies and Equipment

Supplies are expendable and usually are for injury prevention, first aid, and management. Examples of supplies are athletic tape, germicides, and massage lotion. The term *equipment* refers to those items that are not expendable. Equipment may be further divided into fixed and nonfixed. Fixed equipment does not necessarily mean that it cannot be moved but that it is not usually removed from the athletic health care facility. Examples of fixed equipment are icemakers, weight equipment, and electrical therapeutic modalities. Nonfixed equipment refers to nonexpendable items that are less fixed, that may be part of an emergency

Equipment may be fixed or nonfixed.

Purchasing may be done through direct buy or competitive bid.

or field kit, or that may be at the sport site. Examples are blankets, scissors, and training kits. Focus Boxes 2-6 and 2-7 provide a list of supplies for the athletic health care facility and for a field kit.

---

**2-6 ⟩ Focus Box**

### Recommended Basic Health Care Facility Supplies

*Tape*
White adhesive, 1½ inch
White adhesive, 1 inch
Liteguard, 2 inch
Elastic, 2 inch
Elastic, 1 inch
Prewrap

*Bandages*
Bandage strips
Telfa, 2 by 3
Band-Aid Clear Patches
Gauze, 4 by 4 (sterile)
Elastic Wraps, 3, 4, 6 inch
Steri Strips, ¼ inch

*Foam and Felt*
1-inch felt
⅛-inch adhesive foam
Moleskin

*Braces and Splints*
Finger splints
Air splint, leg
Velcro, 1 inch (both sides)
Knee immobilizer
Ankle brace, left
Ankle brace, right
Thermoplastic material, 4 inch
Cervical collar (small, medium, large)
Heel cups (medium, large)
Patella strap, large
Wrist immobilizer (left, right, universal)
Ankle braces (xx-small, x-small, small, medium, large, x-large)

Triangular bandage
Slings
Nose guard
Elbow sleeves
Thigh sleeves
Back support (x-small, small, medium, large, x-large)
Knee sleeves
Stockinet, 3 inch

*Modalities*
Flex All, 1 gallon
Topical analgesic, 5 lb tub
Skin lubricant, 5 lb tub
Gray T-band
Black T-band
Heat packs (medium, large)
Ice bags
Plastic-wrap (small, large)
Lotion, 1 gallon

*First Aid*
Cotton rolls (nose plugs)
Tongue depressors
Cotton tip applicators
Non-latex gloves (medium, large)
Cotton balls
Skin-preps
Save-A-Tooth
Penlights
Biohazard bags
Safety goggles

*Taping Accessories*
Heel and lace pads
Tape adherent spray
Tape remover

*Sharps*
Scissors
Tweezers
Nail clippers (large, small)
Tape cutters
Shark refill blades

*Antiseptics*
Hydrogen Peroxide
Rubbing alcohol
Sterile water

*Skin Treatments*
Antibiotic ointment
Second Skin
Baby powder

*Eye Treatment*
Eye wash
Penlights

*Crutches*
Large
Medium
Small
Large aluminum

*Water*
Bottle carriers
Water bottles
Coolers (3, 7, 10 gallon)
Chest

*Other*
Stools
Spray bottles
Bucket
Cloth towels

2-7 ⟩ *Focus Box*

**Recommended Basic Field Kit Supplies**

Adhesive bandages

Tape cutters

Scissors

Eye cover

Tooth saving kit

Petroleum jelly

Razor blades

Sterile eye irrigating solution

Non-latex gloves

Biohazard bags

Tape spray

Skin lubricant

Gauze pads: 2 by 2, 3 by 3,
or 4 by 4

Heel cup

Sling

Hydrogen peroxide

Finger splints

Cotton-tipped applicators

Tongue depressors

Topical analgesic

Lotion

Sunscreen

Tape supplies:
   white adhesive
      1 inch, 1½ inch
   heel and lace pads
   prewrap
   elastic adhesive
      1 inch, 2 inch, 3 inch

Elastic wraps:
   2 inch, 3 inch, 4 inch,
   6 inch double 4 inch,
   double 6 inch

Alcohol

Reusable elastic wrap

Adhesive foam

Adhesive felt

Penlight

Contact lens cases

Contact lens wetting solution

Mirror

### Purchasing Systems

Purchasing of supplies and equipment must be done through either direct buy or competitive bid. For expensive purchases, an institutional purchasing agent is sent out to competing vendors who quote a price on specified supplies or equipment. Orders are generally placed with the lowest bidder. Smaller purchases or emergency purchases may be made directly from a single vendor.

## Additional Budget Considerations

In addition to supplies and equipment, other costs may be included in the operation of an athletic health care program; these costs include telephone and postage, contracts with physicians or clinics for services, ongoing maintenance of equipment (i.e., modalities), professional liability insurance, memberships in professional organizations, the purchase of professional journals or textbooks, travel and expenses for attending professional meetings, and clothing to be worn in the athletic health care facility.

## CONSIDERATIONS IN PLANNING AN ATHLETIC HEALTH CARE FACILITY

For a school or athletic administrator who may have to assume responsibility for planning an athletic health care facility, or for a coach who may not have an athletic trainer, some guidance and understanding of what should be included in that facility is necessary.

Essential to any sports program is the maximum use of facilities and the most effective use of equipment and supplies.[32] The sports medicine or athletic health care facility must be specially designed to meet the many requirements of an athletic injury management program (Figure 2-4).[24] The size and the layout of the athletic health care facility depend on the scope of the athletic program, including the size and number of teams and athletes, what sports are offered, and the daily traffic flow patterns in the athletic health care facility.[10] The athletic health care facility should be designed to meet regulations and guidelines established by the Occupational Safety and Health Administration (OSHA).

Ideally, the athletic health care facility should be designed from a new space. Realistically, it is more likely that an athletic health care

**Figure 2-4**

The ideal athletic health care facility should be well designed to maximize its use.

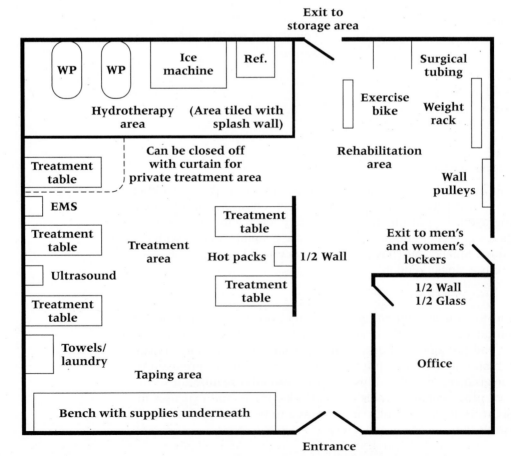

facility in a high school would be constructed in an existing classroom; in an old locker room, weight room, team room, cafeteria, or library; in a corner of the gymnasium; or, in some cases, in a storage or a custodian's closet. Therefore, this new athletic health care facility will need to be designed and adapted based on where power supplies, water supplies, and drains already exist. It should be stressed that regardless of where the athletic health care facility is located, it should be considered a medical care facility and organized appropriately.

An area of less than 1,000 square feet is impractical. An athletic health care facility 1,000 to 1,200 square feet in size is satisfactory for most schools. The 1,200-square-foot area (40 feet by 30 feet) permits handling a number of athletes at one time and allows ample room for the bulky equipment needed. A facility of this size is well suited for pregame preparation. Careful planning will determine whether a larger area is needed or is desirable.[6,14,31]

The athletic health care facility should be located immediately adjacent to the men's and women's locker rooms.[35] The facility should have an outside entrance from the field or court, making it unnecessary to bring injured athletes in through the building. This door also permits access when the rest of the building is not in use.

The athletic health care facility should be organized to provide distinct areas for (1) taping and bandaging; (2) injury treatment using rehabilitative equipment and/or therapeutic modalities; (3) a wet area for whirlpools, a refrigerator, and an ice machine; and (4) an area where a physician or an athletic trainer can conduct evaluations in privacy. This could be either a separate room or an area separated from the rest of the athletic health care facility by a curtain or screen. An office for the athletic trainer should provide for secure storage of medical records and patient files.

*The athletic health care facility is a multipurpose area used for first aid, therapy and exercise rehabilitation, injury prevention, medical procedures such as the physical examination, and athletic training administration.*

## Storage Facilities

Many athletic health care facilities lack adequate storage space (Figure 2-5). Often storage facilities are located a considerable distance away, which is extremely inconvenient. Each of the four special service areas should contain storage cabinets and shelves for storing general supplies and the small specialized equipment used in the respective areas. A large walk-in closet is a necessity for storing bulky equipment, medical supplies, adhesive tape, bandages, and protective devices. Another important piece of equipment is a refrigerator for storing frozen water in styrofoam cups for ice massage and other necessities.[25]

*It is essential to have sufficient storage space for supplies and equipment.*

## HIRING A CERTIFIED ATHLETIC TRAINER IN SECONDARY SCHOOLS

It would be ideal to have certified athletic trainers serve every secondary school in the United States.[11] Many of the physical problems that occur later from improperly managed sports injuries could be avoided if proper care from an athletic trainer had been provided initially. Many

**Figure 2-5**

An effective athletic health care program must have appropriate storage facilities that are highly organized.

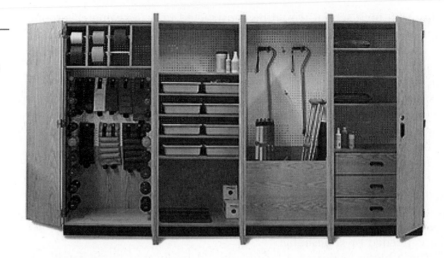

times a coach is in a situation without an athletic trainer and by default must assume the responsibility for athletic health care. In some cases, a coach assumes additional athletic training responsibilities and is assisted by a high school student who is interested in becoming an athletic trainer.

---

**2-8   Focus Box**

**Looking to Hire a Certified Athletic Trainer?**

1. *Hiring a certified athletic trainer in a faculty-athletic trainer capacity.* This individual is usually employed as a teacher in one of the school's classroom disciplines and performs athletic training duties on a part-time or extracurricular basis. In this instance compensation usually is on the basis of released time from teaching, a stipend as a coach, or both.

2. *Using a certified graduate student from a nearby college or university.* The graduate student receives a graduate assistantship with a stipend paid by the secondary school or community college. In this situation both the graduate student and the school benefit. However, this practice may prevent a school from employing a certified athletic trainer on a full-time basis.

3. *Employing a centrally placed certified athletic trainer for a school district.* In this case the athletic trainer, who may be full- or part-time, is a nonteacher who serves a number of schools. The advantage is savings; the disadvantage is that one individual cannot provide the level of service usually required by a typical school.

4. *Contracting with a clinic to provide a certified athletic trainer.* Most clinical athletic trainers see patients with sports-related injuries during the morning hours in the clinic. In the afternoons, athletic trainers' services are contracted out to local high schools or small colleges for game or practice coverage.

In 1995, the National Athletic Trainers Association adopted the following position on hiring athletic trainers in secondary schools:

> *The National Athletic Trainers' Association, as a leader in healthcare for the physically active, believes that the prevention and treatment of injuries to student-athletes are a priority. The recognition and treatment of injuries to student athletes must be immediate. The medical delivery system for injured student-athletes needs a coordinator within the local school community who will facilitate the prevention, recognition, treatment and reconditioning of sports related injuries. Therefore, it is the position of the National Athletic Trainers' Association that all secondary schools should provide the services of a full-time, on-site, certified athletic trainer (ATC) to student athletes.*

Based on a proposal from the American Academy of Pediatrics, in 1998 the American Medical Association adopted a policy calling for certified athletic trainers to be employed in all high-school athletic programs. Although this policy was simply a recommendation and not a requirement, it was a very positive statement supporting the efficacy of athletic trainers in the secondary schools.

Focus Box 2-8 explains how athletic trainers are employed in secondary schools.

### Athletic Injury Management Checklist

The following is a checklist of things that should be done in organizing and administering an athletic health care program.

☐ Establish rules and policies for the athletic health care facility.
☐ Arrange for the facilities to be cleaned and maintained in cooperation with the maintenance staff.
☐ Establish health habits for the athletes.
☐ Arrange for the availability or purchase of emergency phones.
☐ Arrange for preparticipation exams for all athletes.
☐ Maintain appropriate and necessary injury records (injury reports, medical history, etc.).
☐ Develop a budget for purchasing supplies and equipment.
☐ Put together a field kit with the appropriate supplies.
☐ Find a space of reasonable proportions that can be used for an athletic training room.

## SUMMARY

- Organization and administration of the athletic health care program demands significant time and effort on the part of those overseeing the program.
- The athletic health care program best serves the athlete by establishing specific policies and regulations governing the use of available services.

- Preparticipation exams must be given to athletes and should include a medical history, a general physical examination, and an orthopedic screening.
- The individual overseeing the athletic health care program must maintain accurate and up-to-date medical records in addition to the other paperwork necessary for the operation of the athletic training program.
- Budgets should allow for the purchase of equipment and supplies essential for providing appropriate preventive and rehabilitative care for the athlete.
- The athletic health care program can be enhanced by designing or renovating a facility to maximize the potential use of the space available.

---

### Solutions to Critical Thinking Exercises

**2-1** The athletic health care facility should have specific areas designated for taping and preparation, treatment and rehabilitation, and hydrotherapy, and should have adequate storage facilities that are positioned within the space to allow for an efficient traffic flow. Equipment purchases might include four to five treatment tables and two to three taping tables (these could be made in-house if possible), a large-capacity ice machine, a combination ultrasound/electrical simulating unit, a whirlpool, and various free weights and exercise tubing.

**2-2** The preparticipation examination should consist of a medical history, a physical examination, and a brief orthopedic screening. The preparticipation physical may be effectively administered using a station examination system with a team of examiners. A station examination can provide the athlete with a detailed examination in a short time. A team of people is needed to examine this many athletes. The team should include physicians, medically trained nonphysicians (nurses, athletic trainers, physical therapists, or physician's assistants), and managers, student coaches, or assistant coaches.

**2-3** The individual overseeing the athletic health care system should keep a record of the medical history, injury reports, a personal individual information card, treatment logs, injury evaluations and progress notes, and a form for release of medical records.

## REVIEW QUESTIONS AND CLASS ACTIVITIES

1. What major administrative functions must be performed in overseeing an athletic health care program?
2. Design two athletic health care facilities—one for a medium-sized high school and one for a large university.
3. Observe the activities in the athletic health care facility. Pick both a slow time and a busy time to observe.
4. Why do hygiene and sanitation play an important role in athletic health care? How should the athletic training facility be maintained?
5. Fully equip a new medium-sized high school or college athletic health care facility or a clinical facility. Pick equipment from current catalogs.

6. Establish a reasonable health care budget for a small high school, a large high school, and a large college or university.
7. Identify the groups of individuals to be served in the athletic health care facility.
8. Organize a preparticipation health examination for ninety football players.
9. Record keeping is a major function in athletic health care. What records are necessary to keep?
10. Debate what conditions constitute good grounds for medical disqualification from a sport.

## REFERENCES

1. Allan, DC: 2000. Management strategies in athletic training. (Review) 2nd ed (Review), *Journal of sports chiropractic and rehabilitation* 14(4):132.
2. American Academy of Family Physicians: 2005. *Preparticipation physical evaluation.* 3rd ed, Minneapolis, McGraw-Hill Healthcare Information.
3. Ammon, R, Mulrooney, A, Southall, R: 2003. *Sport facility management: organizing events and mitigating risks.* Morgantown, WV, Fitness Information Technology, Incorporated.
4. Anderson, B: 2006. Policies and philosophies related to risk management in the athletic setting, *Athletic therapy today* 11(1):10.
5. Anderson, J, Courson, R, Kleiner, D, McLoda, T: 2002. National Athletic Trainers' Association Position statement: Emergency planning in athletics, *Journal of athletic training,* 37(1):99–104, 2002.
6. Ashley, FB, Courtney, S, Hicks, VL: 1997. Fitness and health-related areas. In Walker, ML, Stotlar, DK, editors: *Sports facility management,* Sudbury, Mass, 1997, Jones & Bartlett.
7. Bagnall, D: 2001. Budget planning key in secondary schools, *NATA News,* January 15.
8. Barker, Anita: 2005. Developing a crisis management plan, *Athletics administration* 40(2):41.
9. Blair, S.A.: 2003. Implementing HIPAA.; *ACSM's health & fitness journal* 7(5)25–27, NCAA; Privacy rules affect exchange of student-athlete medical records, *NCAA news* 40(5):10, 2003.
10. Brown, J: 2005. Athletic training facilities. In Sawyer, T, editor: *Facilities planning for health, fitness, physical activity, recreation & sports,* Champaign, IL, Sagamore Publishing.
11. Claiborne, T, Su-I, H, Cappaert, T: 2007. Certified athletic trainers provide effective care in the high school setting, *Athletic therapy today* 12(2):34.
12. Curtis, N: 2006. Risk management, *Athletic therapy today* 11(1):34.
13. Davidson, D, Eickoff-Shemek, J: 2006. Is your emergency action plan complete? *ACSM's health & fitness journal* 10(1):29–31.
14. Doyle, M: 2002. A new dimension for the athletic training room: the spirit of the room, *Athletic therapy today* 7(1):34–35.
15. Goforth, M, Almquist, J, Matney, M: 2007. Understanding organization structures of the college, university, high school, clinical, and professional settings, *Clinics in sports medicine* 26(2):201.
16. Herbert, D: 2007. Emergency preparedness recommendations for high school and college athletic programs, *Sports, parks & recreation law reporter* 21(1):71.
17. Herbert D: 1994. Professional considerations related to conduct of preparticipation exams, *Sports Med Stand Malpract Report* 6(4):49.

18. Hunt, V: 2002. A general look at the preparticipation exam, *NATA News,* May 15.

19. Hunt, V: 2003. Meeting clarifies HIPAA restrictions, *NATA News,* February 10–12.

20. Johnson MD, Kibler B, Smith D: 1993. Keys to successful preparticipation exams, *Physician Sportsmed* 21(9):108.

21. Knells S: 1994. Leadership and management techniques and principles for athletic training, *Ath Train* 29(4):328.

22. Knight, KL: 2001. Athletic training clinic operations. In Knight, KL (ed), *Assessing clinical proficiencies in athletic training: a modular approach,* 3rd edition, Champaign, IL., Human Kinetics, pp. 14–19.

23. Konin J, Donley P: 1997. The athletic trainer as a personnel manager. In Konin J: *The clinical athletic trainer,* Gaithersburg, MD, Slack.

24. Moyer-Knowles J: 1997. Planning a new athletic facility. In Konin J: *The clinical athletic trainer,* Gaithersburg, MD, Slack.

25. Oliver, C, Schroeder, T: 2002. Athletic training room essentials, *Interscholastic athletic administration* 28(4):21.

26. Peterson E: 1999. Insult to injury: feeling understaffed, underequipped and undervalued, athletic trainers say a minimum of space and equipment will yield extensive benefits, *Ath Bus* 23(1):57.

27. Rankin J: 1992. Financial resources for conducting athletic training programs in the collegiate

and high school settings, *J Ath Train* 27(4):344.

28. Rankin J, Ingersoll C: 2005. *Athletic training management: concepts and applications,* St Louis, McGraw-Hill.

29. Ray, R: 2005. Where athletic trainers work: facility design and planning. In Ray, R (ed), *Management strategies in athletic training,* 3rd ed, Champaign, IL, Human Kinetics.

30. Sabo J: 1999. Athletic training room design and layout, Proceedings of National Athletic Trainers' Association fiftieth annual meeting and clinical symposia, June 16–19, Kansas City, MO, Human Kinetics.

31. Sabo, J: 2001. Design and construction of an athletic training facility, *NATA News,* May 10–23.

32. Sawyer, T: 2005. *Facility design and management for health, fitness, physical activity, recreation and sports facility development.* Champaign, IL, Sagamore Publishing, Inc.

33. Swander H: 1992. *Preparticipation physical examination,* Kansas City, American Academy of Family Physicians, American Academy of Pediatrics, American Orthopedic Society for Sports Medicine, American Osteopathic Academy for Sports Medicine.

34. Walker, M, Stotlar, D (eds.): 1997. *Sports facility management,* Sudbury, Mass., Jones & Bartlett Publishers.

35. Wiese-Bjornstal, D: 2000. Gender in the athletic training room, *Athletic therapy today* 5(5):2627.

36. Tanner M: 1962. *Growth of adolescence,* ed 2, Oxford, England, Blackwell Scientific.

### ANNOTATED BIBLIOGRAPHY

Rankin J, Ingersoll C: 2005. *Athletic training management: concepts and applications,* ed 3, St Louis, McGraw-Hill.

*This text is designed for upper-division undergraduate or graduate students interested in all aspects of organization and administration of an athletic training program. The second edition has been expanded to include coverage of sports medicine clinics, industrial athletic training, the process of seeking employment, third-party reimbursement, financial management, risk management, and information technology, including distance learning and the Web.*

Ray R: 2005. *Management strategies in athletic training,* 3rd ed, Champaign, IL, Human Kinetics.

*This was the first text available to cover the principles of organization and administration as they apply to many different employment settings in athletic training. The third edition contains many examples and case studies based on principles of administration presented in the text.*

# Legal Liability and Insurance

## CHAPTER 3

*When you finish this chapter you will be able to:*

- Explain legal considerations for anyone acting as a health care provider.
- Define the legal concepts of liability, negligence, torts, assumption of risk.
- Identify measures that can be taken to minimize chances of litigation.
- Describe product liability.
- Identify the essential insurance requirements for protection of the athlete.
- Describe the types of insurance necessary to protect an individual who provides health care to anyone who is injured.

## LEGAL CONCERNS

In recent years negligence suits against physical education teachers, fitness professionals, coaches, athletic trainers, school administrators, and physicians arising out of sports injuries have increased both in frequency and in the amount of damages awarded.[8,9] An increasing awareness of the many risk factors present in physical activities is essential.

**This chapter is intended to provide basic information about things that can be done to avoid litigation and to briefly discuss the types of insurance needed to protect both the athlete and the coach, fitness professional and administrator. Liability** means being legally responsible for the harm one causes another person.[12] A great deal of care must be taken in following policies and procedures to reduce the risk of being sued by an athlete and being found liable for negligence.[15] It is important to reemphasize that **it is essential for everyone to know the legal limitations of their responsibilities in providing athletic health care as dictated by the laws and statutes in the specific state where that individual is employed.**

### The Standard of Reasonable Care

**Negligence** is the failure to use ordinary or reasonable care—care that persons would normally exercise to avoid injury to themselves or to others under similar circumstances. The **standard of reasonable care** assumes that an individual is neither exceptionally skillful nor extraordinarily cautious, but is a person of reasonable and ordinary prudence. Put another way, it is expected that an individual will bring a commonsense

---

**liability**
The state of being legally responsible for the harm one causes another person.

**negligence**
The failure to use ordinary or reasonable care.

**standard of reasonable care**
Assumes that an individual is a person of reasonable and ordinary prudence.

approach to the situation at hand and will exercise due care in its handling. In most cases in which someone has been sued for negligence, the actions of a hypothetical, reasonably prudent person are compared with the actions of the defendant to ascertain whether the course of action followed by the defendant was in conformity with the judgment exercised by such a reasonably prudent person.

The standard of reasonable care requires that anyone providing health care must act according to the standard of care of an individual with similar educational background or training.[21] An individual who has many years of experience, who is well educated in his or her field, and who is certified or licensed must act in accordance with those qualifications (Figure 3-1).

To establish negligence, an individual making the complaint must establish three things: (a) a **duty of care** existed between the person injured and the person responsible for that injury; (b) conduct of the defendant fell short of that duty of care; and (c) resultant damages.

## Torts

**Torts** are legal wrongs committed against the person or property of another.[12] Every person is expected to conduct themselves without injuring others. When they do so, either intentionally or by negligence, they can be required by a court to pay money to the injured party ("damages") so that, ultimately, they will suffer the pain caused by their action. A tort also serves as a deterrent by sending a message to the community as to what is unacceptable conduct.

Such wrongs may emanate from **nonfeasance** (also referred to as an *act of omission*), wherein the individual fails to perform a legal duty; from **malfeasance** (also referred to as an *act of commission*), wherein he or she commits an act that is not legally his or hers to perform; or from **misfeasance,** wherein an individual improperly does something that they have the legal right to do. In any instance, if injury results, the person can be held liable. In the case of nonfeasance an individual may fail to

**duty of care**
An individual who has the responsibility of caring for an injury.

**torts**
Legal wrongs committed against a person.

**nonfeasance or an act of omission**
When an individual fails to perform a legal duty.

**malfeasance or an act of commission**
When an individual commits an act that is not legally his to perform.

**misfeasance**
When an individual improperly does something they have the legal right to do.

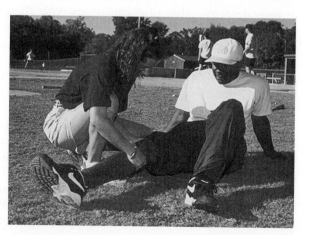

**Figure 3-1**

The chances of litigation can be minimized by providing reasonable and prudent care to an injured athlete.

refer a seriously injured athlete for the proper medical attention. In the case of malfeasance, an individual may perform a medical treatment not within his or her legal province and from which serious medical complications develop. In a case of misfeasance, an individual incorrectly administers a first aid procedure they have been trained to perform.

## Negligence

When an individual is sued by an athlete, the complaint typically is for the tort of negligence. Negligence is alleged when an individual (1) does something that a reasonably prudent person would not do; or (2) fails to do something that a reasonably prudent person would do under circumstances similar to those shown by the evidence.[8] To be successful in a suit for negligence, an athlete must prove that an individual had a duty to exercise reasonable care, breached that duty by failing to use reasonable care, and that there is a reasonable connection between the failure to use reasonable care and the injury suffered by the athlete or that an individual's action made the injury worse. If an individual breaches a duty to exercise reasonable care, but there is no reasonable connection between the failure to use reasonable care and the injury suffered by the athlete, the athlete's suit for negligence will not succeed.

An example of negligence that occurs all too often in sports is when someone moves a possibly seriously injured athlete from the field of play to permit competition or practice to continue and does so either in an improper manner or before consulting those qualified to know the proper course of action. Should a serious or disabling injury result, that person may be found liable.

Individuals employed as health care providers by an institution have a duty to provide athletic health care to athletes at that institution. Once a person assumes the duty of caring for an athlete, that person has an obligation to make sure that appropriate care is given. It should be made clear that no one is obligated to provide first aid care for an injured person outside their scope of employment. However, if they choose to become involved as a caregiver for an injured person, they are expected to provide reasonable care consistent with their level of training. The **Good Samaritan Law** has been enacted in most states to provide limited protection against legal liability to any individual who voluntarily chooses to provide first aid, should something go wrong. As long as the first aid provider does not overstep the limits of his or her professional training, and exercises what would be considered reasonable care in the situation, the provider will not be held liable.

It is expected that a person possessing more training in a given field or area will possess a correspondingly higher level of competence than, for example, a student. An individual will therefore be judged in terms of his or her performance in any situation in which legal liability may be assessed. It must be recognized that liability per se in all of its various aspects is not assessed at the same level nationally but varies in interpretation from state to state and from area to area. It is therefore good

**3-1 Critical Thinking**
Exercise

A softball batter was struck with a pitched ball directly in the orbit of the right eye and fell immediately to the ground. The physical education teacher ran to the player to examine the eye. There was some immediate swelling and discoloration around the orbit; however, the eye appeared to be normal. The player insisted that he was fine and told the teacher that he could continue to bat. After the game, the teacher told the athlete to go back to his room, put ice on his eye, and check in tomorrow. That night the baseball player began to hemorrhage into the anterior chamber of the eye and suffered irreparable damage to his eye.

**?** An ophthalmologist stated that if the athlete's eye had been examined immediately after injury, the bleeding could have been controlled and the athlete would not have suffered any damage to his vision. If the athlete brings a lawsuit against the physical education teacher, what must he prove to win a judgment?

---

**Good Samaritan Law**
Provides limited protection to someone who voluntarily chooses to provide first aid.

to know and to acquire the level of competence expected in a particular area. In essence, negligence is conduct that results in the creation of an "unreasonable risk of harm to others."[2]

## Statute of Limitations

A **statute of limitation** sets a specific length of time that individuals may sue for damages from negligence.[1] The length of time to bring suit varies from state to state, but in general, plaintiffs have between 1 and 3 years to file suit for negligence. The statute of limitations begins to run on a plaintiff's time to file a lawsuit for negligence from either the time of the negligent act or omission that gives rise to the suit, or the discovery of an injury caused by the negligent act or omission. Some states permit an injured minor to file suit up to 3 years after the minor reaches the age of eighteen. Therefore, an injured minor athlete's cause of action for negligence remains valid for many years after the negligent act or omission occurred or the discovery of an injury caused by the negligent act or omission.

## Assumption of Risk

An athlete assumes the risk of participating in an activity when he or she knows of and understands the dangers of that activity, and voluntarily chooses to be exposed to those dangers.[2] An **assumption of risk** can be expressed in the form of a waiver signed by an athlete or his or her parents or guardian, or implied from the conduct of an athlete under the circumstances of his or her participation in an activity.[4,12]

Assumption of risk may be asserted as a defense to a negligence suit brought by an injured athlete. It can be proven that an athlete assumed the risk by producing the document signed by the athlete or his or her

> **statute of limitation**
> A specific length of time to sue for damages from negligence.

> **assumption of risk**
> The individual, through expressed or implied agreement, assumes that some risk or danger will be involved in the particular undertaking. In other words, a person takes his or her own chances.

### 3-2 Critical Thinking
#### Exercise

An administrative assistant is cleaning out a filing cabinet with records from past teams and decides to throw some older medical files away. Concern is expressed about how long these files should be maintained for legal purposes.

**?** What is the statute of limitations for a minor to file suit?

## Athletic Injury Management Checklist

You can significantly decrease risk of litigation by paying attention to several key points.[12] The following is a checklist of things that can be done to decrease the risk of litigation.

☐ Warn the athlete of the potential dangers inherent in the sport.
☐ Supervise constantly and attentively.
☐ Properly prepare and condition the athlete.
☐ Properly instruct the athlete in the skills of the sport.
☐ Ensure that proper and safe equipment and facilities are used by the athlete at all times.
☐ Work to establish good personal relationships with the athletes, parents, and coworkers.
☐ Establish specific policies and guidelines for the operation of an athletic training facility and maintain qualified and

adequate supervision of the athletic training room, its
environs, facilities, and equipment at all times.[4]

☐ Develop and carefully follow an emergency action plan.

☐ Make it a point to become familiar with the health status and
medical history of the athletes under his or her care so as to be
aware of any problems that could present a need for additional
care or caution and keep a file that contains medical history,
preparticipation exams, and any injury records.

☐ Keep good records that document all injuries and
rehabilitation steps.

☐ Document efforts to create a safe playing environment.

☐ Have a detailed job description in writing.

☐ Obtain written consent for providing health care, particularly
when minors are involved.

☐ Maintain confidentiality of medical records.

☐ Don't dispense prescription drugs, and if allowed by law,
exercise extreme caution in the administration of nonprescription medications.

☐ Use only those therapeutic methods that you are qualified to
use and that the law states may be used.

☐ Don't use or permit the presence of faulty or hazardous
equipment.

☐ Work cooperatively with the team physician and/or athletic
trainer in the selection and use of sports protective
equipment, and insist that the best equipment be obtained,
properly fitted, and properly maintained.

☐ Don't permit injured players to participate unless cleared by
the team physician. Players suffering a head injury should not
be permitted to reenter the game. In some states a player
who has suffered a concussion may not continue in the sport
for the balance of the season.

☐ Develop an understanding that an injured athlete will not
be allowed to reenter competition until, in the opinion of
the team physician or the athletic trainer, he or she is
psychologically and physically able. Coaches should not allow
themselves to be pressured to clear an athlete until he or she
is fully cleared by the physician.

☐ Follow the express orders of the team physician or athletic
trainer at all times.

☐ Purchase liability insurance to protect against litigation and be
aware of the limitations of the policy.

☐ Know the limitations of expertise and the applicable state
regulations and restrictions limiting the scope of practice.

☐ Use common sense in making decisions about the athlete's
health and safety.

parents or guardian, or showing that the athlete knew the risk of the activity, understood, and voluntarily accepted those risks.[3]

Assumption of risk, however, is subject to many and varied interpretations by courts, especially when a minor is involved, because he or she is not considered able to render a mature judgment about the risks inherent in the situation. Although athletes participating in a sports program are considered to assume a normal risk, this in no way excuses those in charge from exercising reasonable care and prudence in the conduct of such activities or from foreseeing and taking precautionary measures against accident-provoking circumstances. In general, courts have been fairly consistent in upholding waivers and releases of liability for adults unless there is evidence of fraud, misrepresentation, or duress.[12]

*In the case of an injury, an individual must use reasonable care to prevent further injury until medical care is obtained.*

## PRODUCT LIABILITY

Product liability refers to the liability of any or all parties along the chain of manufacture of any product for damage caused by that product.[10] This includes the manufacturer of component parts, an assembling manufacturer, the wholesaler, and the retail store owner. Products containing inherent defects that cause harm to a consumer of the product, or someone to whom the product was loaned, given, etc., are the subjects of product liability suits. Product liability claims can be based on negligence, strict liability, or breach of warranty of fitness depending on the jurisdiction within which the claim is based. Many states have enacted comprehensive product liability statutes and these statutory provisions can be very diverse. There is no federal product liability law.

Manufacturers of all types of athletic and fitness equipment have a duty to design and produce equipment that will not cause injury as long as it is used as intended. An express warranty is the manufacturer's written guarantee that a product is safe. Warning labels placed on football helmets inform the player of possible dangers inherent in using the product. Athletes must read and sign a form indicating that they have read and understand the warning. The National Operating Committee on Standards for Athletic Equipment (NOCSAE) establishes minimum standards for equipment that must be met to ensure its safety.

## WHAT TYPES OF INSURANCE ARE NECESSARY TO PROTECT THE ATHLETE?

Because of the high cost of medical care, every athlete should be covered by appropriate insurance policies that maximize the benefits should injury occur.[17] During the past 40 years the insurance industry has undergone a significant evolutionary process. Health care reform initiated in the 1990s has focused on the concept of **managed care** in which costs of a health care provider's medical care are closely monitored and scrutinized by insurance carriers. Often preapproval is required before health care is

---

**3-3 Critical Thinking**
Exercise

During a high school gymnastics meet, a gymnast fell off the uneven parallel bars, landing on her forearm. The coach suspected a fracture and decided an x ray was needed. The gymnast's parents have general health insurance through a PPO but because the gymnast was in severe pain she was sent to the nearest emergency room to be treated. Unfortunately the emergency facility was not on the list of preferred providers so the insurance company denied the claim. The coach assured the parents that the school would take care of whatever medical costs were not covered by their insurance policy.

? Because the PPO denied the claim, what type of insurance policy should the school carry to cover the medical costs?

---

**managed care**
Costs of health care are monitored closely by insurance carriers.

---

**medical insurance**
Medical insurance is a
contract between the
insurance company and
policyholder.

---

delivered. Since 1971 there has been a significant increase in the number of lawsuits filed, caused in part by the steady increase in individuals who have become active in sports. The costs of insurance have also significantly increased during this period. More lawsuits and much higher medical costs are creating a crisis in the insurance industry.[13] **Medical insurance** is a contract between an insurance company and a policyholder in which the insurance company agrees to reimburse a portion of the total medical bill after some deductible has been paid by the policyholder. The major types of insurance that coaches should be familiar with are general health insurance, catastrophic insurance, accident insurance, and liability insurance, as well as insurance for errors and omissions. All sports health and safety personnel need to be adequately insured.

## General Health Insurance

Every athlete should have a
general health insurance
policy that covers illness,
hospitalization, and
emergency care.

Secondary insurance pays the
athlete's remaining medical
bills after a general health
insurance plan has made its
payment.

All athletes should have a general health insurance policy as their primary policy that covers illness, hospitalization, and emergency care. Most institutions offer **secondary insurance** coverage that pays the athlete's remaining medical bills once the athlete's personal insurance company has made its payment. Secondary insurance always includes a deductible that will not be covered by the plan. Some institutions offer insurance coverage in which all medical expenses are paid for by the athletic department. The institutions pay an extremely high premium for this type of coverage.

Many athletes are covered under some type of family health insurance policy. However, the school must make certain that personal health insurance is arranged for or purchased by athletes not covered under family policies.[18] A form letter directed to the parents of all athletes should be completed and returned to the institution to make certain that appropriate coverage is provided (Figure 3-2). Some

**Figure 3-2**

---

Sample insurance
information form

---

Insurance Information on Student Athletes
Student's Name _____ Date of Birth _____
Address _____
_____ Sex: M _____ F _____
Names of Insurance Companies _____
Address of Insurance Company _____
Certificate Number _____ Group _____ Type _____
Policy Holder _____ Relationship to Student _____
Employer or Policyholder _____
Is preauthorization required for medical procedures? _____   _____
                                                           Yes      No

Should my son/daughter require services beyond those covered by the Sports Medicine Program, I give permission to the Division of Sports Medicine to file a claim for such services with the above health care insurer.
According to NCAA regulations, I understand that any insurance payments I receive must be returned to be placed on my child's account.
Date _____   _____
                                                     Parent's Signature

so-called comprehensive plans do not cover every health need. For example, such plans may cover physicians' care but not hospital charges. Many of these plans require large prepayments before the insurance takes effect. Supplemental policies such as accident insurance and catastrophic insurance are designed to take over where general health insurance stops.

### Reimbursement

Reimbursement is the primary mechanism of payment for medical services in the United States.[15,19] Health care professionals are reimbursed by the policyholder's insurance company for services performed. Medical insurance companies may provide group and individual coverage for employees and dependents. To cut payout costs, many insurance companies have begun to pay for preventive care (to reduce the need for hospitalization) and to limit where the individual can go for care. Managed care involves a prearranged system for delivering health care that is designed to control costs while continuing to provide quality care. A number of different health care systems have been developed to contain costs.[5]

*Reimbursement comes from the policyholder's insurance company for services performed.*

**Health maintenance organizations**   Health maintenance organizations (HMOs) provide preventive measures and limit where the individual can receive care. With the exception of an emergency, permission must be obtained before the individual can go to another provider. HMOs generally pay 100 percent of medical costs as long as care is rendered at an HMO facility. Many supplemental policies will not cover medical costs that would normally be paid by the general policy. Therefore an athlete treated outside the HMO may be ineligible for any insurance benefits. Many HMOs determine fees using a capitation system that limits the amount that is reimbursed for a specific service. Athletic trainers must understand the limits of and restrictions on coverage at their individual institutions.

*Third-party payers:*
- *private insurance carriers*
- *HMOs*
- *PPOs*

*HMO—Preapproved except in emergency and at HMO facility*

**Preferred provider organizations**   Preferred provider organizations (PPOs) provide discount health care but also limit where a person can go for treatment of an illness. The coach and/or athletic trainer must be apprised in advance where the ill athlete should be sent. Athletes sent to a facility not on the approved list may be required to pay for care, but if they are sent to a preferred facility, all costs are paid.[5] Added services such as physical therapy may be more easily obtained and at no cost or at a much lower cost than with other insurance policies. PPOs pay on a fee-for-service basis.

*PPO—From approved provider list*

**Point of service plan**   The point of service plan is a combination of HMO and PPO plans. It is based on an HMO structure, yet it allows members to go outside the HMO to obtain services. This flexibility is allowed only with certain conditions and under special circumstances.

**Indemnity plan**   The indemnity plan, although not a type of managed care, is the most traditional form of billing for health care, in which the provider charges the patient or a third-party payer a fee for services provided. Charges are based on a set fee schedule.

**Capitation**  Capitation is a form of reimbursement used by managed care providers in which members make a standard payment each month regardless of how much service is rendered to the member by the provider. A therapist in a clinical setting usually treats a patient three times per week. In an athletic training setting an injured athlete may be treated in some instances twice a day every day of the week. Some high schools are going to a capitated health fee for students that goes toward providing athletic health care services.

## Accident Insurance

Besides general health insurance, low-cost accident insurance is available to the student. This insurance covers accidents on school grounds while the student is in attendance. The purpose of this insurance is to protect the student against financial loss from medical and hospital bills, to encourage an injured student to receive prompt medical care, to encourage prompt reporting of injuries, and to relieve a school of financial responsibility.

The school's general insurance may be limited; thus accident insurance for a specific activity such as sports may be needed to provide additional protection.[13] This type of coverage is limited and does not require knowledge of fault, and the amount it pays is limited. For serious sport injuries requiring surgery and lengthy rehabilitation, accident insurance is usually not adequate. This inadequacy can put families with limited budgets into a real financial bind. Of particular concern is insurance that does not adequately cover catastrophic injuries.

## Catastrophic Insurance

Although catastrophic injuries in sports participation are relatively uncommon, if they do occur, the consequences to the athlete, family, institution, and society can be staggering. In the past, when available funds had been completely depleted, the family was forced to seek funding elsewhere, usually through a lawsuit. Organizations such as the NCAA and NAIA provide plans that deal with the problem of a lifetime of extensive medical and rehabilitative care because of a permanent disability.[9] Benefits begin when expenses have reached $75,000 and are then extended for a lifetime. At the secondary school level, a program is offered to districts by the National Federation of State High School Associations (NFSHSA). This plan provides medical, rehabilitation, and transportation costs in excess of $10,000 not covered by other insurance benefits.[18] Costs for catastrophic insurance are based on the number of sports and the number of hazardous sports offered by the institution.

As indicated, insurance that covers the athlete's health and safety can be very complex. Administrators must be concerned that every athlete is adequately covered by a good, reliable insurance company. Because of the intricacies and time involved with filing claims and follow-up communications with parents, doctors, and vendors, a staff person should be assigned this responsibility. In some athletic programs filing claims becomes the responsibility of the athletic trainer. This task can be highly time consuming, taking the athletic trainer away from his or her major role of directly working with the athlete.

## INSURANCE BILLING

It is essential that insurance claims be filed immediately and correctly.[13] The individual or administrator overseeing the athletic health care program working in an educational setting can facilitate this process by collecting insurance information on every athlete at the beginning of the year. A letter should also be drafted to the parents of the athlete, explaining the limits of the school insurance policy and what the parents must do to file a claim if injury does occur. Schools that have secondary policies should stress to the parents that they must submit all bills to their insurance company before submitting the remainder to the school. In educational institutions, most claims will be filed with a single insurance company, which will pay for medical services provided by individual health care providers.

## INSURANCE TO PROTECT THE PROFESSIONAL

### Personal Liability Insurance

Most individual schools and school districts have general liability insurance to protect against damages that may arise from injuries occurring on school property. Liability insurance covers claims of negligence on the part of individuals. Its major concern is whether supervision was reasonable and whether unreasonable risk of harm was perceived by the sports participant.[18]

Because of the amount of litigation based on alleged negligence, premiums have become almost prohibitive for some schools. Typically, when a victim sues, the lawsuit is a "shotgun approach," with the coach, athletic trainer, physician, school administrator, and school district all named. If a protective piece of equipment is involved, the product manufacturer is also sued.

All personnel should carry professional liability insurance and must clearly understand the limits of coverage.[5,7] Liability insurance typically covers negligence in a civil case. If a criminal complaint is also filed, liability insurance will not cover the individual.

Policy, errors, and omissions liability insurance has evolved to offset the shotgun mentality and to cover what is not covered by a general liability. This insurance is designed to cover school employees, officers, and the district against suits claiming malpractice, wrongful actions, errors and omissions, and acts of negligence.[18] Even when working in a program that has good liability coverage, each person within that program who works directly with students must have his or her own personal liability insurance.

Because of the amount of litigation for alleged negligence, all professionals involved with the sports program must be fully protected by personal liability insurance.

**Athletic Injury Management Checklist**

This checklist contains types of insurance that an administrator should look into to protect both the athlete and the personnel involved in athletic health care.

☐ General health insurance
☐ Accident insurance
☐ Product liability insurance
☐ Catastrophic injury insurance
☐ Personal liability insurance

## SUMMARY

- A great deal of care must be taken in an athletic environment to follow policies and procedures that conform to the legal guidelines governing liability.

- Liability is the state of being legally responsible for the harm one causes another person. The standard of reasonable care assumes that an individual acts according to the reasonable standards of care of any individual with similar educational background or training.

- A person who fails to use ordinary or reasonable care—care that persons would normally exercise to avoid injury to themselves or to others under similar circumstances—is deemed negligent.

- Although athletes participating in a sports program are considered to assume a normal risk, this assumption in no way exempts those in charge from exercising reasonable care.

- Individuals can significantly decrease risk of litigation by making certain that they have done everything possible to provide a reasonable degree of care to the injured athlete.

- The major types of insurance are general health insurance, catastrophic insurance, accident insurance, and liability insurance, as well as insurance for errors and omissions.

- Reimbursement is the primary mechanism of payment for medical services in the United States. A number of different health care systems—including health maintenance organizations, preferred provider organizations, point of service plans, indemnity plans, and capitation plans—have been developed to contain costs.

- It is essential that the individual overseeing the athletic health care program file insurance claims immediately and correctly.

*Solutions to Critical Thinking* Exercises

**3-1** When a teacher assumes the duty of caring for an athlete, that teacher is also under the obligation to make sure that appropriate care is given. A coach who fails to provide an acceptable standard of care has committed a breach of duty, and the athlete must prove that this breach caused the injury or made the injury worse.

**3-2** The athlete typically has between 1 and 3 years to file suit for negligence. However, a minor may have up to 3 years after the minor reaches the age of 18 to file.

**3-3** Besides general health insurance, low-cost accident insurance often covers accidents on school grounds while the athlete is competing. The purpose of this insurance is to protect the athlete against financial loss from medical and hospital bills, to encourage an injured athlete to receive prompt medical care, to encourage prompt reporting of injuries, and to relieve a school of financial responsibility.

## REVIEW QUESTIONS AND CLASS ACTIVITIES

1. What are the major legal concerns in terms of liability, negligence, assumption of risk, and torts?
2. What measures can be taken to minimize the chances of litigation should an athlete be injured?
3. Invite an attorney who is familiar with sport litigation to class to discuss how you can protect yourself from a lawsuit.
4. Discuss how an individual provides reasonable and prudent care in dealing with an injured athlete.
5. Why is it necessary for an athlete to have both general health insurance and accident insurance?
6. Briefly discuss the various methods of third-party reimbursement.
7. Why should an individual carry individual liability insurance?
8. What are the critical considerations for filing insurance claims?

## REFERENCES

1. Administrative and legal concerns: 2005. In American Academy of Family Physicians, *Preparticipation physical evaluation.* 3rd ed, Minneapolis, Minn.
2. Connaughton, D.; Eickhoff, Shemek, J.A.: 2003. Law for the health/fitness professional: part II, *ACSM's health & fitness journal* 7(1): 12–16.
3. Cotten, DJ: 2005. Are you safe? Courts in an increasing number of states are enforcing liability waivers signed by parents on behalf of minors, *Athletic business* 29(3):66–68; 70–72, 2005.
4. Cotten, DJ: 2004. Waivers and releases can protect against liability, *Fitness management* 20(4):24.
5. Cotten, DJ: 2001. What is covered by your liability insurance policy? A risk management essential, *Exercise standards and malpractice reporter* 15(4):54–56, 2001.
6. Cozillio, M, Levinstein, M: 2007. *Sports law: cases and materials,* Durham, NC, Carolina Academic Press.

7. Eickhoff, Shemek, J.A.: 2003. Distinguishing "general" and "professional" liability insurance, *ACSM's health & fitness journal* 7 (1): 28–30.

8. Frenkel, DA: 2001. Medico-legal aspects in sport. (Abstract), *Exercise & society journal of sport science* (28):90.

9. Gallup E: 1995. *Law and the team physician*, Champaign, IL, Human Kinetics.

10. Gorman, L: 1999. Product liability in sports medicine, *Athletic therapy today* 4(4):36–37.

11. Halvorson, R: 2008. Insurance tips for fitness pros., *IDEA Fitness Journal* 5(6):14.

12. Hawkins J, Appenzeller H: 1991. Legal aspects of sports medicine. In Mueller F, Ryan A: *Prevention of athletic injuries: the role of the sports medicine team*, Philadelphia, FA Davis.

13. Health Insurance Association of America: 1997. *Fundamentals of health insurance*, Washington, DC, HIAA.

14. Herbert, DL, Herbert, WG: 2002. *Legal aspects of preventive, rehabilitative and recreational exercise programs*, 4th ed. Canton, OH, PRC Publishing.

15. Hunt, V: 2002. Reimbursement efforts continue steady progress, *NATA News*, October 10–12.

16. Jacobs, J: 2003. Dodging the liability bullet. *Association Management* 55(9):65.

17. Polanshek, Kathy: 2004. Combat the increasing cost of athletics accident insurance, *Athletics administration* 39(3):60.

18. Rankin J, Ingersoll C: 2005. *Athletic training management: concepts and applications*, St. Louis, McGraw-Hill.

19. Ray R: 2005. *Management strategies in athletic training*, Champaign, IL, Human Kinetics.

20. Sawyer, T: 2003. Torts, negligence, duty, and sports injuries. *Journal of physical education, recreation & dance* 74(4):18–19.

21. Wong, GM: 2002. *Essentials of sports law*. 3rd ed, Westport, Conn., Greenwood Press.

## ANNOTATED BIBLIOGRAPHY

Appenzeller H: 2000. *Youth sports and the law: a guide to legal issues*, Chapel Hill, NC, Carolina Academic Press.

*Studies various court cases to understand the legal principles involved in sport participation. The objective of the book is to provide better and safer sporting experiences for today's children.*

Appenzeller, H: 2005. *Risk management in sport: issues and strategies*, Chapel Hill, NC, Carolina Academic Press.

*Discusses risk management in sport law and industry. Topics include tort liability, medical, event, and facility issues; warnings, waivers, and informed consent; youth sport and the law.*

Champion, W: 2005. *Fundamentals of sports law*, St. Paul, MN, Thomson/West.

*This introductory text lays out the basic ideas and legal documents important to attorneys, compliance officers, agents, athletic directors, and sports administrators.*

Gayson E: 1999. *Ethics, injury and the law in sports medicine*, New York, Heinnman-Butterworth.

*Provides an up-to-date review of the status of sports medicine and the law. Addresses the key legal and ethical issues in sports and exercise medicine. For practitioners and students preparing for sport and exercise medicine exams.*

Herbert D: 1995. *Legal aspects of sports medicine,* Canton, OH, Professional Reports Corporation.

*A discussion of sports medicine, policies, procedures, responsibilities of the sports medicine team, informed consent, negligence, insurance and risk management, medication, drug testing, and other topics.*

Rowell JC: 1994. *Understanding medical insurance: a step-by-step guide,* Albany, NY, Delmar.

*Provides a comprehensive resource for dealing with issues related to insurance.*

## WEB SITES

Duhaime & Co. Legal Dictionary: www.duhaime.org/dictionary
   *This is a site that has put together an extensive list of legal terms with clear definitions and explanations.*
Health Insurance Association of America: www.hiaa.org
   *The nation's most prominent trade association representing the private health care system. It is the nation's premier provider of self-study courses on health insurance and managed care.*
Legal Information Institute at Cornell: http://topics.law.cornell.edu/wex/ Sports_law

   *Part of a series of legal information, this site specifically addresses law in sport, but is rather technical. The relevant area to sports medicine is addressed in the area titled torts.*
Sports Lawyers Journal: www.law. tulane.edu/tlsjournals/slj/index.aspx
   *Specialized academic and professional publication on legal aspects of sports.*
The Center for Sports Law & Policy Duke University School of Law: www.law.duke.edu/sportscenter/

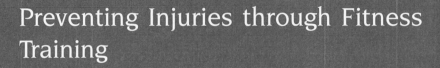

# Preventing Injuries through Fitness Training

## CHAPTER 4

*When you finish this chapter you will be able to:*

- Identify the concept of periodization and the types of exercise that are performed in each phase.
- Identify the principles of conditioning.
- Explain the importance of the warm-up and cooldown periods.
- Describe the importance of flexibility, strength, and cardiorespiratory endurance in injury prevention.
- Identify specific techniques and principles for improving flexibility, muscular strength, and cardiorespiratory endurance.

I t is obvious that for an athlete to compete successfully at a high level, the athlete must be fit. But it is also true that an athlete who is not fit is more likely to sustain an injury. Improper conditioning is one of the major causes of sports injuries. Improving flexibility, muscular strength, endurance, and power, and cardiorespiratory endurance through a well-designed conditioning program can help to reduce the likelihood of injury in the competitive athlete. Fitness does not develop overnight. It takes time and careful preparation to bring an athlete into competition at a level of fitness that will preclude early-season injury. Training and conditioning programs should minimize the possibility of injury and maximize performance.

## CONDITIONING SEASONS AND PERIODIZATION

No longer do serious athletes engage only in preseason conditioning and in-season competition. Sports conditioning is a year-round endeavor. The concept of **periodization** is an approach to conditioning that attempts to bring about peak performance while reducing injuries and overtraining in the athlete by developing a training and conditioning program to be followed throughout the various seasons.[37] Periodization takes into account athletes' different training and conditioning needs during different seasons and modifies the program according to individual needs (Table 4-1).

**periodization**
Allows athletes to train year-round with less risk of injury and staleness.

Periodization organizes a training and conditioning program into cycles. The complete training period, which could be a year in the case of seasonal sports or perhaps 4 years for an Olympic athlete, can be divided into a preseason, an in-season, and an off-season. Throughout the course of this cycle, intensity, volume, and specificity of training are

**TABLE 4-1** Periodization Training

| Season | Period/Phase | Type of Training Activity |
|---|---|---|
| Off-season sports | Transition period (postseason) | Unstructured<br>Recreational |
| | Preparatory period | Cross training |
| | Hypertrophy/endurance phase | Low intensity<br>High volume<br>Non–sport-specific |
| | Strength phase | Moderate intensity<br>Moderate volume<br>More sport-specific |
| Preseason | Power phase | High intensity<br>Decreased volume<br>Sport-specific |
| In-season | Competition period | High intensity<br>Low volume<br>Skill training<br>Strategy<br>Maintenance of strength and<br>power gained during off-season |

altered so that an athlete can achieve peak levels of fitness for competition. As competition approaches, training sessions change gradually and progressively from high volume, low intensity, non–sport-specific activity to low volume, high intensity, sport-specific training.[37]

Within the year round training cycle are a series of periods or phases, each of which may last for several weeks or even months including preparatory, competition, and transition periods.[7]

**Transition period**  The transition period (postseason) begins after the last competition and comprises the early part of the off-season. The transition period is generally unstructured and the athlete is encouraged to participate in sport activities on a recreational basis. The idea is to allow the athlete to escape both physically and psychologically from the rigor of a highly organized training regimen. The value of a period of rest and relaxation after a long competitive season should never be underestimated.

**Preparatory period**  The preparatory period occurs primarily during the off-season when there are no upcoming competitions. The preparatory period has three phases; the hypertrophy/endurance phase, the strength phase, and the power phase.

During the hypertrophy/endurance phase, which occurs in the early part of the off-season, training is at a low intensity with a high volume of repetitions, using activities that may or may not be directly related to a specific sport. The goal is to develop a base of endurance, on which more intense training can occur. This phase may last from several weeks to 2 months.

During the strength phase, which also occurs during the off-season, the intensity and volume progress to moderate levels. Weight training activities should become more specific to the sport or event.

The third phase or power phase occurs in the preseason. The athlete trains at a high intensity at or near the level of competition. The volume of training is decreased so that full recovery is allowed between sessions.

**Competition period**   In certain cases the competition period may last for only a week or less. However, with seasonal sports the competition period may last for several months. In general this period involves high intensity training at a low volume. As training volume decreases, an increased amount of time is spent on skill training or strategy sessions and in maintaining levels of flexibility, strength, and cardiorespiratory endurance established in the off-season. During the competition period it may be necessary to establish weekly training cycles. During a weekly cycle, training should be intense early in the week, progressing to moderate, and finally light the day before a competition. The goal is to make sure that the athlete is at peak levels of fitness and performance on days of competition.[7]

### Cross Training

The concept of cross training is an approach to training and conditioning for a specific sport that involves substitution of alternative activities that have some carryover value to that sport. For example, a swimmer can engage in jogging, running, or aerobic exercise to maintain levels of cardiorespiratory conditioning. Cross training is particularly useful in both the postseason and the off-season to help athletes maintain fitness levels and avoid the boredom that typically occurs from following the same training regimen and using the same techniques for conditioning as during the preseason and competitive season.

## FOUNDATIONS OF CONDITIONING

The SAID principle indicates that the body will gradually adapt to the specific demands imposed on it.

The **SAID principle** relates to the process of training and conditioning. SAID is an acronym for Specific Adaptation to Imposed Demands. The SAID principle states that when the body is subjected to stresses and overloads of varying intensities, it will gradually adapt over time to overcome whatever demands are placed on it and, in doing so, minimize the potential for injury.

Although overload is a critical factor in training and conditioning, the stress must not be great enough to produce damage or injury before the body has had a chance to adjust specifically to the increased demands. Therefore, to reduce the likelihood of injury, the principles of training and conditioning should be emphasized. See Focus Box 4-1.

4-1  *Focus Box*

**Principles of Conditioning**

1. *Warm-up/cooldown.* Give the athletes time to do an appropriate warm-up before engaging in any activity. Do not neglect the cooldown period following a training bout.
2. *Motivation.* Athletes are generally highly motivated to work hard because they want to be successful in their sport. By varying the training program and incorporating different aspects of conditioning, the program can remain enjoyable rather than becoming routine and boring.
3. *Overload.* To see improvement in any physiological component, the system must work harder than it is accustomed to working. Gradually, that system will adapt to the imposed demands.
4. *Consistency.* The athlete must engage in a training and conditioning program on a consistent, regularly scheduled basis if the program is to be effective.
5. *Progression.* Increase the intensity of the conditioning program gradually and within the individual athlete's ability to adapt to increasing workloads.
6. *Intensity.* Stress the intensity of the work rather than the quantity. It is easy to confuse working hard with working for long periods. Prolonging the workout rather than increasing tempo or workload may be a mistake. The tired athlete is prone to injury.
7. *Specificity.* Specific goals for the training program must be identified. The program must be designed to address specific components of fitness (i.e., strength, flexibility, cardiorespiratory endurance) relative to the sport in which the athlete is competing.
8. *Individuality.* The needs of individual athletes vary considerably. A successful coach is one who recognizes these individual differences and adjusts or alters the training and conditioning program accordingly to best accommodate the athlete.
9. *Stress.* Expect that athletes will train as close to their physiological limits as possible. Push the athletes but consider other stressful aspects of their lives; allow them time to be away from the conditioning demands of their sport.
10. *Safety.* Make the training environment as safe as possible. Take time to educate athletes about proper techniques, how they should feel during the workout, and when they should push harder or back off.

## WARM-UP AND COOLDOWN

### Warm-Up

A period of warm-up exercises should take place before a training session begins.[33] The warm-up increases body temperature, stretches muscles, increases ligament elasticity, and increases flexibility. Related warm-ups, those similar to the activity engaged in, are preferable to unrelated ones because of the rehearsal or practice effect that results.

An effective, quick warm-up can be an effective motivator. If athletes derive satisfaction from a warm-up, they probably will have a stronger desire to participate in the activity. By contrast, a poor warm-up can lead to fatigue and boredom, limiting athletes' attention and ultimately resulting in a poor program. A good warm-up may also improve certain aspects of performance.[40]

The function of the warm-up is to prepare the body physiologically for some upcoming physical work bout. The purpose is to very gradually

**4-1 *Critical Thinking* Exercise**

A track athlete constantly complains of tightness in her lower extremities during workouts. She states that she has a difficult time during her warm-up and cannot seem to "get loose" until her workout is almost complete. She feels that she is always on the verge of "pulling a muscle."

? What should be recommended as a specific warm-up routine that this athlete should consistently perform before she begins her workout?

stimulate the cardiorespiratory system to a moderate degree, thus producing an increased blood flow to working skeletal muscles and resulting in an increase in muscle temperature.[33]

Moderate activity speeds up the metabolic processes that produce an increase in core body temperature. An increase in the temperature of skeletal muscle facilitates speed of contraction and relaxation. The elastic properties (the length of stretch) of the muscle are increased, whereas the viscous properties (the rate at which the muscle can change shape) are decreased.

Every workout should be preceded by a warm-up. This activity should include a general warm-up followed by a specific warm-up. The general warm-up elevates the core temperature and then uses stretching exercises. The specific warm-up involves actions related to the activity to be performed. These actions are sport specific and should gradually increase in intensity. For example, soccer players use the upper extremity considerably less than the lower extremity, so their general warm-up should be directed more toward the lower extremity, perhaps by adding some stretching exercises for the lower extremity. The specific warm-up also relates to the sport: A basketball player should warm up by shooting layups and jump shots and by dribbling, for example, or a tennis player should hit forehand and backhand shots and serves.

The warm-up should last approximately 10 to 15 minutes. Athletes should not wait longer than 15 minutes after the warm-up to get started in the activity, although the effects will generally last up to about 45 minutes. Thus the third-string football player who warms up before the game and then does nothing more than stand around until he gets into the game during the fourth quarter is running a much higher risk of injury. This player should be encouraged to stay warmed up and ready to play throughout the course of a game. In general, sweating is a good indication that the body has been sufficiently warmed up and is ready for more strenuous activity.

The warm-up should begin with 2 or 3 minutes of light jogging to increase metabolic rate and core temperature. The jogging should be followed by flexibility exercises in which the muscles are stretched to take advantage of the increase in muscle elasticity and decreased viscosity.[2] Finally, the intensity of the warm-up should be increased gradually by performing body movements and skills associated with the specific activity in which the athlete is going to participate.

## Cooldown

After a vigorous workout, a cooldown is essential.[2] This part of the training program helps in returning the blood to the heart for reoxygenation, thus preventing the blood from pooling in the muscles of the arms and the legs. Pooling of the blood in the extremities places additional unnecessary stress and strain on the heart. After vigorous activity, enough blood may not circulate back to the brain, heart, and intestines, and symptoms such as dizziness or faintness may occur without a

Warming up involves general body warming and warming specific body areas for the demands of the sport.

A warm-up helps reduce injuries by progressively increasing:
- flexibility
- strength
- power
- endurance

Properly cooling down decreases blood and muscle lactic acid levels more rapidly.

cooldown period. The cooldown enables the body to cool and return to a resting state. Such a period should last about 5 to 10 minutes.

Although the value of warm-up and workout periods is well accepted, the importance of a cooldown period afterward is often ignored. Stretching exercises should be an important part of the cooldown periods. Persons who stretch during the cooldown period tend to have fewer problems with muscle soreness following strenuous activity.[2]

## WHY IS IT IMPORTANT TO HAVE GOOD FLEXIBILITY?

*Flexibility* may best be defined as the range of motion possible about a given joint or series of joints.[19] Flexibility can be discussed in relation to movement involving only one joint, such as in the knees, or movement involving a whole series of joints, such as the spinal vertebral joints, which must all move together to allow smooth bending, or rotation, of the trunk. Flexibility is specific to a given joint or movement. A person may have good range of motion in the ankles, knees, hips, back, and one shoulder joint. However, if the other shoulder joint lacks normal movement, then this person has a problem that needs to be corrected before he or she can function normally.

For many years it has been generally accepted that increasing flexibility promotes performance. A lack of flexibility in an athlete will potentially impair performance. For example, a sprinter with tight, inelastic hamstring muscles may have a problem sprinting at maximum speed because tight hamstrings restrict the ability to flex the hip joint, thus shortening stride length. Most activities in sport require relatively normal amounts of flexibility. However, some athletic activities, such as gymnastics, ballet, diving, karate, and yoga, require increased flexibility for superior performance (Figure 4-1). Increased flexibility may increase an athlete's performance through improved balance and reaction time. Experts in the field of training and conditioning generally agree that good flexibility is essential to successful physical performance.[1] However there is some evidence to suggest that stretching is only beneficial to performance in those sports which are dynamic and not as effective in less dynamic activities like swimming and distance running.[31,38]

It has also been generally accepted that stretching has a beneficial effect on injury prevention. However, recent clinical evidence has suggested that stretching before exercise does not necessarily prevent injuries.[38]

The type of sports activity in which an individual is participating significantly affects this relationship. Dynamic sport activities like soccer and basketball that involve bouncing and jumping with a high intensity of muscle stretch-shortening cycles (SSCs) require that the muscle-tendon unit be compliant enough to store and release the high amount of elastic energy required for successful performance. If this is not the case, the demands in energy absorption and release may exceed the capacity of the muscle-tendon unit leading to an increased risk for injury. In these types of sports, it has been shown that stretching can

Conditioning should be performed gradually, with work added in small increments.

Good flexibility is important in injury prevention.

Stretching does not necessarily improve performance, nor does it help to prevent injury.

**Figure 4-1**

Certain athletic activities require extreme flexibility for successful performance.

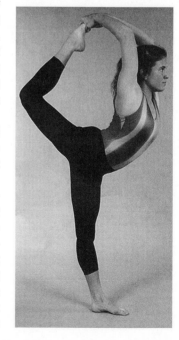

significantly influence the viscosity of the tendon making it more compliant, thus reducing the likelihood of injury.

In contrast, in sports like jogging and cycling that involve low-intensity, or limited stretch-shortening cycles, it is not as critical for the muscle-tendon unit to be compliant since most of its power generation is a consequence of active muscle contraction that needs to be directly transferred, via the tendon, to the articular system to generate motion. Thus stretching is not as essential in reducing the chance of injury.

Currently, no scientifically based conclusive statements can be made about the relationship between stretching and the occurrence of athletic injuries.

## What Structures in the Body Can Limit Flexibility?

A number of different anatomical structures may limit the ability of a joint to move through a full, unrestricted range of motion. Normal bone structure, fat, and skin or scar tissue may limit the ability to move through a full range of motion.

Muscles and their tendons are most often responsible for limiting range of motion. Performing stretching exercises for the purpose of improving a particular joint's flexibility is an attempt to take advantage of the highly elastic properties of a muscle. Over time it is possible to increase the elasticity, or the length, that a given muscle can be stretched. Athletes who have a good range of motion at a particular joint tend to have highly elastic and flexible muscles.

Connective tissue surrounding the joint, such as ligaments or the joint capsule, may be subject to contractures. Ligaments and joint capsules do have some elasticity; however, if an injured joint is immobilized for a time, these structures tend to lose some elasticity and actually shorten. This condition is most commonly seen after surgical repair of an unstable joint, but it can also result from long periods of inactivity.

On the other hand, it is also possible for an athlete to have slack ligaments and joint capsules. These individuals are generally referred to as being loose-jointed. An example of this condition is an elbow or knee that extends beyond being straight. Frequently the instability associated with loose-jointedness may present as great a problem in movement as a joint that is too tight.

## Active and Passive Range of Motion

When a muscle actively contracts, it produces a joint movement through a specific range of motion. However, if passive force is applied to an extremity, it is capable of moving farther in the range of motion. *Active range of motion* refers to that portion of the total range of motion through which a joint can be moved by an active muscle contraction. The ability to move through the active range of motion is not necessarily a good indicator of the stiffness or looseness of a joint because it applies to the ability to move a joint efficiently, with little resistance to motion. *Passive range of motion* refers to the portion of the total range of motion through which a joint may be moved passively. No muscle contraction is needed to move a joint through a passive range of motion. Passive range of motion begins at the end of and continues beyond active range of motion.

In sport activities an extremity should be capable of moving through a nonrestricted range of motion both to reduce the likelihood of injury and to enhance performance.[35] For example, a hurdler who cannot fully extend the knee joint in a normal stride is at a considerable disadvantage because stride length and thus speed are reduced significantly. Passive range of motion is important for injury prevention. Sports contain many situations in which a muscle is forced to stretch beyond its normal active limits. If the muscle does not have enough elasticity to compensate for this additional stretch, the muscle or its tendon will likely be injured.

### Agonist versus Antagonist Muscles

Before discussing the three different stretching techniques, it is essential to define the terms *agonist muscle* and *antagonist muscle*. Most joints in the body are capable of more than one movement. The knee joint, for example, is capable of flexion and extension. Contraction of the quadriceps group of muscles on the front of the thigh causes knee extension, whereas contraction of the hamstring muscles on the back of the thigh produces knee flexion. In knee extension, the quadriceps muscle that contracts to extend the knee is referred to as the agonist muscle. Conversely, the muscle being stretched in response to contraction of the agonist muscle is called the antagonist muscle. In this example of knee extension, the antagonist muscle is the hamstring group.

Some degree of balance in strength must exist between agonist and antagonist muscle groups. This balance is necessary for normal, smooth, coordinated movement and for reducing the likelihood of muscle strain caused by the muscular imbalance. Understanding the relationship between agonist and antagonist muscles facilitates understanding of the three techniques of stretching (see Focus Box 4-2).

### What Are the Different Stretching Techniques?

Maintaining a full, nonrestricted range of motion has long been recognized as an essential component of being fit and preventing injury. Flexibility is important not only for successful physical performance but also in the prevention of injury. The goal of any effective flexibility program should be to improve the range of motion around a given joint by altering the extensibility of the muscles and tendons that produce movement at that joint. Exercises that stretch these muscles and tendons over time will increase the range of movement possible about a given joint.

#### Ballistic Stretching

**Ballistic stretching** involves a bouncing movement in which repetitive contractions of the agonist muscle are used to produce quick stretches of the antagonist muscle. The ballistic stretching technique, although apparently effective in improving range of motion, has been

> **ballistic stretching**
> Stretching technique that uses repetitive bouncing motions.

**Guidelines and Precautions for Stretching**

The following guidelines and precautions should be incorporated into a sound stretching program:

- Warm up using a slow jog or fast walk before stretching vigorously.
- To increase flexibility, the muscle must be overloaded or stretched beyond its normal range but not to the point of pain.
- Stretch only to the point at which tightness or resistance to stretch or perhaps some discomfort is felt. Stretching should not be painful.
- Increases in range of motion will be specific to whatever joint is being stretched.
- Exercise caution when stretching muscles that surround painful joints. Pain is an indication that something is wrong; it should not be ignored.
- Avoid overstretching the ligaments and capsules that surround joints.
- Exercise caution when stretching the low back and neck. Exercises that compress the vertebrae and their disks may cause damage.
- Stretching from a seated position rather than a standing position takes stress off the low back and decreases the chances of back injury.
- Stretch those muscles that are tight and inflexible.
- Strengthen those muscles that are weak.
- Always stretch slowly and with control.
- Be sure to continue normal breathing during a stretch.
- Static and PNF techniques are most often recommended for individuals who want to improve their range of motion.
- Dynamic stretching should be done by those who are already flexible and/or are accustomed to stretching and should be done only after static stretching.
- Stretching should be done at least three times per week to see minimal improvement, between five and six times per week to see maximum results.

criticized in the past because increased range of motion is achieved through a series of jerks or pulls on the resistant muscle tissue.[4] The concern was that if the forces generated by the jerks are greater than the tissues' extensibility, muscle injury may result.

### Dynamic Stretching

Certainly successive forceful contractions of the agonist muscle that result in stretching of the antagonist muscle may cause muscle soreness. For example, forcefully kicking a soccer ball fifty times may result in muscular soreness of the hamstrings (antagonist muscle) as a result of eccentric contraction of the hamstrings to control the dynamic movement of the quadriceps (agonist muscle). Stretching that is controlled usually does not cause muscle soreness.[63] This is the difference between ballistic stretching and dynamic stretching. In fact, in the athletic population, *dynamic stretching* has become the stretching technique of choice. The argument has been that dynamic stretching exercises are more closely related to the types of activities that athletes engage in and should be considered more functional.[31,63] So dynamic stretching exercises are routinely recommended for athletes prior to beginning an activity (Figure 4-21A).

### Static Stretching

The **static stretching** technique is an extremely effective and perhaps the most widely used technique of stretching. This technique involves passively stretching a muscle by placing it in a maximal position of stretch and holding it there for an extended time.[39] Recommendations for the optimal time for holding this stretched position vary, ranging from as short as 3 seconds to as long as 60 seconds. It appears that 20 to 30 seconds may be the best length of time to hold a stretch. The static stretch of each muscle should be repeated three or four times. Much research has been done comparing dynamic and static stretching techniques for the improvement of flexibility. Both static and dynamic stretching are effective in increasing flexibility, and there is no significant difference between the two. However, static stretching offers less danger of exceeding the extensibility limits of the involved joints because the stretch is more controlled. Dynamic stretching may cause muscular soreness (if an individual is not fit), whereas static stretching generally does not and is commonly used in injury rehabilitation of sore or strained muscles.

Static stretching is certainly a much safer stretching technique, especially for unfit individuals. However, many physical activities involve dynamic movement. Thus, stretching as a warm-up for these types of activities should begin with static stretching followed by dynamic stretching, which more closely resembles the dynamic activity.

> **static stretching**
> Passively stretching an antagonist muscle by placing it in a maximal stretch and holding it there.

### Proprioceptive Neuromuscular Facilitation (PNF) Techniques

PNF techniques were first used by physical therapists for treating patients who had various types of neuromuscular paralysis.[21] More recently PNF stretching exercises have been used as a stretching technique for increasing flexibility. A number of different PNF techniques are currently being used for stretching, including *slow-reversal-hold-relax, contract-relax,* and *hold-relax* techniques. All involve some combination of alternating contraction and relaxation of both agonist and antagonist muscles (a 10-second pushing phase followed by a 10-second relaxing phase).

Using a hamstring stretching technique as an example (Figure 4-2), the slow-reversal-hold-relax technique is done as follows. With the athlete lying supine with knee extended and the ankle flexed to 90 degrees, a partner passively flexes the leg at the hip joint to the point at which the athlete feels slight discomfort in the muscle. At this point the athlete begins pushing against the partner's resistance by contracting the hamstring muscle. After pushing for 10 seconds, the athlete relaxes the hamstring muscles and contracts the quadriceps muscle while the partner applies passive pressure to further stretch the hamstrings. This pressure should move the leg so that the hip joint flexion is increased. The relaxing phase lasts for 10 seconds, at which time the athlete again pushes against the partner's resistance, beginning at this new joint angle. The push-relax sequence is repeated at least three times.[19]

> **proprioceptive neuromuscular facilitation (PNF)**
> Stretching techniques that involve combinations of alternating contractions and stretches.

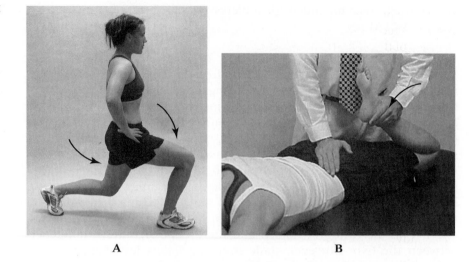

A

B

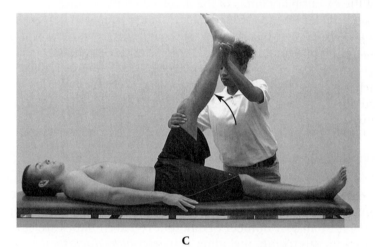

C

**Figure 4-2**

(A) Dynamic stretch for hip
flexors.

(B) Static stretch for
quadriceps.

(C) The slow-reversal-hold-
relax technique to stretch
hamstring muscles.

The contract-relax and hold-relax techniques are variations on the slow-reversal-hold-relax method. In the contract-relax method, the hamstrings are isotonically contracted so that the leg actually moves toward the floor during the push phase. The hold-relax method involves an isometric hamstring contraction against immovable resistance during the push phase. During the relax phase, both techniques involve relaxation of hamstrings and quadriceps while the hamstrings are passively stretched. This same basic PNF technique can be used to stretch any muscle in the body. PNF stretching techniques are perhaps best performed with a partner, although they may also be done using a wall as resistance.[19]

## Practical Application

Although all three stretching techniques have been demonstrated to effectively improve flexibility, there is still considerable debate as to which technique produces the greatest increases in range of movement.[33,39] The dynamic technique is seldom recommended in sedentary individuals because of the potential for causing muscle soreness. However, most sport activities are ballistic in nature (i.e., kicking, running). In highly trained individuals, it is unlikely that dynamic stretching will result in muscle soreness.[29] Static stretching is perhaps the most widely used technique. It is a simple technique and does not require a partner. A fully nonrestricted range of motion can be attained through static stretching over time.

PNF stretching techniques are capable of producing dramatic increases in range of motion during one stretching session. Studies comparing static and PNF stretching suggest that PNF stretching is capable of producing greater improvement in flexibility over an extended training period.[10] The major disadvantage of PNF stretching is that a partner is required, although stretching with a partner may have some motivational advantages.

## Stretching Exercises

Figures 4-3 to 4-14 illustrate stretching exercises that may be used to improve flexibility at specific joints throughout the body. The exercises described may be done statically, or with slight modification they may also be done with a partner using a PNF technique.

Each of these exercises has many possible variations. The exercises selected are those that seem to be the most effective for stretching various muscle groups.

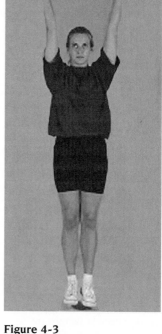

**Figure 4-3**

**Arm hang exercise**

*Muscles stretched:* Entire shoulder girdle complex

*Instructions:* Using a chinning bar, simply hang with shoulders and arms fully extended for 30 seconds. Repeat five times.

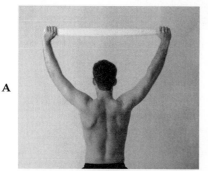

A

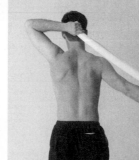

B

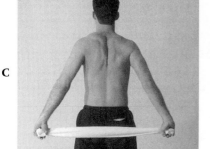

C

**Figure 4-4**

**Shoulder towel stretch exercise**

*Muscles stretched:* Internal and external rotators

*Instructions:* Begin by holding towel above head with hands shoulder width apart. (A) Try to pull towel down behind back, first with right hand then with left. (B) You should end up with elbows extended and hands below waist. (C) Reverse order to get back to position A. Repeat five times on each side.

**Figure 4-5**

### Chest and shoulder stretch exercise

*Muscles stretched:* Pectoralis and deltoid

*Instructions:* Stand in a corner, hands and arms on walls, and lean forward. Hold for 30 seconds. Repeat three times.

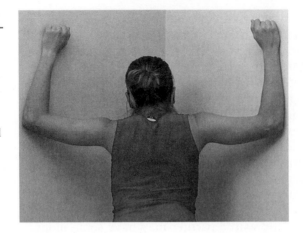

**Figure 4-6**

### Abdominal and anterior chest wall stretch exercise

*Muscles stretched:* Muscles of respiration in thorax and abdominal muscles

*Instructions:* Extend upper trunk, support weight on elbows, keeping pelvis on the table. If possible, lift the feet off the table. Hold for 30 seconds. Repeat three times.

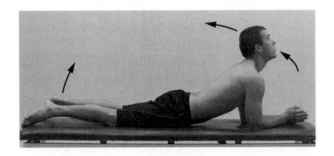

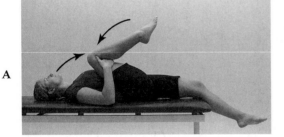
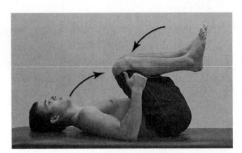

A
B

**Figure 4-7**

### Williams's flexion exercise

*Muscles stretched:* Low back and hip extensors

*Instructions:* (A) Touch chin to right knee and hold, then to left knee and hold. (B) Touch chin to both knees and hold. Hold each position for 30 seconds.

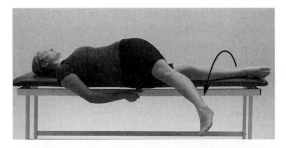

**Figure 4-8**

**Low back twister exercise**

*Muscles stretched:* Rotators of lower back and hip abductors

*Instructions:* Lie on back on edge of bed or table. Keep shoulders and arms flat on surface. Cross leg farthest from edge over the top and let it hang off the side of table, keeping knee straight; hold for 30 seconds. Repeat with other leg. Repeat three times with each leg.

Caution: If keeping the leg straight produces pain, this exercise may be done with the leg bent. Be sure to exercise caution in returning the leg to the starting position.

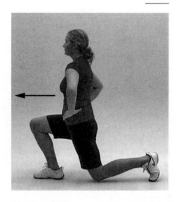

**Figure 4-9**

**Forward lunge exercise**

*Muscles stretched:* Hip flexors and quadriceps

*Instructions:* In a kneeling position with one knee on the ground, thrust pelvis forward. Hold for 30 seconds. Repeat three times.

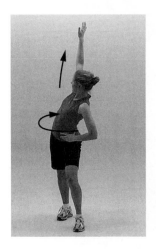

**Figure 4-10**

**Lateral trunk stretch exercise**

*Muscles stretched:* Lateral abdominals and intercostals

*Instructions:* Standing with a tandem stance, extend right arm straight up and reach for the ceiling twist to the right. Hold for 30 seconds. Repeat three times on each side.

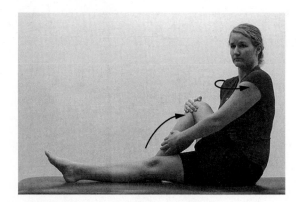

**Figure 4-11**

**Trunk twister exercise**

*Muscles stretched:* Trunk and hip rotators

*Instructions:* Place one foot over opposite knee. Rotate trunk to bent knee side.

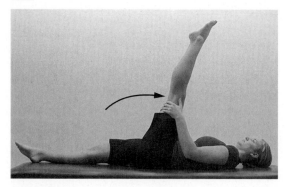

**Figure 4-12**

**Hamstring stretch exercise**

*Muscles stretched:* Hip extensors and knee flexors

*Instructions:* Lie flat on back. Raise one leg straight up with knee extended. Grasp leg around the hamstring and pull toward head; hold for 30 seconds. Repeat with opposite leg. Repeat three times with each leg.

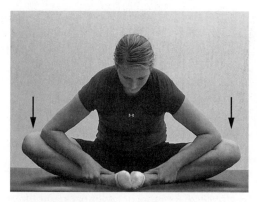

**Figure 4-13**

**Groin stretch exercise**

*Muscles stretched:* Hip adductors in groin

*Instructions:* Sit with knees flexed and soles of feet together. Try to press knees flat on the floor; if they are flat to begin with, try to touch face to floor. Hold for 30 seconds. Repeat three times.

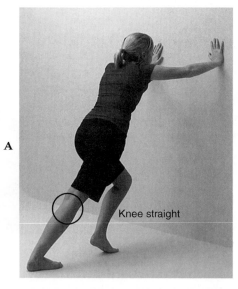

A

Knee straight

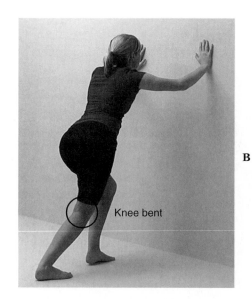

B

Knee bent

**Figure 4-14**

**Achilles heel cord stretch exercise**

*Muscles stretched:* Foot plantar flexors. (A) Gastrocnemius; (B) Soleus

*Instructions:* (A) Stand facing wall with toes pointing straight ahead and with the knee straight. Lean forward toward wall, keeping heels flat on floor. You should feel stretching high in calf. (B) Stand facing wall with toes pointing straight ahead and with the knee flexed. Lean forward toward wall, keeping heels flat on floor. You should feel stretching low in calf. Hold each position for 30 seconds. Repeat each position three times for each leg.

## Assessment of Flexibility

A general estimation of an athlete's flexibility can be obtained by using the trunk hip flexion test (Figure 4-15), the trunk extension test (Figure 4-16), and the shoulder extension test (Figure 4-17). Each of these tests may be easily performed on either individuals or a group of athletes.

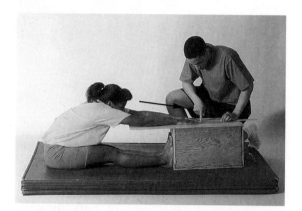

**Figure 4-15**

**Trunk and hip flexion test**

*Instructions to athlete:* Sit with legs together, knees flat on the floor, and feet against some vertical surface. Bend forward and reach as far forward as possible with the fingers.

*Measurement:* Measure the number of inches either in front of or beyond the vertical surface.

*Normal Range:* 3–8 inches past vertical.

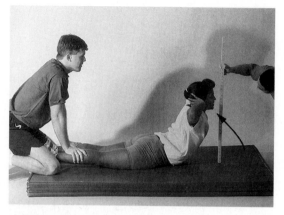

**Figure 4-16**

**Trunk extension test**

*Instructions to the athlete:* Lie in the prone position on the floor. Have a partner hold your legs just below the knees holding you to the ground. Grasp your hands behind your neck, inhale, lift your upper trunk as high off the floor as possible.

*Measurement:* Measure the distance from the chin to the floor.

*Normal Range:* 19–24 inches.

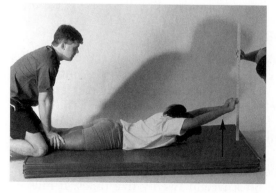

**Figure 4-17**

**Shoulder extension test**

*Instructions:* Lie prone on the floor with arms extended over head, while holding a stick or pencil in the hands. Raise the stick as high as possible with the face and chest kept flat on the floor.

*Measurement:* Measure the distance from the stick to the ground.

*Normal Range:* 23–27 inches.

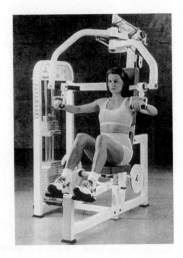

**Figure 4-18**

If strength training is combined with flexibility
exercise, a full range of motion may be
maintained.

## Is There a Relationship between Strength and Flexibility?

It is often said that strength training has negative effects on flexibility. For example, someone who develops a great deal of bulk through strength training is often referred to as muscle-bound. The expression "muscle-bound" has negative connotations in terms of the ability of that person to move. People who have highly developed muscles are thought to have lost much of their ability to move freely through a full range of motion.

Occasionally a person develops so much bulk that the physical size of the muscle prevents a normal range of motion. When strength training is not properly done, movement can be impaired. However, weight training, if done properly through a full range of motion, will not impair flexibility. Proper strength training probably improves dynamic flexibility and, if combined with a rigorous stretching program, can greatly enhance powerful and coordinated movements that are essential for success in many athletic activities.[19] In all cases a heavy weight-training program should be accompanied by a strong flexibility program (Figure 4-18).

## WHY ARE MUSCULAR STRENGTH, ENDURANCE, AND POWER IMPORTANT FOR ATHLETES?

The development of muscular strength is an essential component of a training program for every athlete.[23] Athletes who do not possess sufficient levels of muscle strength, endurance, and power are more susceptible to injury. By definition, **muscular strength** is the ability of a muscle to generate force against some resistance. **Muscular endurance** is the ability to perform repetitive muscular contractions against some resistance for an extended time. As muscular strength increases, there tends to be a corresponding increase in endurance. For example, an athlete can lift a weight twenty-five times. If muscular strength is increased by 10 percent through weight training, the

---

**muscular strength**
The maximum force that can be applied by a muscle during a single maximum contraction.

---

**muscular endurance**
The ability to perform repetitive muscular contractions against some resistance.

maximal number of repetitions is increased because it is easier for the athlete to lift the weight.

Most movements in sports are explosive and must include elements of both strength and speed if they are to be effective. If a large amount of force is generated quickly, the movement can be referred to as a **power** movement. Without the ability to generate power, an athlete is limited in his or her performance capabilities. It is difficult to hit a baseball, drive a golf ball, or kick a soccer ball without generating power. For most athletes, the ability to generate power is more critical for successful performance than simply having great strength or muscular endurance.

> **power**
> The ability to generate force rapidly.

## Types of Skeletal Muscle Contraction

Skeletal muscle is capable of three different types of contraction: (1) an *isometric contraction*, (2) a *concentric*, or positive, contraction, and (3) an *eccentric*, or negative, contraction. An isometric contraction occurs when the muscle contracts to produce tension, but there is no change in length of the muscle. Considerable force can be generated against some immovable resistance, even though no movement occurs. In a concentric contraction, the muscle shortens while tension is developed to overcome or move some resistance. In an eccentric contraction, the resistance is greater than the muscular force being produced, and the muscle lengthens while producing tension. For example, when lifting a weight in the hand the biceps muscle in the upper arm is shortening as it contracts, which is a concentric contraction. As the weight is lowered, the biceps muscle is still contracting but now it is lengthening. This movement is an eccentric contraction. Concentric and eccentric contractions must occur to allow most movements.

## What Determines the Amount of Strength?

### Size of the Muscle

Muscular strength is proportional to the size of a muscle as determined by the cross-sectional diameter of the muscle fibers.[16] The greater the cross-sectional diameter or the bigger a particular muscle, the stronger it is, and thus, the more force it is capable of generating. The size of a muscle tends to increase in cross-sectional diameter with weight training. This increase in muscle size is referred to as *hypertrophy*. Conversely, a decrease in the size of a muscle is referred to as *atrophy*.

### Number of Muscle Fibers

Strength is a function of the number and diameter of muscle fibers comprising a given muscle. The number of fibers is an inherited characteristic; a person with a large number of muscle fibers to begin with has the potential to hypertrophy to a much greater degree than does someone with relatively few fibers. But anyone can increase his or her strength through exercise.

### Neuromuscular Efficiency

Strength is also directly related to the efficiency of both the nervous and muscular systems (or the neuromuscular system) and the function of the motor unit in producing muscular force. Initial increases in strength during a weight-training program can be attributed primarily to increased neuromuscular efficiency. For a muscle to contract, a nerve impulse must be transmitted from the nervous system to the muscle. Each muscle fiber is innervated by a specific *motor unit.* By overloading a particular muscle, as in weight training, the muscle is forced to work efficiently. Efficiency is achieved by getting more motor units to fire, causing a stronger contraction of the muscle.[12]

### Biomechanical Factors

Strength in a given muscle is determined not only by the physical properties of the muscle but also by biomechanical factors. Bones along with muscles and their tendons form a system of levers and pulleys that collectively generate force to move an external object. The position of attachment of a particular muscle tendon on the bone will largely determine how much force this muscle is capable of generating.

### Fast-Twitch versus Slow-Twitch Muscle Fibers

There are two basic types of muscle fibers:
- Slow-twitch
- Fast-twitch

The fibers that make up a muscle are either slow-twitch fibers or fast-twitch fibers.[16] Within a particular muscle, both types of fibers exist, and the ratio in an individual muscle varies with each person. Those muscles that have a primary function of maintaining posture against the pull of gravity require more endurance and have a higher percentage of slow-twitch fibers. Muscles that produce powerful, explosive, and strength movements tend to have a much greater percentage of fast-twitch fibers.

Because this ratio is genetically determined, it may play a large role in determining ability for a given sport activity. For example, sprinters and weight lifters have a large percentage of fast-twitch fibers in relation to slow-twitch ones. One study has shown that sprinters may have as many as 95 percent fast-twitch fibers in certain muscles. Conversely, marathon runners generally have a higher percentage of slow-twitch fibers. The question of whether fiber types can change as a result of training has not been completely resolved.[16] However, both types of fibers can improve their metabolic capabilities through specific strength and endurance training.

### Level of Physical Activity

Loss in muscle strength is definitely related to individual levels of physical activity. Those people who are more active, or perhaps those who continue to strength train, considerably reduce this tendency toward declining muscle strength. In addition, exercise may also have an effect in slowing the decrease in cardiorespiratory endurance and flexibility as well as slowing increases in body fat that tend to occur with aging. Therefore, if total wellness and health is an ultimate goal, strength maintenance is important for all individuals regardless of age or the level of competition.

### Overtraining

Overtraining can have a negative effect on the development of muscular strength. The statement "If you abuse it you will lose it" is very applicable. Overtraining can result in **staleness,** which involves both psychological breakdown and physiological breakdown. With deterioration in the usual standard of performance, staleness may result in musculoskeletal injury, chronic fatigue, sickness, apathy, loss of appetite, indigestion, weight loss, and inability to sleep or rest properly. Engaging in proper and efficient resistance training, eating a proper diet, and getting appropriate rest can all minimize the potential negative effects of overtraining.[30]

Gains in muscular strength resulting from resistance training are reversible. Individuals who interrupt or stop resistance training altogether will see rapid decreases in strength gains. "If you don't use it, you'll lose it."

> **staleness**
> Deterioration in usual standard of performance.

## WHAT PHYSIOLOGICAL CHANGES OCCUR TO CAUSE INCREASED STRENGTH?

Weight training to improve muscular strength results in an increased size, or hypertrophy, of a muscle. What causes a muscle to hypertrophy? Over the years, a number of theories have been proposed to explain this increase in muscle size, the majority of which have been discounted.

The primary explanation for this hypertrophy is best attributed to an increase in the size and number of small contractile protein filaments within the muscle, called *myofilaments*. Increases in both size and number of the myofilaments as a result of strength training cause the individual muscle fibers to increase in cross-sectional diameter.[16] This increase is particularly true in men, although women also see some increase in muscle size. More research is needed to further clarify and determine the specific causes of muscle hypertrophy.

## CORE STABILIZATION TRAINING

A dynamic core stabilization training program should be an important component of all comprehensive strengthening programs. The **core** is defined as the lumbo-pelvic-hip complex. The core is where the center of gravity is located and where all movement begins. There are 29 muscles in the lumbar spine, the abdomen, and around the hip and pelvis that have their attachment to the lumbo-pelvic-hip complex.[12]

A core stabilization program will improve dynamic postural control; ensure appropriate muscular balance and joint movement around the lumbo-pelvic-hip complex; allow for the expression of dynamic functional strength; and improve neuromuscular efficiency throughout the entire body allowing for optimal acceleration, deceleration, and dynamic

**4-1 Critical Thinking**
Exercise

A swimmer has been engaged in an off-season weight-training program to increase her muscular strength and endurance. Although she has seen some improvement in her strength, she is concerned that she also seems to be losing flexibility in her shoulders, which she feels is critical to her performance as a swimmer. She has also noticed that her muscles are hypertrophying to some degree and is worried that that may be causing her to lose flexibility. She has just about decided to abandon her weight-training program altogether.

**?** What can be recommended that will allow her to continue to improve her muscular strength and endurance while maintaining or perhaps even improving her flexibility?

stabilization of the entire kinetic chain during functional movements. It also provides proximal stability for efficient lower extremity movements.[12]

Many individuals work on developing the functional strength, power, neuromuscular control, and muscular endurance in specific muscles that enable them to perform functional activities. However, relatively few individuals have developed the muscles required for stabilization of the spine. The body's stabilization system has to be functioning optimally to effectively utilize the strength, power, neuromuscular control, and muscular endurance that they have developed in their prime movers. If the extremity muscles are strong and the core is weak, then there will not be enough force created to produce efficient movements. A weak core is a fundamental problem of inefficient movements, which leads to injury.[27]

A core stabilization training program is designed to help an individual gain strength, neuromuscular control, power, and muscle endurance of the lumbo-pelvic hip complex. A comprehensive core stabilization training program should be systematic, progressive, and functional. When designing a functional core stabilization training program, you should select the appropriate exercises to elicit a maximal training response. The exercises must be safe, challenging, stress multiple planes, incorporate a variety of resistance equipment (physioball, medicine ball, dumbbells, tubing, etc.), be derived from fundamental movement skills, and be activity specific.[32] Figure 4-19 shows examples of exercises that may be used to improve core stability. You should start with exercises in which you can maintain stability and optimal neuromuscular control.

## WHAT ARE THE TECHNIQUES OF RESISTANCE TRAINING?

A number of different techniques of resistance training can be used for strength improvement, including *isometric exercise, progressive resistance exercise, isokinetic training, circuit training, plyometric exercise,* and *calisthenic exercise.* Regardless of which technique is used, one basic principle of training is extremely important: *For a muscle to improve in strength, it must be forced to work at a higher level than that to which it is accustomed.* In other words, the muscle must be *overloaded.*[30] Without overload the muscle will be able to *maintain* strength as long as training is continued against a level of resistance to which the muscle is accustomed. However, *no additional* strength gains will be realized. This maintenance of existing levels of muscular strength may be more important in weight-training programs that emphasize muscular endurance rather than strength gains. Many individuals can benefit more in terms of overall health by concentrating on improving muscular endurance. However, to most effectively build muscular strength, weight training requires a consistent, increasing effort against progressively increasing resistance. Progressive resistance exercise is based primarily on the principles of overload and progression, although the principle of overload also applies to isometric and plyometric exercise. All three training techniques produce improvement of muscular strength over time. Table 4-2 summarizes the seven different techniques for improving muscular strength.

**Figure 4-19**

## Core Stabilization Strengthening Exercises

(A) Bridging (B) Prone cobra (C) Side lying iso-abdominal (D) Human arrow
(E) Quadriped opposite arm/leg raise (F) Diagonal crunch (G) Stability ball
hip extension (H) Stability ball straight leg raise

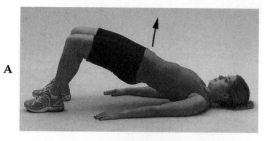

A

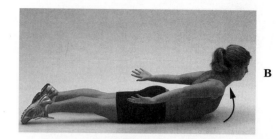

B

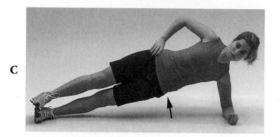

C

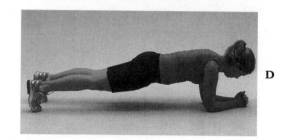

D

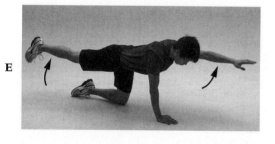

E

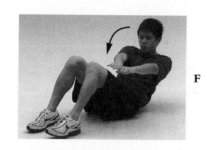

F

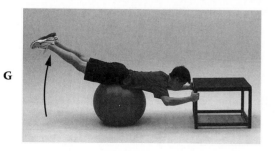

G

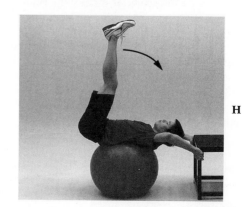

H

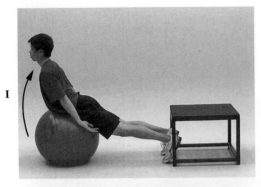

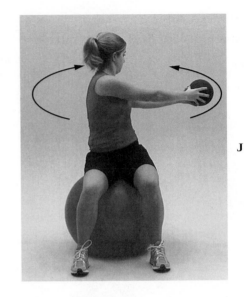

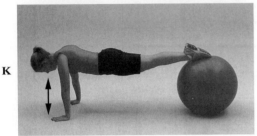

**Figure 4-19** (*continued*)

## Core Stabilization Strengthening Exercises

(I) Stability ball trunk extension (J) Stability ball rotation with power ball (K) Stability ball pushup

**TABLE 4-2** Techniques for Improving Muscular Strength

| Technique | Action | Equipment/Activity |
|---|---|---|
| Isometric exercise | Force develops while muscle length remains constant | Any immovable resistance |
| Progressive resistance exercise (PRE) | Force develops while the muscle shortens or lengthens | Free weights, Universal, Nautilus, Cybex, Eagle, Body Master Free Motion Fitness |
| Isokinetic training | Force develops while muscle is contracting at a constant velocity | Kincom, Biodex |
| Circuit training | Uses a combination of isometric, PRE, or isokinetic exercises organized into a series of stations | May use any of the equipment listed above |
| Plyometric exercise | Uses a rapid eccentric stretch of the muscle to facilitate an explosive concentric contraction | Hops, bounds, and depth jumping |
| Calisthenics | Uses body weight for resistance | No equipment needed (Sit-ups, push-ups, etc.) |
| Functional strength training | Uses functional concentric, eccentric, and isometric muscle contractions in 3 planes of motion simultaneously | Uses body weight for resistance on different stable and unstable surfaces |

## Isometric Exercise

An **isometric exercise** involves a muscle contraction in which the length of the muscle remains constant while tension develops toward a maximum force against an immovable resistance[22] (Figure 4-20). To develop strength, the muscle should generate a maximum force for 10 seconds at a time, and this contraction should be repeated five to ten times per day.

Isometric exercises are capable of increasing muscular strength; unfortunately, strength gains in a particular muscle will occur only in the position in which resistance is applied. At other positions in the range of motion, the strength curve drops off dramatically because of a lack of motor activity at those angles, and there is no corresponding increase in strength.

Another major disadvantage of isometric exercises is that they tend to produce a spike in blood pressure that can result in potentially life-threatening cardiovascular accidents. This sharp increase in blood pressure results from holding the breath and increasing pressure within the chest cavity. Consequently, the heart experiences a significant increase in blood pressure. This spike has been referred to as the *Valsalva effect.* To avoid or minimize this effect, breathing should be done during the maximum contraction.

Isometric exercises certainly have a place in a conditioning program. In certain instances, an isometric contraction can greatly enhance a particular movement.[22] A common use for isometric exercises is in injury rehabilitation or reconditioning. Many conditions or ailments resulting from either trauma or overuse must be treated with strengthening exercises. Unfortunately, these problems may get worse with full range-of-motion strengthening exercises. It may be more desirable to make use of isometric exercises until the injury has healed to the point that full-range activities can be performed.

## Progressive Resistance Exercise

Progressive resistance exercise is perhaps the most commonly used and most popular technique for improving muscular strength. Progressive resistance exercise training uses exercises that strengthen muscles through a contraction that overcomes some fixed resistance produced by equipment such as dumbbells, barbells, various weight machines, or exercise tubing (Theraband). Progressive resistance exercise uses isotonic contractions in which force is generated while the muscle is changing in length.[14]

Isotonic contractions may be either *concentric* or *eccentric.* Suppose an athlete is going to perform a biceps curl (see Figure 4-31). To lift the weight from the starting position, the biceps muscle must contract and shorten (**concentric,** or **positive, contraction**). If the biceps muscle does not remain contracted when the weight is being lowered, gravity causes this weight to simply fall back to the starting position. Thus, to control the weight as it is being lowered, the biceps muscle must continue to contract while gradually lengthening (**eccentric,** or **negative, contraction**).

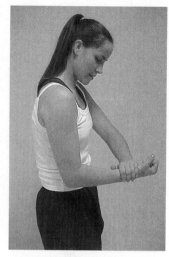

**Figure 4-20**

An isometric exercise involves a maximum force against an immovable resistance.

---

**isometric exercise**
Contracts the muscle statically without changing its length.

---

**concentric (positive) contraction**
The muscle shortens while contracting against resistance.

---

**eccentric (negative) contraction**
The muscle lengthens while contracting against resistance.

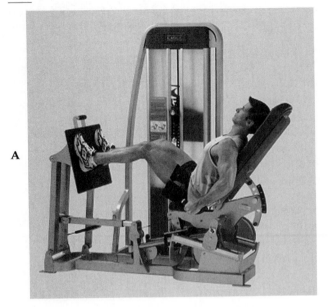

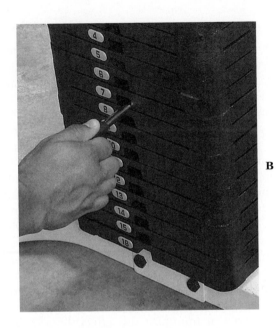

A

B

**Figure 4-21**

(A) This exercise machine is isotonic. (B) Resistance may be easily altered by changing the key in the stack of weights.

Various types of exercise equipment can be used with progressive resistive exercise, including free weights (barbells and dumbbells) or exercise machines such as Universal, Cybex, Tough Stuff, Icarian Fitness, King Fitness, Body Solid, Pro-Elite, Life Fitness, Nautilus, BodyCraft, Yukon, Flex, Cam-Bar, GymPros, Nugym, Body Works, DP, Soloflex, Eagle, Free Motion Fitness, and Body Master, to name a few (Figure 4-21A). Dumbbells and barbells require the use of iron plates of varying weights that can be easily changed by adding or subtracting equal amounts of weight to both sides of the bar.

Weight machines have a stack of weights that is lifted through a series of levers or pulleys. The stack of weights slides up and down on a pair of bars that restrict the movement to only one plane (Figure 4-21B). Weight can be increased or decreased simply by changing the position of a weight key.

Both the free weights and the machines have advantages and disadvantages.[18] The weight machines are safer to use than free weights are. For example, athletes who are doing a bench press with free weights must have someone spot (help them lift the weights back onto the support racks if they don't have enough strength to complete the lift); otherwise the weights may be dropped on the chest. The weight machines allow an athlete to easily and safely drop the weight without fear of injury. It is also a simple process to increase or decrease the weight on the weight machines by moving a single weight key, although changes can generally be made only in increments of 10 or 15 pounds. With free weights, iron plates must be added or removed from each side of the barbell.

Athletes will find a difference in the amount of weight that can be lifted with free weights versus the weight machines. Unlike the weight machines, free weights have no restricted motion and can thus move in many different directions, depending on the forces applied. Also, with free weights, an element of muscular control on the part of the lifter is required to prevent the weight from moving in any direction other than vertical. This control will usually decrease the amount of weight that can be lifted. Regardless of which type of equipment is used, the same principles of **isotonic** training may be applied.[18]

Surgical tubing or Theraband, as a means of providing resistance, has been widely used in training and conditioning. The advantage of exercising with surgical tubing or Theraband is that the direction of movement is less restricted than with free weights or exercise machines. Thus exercise can be done against resistance in more functional movement planes. The use of surgical tubing exercise in plyometrics and PNF strengthening techniques, as well as with the majority of the strengthening exercises shown in this chapter, is very popular.

Progressive resistance exercise must incorporate both concentric and eccentric contractions.[14] It is possible to generate greater amounts of force against resistance with an eccentric contraction than with a concentric contraction. Eccentric contractions are more resistant to fatigue than are concentric contractions. The mechanical efficiency of eccentric exercise may be several times higher than that of concentric exercise. Research has clearly demonstrated that the muscle should be overloaded and fatigued both concentrically and eccentrically for the greatest strength improvement to occur.

For athletes training specifically for the development of muscular strength, the concentric, or positive, portion of the exercise should require 1 to 2 seconds, whereas the eccentric, or negative, portion of the lift should require 2 to 4 seconds. The ratio of negative to positive should be approximately 2 to 1. Physiologically the muscle will fatigue much more rapidly concentrically than eccentrically.

One suggested disadvantage of any type of isotonic exercise is that the force required to move the resistance is constantly changing throughout the range of movement. Several years ago, Nautilus attempted to address this problem of changing force capabilities by using a cam in its pulley system (Figure 4-22). The cam has been individually designed for each piece of equipment so that the resistance is variable throughout the movement. This change in resistance at different points in the range has been labeled *accommodating resistance,* or **variable resistance.** Whether this design does what it claims to do is debatable. In real-life situations, it does not matter whether the resistance is changing.

### Progressive Resistance Exercise Techniques

Perhaps the most confusing aspect of progressive resistance exercise is the terminology used to describe specific programs. Table 4-3 lists specific terms and their operational definitions, which may provide some clarification.

> **isotonic exercise**
> Shortens and lengthens the muscle through a complete range of motion.

> **variable resistance**
> Resistance is varied throughout the range of motion.

**Figure 4-22**

The cam on this Nautilus machine is designed to equalize resistance throughout the full range of motion.

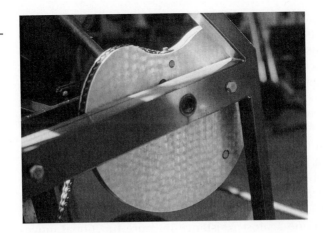

A considerable amount of research has been done in the area of resistance training to determine optimal techniques in terms of (1) the intensity or the amount of weight to be used, (2) the number of repetitions, (3) the number of sets, (4) the recovery period, and (5) the frequency of training.[22]

There is no such thing as an optimal strength-training program.[4] Achieving total agreement on a program of resistance training that includes specific recommendations relative to repetitions, sets, intensity, recovery time, and frequency among researchers and/or other experts in resistance training is impossible. However, the following general recommendations provide an effective resistance training program.

For any given exercise, the amount of weight selected should be sufficient to allow at most six to eight repetitions in each of three sets, with a recovery period of 60 to 90 seconds between sets. Initial selection of a starting weight may require some trial and error to achieve this six to eight repetitions maximum (RM) range. If at least three sets of six repetitions cannot be completed, the weight is too heavy and should be reduced. If it is possible to do more than three sets of eight

**TABLE 4-3** Progressive Resistance Exercise Terminology

| Terms | Definitions |
| --- | --- |
| Repetitions | Number of times a specific movement is repeated |
| Repetitions maximum (RM) | Maximum number of repetitions at a given weight |
| Set | A particular number of repetitions |
| Intensity | The amount of weight or resistance lifted |
| Recovery period | The rest interval between sets |
| Frequency | The number of times an exercise is done in a week's period |

repetitions, the weight is too light and should be increased. Progression to heavier weights is determined by the ability to perform at least eight RM in each of three sets. When progressing weight, an increase of about 10 percent of the current weight being lifted should still allow at least six RM in each of three sets.[4]

Muscular endurance is defined as the ability to perform repeated muscle contractions against resistance for an extended period. Most weight-training experts believe that muscular strength and muscular endurance are closely related. As one factor improves, the tendency is for the other factor to improve also. When weight training for strength, heavier weights with a lower number of repetitions should be used. Conversely, endurance training uses lighter weights with a greater number of repetitions.[4]

Endurance training should consist of three sets of ten to fifteen repetitions using the same criteria for weight selection, progression, and frequency as recommended for progressive resistance exercise.[24] Thus, training regimens for both muscular strength and endurance are similar in terms of sets and numbers of repetitions. Athletes who possess great strength levels tend to also exhibit greater muscular endurance when asked to perform repeated contractions against resistance.[4]

A particular muscle or muscle group should be exercised consistently every other day. Thus, the frequency of weight training should be at least three times per week but no more than four times per week. Serious weight trainers commonly lift every day; however, they exercise different muscle groups on successive days. For example, Monday, Wednesday, and Friday may be used for upper body muscles, whereas Tuesday, Thursday, and Saturday are used for lower body muscles.

**Regardless of what technique is used, to improve strength in a muscle, it must be overloaded in a progressive manner.**[30] This criterion is the basis of progressive resistance exercise. The amount of weight used and the number of repetitions performed must be sufficient to make the muscle work at a higher intensity than it is used to. This is the single most critical factor in any strength-training program.

Figures 4-23 to 4-46 describe exercises for strength improvement of shoulder, hip, knee, and ankle joint movements. These exercises are

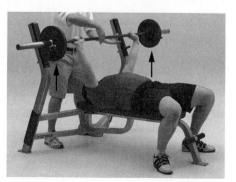

**Figure 4-23**

---

**Bench press**

*Joints affected:* Shoulder, elbow

*Movement:* Pushing away

*Position:* Supine, feet flat on floor, back flat on bench

*Primary muscles:* Pectoralis major, tricep

**Figure 4-24**

**Incline press**

*Joints affected:* Shoulder, elbow

*Movement:* Pushing upward and away

*Position:* Supine at an inclined angle, feet flat on floor or support back flat against bench

*Primary muscles:* Pectoralis major, triceps

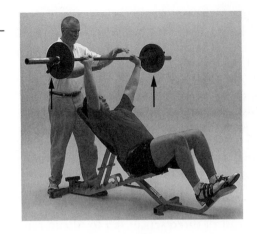

**Figure 4-25**

**Shoulder rotation**

*Joint affected:* Shoulder

*Movement:* External rotation

*Position:* Sidelying arm at side and elbow flexed at 90-degree angle

*Primary muscles:* Infraspinatus, teres minor

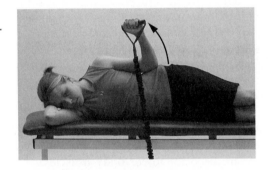

**Figure 4-26**

**Military press**

*Joints affected:* Shoulder, elbow

*Movement:* Pressing the weight overhead

*Position:* Seated, back straight

*Primary muscles:* Deltoid, trapezius, tricep

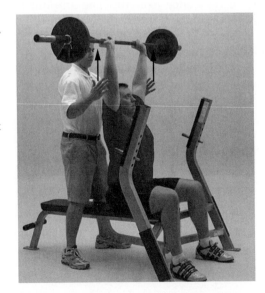

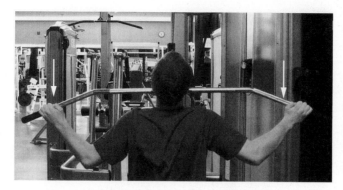

**Figure 4-27**

**Lat pull-downs**

*Joints affected:* Shoulder, elbow

*Movement:* Pulling the bar down in front of head

*Position:* Sitting, back straight, head up

*Primary muscles:* Latissimus dorsi, biceps

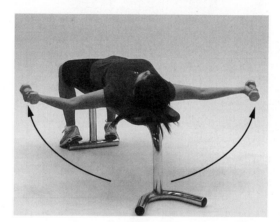

**Figure 4-28**

**Flys**

*Joint affected:* Shoulder

*Movement:* Horizontal flexion, bringing arms together over head

*Position:* Lying on back, feet on floor, back flat on bench

*Primary muscles:* Deltoid, pectoralis major

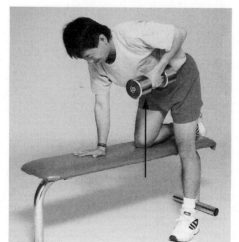

**Figure 4-29**

**Bent-over rows**

*Joint affected:* Shoulder

*Movement:* Shoulder extension, elbow flexion

*Position:* Standing bent over at waist, knee on bench

*Primary muscles:* Trapezius, rhomboids, latissimus dorsi

**Figure 4-30**

### Shoulder medial rotation

*Joint affected:* Shoulder

*Movement:* Internal rotation, lifting weight off the floor

*Position:* Supine, shoulder abducted and elbow flexed

*Primary muscles:* Subscapularis

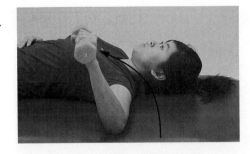

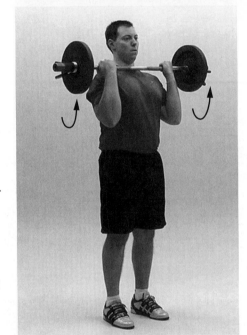

**Figure 4-31**

### Bicep curls

*Joint affected:* Elbow

*Movement:* Elbow flexion, curling the weight up to the shoulder

*Position:* Standing feet spread at shoulder width, back straight, arms extended

*Primary muscles:* Biceps

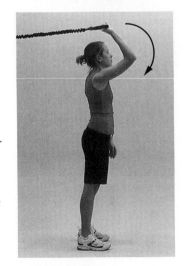

**Figure 4-32**

### Tricep extensions

*Joint affected:* Elbow

*Movement:* Elbow extension against cable or tube resistance

*Position:* Standing, elbow pointing upward

*Primary muscles:* Triceps

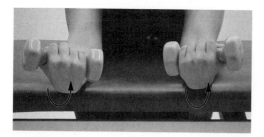

**Figure 4-33**

**Wrist curls**

*Joint affected:* Wrist

*Movement:* Wrist flexion, curling weight upward

*Position:* Seated, forearms on table, palms up

*Primary muscles:* Long flexors of forearm

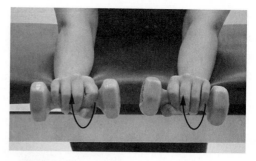

**Figure 4-34**

**Wrist extensions**

*Joint affected:* Wrist

*Movement:* Extension, curling weight upward

*Position:* Seated, forearms on table, palms down

*Primary muscles:* Long extensors of forearm

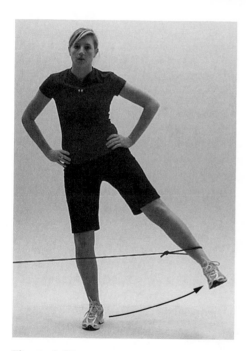

**Figure 4-35**

**Leg lifts**

*Joint affected:* Hip

*Movement:* Hip abduction, lifting leg up against resistance

*Position:* Standing, resistance on lower leg

*Primary muscles:* Hip Abductors

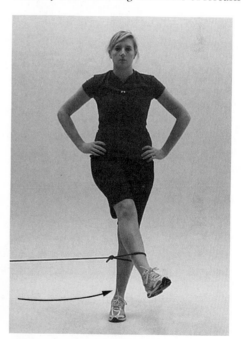

**Figure 4-36**

**Leg pulls**

*Joint affected:* Hip

*Movement:* Hip adduction, pulling down against resistance

*Position:* Standing, resistance on inside of lower leg

*Primary muscles:* Hip adductors

**Figure 4-37**

## Bent-knee leg lifts

*Joint affected:* Hip

*Movement:* Hip flexion, lifting leg up

*Position:* Standing, knee extended, resistance on shin

*Primary muscles:* Iliopsoas

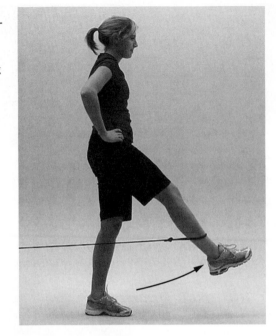

**Figure 4-38**

## Reverse leg lifts

*Joint affected:* Hip

*Movement:* Hip extension, lifting leg up against resistance

*Position:* Standing, knee extended, resistance behind lower leg

*Primary muscles:* Gluteus maximus, hamstrings

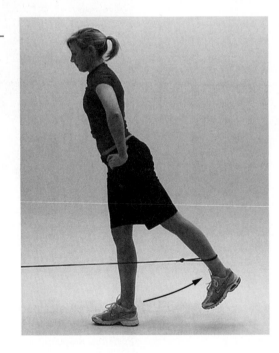

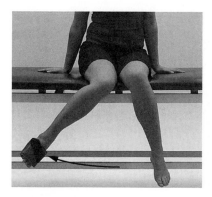

**Figure 4-39**

**Hip medial rotation**

*Joint affected:* Hip

*Movement:* Internal rotation, rotating lower leg outward

*Position:* Sitting, knee flexed, weight on ankle

*Primary muscles:* Medial rotators

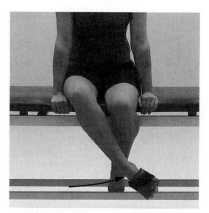

**Figure 4-40**

**Hip lateral rotation**

*Joint affected:* Hip

*Movement:* Lateral rotation, rotating lower leg inward

*Position:* Sitting, knee flexed, weight on ankle

*Primary muscles:* Lateral rotators

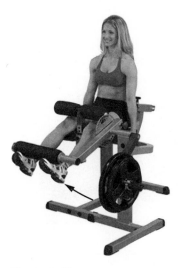

**Figure 4-41**

**Quadricep extensions**

*Joint affected:* Knee

*Movement:* Extension, straightening knee

*Position:* Sitting, on knee machine

*Primary muscles:* Quadriceps group

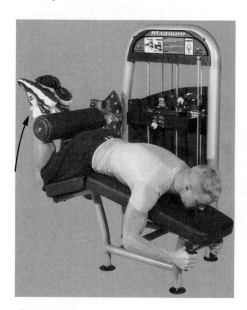

**Figure 4-42**

**Hamstring curls**

*Joint affected:* Knee

*Movement:* Flexion, bending knee and lifting weight up

*Position:* Prone, on knee machine

*Primary muscles:* Hamstring group

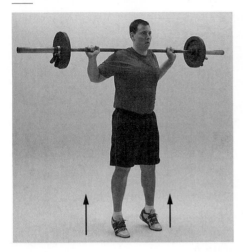

**Figure 4-43**

**Toe raises**

*Joint affected:* Ankle

*Movement:* Plantar flexion, pressing up on toes

*Position:* Standing on both legs and lifting body weight

*Primary muscles:* Gastrocnemius with knees fully extended. If knees are bent the primary muscle becomes the soleus

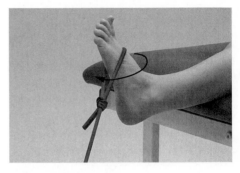

**Figure 4-44**

**Ankle inversion**

*Joint affected:* Ankle

*Movement:* Inversion, turning the sole of the foot up and in

*Position:* Sitting, knee flexed, instep up

*Primary muscles:* Anterior tibialis

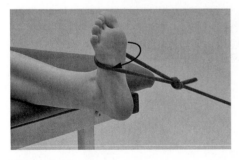

**Figure 4-45**

**Ankle eversion**

*Joint affected:* Ankle

*Movement:* Eversion, lifting the sole of the foot up and out

*Position:* Sitting, knee flexed, instep down

*Primary muscles:* Peroneals

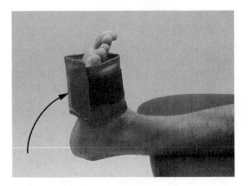

**Figure 4-46**

**Ankle dorsiflexion**

*Joint affected:* Ankle

*Movement:* Dorsiflexion, lifting the toes upward

*Position:* Sitting, knee flexed, heel on edge of table, weight on foot

*Primary muscles:* Dorsiflexors in shin

demonstrated using free weights (barbells, dumbbells, weights, and some machine weights). Any of these exercises may be performed on various commercial weight machines such as Cybex or Body Master. All of these exercises can also be done using exercise tubing or elastic resistance. Positions may differ slightly when different pieces of equipment are used. However, the joint motions that affect the various muscles are still the same.

### Open versus Closed-Kinetic Chain Exercises

The concept of the kinetic chain is based on the anatomical functional relationships which exist in the upper and lower extremities. An open-kinetic chain exists when the foot or hand is not in contact with the ground or some other surface. In a closed-kinetic chain, the foot or hand is weight-bearing (Figure 4-47). In training and conditioning, the use of closed-chain strengthening techniques has become a widely used technique because these exercises tend to be more functional since most sports

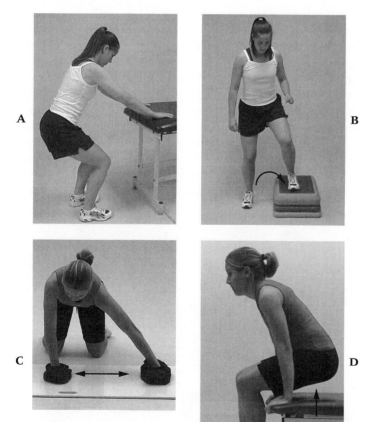

**Figure 4-47**

**Closed-kinetic chain exercises**

(A) Minisquats (B) Lateral Step-ups (C) Slide board upper extremity slides (D) Seated push-ups

activities are weight-bearing. Closed-kinetic chain exercises use varying combinations of isometric, concentric, and eccentric contractions which must occur simultaneously in different muscle groups within the chain.

### Isokinetic Exercise

> **isokinetic exercise**
> Resistance is given at a fixed velocity of movement with accommodating resistance.

An **isokinetic exercise** involves a muscle contraction in which the length of the muscle is changing while the contraction is performed at a constant velocity. In theory, the machine provides maximum resistance throughout the range of motion. The resistance provided by the machine will move only at some preset speed, regardless of the force applied to it by the individual. Thus, the key to isokinetic exercise is not the resistance but the speed at which resistance can be moved.[9]

Isokinetic exercise has never been widely used as a training and conditioning technique. In recent years, isokinetic exercise has also lost popularity as a rehabilitation tool. Currently only Biodex and KinCom still manufacture isokinetic exercise equipment (Figure 4-48).

### Circuit Training

> **circuit training**
> Exercise stations that consist of various combinations of weight training, flexibility, calisthenics, and aerobic exercises.

**Circuit training** uses a series of exercise stations that consist of various combinations of weight training, flexibility, calisthenics, and brief aerobic exercises. Circuits may be designed to accomplish many different training goals. With circuit training, the athlete moves rapidly from one station to the next and performs whatever exercise is to be done at that station within a specified time. A typical circuit consists of eight to twelve stations, and the entire circuit is repeated three times.

Circuit training is definitely an effective technique for improving strength and flexibility. Certainly if the pace or the time interval between stations is rapid and if workload is maintained at a high level of intensity with heart rates at or above target training levels, the

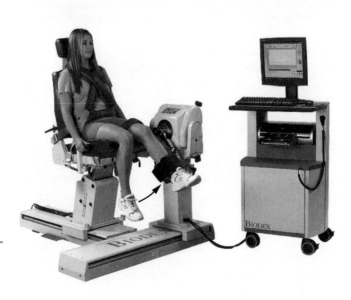

**Figure 4-48**

Biodex is an example of isokinetic exercise equipment.

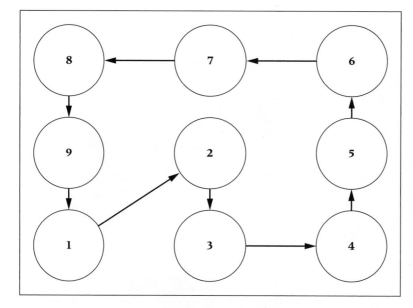

**Figure 4-49**

**Sample circuit program**

Station 1, squat thrusts, 75% maximum number of repetitions performed in 1 minute; Station 2, general flexion exercise, performed for 1 minute; Station 3, jump rope for 1 minute; Station 4, abdominal curls with weights, 75% maximum number of repetitions; Station 5, two-arm curls, 75% maximum number of repetitions; Station 6, vertical jump (sargent), 75% maximum number of repetitions performed in 1 minute; Station 7, wrist curls with weight for 1 minute; Station 8, half squat, heels raised, exercise with weight, 75% maximum number of repetitions; Station 9, general flexion exercises.

cardiorespiratory system benefits from this circuit. However, little research evidence shows that circuit training is very effective in improving cardiorespiratory endurance. It should be and is most often used as a technique for developing and improving muscular strength and endurance. Figure 4-49 provides an example of a simple circuit training setup.

## Plyometric Exercise

**Plyometric exercise** is a technique of exercise that involves a rapid eccentric (lengthening) stretch of a muscle, followed immediately by a rapid concentric contraction of that muscle for the purpose of producing a forceful explosive movement over a short period.[11] Plyometric exercises involve hops, bounds, and depth jumping for the lower extremity and the use of medicine balls and other types of weighted equipment for the upper extremity. Depth jumping is an example of a plyometric exercise in which an individual jumps to the ground from a specified height and then quickly jumps again as soon as ground contact is made (Figure 4-50).

The greater the stretch put on the muscle from its resting length immediately before the concentric contraction, the greater the resistance the muscle can overcome. Plyometrics emphasize the speed of the stretch phase. **The rate of stretch is more critical than the magnitude of the stretch.** An advantage to using plyometric exercise is that it can help develop eccentric control in dynamic movements. Plyometrics tend to place a great deal of stress on the musculoskeletal system. The coach who is implementing a plyometric exercise program should be aware that it is very likely that the athlete will develop muscle soreness in the early stages of a plyometric exercise program. This occurs primarily due to the

**plyometric exercise**
Uses a quick eccentric stretch of the muscle to facilitate a concentric contraction.

Plyometric exercise can cause muscle soreness in the early stages of use.

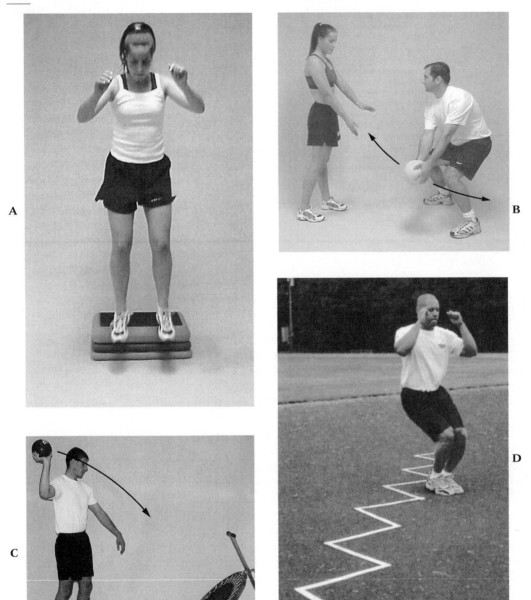

**Figure 4-50**

**Plyometric Exercises.**

**(A)** Depth jump. **(B)** Medicine ball toss to partner with
rotation. **(C)** Shoulder rotation with rebounder.
**(D)** Hopping exercise.

eccentric component of plyometric exercise to which the athlete is un-accustomed. The learning and perfection of specific jumping skills and other plyometric exercises must be technically correct and specific to the athlete's age, activity, and physical and skill development.[34]

Recommendations for plyometric exercise are variable, but the athlete should once again adhere to the three sets of six to eight repetitions rule.

## Calisthenic Strengthening Exercises

Calisthenics, or free exercise, is one of the more easily available means of developing strength. Isotonic movement exercises can be graded according to intensity by using gravity as an aid, ruling gravity out, moving against gravity, or using the body or body part as a resistance against gravity. Most calisthenics require the athlete to support the body or move the total body against the force of gravity. Push-ups are a good example of a vigorous antigravity free exercise. To be considered maximally effective, the isotonic calisthenic exercise, as in all types of exercise, must be performed in an exacting manner and in full range of motion. In most cases, ten or more repetitions are performed for each exercise and are repeated in sets of two or three.

Some free exercises use an isometric or holding phase instead of using a full range of motion. Examples of these exercises are back extensions and sit-ups. When the exercise produces maximum muscle tension, it is held between 6 and 10 seconds and then repeated one to three times. The exercises illustrated in Figures 4-51 to 4-59 are rec-ommended because they work on specific muscle groups and with a specific purpose. The athlete should work quickly and move from one exercise to the next without delay.

*Calisthenic, or free exercise, uses the force of gravity as resistance.*

## Functional Strength Training

Functional strength training is a rapidly evolving technique for improving not only muscular strength but also neuromuscular control.[8] The strength training techniques discussed to this point have traditionally focused on isolated, single-plane exercises used to elicit muscle hypertrophy in a specific muscle. These exercises have a very low neuromuscular demand because they are performed primarily with the rest of the body artificially stabilized on stable pieces of equipment. The central nervous system con-trols the ability to integrate the proprioceptive function of a number of individual muscles that must act simultaneously to produce a specific movement pattern that occurs in three planes of motion. If the body is designed to move in three planes of motion, then isolated training does little to improve functional ability. When strength training using isolated, single-plane, artificially stabilized exercises, the entire body is not being prepared to deal with the imposed demands of normal daily activities (walking up/down stairs, getting groceries out of the trunk, etc.).[12]

Earlier in this chapter it was stated that muscles are capable of three different types of contraction: concentric, eccentric, and isometric.

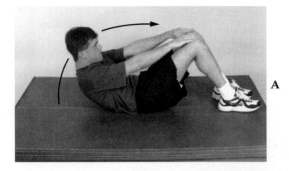
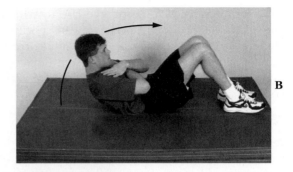
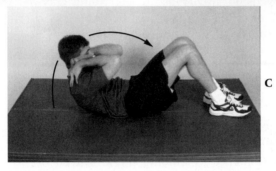

**Figure 4-51**

**Curl-ups. (A) Beginning. (B) Intermediate. (C) Advanced.**

*Joints affected:* Spinal vertebral joints

*Movement:* Trunk flexion

*Instruction:* Lying on back, hands either on chest or behind back, knees flexed to 90-degree angle, feet on floor; curl trunk and head to approximately 45-degree angle.

*Primary muscles:* Rectus abdominis.

**Figure 4-52**

**(A) Push-ups.**
**(B) Modified push-ups.**

*Purpose:* Strengthening

*Muscles:* Triceps and pectoralis major

*Repetitions:* Beginner, 10; intermediate, 20; advanced, 30

*Instructions:* Keep the upper trunk and legs extended in a straight line; touch floor with chest.

*Caution:* Avoid hyperextending the back, especially in modified push-ups.

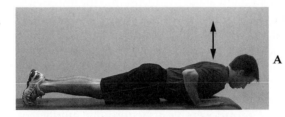
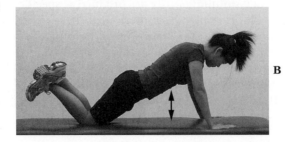

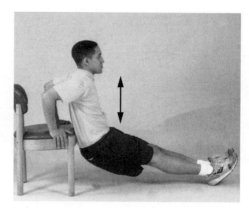

**Figure 4-53**

**Tricep extensions**

*Purpose:* Strengthening and range of motion at shoulder joint

*Muscles:* Triceps and trapezius

*Repetitions:* Beginner, 7; intermediate, 12; advanced, 18

*Instructions:* Begin with arms extended and body straight; lower buttocks until they touch the ground, then press back up.

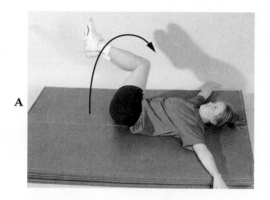

A

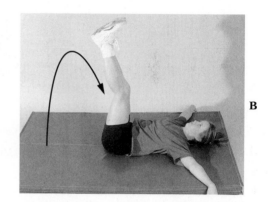

B

**Figure 4-54**

**Trunk rotation. (A) Beginner. (B) Advanced.**

*Muscles:* Internal and external obliques

*Repetitions:* Beginner, 10 each direction; intermediate, 15 each direction; advanced, 20 each direction

*Instructions:* Rotate trunk from side to side until knees touch the floor, keeping knees slightly bent.

*Caution:* This exercise should be done only by those who already have strong abdominals.

**Figure 4-55**

**Sitting tucks**

*Purpose:* Strengthen abdominals and stretch low back

*Muscles:* Rectus abdominis and erector muscles in low back

*Repetitions:* Beginner, 10; intermediate, 20; advanced, 30

*Instructions:* Keep legs and upper back off the ground and pull knees to chest.

*Caution:* This exercise should be done only by those who have strong abdominals.

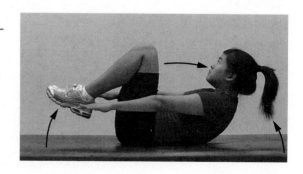

**Figure 4-56**

**Bicycle**

*Purpose:* Strengthen hip flexors and stretch lower back

*Muscles:* Iliopsoas

*Repetitions:* Beginner, 10 each side; intermediate, 20 each side; advanced, 30 each side

*Instructions:* Alternately flex and extend legs as if you were pedaling a bicycle.

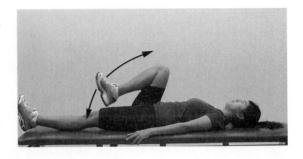

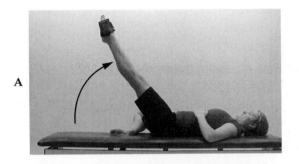

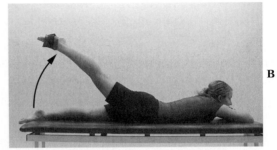

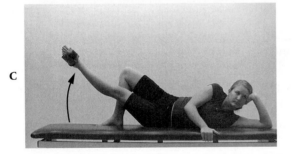

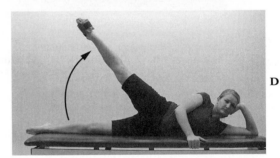

**Figure 4-57**

**Leg lifts. (A) Front. (B) Back. (C) Side (leg up). (D) Side (leg down).**

*Purpose:* Strengthen (A) hip flexors; (B) hip extensors; (C) hip adductors; (D) hip abductors.

*Muscles:* (A) Iliopsoas; (B) gluteus maximus; (C) adductor group; (D) gluteus medius.

*Repetitions:* Beginner, 10 each leg; intermediate, 15 each leg; advanced, 20 each leg

*Instructions:* Raise the exercising leg up as far as possible in each position.

*Caution:* If position A causes low back pain, bend the opposite leg.

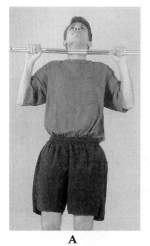
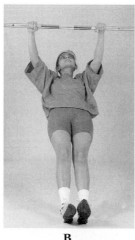
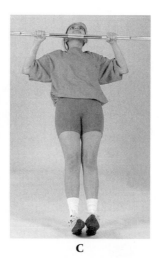

**A**  **B**  **C**

**Figure 4-58**

**(A) Chin-ups. (B) Modified chin-ups.**

*Purpose:* Strengthening and stretch of shoulder joint

*Muscles:* Biceps, brachialis, and latissimus dorsi

*Repetitions:* Beginner, 7; intermediate, 10; advanced, 15

*Instructions:* Pull up until chin touches top of bar. (C)

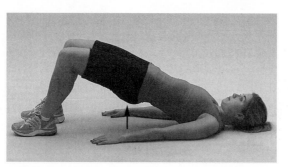

**Figure 4-59**

**Buttock tucks**

*Purpose:* Strengthen muscles of buttocks

*Muscles:* Gluteus maximus and hamstrings

*Repetitions:* Beginner, 10; intermediate, 15; advanced, 20

*Instructions:* Lying flat on back with knees bent, arch back and thrust the pelvis upward.

During functional movements, some muscles are contracting concentrically (shortening) to produce movement, others are contracting eccentrically (lengthening) to allow movement to occur, and still other muscles are contracting isometrically to create a stable base on which the functional movement occurs.

Since all muscles involved in a movement function either eccentrically, concentrically, or isometrically in three planes of motion simultaneously, **functional strength training** uses integratred exercises designed to improve functional movement patterns in terms of both increased strength and improved neuromuscular control.[12] When using functional strengthening exercises, individuals develop not only functional strength and neuromuscular control, but also high levels of core stabilization strength and flexibility. Figure 4-60 provides examples of functional strengthening exercises.

## Strength Training Considerations for Female Athletes

Strength is just as important to the female athlete as it is to the male athlete for preventing injury and maximizing performance.[14] The average female is incapable of building significant muscle bulk through weight

| **functional strength training** |
|---|
| Trains muscles to function concentrically, eccentrically, and isometrically in three planes simultaneously. |

Perhaps the most critical performance difference between men and women is the ratio of strength to weight.

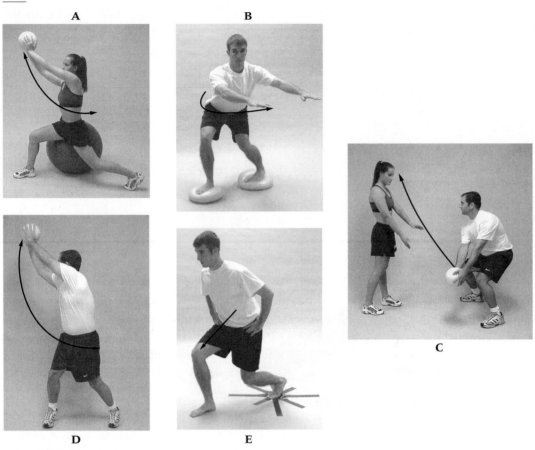

A

B

C

D

E

**Figure 4-60**

Functional strengthening exercises use simultaneous, concentric, eccentric and isometric contractions in three planes on stable or unstable surfaces.

training. Significant muscle hypertrophy depends on the presence of a hormone called *testosterone*. Testosterone is considered a male hormone, although all females possess some testosterone in their systems. Females with higher testosterone levels tend to have more masculine character-istics such as increased facial and body hair, a deeper voice, and the potential to develop a little more muscle bulk.

The average female does not need to worry about developing large bulky muscles with strength training. What does happen is that muscle tone is improved. Muscle tone refers to the firmness, or tension, of the muscle during a resting state. For example, doing sit-ups increases the firmness of the abdominal muscles and makes them more resistant to fatigue.

A female in weight training will probably see some remarkable gains in strength initially, even though her muscle bulk does not increase. How is this possible? These initial strength gains, which can be attributed to improved neuromuscular system efficiency, begin to plateau, and in the female, more limited improvement in muscular strength will be realized during a continuing strength-training program.

These initial neuromuscular strength gains will also be seen in men, although their strength will continue to increase with appropriate training. Females who do possess higher testosterone levels have the potential to further increase their strength because of the development of greater muscle bulk.

Perhaps the most critical difference between males and females regarding physical performance is the ratio of strength to body weight. The reduced *strength/body weight ratio* in females is the result of their higher percentage of body fat.[14] The strength/body weight ratio may be significantly improved through weight training by decreasing the body fat percentage while increasing lean weight. Strength training programs for females should follow the same guidelines as those for males.

## WHY IS CARDIORESPIRATORY FITNESS IMPORTANT FOR AN ATHLETE?

A healthy cardiorespiratory system is critical both for performance and for preventing undue fatigue that may predispose an athlete to injury.[36] By definition, cardiorespiratory endurance is the ability to perform whole-body large muscle activities for extended periods. The cardiorespiratory system provides a means by which oxygen is supplied to the various tissues of the body.

*Aerobic* exercise is great for building cardiorespiratory fitness. An aerobic activity is one in which the intensity of the activity is low enough that the cardiovascular system can supply enough oxygen to continue the activity for long periods. An activity in which the intensity is so great that the demand for oxygen is greater than the body's ability to deliver oxygen is called an *anaerobic* activity. Short bursts of muscle contraction, as in running or swimming sprints or lifting weights, use predominantly the anaerobic system. However, endurance-type activities that last for a longer time depend a great deal on the aerobic system. In most activities both aerobic and anaerobic systems function simultaneously. Table 4-4 provides a comparison summary between aerobic and anaerobic activities.

Cardiorespiratory endurance is essential to reduce fatigue, which can lead to injury.

Cardiorespiratory endurance refers to the body's ability to transport and use oxygen efficiently.

**TABLE 4-4** Comparison of Aerobic versus Anaerobic Activities

|  | Mode | Relative Intensity | Intensity | Frequency | Duration | Miscellaneous |
|---|---|---|---|---|---|---|
| Aerobic activities | Continuous, long-duration, sustained activities | Less intense | 60%–90% of MHR | At least three but not more than six times per week | 20–60 min | Less risk to sedentary or older individuals |
| Anaerobic activities | Explosive, short-duration, burst-type activities | More intense | 90%–100% of MHR | Three to four times per week | 10 sec–2 min | Used in sport and team activities |

Organizing and Establishing
an Effective Athletic Health
Care System

A high school shot-putter has
been working intensely on
weight training to improve his
muscular power. In particular he
has been concentrating on lifting
extremely heavy free weights using a low number of repetitions
(three sets of six to eight reps).
Although his strength has improved significantly over the last
several months, he is not seeing
the same degree of improvement
in his throws even though his
technique is very good.

? The athlete is frustrated with
his performance and wants to
know if he can add anything to
his training program that might
enhance his performance.

The capacity of the cardiorespiratory system to carry oxygen throughout the body depends on the coordinated function of four components:
(1) the heart, (2) the blood vessels, (3) the blood, and (4) the lungs.
Improvement of cardiorespiratory endurance through exercise occurs
because of an increase in the capability of each of these four components in providing necessary oxygen to the working tissues.[3] A basic
discussion of the training effects and responses to exercise that occur in
the heart should make it easier to understand why the training techniques to be discussed later are effective in improving cardiorespiratory
endurance.

### How Does Exercise Affect the Function of the Heart?

The heart is the main pumping mechanism and circulates oxygenated
blood throughout the body to the various tissues. The heart receives
oxygen-poor blood from the venous system and pumps that blood
through the pulmonary vessels to the lungs, where carbon dioxide is
exchanged for oxygen. The oxygen-rich blood then returns to the
heart, from which it exits through the aorta to the arterial system
and is circulated throughout the body, supplying oxygen to the tissues
(Figure 4-61).[3]

During exercise, muscles use oxygen at a much higher rate, and
thus the heart must pump more oxygenated blood to meet this
increased demand.

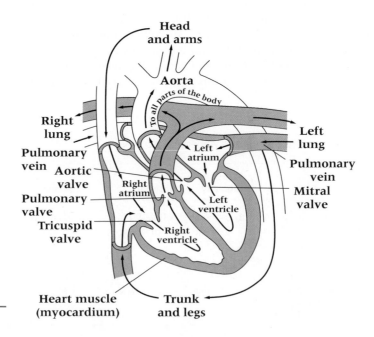

**Figure 4-61**

Anatomy of the heart

## WHAT DETERMINES HOW EFFICIENTLY THE BODY IS USING OXYGEN?

The greatest rate at which oxygen can be taken in and used during exercise is referred to as *maximum aerobic capacity.*[5] Maximum aerobic capacity determines how much oxygen can be used during 1 minute of maximal exercise. This rate is most often presented in terms of the volume of oxygen used relative to body weight per unit of time (ml/kg/min). Normal maximum oxygen utilization for most men and women aged 15 to 25 years falls in the range of 38 to 46 ml/kg/min. A world-class male marathon runner may have a maximum aerobic capacity in the 70 to 80 ml/kg/min range whereas a female marathoner may have a 60 to 70 ml/kg/min range.

The performance of any activity requires a certain rate of oxygen use that is about the same for everybody. Generally the greater the rate or intensity of the activity, the greater the oxygen demand. Each person has his or her own maximum rate of oxygen consumption, and the ability to perform an activity is closely related to the amount of oxygen required by that activity.

The maximum rate at which oxygen can be used is to a large extent a genetically determined characteristic. Each person's maximum aerobic capacity falls within a given range. The more active the athlete, the higher the existing maximum aerobic capacity will be within that range. The less active the athlete, the lower the maximum aerobic capacity will be in that range. Thus, athletes engaging in a serious training program can increase aerobic capacity to its highest limit within their range.

The range of maximum aerobic capacity inherited is to a large extent determined by the ratio of fast-twitch to slow-twitch muscle fibers. Athletes with a high percentage of slow-twitch muscle fibers are more resistant to fatigue and are able to use oxygen more efficiently; thus maximum aerobic capacity will be higher.

Fatigue is closely related to the percentage of maximum aerobic capacity that a particular activity demands. The greater the percentage of maximum aerobic capacity that is required during an activity, the less time the activity can be performed. Fatigue occurs in part when insufficient oxygen is supplied to muscles. For example, Figure 4-62 presents two athletes, A and B. A has a maximum aerobic capacity of 50 ml/kg/min, whereas B has a maximum aerobic capacity of only 40 ml/kg/min. If A and B are exercising at the same intensity, then A will be working at a much lower percentage of maximum aerobic capacity than B is. Consequently, A should be able to sustain his or her activity over a much longer time. Everyday activities such as walking up stairs or running to catch a bus may be adversely affected if a person's ability to use oxygen efficiently is impaired. Certainly the ability to perform a sport activity is hindered if an athlete's level of cardiorespiratory endurance is not what it should be. Thus improvement of cardiorespiratory endurance must be an essential component of any fitness program.

**Figure 4-62**

Athlete A should be able to work longer than Athlete B as a result of using a lower percentage of maximum aerobic capacity.

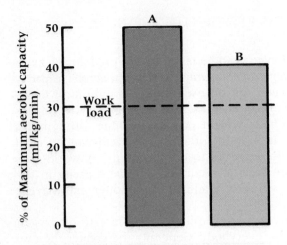

## How Is Maximum Aerobic Capacity Determined?

The most accurate technique for measuring aerobic capacity must be done in a laboratory. This technique involves exercising a subject on a treadmill or bicycle ergometer at a specific intensity and then monitoring heart rate and collecting samples of expired air using somewhat expensive and sophisticated equipment. Obviously for the typical person this technique is somewhat impractical. Therefore, the technique used most often is to monitor heart rate as a means of estimating a percentage of maximum aerobic capacity.[5]

Monitoring heart rate is an indirect method of estimating maximum aerobic capacity. In general, heart rate and aerobic capacity have a linear relationship, although at very low intensities and at high intensities this linear relationship breaks down (Figure 4-63). The greater the intensity of the exercise, the higher the heart rate. Because of this existing relationship, the rate of oxygen utilization can be estimated by taking the heart rate.[21]

### Monitoring Heart Rate

Heart rate can be determined by taking a pulse rate at specific sites. The most accurate site for measuring the pulse rate is the radial artery located on the thumb side of the wrist joint (Figure 4-64). An accurate heart rate can be determined by counting the number of beats that occur in 30 seconds and then multiplying that number by two. Heart rate should be monitored within 15 seconds after stopping exercise.

## WHAT TRAINING TECHNIQUES CAN IMPROVE CARDIORESPIRATORY ENDURANCE?

There are a number of different methods through which cardiorespiratory endurance may be improved, including (1) continuous training, (2) interval training, and (3) fartlek training. Regardless of the training technique used for the improvement of cardiorespiratory endurance,

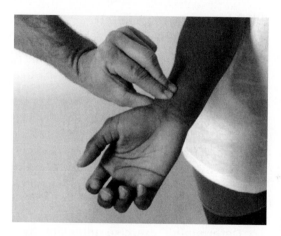

**Figure 4-63**

Maximum heart rate is achieved at about the same time as maximum aerobic capacity.

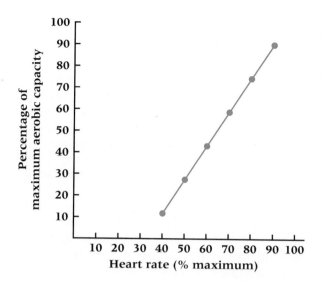

**Figure 4-64**

The radial artery provides the most accurate estimation of pulse rate.

one principal goal remains the same: to increase the ability of the cardiorespiratory system to supply a sufficient amount of oxygen to working muscles. Without oxygen, the body is incapable of producing energy for an extended time.

## Continuous Training

Continuous training is a technique that uses exercises performed at the same level of intensity for long periods. Continuous training has four considerations:

- The type of activity
- The frequency of the activity
- The intensity of the activity
- The duration of the activity

### Type of Activity

The type of activity used in continuous training must be aerobic. Aerobic activities are any activities that use large amounts of oxygen, elevate the heart rate, and maintain it at that level for an extended time. Aerobic activities generally involve repetitive, whole body, large-muscle movements performed over an extended time. Examples of aerobic activities include walking, running, swimming, cycling, rowing, cross-country skiing, and so on. The advantage of these aerobic activities as opposed to more intermittent activities, such as racquetball, squash, basketball, or tennis, is that with aerobic activities it is easy to regulate intensity by either speeding up or slowing down the pace. Because it is already known that the given intensity of the workload elicits a given heart rate, these aerobic activities allow athletes to maintain heart rate at a specified *target level*. Intermittent activities involve variable speeds and intensities that cause the heart rate to fluctuate considerably. Although these intermittent activities will improve cardiorespiratory endurance, they are much more difficult to monitor in terms of intensity.

### Frequency of Activity

To see at least minimal improvement in cardiorespiratory endurance, it is necessary for the average person to engage in no less than three exercise sessions per week. A competitive athlete should be prepared to train as often as six times per week. Everyone should take off at least one day per week to give damaged tissues a chance to repair themselves.

### Intensity of Activity

The intensity of the exercise is also a critical factor, although recommendations regarding training intensities vary. This is particularly true in the early stages of training, when the body is forced to make a lot of adjustments to increased workload demands.

**Determining exercise intensity by monitoring heart rate** The objective of aerobic exercise is to elevate heart rate to a specified target rate and maintain it at that level during the entire workout. Because heart rate is directly related to the intensity of the exercise and to the rate of oxygen utilization, it becomes a relatively simple process to identify a specific workload (pace) that will make the heart rate plateau at the desired level. By monitoring heart rate, athletes know whether the pace is too fast or too slow to get the heart rate into a target range.[21]

Heart rate can be increased or decreased by speeding up or slowing down pace. As mentioned, heart rate increases proportionately with the intensity of the workload and will plateau after 2 to 3 minutes of activity. Thus the athlete should be actively engaged in the workout for 2 to 3 minutes before measuring his or her pulse.

Several formulas can be used to identify a training *target heart rate*.[36] To calculate a specific target heart rate, maximum heart rate must first be calculated. Exact determination of maximum heart rate involves exercising an individual at a maximal level and monitoring the heart rate using an electrocardiogram. This process is difficult outside a laboratory. An approximate estimate of maximum heart rate for both males and females in the population is about 220 beats per minute. Maximum heart rate is related to age. As age increases, maximum heart rate decreases. A simple estimate of maximum heart rate (HR) is Maximum HR = 220 − Age. For a 20-year-old individual, maximum heart rate is about 200 beats per minute (220 − 20 = 200). Thus if training intensity is to be at 70 percent of maximum heart rate, the target heart rate can be calculated by multiplying 0.7 × (220 − Age).

Another commonly used formula that takes into account current levels of fitness is the Karvonen equation:[20]

*Target HR = Resting HR\* + (0.6 [maximum HR − Resting HR])*

Resting heart rate generally falls between 60 and 80 beats per minute. A 20-year-old athlete with a resting pulse of 70 beats per minute, according to the Karvonen equation, has a target training heart rate of 148 beats per minute (70 + 0.6 [200 − 70] = 148).

Regardless of the formula used, the American College of Sports Medicine recommends that young healthy individuals train with a target heart rate in the 60 percent to 85 percent range when training continuously. Exercising at a 70 percent level is considered a moderate level because activity can be continued for a long time with little discomfort and still produce a **training effect.** A highly trained athlete will not find it difficult to sustain a heart rate at the 85 percent level.

**Determining exercise intensity through rating of perceived exertion** *Rating of perceived exertion* (RPE) can be used in addition to heart rate monitoring to indicate exercise intensity.[25] During exercise, individuals are asked to rate subjectively on a numerical scale from 6 to 20 exactly how they feel relative to their level of exertion (Table 4-5). More intense exercise that requires a higher level of oxygen consumption and energy expenditure is directly related to higher subjective ratings of perceived exertion. Over time, individuals can be taught to exercise at a specific RPE that relates directly to more objective measures of exercise intensity.

### Duration of Activity

For minimal improvement to occur, the American College of Sports Medicine recommends 20 to 60 minutes of workout/activity with the heart rate elevated to training levels.[17] Generally, the greater the

**training effect**
Stroke volume increases while heart rate is reduced at a given exercise load.

**TABLE 4-5** Rating of perceived exertion

| Scale | Verbal Rating |
|-------|---------------|
| 6 | |
| 7 | Very, very light |
| 8 | |
| 9 | Very light |
| 10 | |
| 11 | Fairly light |
| 12 | |
| 13 | Somewhat hard |
| 14 | |
| 15 | Hard |
| 16 | |
| 17 | Very hard |
| 18 | |
| 19 | Very, very hard |
| 20 | |

\* True resting heart rate should be monitored with the subject lying down.

duration of the workout, the greater the improvement in cardiorespiratory endurance. The competitive athlete should train for at least 45 minutes per session.

### Interval Training

interval training
Alternating periods of work
with active recovery.

Unlike continuous training, **interval training** involves activities that are more intermittent. Interval training consists of alternating periods of relatively intense work and active recovery. It allows for performance of much more work at a more intense workload over a longer period than does working continuously.[6] In continuous training, the athlete strives to work at an intensity of about 60 to 85 percent of maximum heart rate. Obviously, sustaining activity at the higher intensity over a 20-minute period is extremely difficult. The advantage of interval training is that it allows work at the 80 percent or higher level for a short period followed by an active period of recovery during which the athlete may be working at only 30 to 45 percent of maximum heart rate. Thus the intensity of the workout and its duration can be greater than with continuous training.

Most sports are anaerobic, involving short bursts of intense activity followed by a sort of active recovery period (for example, football, basketball, soccer, or tennis).[26] Training with the interval technique allows the athlete to be more sport specific during the workout. With interval training, the overload principle is applied by making the training period much more intense. There are several important considerations in interval training. The *training period* is the amount of time that continuous activity is actually being performed, and the *recovery period* is the time between training periods. A *set* is a group of combined training and recovery periods, and a *repetition* is the number of training/recovery periods per set. *Training time* or *distance* refers to the rate or distance of the training period. The training/recovery ratio indicates a time ratio for training versus recovery.

An example of interval training is a soccer player running sprints. An interval workout would involve running ten 120-yard sprints in under 20 seconds each, with a 1-minute walking recovery period between each sprint. During this training session, the soccer player's heart rate will probably increase to 85 to 90 percent of maximum level during the sprint and will probably fall to the 35 to 45 percent level during the recovery period.

### Fartlek Training

*Fartlek*, a training technique that is a type of cross-country running, originated in Sweden. Fartlek literally means "speed play." It is similar to interval training in that the athlete must run for a specified period; however, specific pace and speed are not identified. The course for a fartlek workout should be a varied terrain with some level running, some uphill and downhill running, and some running through obstacles such as trees or rocks. The object is to put surges into a running work-out, varying the length of the surges according to individual purposes. One big advantage of fartlek training is that because the pace and ter-rain are always changing, the training session is less regimented and al-lows for an effective alternative in the training routine. Most people who jog or walk around the community are really engaging in a fartlek-type workout.

Again, if fartlek training is going to improve cardiorespiratory endurance, it must elevate the heart rate to at least minimal train-ing levels (60%–85%). Fartlek may best be used as an off-season conditioning activity or as a change-of-pace activity to counteract the boredom of a training program that uses the same activity day after day.

### Athletic Injury Management Checklist

The following is a checklist of factors in a training and conditioning program to make sure the athlete is fit and to prevent injuries.

☐ Incorporate the concept of periodization into the year-round training and conditioning plan.
☐ Make sure the athlete does a proper warm-up before training and a cooldown afterwards.
☐ Incorporate flexibility training.
☐ Use dynamic, static, or PNF stretching techniques.
☐ Select specific and appropriate stretching exercises to improve flexibility.
☐ Incorporate training techniques to improve muscular strength, endurance, or power.
☐ Use isometric, progressive resistance exercise, isokinetic, plyometric, or calisthenic techniques or some combination of these to achieve the goal of strength development.
☐ Select specific strengthening exercises to be included in a workout.
☐ Incorporate training techniques to improve cardiorespiratory fitness.
☐ Use continuous training to improve aerobic capacity.
☐ Use interval training or fartlek training to improve anaerobic function.

## SUMMARY

• Proper physical conditioning for sports participation should prepare the athlete for a high-level performance while helping to prevent injuries inherent to that sport.

- Year-round conditioning is essential in most sports to assist in preventing injuries. Periodization is an approach to conditioning that attempts to bring about peak performance while reducing injuries and overtraining in the athlete by developing a training and conditioning program to be followed throughout the various seasons.

- Physical conditioning must follow the SAID principle—an acronym for specific adaptation to imposed demands.

- It is generally accepted that for preventing injuries, a proper warm-up should precede conditioning, and a proper cooldown should follow. It takes at least 15 to 30 minutes of gradual warm-up to bring the body to a state of readiness for vigorous sports training and participation. Warming up consists of general, unrelated activities followed by specific, related activities.

- Optimum flexibility is necessary for preventing injury in most sports. Too much flexibility can allow joint trauma to occur, whereas too little flexibility can result in muscle tears or strains. The safest and most effective means of increasing flexibility are static stretching and the PNF techniques.

- A dynamic core stabilization program should be an important component of all programs designed to improve muscular strength.

- Strength is that capacity to exert a force or the ability to perform work against a resistance. There are numerous means to develop strength, including isometric exercise, progressive resistance exercise, isokinetic exercise, circuit training, plyometric exercise, calisthenics, and functional strength training.

- Cardiorespiratory endurance is the ability to perform whole-body, large-muscle activities repeatedly for long periods. Maximum aerobic capacity is the greatest determinant of the level of cardiorespiratory endurance. Improvement of cardiorespiratory endurance may be accomplished through continuous, interval, or fartlek training.

---

### Solutions to Critical Thinking Exercises

**4-1** The warm-up should begin with a 5- to 7-minute slow jog during which the athlete should break into a light sweat. At that point, she should engage in stretching (using either static or PNF techniques), concentrating on quadriceps, hamstrings, groin, and hip abductor muscles. She should repeat each specific stretch four times, holding the stretch for 15 to 20 seconds. Once her workout begins, she should gradually and moderately increase the intensity of the activity. The importance of stretching during the cooldown that follows the workout should also be stressed.

**4-2** Weight training will not have a negative effect on flexibility as long as the lifting technique is done properly. Lifting the weight through a complete and full range of motion will improve strength and simultaneously maintain range of motion. This female swimmer is not likely to bulk up to the point at which range of motion will be affected by muscle size. She should also continue to incorporate active stretching into her training regimen.

**4-3** The shot put, like many other dynamic movements in sport, requires not only great strength, but also the ability to generate that strength very rapidly. To develop muscular power, the athlete must engage in dynamic, explosive training techniques that will help him develop his ability. Power-lifting techniques such as squats and power cleans should be helpful. In addition, plyometric exercises using weights for added resistance will help him learn to improve his speed of muscular contraction against some resistive force.

**4-4** Alternative activities such as swimming or riding a stationary exercise bike should be incorporated into this athlete's rehabilitation program immediately. If the pressure on the ankle when riding an exercise bike is initially too painful, she should use a bike that incorporates upper extremity exercise. The soccer player should engage in a minimum of 30 minutes of continuous training and some higher intensity interval training to maintain both aerobic and anaerobic fitness.

## REVIEW QUESTIONS AND CLASS ACTIVITIES

1. Why is year-round conditioning so important for injury prevention?
2. In terms of injury prevention, list as many advantages as you can for conditioning.
3. How does the SAID principle relate to sports conditioning and injury prevention?
4. What is the value of proper warm-ups and cooldowns to sports injury prevention?
5. Critically observe how a variety of sports use warm-up and cooldown procedures.
6. Compare ways to increase flexibility and how those ways may decrease or increase the athlete's susceptibility to injury.
7. How may increasing strength decrease susceptibility to injury?
8. Compare different techniques of increasing strength. How may each way be an advantage or a disadvantage to the athlete in terms of injury prevention?
9. Discuss the relationship between maximum aerobic capacity and heart rate.
10. Differentiate between aerobic and anaerobic training methods.
11. How is continuous training different from interval training?
12. Design a preseason training and conditioning program.

**REFERENCES**

1. Anderson B: 2008. *Stretching,* 20th ed, Bolinas, Calif, 2000, Shelter Publishers.
2. Andersen, J.C.; 2005. Stretching before and after exercise: Effect on muscle soreness and injury risk, *Journal of athletic training* 40(3): 218–220.
3. Bassett DR, Howley ET: 2000. Limiting factors for maximum oxygen uptake and determinants of endurance performance, *Med Sci Sports Exerc* 32(1):70.
4. Berger R: 1973. *Conditioning for men,* Boston, Allyn & Bacon.

5. Bergh U, Ekblom B, Astrand PO: 2000. Maximal oxygen uptake "classical" versus "contemporary" viewpoints, *Med Sci Sports Exerc* 32(1):85.

6. Billat, LV: 2001. Interval training for performance: a scientific and empirical practice. Special recommendations for middle- and long-distance running. Part I: aerobic interval training. *Sports medicine* 31(1), 13–31.

7. Bompa TO: 2005. *Periodization training for sports*, Champaign, IL, Human Kinetics.

8. Boyle, M: 2004. *Functional training for sports*, Champaign, Ill., Human Kinetics.

9. Brown LE: 2000. *Isokinetics in human performance*, Champaign, IL, Human Kinetics.

10. Burke, DG, Culligan, CJ, Holt, LE: 2000. The theoretical basis of proprioceptive neuromuscular facilitation. *Journal of strength and conditioning research* 14(4): 496–500.

11. Chu DA: 1999. Plyometrics in sports injury rehabilitation and training, *Ath Ther Today* 4(3):7.

12. Clark, M: 2001. *Integrated training for the new millennium*, Calabasas, CA, National Academy of Sports Medicine.

13. Decoster, L: 2005. The effects of hamstring stretching on range of motion: A systematic literature review, *The journal of orthopaedic & sports physical therapy* 3(6): 377–387.

14. De Lorme TL, Watkins AL: 1951. *Progressive resistance exercise*, New York, Appleton-Century-Crofts.

15. Goldenberg, L, Twist, P: 2002. Core stabilization. In Goldenberg, L. (ed.), *Strength ball training*, Champaign, IL, Human Kinetics, pp. 65–97; 187.

16. Gravelle BL, Blessing DL: 2000. Physiological adaptation in women concurrently training for strength and endurance, *J Streng Cond Res* 14(1):5.

17. Haywood, KM, Getchell, N: 2001. Development of cardiorespiratory endurance. In Haywood, KM (ed), *Learning activities for life span motor development*. 3rd ed, Champaign, IL, Human Kinetics, pp. 181–186; 212–223.

18. Hilbert S, Plisk SS: 1999. Free weights versus machines, *Streng Cond J* 21(6):66.

19. Holcomb WR: 2000. Improved stretching with proprioceptive neuromuscular facilitation, *Streng Cond J* 22(1):59.

20. Karvonen MJ, Kentala E, Mustala O: 1957. The effects of training on heart rate: a longitudinal study, *Ann Med Exp Biol* 35:305.

21. Klinger, T. McConnell, T. Gardner, J. 2001. Prescribing target heart rates without the use of a graded exercise test, *Clinical exercise physiology* 3(4):207–212.

22. Knight, KL, Ingersoll, CD, Bartholomew, J: 2001. Isotonic contractions might be more effective than isokinetic contractions in developing muscle strength. *Journal of sport rehabilitation* 10(2), May: 124–131.

23. Kraemer, W, Hakkinen, K, Kraemer W: 2001. *Strength training for sport*, Cambridge, MA, Blackwell Science.

24. Kubukeli, ZN, Noakes, TD, Dennis, SC: 2002. Training techniques to improve endurance exercise performances. *Sports medicine* 32(8), 489–509.

25. Lagally, KM, Robertson, RJ, Gallagher, KI, Gearhart, R, Goss, FL: 2002. Ratings of perceived exertion during low- and high-intensity resistance exercise by young adults. *Perceptual and motor skills* 94(3 Part I), June: 723–731.

26. Laursen, PB, Jenkins, DG: 2002. The scientific basis for high-intensity interval training: optimising training programmes and

maximising performance in highly trained endurance athletes. *Sports medicine* 32(1), 53–73.

27. Leetun, D, Ireland, M, Wilson, J: 2005. Core stability measures as risk factors for lower extremity injury in athletes, *Medicine and science in sports and exercise* 36(6):926–934.

28. Lepretre, P, Koralsztein, J, Billat, V: 2004. Effect of exercise intensity on relationship between VO2max and cardiac output, *Medicine and science in sports and exercise* 36(8): 1357–1363.

29. Mann, D, Whedon, C: 2001. Functional stretching: implementing a dynamic stretching program. *Athletic therapy today* 6(3):10–13.

30. Mannie, K: 2004. Overloading without overtraining, *Coach and athletic director* 74(4):9–12.

31. Marek, S, Cramer, J, Fincher, L: 2005. Acute effects of static and proprioceptive neuromuscular facilitation stretching on muscle strength and power output, *Journal of athletic training* 40(2):94–103.

32. Marshall, P, Murphy, B: 2005. Core stability Exercises on and off a Swiss ball, *Archives of physical medicine and rehabilitation* 86(2): 242–249.

33. Molkin, M: 2004. Warming up, cooling down and stretching: preparing for a workout and recovering afterward deserve a lot more attention than many believe, *Fitness management* 20(2):30–32.

34. Radcliffe JC, Farentinos RC: 2001. *High-powered plyometrics*, Champaign, IL, Human Kinetics.

35. Schilling BK, Stone MH: 2000. Stretching: acute effects on strength and power performance, *Streng Cond J* 22(1):44.

36. Swain, D, Parrott, J, Bennett, A: 2004. Validation of a new method for estimating VO2max based on VO2 reserve, *Medicine and science in sports and exercise* 36(8): 1421–1426.

37. Swanson, J: 2004. Periodization for the multisport athlete, *Strength and conditioning journal* 26(4): 50–58.

38. Thacker, S, Gilchrist, J, Stroup, D: 2004. The impact of stretching on sports injury risk: a systematic review of the literature, *Medicine and science in sports and exercise* 36(3):371–378.

39. Young, W, Elliott, S: 2001. Acute effects of static stretching, proprioceptive neuromuscular facilitation stretching, and maximum voluntary contractions on explosive force production and jumping performance. *Research quarterly for exercise and sport* 72(3), Sept: 273–279.

40. Zentz C: 2000. Warm up to perform up, *Ath Ther Today* 5(2):59.

## ANNOTATED BIBLIOGRAPHY

Alter J: 2004. *The science of flexibility,* Champaign, IL, Human Kinetics.

*This text explains the principles and techniques of stretching and details the anatomy and physiology of muscle and connective tissue. It includes guidelines for developing a flexibility program and illustrated stretching exercises and warm-up drills.*

Anderson B: 2000. *Stretching,* Bolinas, Calif, Shelter.

*An extremely comprehensive best-selling text on stretching exercises for the entire body.*

Baechle T, Earle, R: 2008. *Essentials of strength training and conditioning,* Champaign, IL, Human Kinetics.

*Explains the various concepts of exercise, identifies correct lifting techniques, corrects common weight-training errors, and lists personal goals for weight training.*

Bishop, J: 2004. *Fitness through aerobics,* Philadelphia, Benjaman Cummings.

*This text uses the most up-to-date fitness and wellness information on aerobic dance exercise.*

Brooks G, Baldwin, K, Fahey T: 2004. *Exercise physiology: human bioenergetics and its applications,* 4th ed. Mountain View, Calif, Mayfield.

*An up-to-date advanced text in exercise physiology that contains a comprehensive listing of the most current journal articles relative to exercise physiology.*

Fleck, S. Kraemer, W: 2003. *Designing resistance training programs,* Champaign, IL, Human Kinetics.

*A clear, readable, state-of-the-art guide to developing individualized training programs for both athletes and fitness enthusiasts.*

Moran, G, McGlynn, G: 2000. *Dynamics of strength training,* St. Louis, McGraw-Hill.

*Provides a comprehensive resource using an individualized approach to strength training, including conditioning and cardiorespiratory fitness. Emphasizes the physiological basis of muscle strength and endurance. Illustrates the most efficient and effective training techniques.*

Radcliffe, J, Farentinos, R: 2001. *High powered plyometrics,* Champaign IL, Human Kinetics

*Detailing plyometric exercises for a variety of sports, this guide explains how plyometrics work and how to incorporate plyometrics into a comprehensive strength and power-training program.*

Verstegen, M, Williams, P: 2005. *Core performance: the revolutionary workout program to transform your body and your life,* Mountain View, CA, Rodale Press.

*This text concentrates primarily on core stabilization exercises to improve posture and improve performance in athletes.*

## WEB SITES

Fitness World: www.fitnessworld.com
*Presents information about fitness in general and includes access to Fitness Management magazine.*

National Academy of Sports Medicine: www.nasm.org

National Strength and Conditioning Association: www.nsca.com
*This organization distributes a wealth of information relative to strength training and conditioning.*

Stretching and Flexibility: Everything you never wanted to know: www.cmcrossroads.com/bradapp/docs/rec/stretching/
*Prepared by Brad Appleton, detailed information on stretching and stretching techniques is presented, including normal ranges of motion, flexibility, how to stretch, the physiology of stretching, and the types of stretching including PNF.*

# Sports Nutrition and Supplements

## CHAPTER 5

*When you finish this chapter you will be able to:*

- Identify the six classes of nutrients and describe their major functions.
- Explain the importance of good nutrition in enhancing performance and preventing injuries.
- Describe the advantages or disadvantages of dietary supplementation in the athlete's diet.
- Discuss common eating and drinking practices in the athletic population.
- Explain the distinction between body weight and body composition.
- Explain the principle of caloric balance and how to assess it.
- Describe methods for losing and gaining weight.
- List the signs of disordered eating.

The relation of nutrition, diet, and weight control to overall health and fitness is an important aspect of any training and conditioning program for an athlete.[33] Athletes who practice sound nutritional habits reduce the likelihood of injury by maintaining a higher standard of healthful living.[8] Eating a well-balanced diet can positively contribute to the development of strength, flexibility, and cardiorespiratory endurance.[6] Unfortunately, misconceptions, fads, and, in many cases, superstitions regarding nutrition affect dietary habits, particularly in the athletic population.[8]

Many athletes associate successful performance with the consumption of special foods or supplements.[15] An athlete who is performing well may be reluctant to change dietary habits regardless of whether the diet is physiologically beneficial to overall health. The psychological aspect of allowing the athlete to eat whatever he or she is most comfortable with can greatly affect performance. The problem is that these eating habits tend to become accepted as beneficial and may become traditional when in fact they may be physiologically detrimental to athletic performance. Thus, many nutrition "experts" may disseminate nutritional information based on traditional rather than experimental information.

Although this chapter provides information on basic nutrition, the focus is on how this information relates specifically to the athlete. Despite the fact that there are great differences in what individual athletes like to eat, it is also true that there are many different ways that athletes can obtain the nutrients they need. However, athletes who

Organizing and Establishing
an Effective Athletic Health
Care System

Six classes of nutrients:
• CHO
• fats
• proteins
• vitamins
• minerals
• water

engage in poor nutritional practices and habits are not doing everything possible to optimize their performance.[33]

## THE NUTRIENTS

People usually think of losing weight when they hear the word *diet.* Actually, diet refers to a person's usual food selections. What people choose to eat is their diet. Although people have different food likes and dislikes, everyone must eat to survive. Nutrition is the science of certain food substances, *nutrients,* and what they do in the body.[42] Nutrients perform three major roles:[37]

1. Grow, repair, and maintain all body cells
2. Regulate body processes
3. Supply energy for cells

The various nutrients are categorized into six major classes: *carbohydrates, fats* (often called *lipids*), *proteins, water, vitamins,* and *minerals.* Carbohydrates, proteins, and fats are referred to as the *macronutrients:* the absorbable components of food, from which energy is derived. Vitamins, minerals, and water are considered to be *micronutrients,* which are necessary for normal body functions. They do not provide energy, but without sufficient quantities of micronutrients, the energy from the macronutrients cannot be utilized. Most foods are actually mixtures of these nutrients. Some nutrients can be made by the body, but an *essential nutrient* must be supplied by the diet. Not all substances in food are considered nutrients. There is no such thing as the perfect food; that is, no single natural food contains all of the nutrients needed for health. A summary of current percentages and recommended percentages of calories from carbohydrates, fats, and proteins is shown in Figure 5-1.

It is recommended that the majority, about 55 to 60 percent, of the calories consumed be in the form of carbohydrates. Fat should account for

**Figure 5-1**

Comparison of calories from carbohydrates, fats, and proteins

Source: Wardlaw G. *Perspectives in Nutrition,* St. Louis, 1996, Mosby.

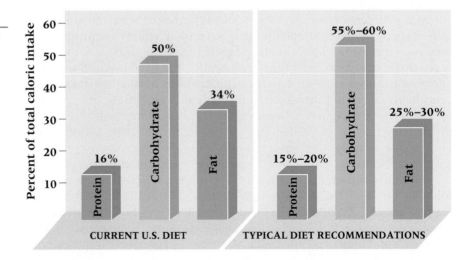

between 25 and 30 percent of the total caloric intake. Only 15 to 20 percent of the caloric intake should be protein. For an athlete who requires additional energy during the course of a day, the extra calories consumed should be in the form of carbohydrates.

## Carbohydrates (CHO)

Athletes have increased energy needs. *Carbohydrates* are the body's most efficient source of energy and should be relied on to fill that need.[14] Carbohydrates should account for at least 55 percent or more of total caloric intake and some recommendations go as high as 60 percent. Carbohydrates may be considered either simple or complex based upon their chemical structure. Both simple and complex carbohydrates can be digested and converted into blood glucose. *Simple carbohydrates* are digested quickly and contain refined sugars and few essential vitamins and minerals (e.g., fruits, fruit juice, milk, yogurt, honey, sugar). *Complex carbohydrates* take longer to digest and are usually packed with fiber, vitamins, and minerals (e.g., vegetables, breads, cereals, and pasta). It is recommended that the athlete consume the bulk of their carbohydrate intake in the form of complex carbohydrates and the majority of the simple carbohydrate intake should come from fruits and milk or yogurt, which also contain vitamins and minerals. Foods high in refined sugar content should be avoided since they are usually low in the nutrients we need to maintain health and energy levels. An inadequate intake of dietary carbohydrate causes the body to use protein to make glucose. Therefore a supply of glucose must be kept available to prevent the use of protein for energy.

## Fats

*Fats* are another essential component of the diet. They are the most concentrated source of energy, providing more than twice the calories per gram when compared to carbohydrates or proteins. Fat is used as a primary source of energy. Some dietary fat is needed to make food more flavorful and for sources of the fat-soluble vitamins. Also, a minimal amount of fat is essential for normal growth and development.[42]

In the United States, dietary fat represents a high percentage of the total caloric intake (see Figure 5-1). For many Americans, a substantial amount of the fat is from saturated fatty acids (primarily from animal sources) and from transfatty acids (found in cookies, dairy products, meats and fast food). This intake is believed to be too high and contributes to the prevalence of obesity, certain cancers, and coronary artery disease. The recommended intake should be limited to less than 25 percent of total calories with saturated fat reduced to less than 10 percent of total calories.

## Proteins

*Proteins* make up the major structural components of the body. They are needed for growth, maintenance, and repair of all body tissues. In addition, proteins are needed to make enzymes, many hormones, and

Dietary recommendations:
- CHO 55–60 percent
- fats 25–30 percent
- proteins 15 percent

Carbohydrates are sugars, starches, or fiber.

### 5-1 *Critical Thinking* Exercise

A female softball player has been told that she is slightly overweight and needs to lose a few pounds. The athlete has been watching television and reading about how important it is to limit the dietary intake of fat for losing weight. She has decided to go on a diet that is essentially fat free and is convinced that this diet will help her lose weight.

? What should the coach tell her about avoiding excessive intake of fat as a means of losing weight?

Saturated fat and transfatty acids are harmful forms of fat.

Organizing and Establishing an Effective Athletic Health Care System

5-2 *Critical Thinking*
Exercise

A volleyball player complains that she constantly feels tired and lethargic even though she thinks that she is eating well and getting a sufficient amount of sleep. A teammate has suggested that she begin taking vitamin supplements, which, the teammate claims, will give her more energy and make her more resistant to fatigue. The athlete comes to the sports nutritionist to ask advice about what kind of vitamins she needs to take.

? What facts should the sports nutritionist explain to the athlete about vitamin supplementation, and what recommendations should be made?

The fat-soluble vitamins:
- vitamin A
- vitamin D
- vitamin E
- vitamin K

The water-soluble vitamins:
- vitamin C
- thiamin
- riboflavin
- niacin
- folate
- biotin
- pantothenic acid
- vitamin $B_6$
- vitamin $B_{12}$

antibodies that help fight infection. In general, the body tends not to use much protein for energy; instead it relies on fats and carbohydrates. Protein intake should be around 15 percent of total calories.

The basic units that make up proteins are called *amino acids.* Most of the body's proteins are made up of about twenty different amino acids. The majority of the amino acids can be produced as needed in the body. The others cannot be made to any significant degree and therefore must be supplied by the diet. These are referred to as the *essential* amino acids. A diet that contains large amounts of protein will not support growth, repair, and maintenance of tissues if the essential amino acids are not available in the proper proportions.[29] Most of the proteins from animal foods contain all the essential amino acids that humans require. Examples are the proteins found in meat, fish, poultry, eggs, milk, and other dairy products.

## Vitamins

Although they are required in very small amounts when compared to carbohydrates, fats, proteins, and water, *vitamins* perform essential roles primarily as regulators of body processes. They also play a critical role in tissue healing and repair. Over the years, researchers have identified thirteen vitamins and determined their specific roles in the body.

People mistakenly think that vitamins provide energy. In fact, the body cannot break them down to release energy. Table 5-1 provides information about vitamins, including rich food sources, deficiency symptoms, and toxicity potential from high doses.

Vitamins are classified into two groups: The *fat-soluble vitamins* are dissolved in fats and stored in the body; the *water-soluble vitamins* are dissolved in watery solutions and are not stored. The fat-soluble vitamins that dissolve in fat rather than water are vitamins A, E, D, and K. Extra amounts of the fat-soluble vitamins are not easy to eliminate from the body in urine, which is mostly water. Instead they are stored in the liver or body fat until needed, making them potentially toxic.[41]

The water-soluble vitamins are vitamin C, known as *ascorbic acid,* and the B-complex vitamins, including thiamin, riboflavin, niacin, $B_6$, folate, $B_{12}$, biotin, and pantothenic acid. Vitamin C is used for building bones and teeth, maintaining the tissues that hold muscles and other tissues together (connective tissues), and strengthening the immune system. Unlike fat-soluble vitamins, the water-soluble ones cannot be stored to any significant extent in the body and should be supplied in the diet each day. Excess amounts of water-soluble vitamins are excreted daily in urine.

### Antioxidant Nutrients

Certain nutrients, called antioxidants, may prevent premature aging, certain cancers, heart disease, and other health problems.[31] An antioxidant protects vital cell components from the destructive effects of certain agents, including oxygen. Vitamins C and E and beta carotene are

**TABLE 5-1** Vitamins

| Vitamin | Major Function | Most Reliable Sources | Deficiency | Excess (Toxicity) |
|---|---|---|---|---|
| A | Maintains skin and other cells that line the inside of the body; bone and tooth development; growth; vision in dim light | Liver, milk, egg yolk, deep green and yellow fruits and vegetables | Night blindness, dry skin, growth failure | Headaches, nausea, loss of hair, dry skin, diarrhea |
| D | Normal bone growth and development | Exposure to sunlight; fortified dairy products; eggs and fish liver oils | Rickets in children—defective bone formation leading to deformed bones | Appetite loss, weight loss, failure to grow |
| E | Prevents destruction of polyunsaturated fats caused by exposure to oxidizing agents; protects cell membranes from destruction | Vegetable oils, some in fruits and vegetables, whole grains | Breakage of red blood cells leading to anemia | Nausea and diarrhea; interferes with vitamin K if vitamin D is also deficient. Not as toxic as other fat-soluble vitamins |
| K | Production of blood-clotting substances | Green leafy vegetables; normal bacteria that live in intestines produce K that is absorbed | Increased bleeding time | |
| thiamin | Needed for release of energy from carbohydrates, fats, and proteins | Cereal products, pork, peas, and dried beans | Lack of energy, nerve problems | |
| riboflavin | Energy from carbohydrates, fats, and proteins | Milk, liver, fruits and vegetables, enriched breads and cereals | Dry skin, cracked lips | |
| niacin | Energy from carbohydrates, fats, and proteins | Liver, meat, poultry, peanut butter, legumes, enriched breads and cereals | Skin problems, diarrhea, mental depression, and eventually death (rarely occurs in U.S.) | Skin flushing, intestinal upset, nervousness, intestinal ulcers |
| B₆ | Metabolism of protein; production of hemoglobin | White meats, whole grains, liver, egg yolk, bananas | Poor growth, anemia | Severe loss of coordination from nerve damage |
| B₁₂ | Production of genetic material; maintains central nervous system | Foods of animal origin | Neurological problems, anemia | |
| Folate (folic acid) | Production of genetic material | Wheat germ, liver, yeast, mushrooms, green leafy vegetables, fruits | Anemia | |
| C (ascorbic acid) | Formation and maintenance of connective tissue; tooth and bone formation; immune function | Fruits and vegetables | Scurvy (rare), swollen joints, bleeding gums, fatigue, bruising | Kidney stones, diarrhea |
| Pantothenic acid | Energy from carbohydrates, fats, and proteins | Widely found in foods | Not observed in humans under normal conditions | |
| Biotin | Use of fats | Widely found in foods | Rare under normal conditions | |

antioxidants. Beta carotene is a plant pigment found in dark green, deep yellow, or orange fruits and vegetables. The body can convert beta carotene to vitamin A.[34] In the early 1980s, researchers reported that smokers who ate large quantities of beta carotene–rich fruits and vegetables were less likely to develop lung cancer than were other smokers. Since that time, more evidence is accumulating about the benefits of a diet rich in the antioxidant nutrients.

Some research has indicated that athletes should increase their intake of antioxidants, even if it means taking supplements. Others are more cautious. Excess beta carotene pigments circulate throughout the body and may turn the skin yellow. However, the pigment is not believed to be toxic like its nutrient cousin, vitamin A. On the other hand, increasing intake of vitamins C and E is not without some risk.[31] Excesses of vitamin C are not well absorbed; the excess is irritating to the intestines and creates diarrhea. Although less toxic than vitamins A or D, too much vitamin E causes health problems.

## Minerals

The antioxidants:
- vitamin C
- vitamin E
- beta carotene

More than twenty *mineral* elements need to be supplied by the diet.[15] Some of these minerals are listed in Table 5-2. Other mineral elements are found in the body. The role of minerals is unclear. Minerals are needed for a variety of jobs such as forming strong bones and teeth, generating energy, activating enzymes, and maintaining water balance. Most minerals are stored in the body, especially in the bones and liver. Although each of these minerals is important in its own way, two minerals, calcium and iron, require special attention and will be discussed later in this chapter.

## Water

Water is the most essential nutrient.[42] A person can live for weeks, months, even years without the other nutrients, but will perish after a few days without water. About 60 percent of the adult's body weight is water. Many materials used in the body are water soluble, that is, dissolved in water. Although water does not supply any calories, an adequate supply of water is needed for energy production. Water also takes part in digestion and maintaining the proper environment inside and outside of cells. When the body burns fuels for energy, it produces a great deal of heat energy. Sweating is how the body uses water to keep itself from overheating.

The average adult requires a minimum of 2.5 liters of water or about ten glasses of water a day.[42] Because water is so vital, the healthy body carefully manages its internal water levels. When body water weight drops by 1 to 2 percent, you begin to feel thirsty. Drinking water causes the internal water levels to return to normal. If thirst signals are ignored and body water continues to decrease, *dehydration* results and heat-related illnesses can result (see Chapter 10). People who are dehydrated cannot generate enough energy and feel weak. Other symptoms include nausea, vomiting, and fainting.

**TABLE 5-2** Major minerals

| Mineral | Major Role | Most Reliable Sources | Deficiency | Excess |
|---|---|---|---|---|
| Calcium | Bone and tooth formation; blood clotting; muscle contraction; nerve function | Dairy products | May lead to osteoporosis | Calcium deposits in soft tissues |
| Phosphorus | Skeletal development; tooth formation | Meats, dairy products, and other protein-rich foods | Rarely seen | |
| Sodium | Maintenance of fluid balance | Salt (sodium chloride) added to foods and sodium-containing preservatives | | May contribute to the development of hypertension |
| Iron | Formation of hemoglobin; energy from carbohydrates, fats, and proteins | Liver and red meats, enriched breads and cereals | Iron-deficiency anemia | Can cause death in children from supplement overdose |
| Copper | Formation of hemoglobin | Liver, nuts, shellfish, cherries, mushrooms, whole grain breads and cereals | Anemia | Nausea and vomiting |
| Zinc | Normal growth and development | Seafood and meats | Skin problems, delayed development, growth problems | Interferes with copper use; may decrease HDL levels |
| Magnesium | Strengthens bones; improves enzyme function and nerve and heart function | Wheat germ, vegetables, nuts, chocolate | Weakness, muscle pain, poor heart function, osteoporosis | Kidney failure |
| Iodine | Production of the hormone thyroxin | Iodized salt, seafood | Mental and growth retardation; lack of energy | |
| Fluorine | Strengthens bones and teeth | Fluoridated water | Teeth are less resistant to decay | Damage to tooth enamel |

Replacing fluid after heavy
sweating is equally as
important as replacing
electrolytes.

Dehydration is more likely to occur when you are outdoors, and sweating heavily while engaging in some strenuous activity. To prevent dehydration make sure to replace the lost water by drinking plenty of fluids. Don't rely on thirst as a signal that it's time to have a drink. By the time thirst develops the body is already slightly dehydrated. Many people ignore their thirst, or if they do heed it, they don't drink enough. Most people replace only about 50 percent of the water they lose through sweating.[25] It is recommended that athletes drink frequently throughout the day, perhaps even carrying a water bottle with them all the time to minimize the chances of dehydration. An athlete should consume fluids before, during, and after practice or competition. Fluids should be either water or sports drinks, which will be discussed in Chapter 10.

### Electrolyte Requirements

Electrolytes: sodium,
chloride, potassium,
magnesium, and calcium

Electrolytes, including sodium, chloride, potassium, magnesium, and calcium, are electrically charged ions in solution. They maintain the balance of water outside the cell. Electrolyte replenishment may be needed when a person is not fit, suffers from extreme water loss, participates in a marathon, or has just completed an exercise period and is expected to perform at near-maximum effort within the next few hours. In most cases, electrolytes can be sufficiently replaced with a balanced diet. Free access to water (ad libitum) before, during, and after activity should be the rule. Electrolyte losses are primarily responsible for muscle cramping and intolerance to heat. Sweating results not only in a body water loss but in some electrolyte loss as well.[28]

## THE PRODUCTION OF ENERGY FROM FOODSTUFFS

Energy is produced when cells break down CHO, fats, or proteins to release energy stored in these compounds. As can be seen in Figure 5-2, carbohydrates provide the major proportion of energy for short-term, high-intensity muscular contractions. As the duration and the intensity of the activity increases, breathing also increases, supplying more oxygen for the cells and maximizing energy production. When the activity is prolonged, such as in an endurance sport, the percentage of fat and carbohydrate used for fuel is similar. Under usual conditions, proteins supply less than about 5 percent of energy. However, athletes engaged in endurance activities receive as much as 10 to 15 percent of their energy needs from protein.[29]

## WHAT IS A NUTRITIOUS DIET?

### MyPyramid*

The USDA's new MyPyramid, introduced in 2005, replaces the Food Guide Pyramid developed in 1992 and is part of an overall food guidance system that emphasizes the need for a more individualized approach to

---

* Modified from United States Department of Agriculture Web site www.mypyramid.gov

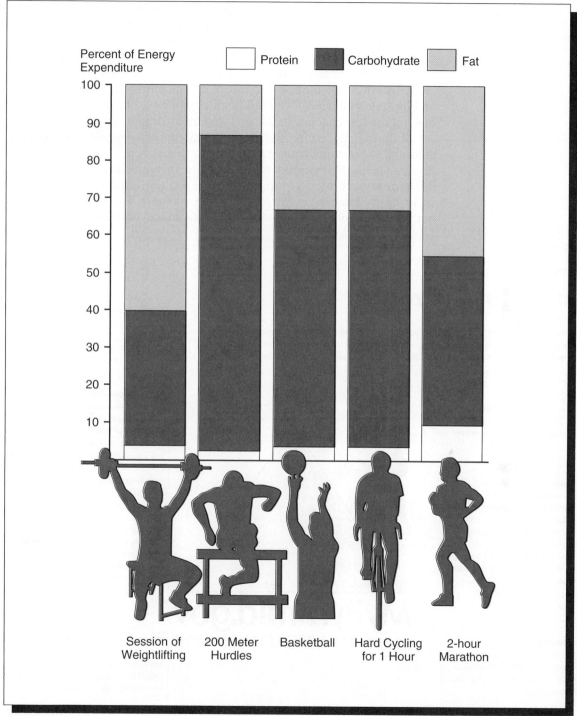

**Figure 5-2**

**The Relative Proportions of CHO, FAT, and Protein Fuels Used for Physical Activity**

improving diet and lifestyle. It allows individuals to personalize their approach when choosing a healthier lifestyle that balances nutrition and exercise. MyPyramid incorporates recommendations from the *2005 Dietary Guidelines for Americans,* and was developed to carry the messages of the dietary guidelines and to make Americans aware of the vital health benefits of simple and modest improvements in nutrition, physical activity, and lifestyle behavior.[46] Overall health can be significantly improved by making modest changes in the diet and by incorporating regular physical activity into daily living. MyPyramid's daily food intake patterns identify amounts to consume from each food group and subgroup at a variety of energy levels. MyPyramid represents the recommended proportion of foods from each food group and focuses on the importance of making smart food choices in every food group, every day. The MyPyramid symbol is meant to encourage consumers to make healthier food choices

**Figure 5-3**

MyPyramid

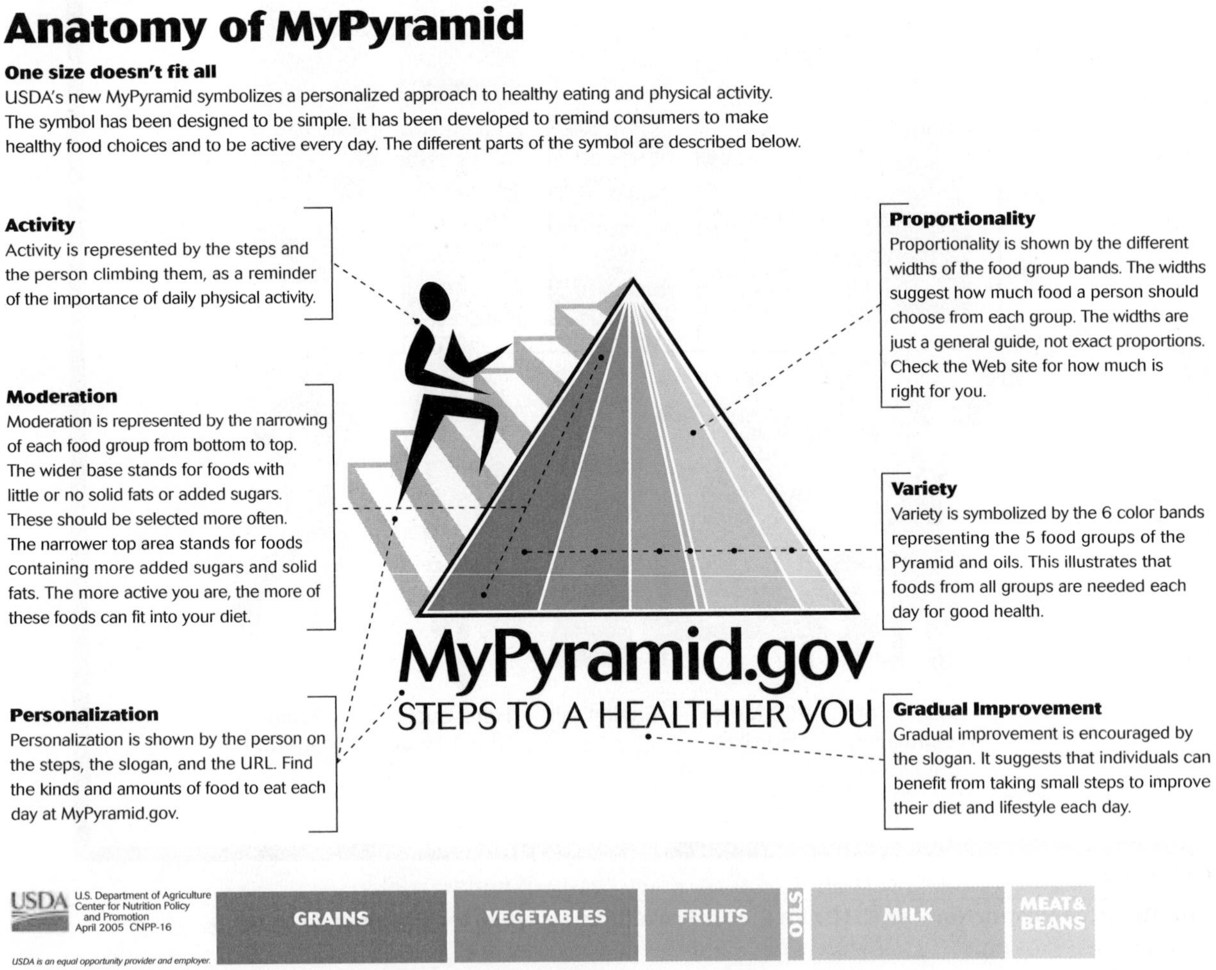

# Anatomy of MyPyramid

**One size doesn't fit all**

USDA's new MyPyramid symbolizes a personalized approach to healthy eating and physical activity. The symbol has been designed to be simple. It has been developed to remind consumers to make healthy food choices and to be active every day. The different parts of the symbol are described below.

**Activity**
Activity is represented by the steps and the person climbing them, as a reminder of the importance of daily physical activity.

**Moderation**
Moderation is represented by the narrowing of each food group from bottom to top. The wider base stands for foods with little or no solid fats or added sugars. These should be selected more often. The narrower top area stands for foods containing more added sugars and solid fats. The more active you are, the more of these foods can fit into your diet.

**Personalization**
Personalization is shown by the person on the steps, the slogan, and the URL. Find the kinds and amounts of food to eat each day at MyPyramid.gov.

**Proportionality**
Proportionality is shown by the different widths of the food group bands. The widths suggest how much food a person should choose from each group. The widths are just a general guide, not exact proportions. Check the Web site for how much is right for you.

**Variety**
Variety is symbolized by the 6 color bands representing the 5 food groups of the Pyramid and oils. This illustrates that foods from all groups are needed each day for good health.

**Gradual Improvement**
Gradual improvement is encouraged by the slogan. It suggests that individuals can benefit from taking small steps to improve their diet and lifestyle each day.

# MyPyramid.gov
## STEPS TO A HEALTHIER YOU

USDA  U.S. Department of Agriculture
Center for Nutrition Policy and Promotion
April 2005 CNPP-16

*USDA is an equal opportunity provider and employer.*

GRAINS  VEGETABLES  FRUITS  OILS  MILK  MEAT & BEANS

and to be active every day (Figure 5-3). The MyPyramid symbol illustrates these goals:

*Gradual improvement,* encouraged by the slogan, "Steps to a Healthier You." It suggests that individuals can benefit from taking small steps to improve their diet and lifestyle each day.

*Physical activity,* represented by the steps and the person climbing them, as a reminder of the importance of daily physical activity.

*Variety,* symbolized by the six color bands representing the five food groups of MyPyramid and oils. Foods from all groups are needed each day for good health.

*Moderation,* represented by the narrowing of each food group from bottom to top. The wider base stands for foods with little or no solid fats, added sugars, or caloric sweeteners. These should be selected more often to get the most nutrition from calories consumed.

*Proportionality,* shown by the different widths of the food group bands. The widths suggest how much food a person should choose from each group. The widths are just a general guide, not exact proportions.

## Nutrient Dense Foods versus Junk Foods

Foods that contain considerable amounts of vitamins, minerals, and proteins in relation to their caloric content are referred to as being *nutrient dense.* Candy, chips, doughnuts, cakes, and cookies are often referred to as junk foods. These foods are not nutrient dense because they provide too many calories from fats and sugars in relation to vitamins and minerals. If an athlete's overall diet is nutritious, and he or she can afford the extra calories, it's okay to eat occasional fatty or sugary foods. However, many people who live on diets that are rich in these kinds of foods displace more nutritious food items in their diets. This behavior is not a healthy one to practice in the long run.[36]

*Nutrient-dense foods supply adequate amounts of vitamins and minerals in relation to caloric value.*

## DIETARY SUPPLEMENTS

### Myths and Misconceptions

Athletes often believe that exercise increases requirements for nutrients such as proteins, vitamins, and minerals and that it is possible and desirable to saturate the body with these nutrients.[26] **There is no scientific basis for ingesting levels of these nutrients above the Dietary Reference Intake (DRI) levels.**[24] Exercise increases the need for energy, not for proteins, vitamins, and minerals.[29] Thus it is necessary to explore some of the more common myths that surround the subject of using dietary supplements to enhance physical performance.[18]

There are probably more myths associated with the contribution of dietary supplements to successful athletic performance than with any other related topic of concern for your athlete. Many popular books and magazine articles about the topic give advice for using dietary supplements designed to enhance performance.[3] Unfortunately, more

*Vitamin requirements do not increase during exercise.*

*DRI helps consumers compare nutritional values of foods.*

Supplements are not
regulated by any government
agency.

unreliable sources of nutrition information are available to the consumer than reliable, fact-filled ones. There is no doubt that if an athlete really believes that some nutritional powder, pill, or drink is the key to success, he or she may be successful. Often the belief that an item will have an effect can actually induce the desired effect, even though the item itself really does not have an effect. This is known as the placebo effect, which can be very powerful. The supplement provides a psychological boost. In many cases no harm is done. However, many people spend considerable amounts of money on such worthless supplements, and the use of some products can actually harm the body.[35] Perhaps the most significant dilemma with dietary supplements is that there is currently no premarket approval or any postmarket surveillance of these products by any regulating agency. **The burden of proof of safety or harm of supplements falls on the Food and Drug Administration (FDA). With the exception of ephedrine, the FDA has not acted to support or ban the use of any supplement.**

Before discussing supplementation, it should be emphatically stated that with the exception of a licensed nutritionist or a physician, **no fitness professional or coach should provide or distribute nutritional supplements of any kind to an athlete.**[2] To do so may be in violation of the laws and statutes in a particular state, and may also be in violation of the rules of national and state sport governing bodies such as the NCAA.

### Vitamin Supplements

Many athletes believe that taking large amounts of vitamin supplements can lead to superior health and performance.[11] A megadose of a nutrient supplement is essentially an overdose; the amount ingested far exceeds the DRI levels. The rationale used for such excessive intakes is that if a pill that contains the DRI for each vitamin and mineral makes an athlete healthy, then taking a pill that has ten times the DRI should make that athlete ten times healthier. There is no truth to this kind of logic. For an athlete eating a balanced diet, vitamin supplementation is probably not really necessary. However, if the athlete is not consuming a good diet, supplementation with a multiple vitamin can be beneficial. Supplementing with excessive amounts of fat-soluble vitamins can produce toxic effects.

### Mineral Supplements

Obtaining adequate levels of certain minerals can be a problem for some athletes. Calcium and iron intakes may be low for athletes whose diets do not include dairy products, red meats, or enriched breads and cereals. However, athletes must first determine whether they need extra minerals to prevent wasting their money and overdosing. The following sections explore some of the minerals that can be low in the diet and some suggestions for improving the quality of the diet so that supplements may not be necessary.

### Calcium Supplements

Calcium is the most abundant mineral in the body. It is essential for bones and teeth and for muscle contraction and conduction of nerve impulses. If calcium intake is too low to meet needs, the body can remove calcium from the bones. Over time, the bones become weakened and appear porous on x-ray films. These bones are brittle and often break spontaneously. This condition is called **osteoporosis** and is estimated to be eight times more common among women than men. Osteoporosis becomes a serious problem for women after menopause.[16]

**osteoporosis**
A decrease in bone density.

Exercise causes calcium to be retained in bones, so physical activity is beneficial. However, younger females who exercise to extremes so that their normal hormonal balance is upset are prone to develop premature osteoporosis. For females who have a family history of osteoporosis, calcium supplementation, preferably as calcium carbonate or citrate rather than phosphate, may be advisable.[32]

Milk products are the most reliable sources of calcium. Many athletes dislike milk or complain that it upsets their stomach. Those athletes may lack an enzyme called *lactase* that is needed to digest milk sugar, lactose. This condition is referred to as lactose intolerance, or **lactase deficiency.** The undigested lactose enters the large intestine, where the bacteria that normally reside there use it for energy. The bacteria produce large quantities of intestinal gas, which causes discomfort and cramps. Many lactose-intolerant people also suffer from diarrhea. Fortunately, scientists have produced the missing enzyme, lactase. Lactase is available without prescription in forms that can be added to foods before eating or taken along with meals.

**lactase deficiency**
Difficulty digesting dairy products.

### Iron Supplements

Iron deficiency is also a common problem, especially for young females. Lack of iron can result in iron-deficiency **anemia.**[17] Iron is needed to properly form hemoglobin. In anemia, the oxygen-carrying ability of the red blood cells is reduced so that muscles cannot obtain enough oxygen to generate energy. An anemic person feels tired and weak. Obviously, athletes cannot compete at their peak level while suffering from an iron deficiency.

**anemia**
Lack of iron.

## Protein Supplements

Athletes often believe that more protein is needed to build bigger muscles. It is true that a relatively small amount of protein is needed for developing muscles in a training program. Many athletes, particularly those who are weight training heavily or body builders, routinely take commercially produced protein supplements. To build muscle, athletes should consume 1 to 1.5 grams of extra protein per kilogram (0.5 to 0.7 grams per pound) of body weight every day.[27] This range goes from slightly above to about double the protein DRI (0.8 grams per kilogram of desirable body weight). Anyone eating a variety of foods, but especially protein-rich foods, can easily meet the higher amounts. Thus protein supplements are not needed for athletes because their diets typically exceed even the most generous protein recommendations.[22]

## Creatine Supplements

Creatine is a naturally occurring organic compound synthesized by the kidneys, liver, and pancreas, 95 percent of which is found in skeletal muscle. The body acquires the creatine it needs mainly from the ingestion of meat and fish. The important role of creatine is in energy metabolism and the contraction of skeletal muscle. With creatine supplementation, depletion is delayed and performance is enhanced through the maintenance of the normal metabolic pathways. There are several problems with supplementing the human body with any of the creatine forms, and specifically creatine monohydrate, including weight gain, occasional muscle cramping, gastrointestinal disturbances, and renal dysfunction. However, there are currently no other known long-term side effects.[38]

The positive physiological effects of creatine include allowing for increased intensity in a workout, prolonging maximal effort and improving exercise recovery time during maximal intensity activities, stimulating protein synthesis, decreasing total cholesterol, and increasing fat-free mass.[21] Oral supplementation with creatine may enhance muscular performance during high-intensity resistance exercise.

In August 2000 the NCAA Committee on Competitive Safeguards and Medical Aspects of Sports banned the distribution to student athletes of all muscle-building substances, including creatine, by NCAA member institutions. The use of creatine itself is not banned by the FDA. It is still being widely used by non-NCAA athletes at all levels and thus warrants discussion.

## Herbal Supplements

The use of herbs as natural alternatives to drugs and medicines has clearly become a trend among American consumers.[23] Despite a lack of evidence to support the use of herbs in the professional literature, their use is widespread among the general population and especially in the athletic population. Thus, a discussion of the most commonly used herbs is necessary. Most herbs, as edible plants, are safe to take as foods, and they are claimed to have few side effects as natural medicines, although occasionally a mild allergy-type reaction may occur. In some cases the use of herbal supplements has resulted in death.

Nutritionally, herbs can offer the body nutrients that are reported to nourish the brain and glands and aid hormone production. Unlike vitamins, which work best when taken with food, it is not necessary to take herbs with other foods.[23]

Herbs in their whole form are not drugs. As medicines, herbs are essentially body balancers that work with the body functions to help the body heal and regulate itself. Herbal formulas can be general for overall strength and nutrient support, or specific to a particular ailment or condition.

Hundreds of herbs are widely available today at all quality levels. They are readily available at health-food stores. However, unlike both food and medicine, there are no federal or governmental controls to regulate the sale and ensure the quality of the products being sold. Thus the consumer of herbal products must exercise extreme caution.

Focus Box 5-1 lists the most popular and widely used herbal products sold in health-food stores. Some additional potent and complex herbs, such as capsicum, lobelia, sassafras, mandrake, tansy, canada snake root, wormwood, woodruff, poke root, and rue may be useful in small amounts and as catalysts, but should not be used alone.

---

**5-1 ⟩ Focus Box**

---

**Most Widely Used Herbs and Purposes for Use**

*cascara*—used as a laxative, can cause dehydration

*cayenne*—used for weight loss

*dong quai*—to treat menstrual symptoms

*echinacea*—to promote wound healing and strengthen the immune system

*feverfew*—to prevent and relieve migraine headaches, arthritis, and PMS

*garlic*—as an antibiotic, antibacterial, antifungal agent to prevent and relieve coronary artery disease by reducing total blood cholesterol and triglyceride levels and raising HDL levels

*garcina cambagia*—used to promote loss of fat

*ginkgo biloba*—to improve blood circulation, especially in the brain

*ginseng*—to reduce impotence, weakness, lethargy, and fatigue

*guarana**—used as a stimulant, contains large amounts of caffeine, often in weight loss products

*kava*—to reduce anxiety, relax muscle tension, produce analgesic effects, act as a local anesthetic, provide antibacterial benefit

*ma huang (ephedrine)**—derived from the ephedra plant, it has been used in China for medicinal purposes including increased energy, appetite suppression, increased fat burning, and preservation of muscle tissue from breaking down. It is a central nervous system stimulant drug which was used in many diet pills. In 1995, the FDA revealed adverse reactions to ephedrine such as heart attacks, strokes, paranoid psychosis, vomiting, fever, palpitations, convulsions, and comas. In 2003 it was banned by the FDA.

*mate*—CNS stimulant

*saw palmetto*—to treat inflamed prostate; also used as a diuretic and as a sexual enhancement agent

*senna*—used as a laxative, can cause water and electrolyte loss

*St. John's wort*—used as an antidepressant; also used to treat nervous disorders, depression, neuralgia, kidney problems, wounds, and burns

*valerian*—to treat insomnia, anxiety, stress

*yohimbe*—to increase libido and blood flow to sexual organs in the male

---

* Banned by some athletic organizations and/or the FDA.

### Ephedrine

Ephedrine is a stimulant that is used as an ingredient in diet pills, illegal recreational drugs, and legitimate over-the-counter medications to treat congestion and asthma.[24] Ephedrine is similar to amphetamine. For several years, the FDA has warned consumers about the potential dangers of using ephedrine. In recent years both the NCAA and minor league baseball have banned the use of ephedrine by their athletes. In December 2003, the FDA banned the use of ephedrine as a dietary supplement. Some companies continue to sell dietary supplements that contain ephedrine and other stimulants. Despite the fact that these ephedrine diet supplements have caused numerous problems, some may still be on the market. Ephedrine can produce the following adverse reactions: heart attack, stroke, tachycardia, paranoid psychosis, depression, convulsions, coma, fever, vomiting, palpitations, hypertension, and respiratory depression.

## Glucose Supplements

Ingesting large quantities of glucose in the form of honey, candy bars, or pure sugar immediately before physical activity has a significant impact on performance. As carbohydrates are digested, large quantities of glucose enter the blood. This increase in blood sugar (glucose) levels stimulates the release of the hormone insulin. Insulin allows the cells to use the circulating glucose so that blood glucose levels soon return to normal. It was hypothesized that this decline in blood sugar levels was detrimental to performance and endurance. However, recent evidence indicates the effect of eating large quantities of carbohydrates is beneficial rather than negative.[14]

Nevertheless, some athletes are sensitive to high carbohydrate feedings and experience problems with increased levels of insulin. Also, some athletes cannot tolerate large amounts of the simple sugar fructose. For these individuals, too much fructose leads to intestinal upset and diarrhea. Athletes should test themselves with various high-carbohydrate foods to see if they are affected, but they should not try this test before a competitive event.[42]

## POPULAR EATING AND DRINKING PRACTICES

### Caffeine Consumption

Caffeine is a central nervous system stimulant. Most people who consume caffeine in coffee, tea, or carbonated beverages are aware of its effect of increasing alertness and decreasing fatigue. Chocolate contains compounds that are related to caffeine and have the same stimulating effects. However, large amounts of caffeine cause nervousness, irritability, increased heart rate, and headaches. Also, headaches are a withdrawal symptom experienced when a person tries to stop consuming caffeinated products.

Although small amounts of caffeine do not appear to harm physical performance, cases of nausea and lightheadedness have been reported.

Caffeine may enhance the use of fat during endurance exercise, thus delaying the depletion of glycogen stores, which would help endurance performance. Caffeine also appears to help make calcium more available to the muscle during contraction, which helps the muscle work more efficiently. However, Olympic officials rightfully consider caffeine to be a drug. It should not be present in an Olympic competitor's blood in levels greater than that resulting from drinking five or six cups of coffee.

## Alcohol Consumption

Alcohol provides energy for the body; each gram of pure alcohol (ethanol) supplies 7 calories. However, sources of alcohol provide very little other nutritional value in regard to vitamins, minerals, and proteins. The depressant effects of alcohol on the central nervous system include decreased physical coordination, slowed reaction times, and decreased mental alertness. Also, this drug increases the production of urine, resulting in body water losses (diuretic effect). Therefore use of alcoholic beverages by the athlete cannot be recommended before, during, or after physical activity.

## Eating Organic, Natural, and Health Foods

Many athletes are concerned about the quality of the foods they eat—not just the nutritional value of the food but also its safety. *Organic* refers to the way farmers grow and process fruits, vegetables, grains, meat, poultry, eggs, and dairy products, according to U.S. Department of Agriculture's organic standards. Chemical fertilizers and insecticides are not used in organic farming. There is significant disagreement as to whether foods grown under organic standards have any nutrional advantage over foods grown by conventional methods. A few studies have shown that while organic foods have more minerals and antioxidants, the amount is insignificant.[10] In comparing data, the British Nutrition Foundation (BNF) found no differences in the products' nutritional profiles with some minor exceptions, suggesting that conventionally grown products are just as nutritious as organic foods.[12] The USDA suggested that organic foods do not have more taste, are not more nutritious, and are not safer than nonorganic products.[20] Nevertheless, for some, the psychological benefit of believing that they are doing something "good" for their bodies justifies the extra cost.

Natural foods have been subjected to very little processing and contain no additives such as preservatives or artificial flavors. Processing can protect nutritional value. Preservatives save food that would otherwise spoil and have to be destroyed. Furthermore, many foods in their natural form are quite poisonous. The green layer often found under the skin of potatoes is poisonous if eaten in large amounts. There are poisonous mushrooms, and molds in peanuts can cause liver cancer.

Both organic and natural foods could be described as health foods. However, no benefit is derived from eating a diet consisting of health foods, even for the athlete.

## Vegetarianism

Many athletes are health conscious and try to do things that are good for their bodies. *Vegetarianism* has emerged as an alternative to the usual American diet. All vegetarians use plant foods to form the foundation of their diet; animal foods are either totally excluded or included in a variety of eating patterns. Athletes who choose to become vegetarians do so for economic, philosophical, religious, cultural, or health reasons. Vegetarianism is no longer considered to be a fad if it is practiced intelligently. However, the vegetarian diet may create deficiencies if nutrient needs are not carefully considered. Athletes who follow this eating pattern need to plan their diet carefully so that their calorie needs are met.

## Preevent Nutrition

The importance and content of the preevent meal have been heatedly debated among coaches, athletic trainers, and athletes. Sometimes competitors ignore logical thinking about what they should eat before competition because of the tradition of "rewarding" the athlete for hard work with foods that may hamper performance. The important point is that too often people are concerned primarily with the preevent meal and fail to realize that those nutrients consumed over several days before competition are much more important than what is eaten 3 hours before an event. The purpose of the preevent meal should be to provide the competitor with sufficient nutrient energy and fluids for competition while taking into consideration the digestibility of the food and, most important, the eating preferences of the individual athlete. Figure 5-4 gives examples of preevent meals.

**Figure 5-4**

Sample preevent meals

**MEAL 1**

| | |
|---|---|
| ³/₄ c Orange juice | ³/₄ c Orange juice |
| ¹/₂ c Cereal with 1 tsp sugar | 1–2 Pancakes with: |
| 1 slice whole wheat toast with: |   1 tsp Margarine |
|   1 tsp Margarine |   2 tbsp Syrup |
|   1 tsp Honey or jelly    or | 8 oz Skim or lowfat milk |
| 8 oz Skim or lowfat milk | Water |
| Water | (Approximately 450–500 kcal) |
| (Approximately 450–500 kcal) | |

**MEAL 2**

| | |
|---|---|
| 1 c Vegetable soup | 1 c Spaghetti with tomato sauce and cheese |
| 1 Turkey sandwich with: | ¹/₂ c Sliced pears (canned) on ¹/₄ c cottage cheese |
|   2 Slices bread | 1–2 Slices (Italian) bread with 1–2 tsp margarine |
|   2 oz Turkey (white or dark) | (avoid garlic) |
|   1 oz Cheese slice    or | ¹/₂ c Sherbet |
|   2 tsp Mayonnaise | 1–2 Sugar cookies |
| 8 oz Skim or lowfat milk | 4 oz Skim or lowfat milk |
| Water | Water |
| (Approximately 550–600 kcal) | (Approximately 700 kcal) |

The athlete should be encouraged to be conscious of his or her diet. However, no experimental evidence indicates that performance may be enhanced by altering a diet that is basically sound. A nutritious diet may be achieved in several ways, and the diet that is optimal for one athlete may not be the best for another. In many instances, the individual is the best judge of what he or she should or should not eat in the preevent meal or before exercising. A person's best guide is to eat whatever he or she is most comfortable with.

### Liquid Food Supplements

Liquid food supplements have been recommended as extremely effective preevent meals and are being used by high school, college, university, and professional teams with some indications of success. These supplements supply from 225 to 400 calories per average serving. Athletes who have used these supplements have reported elimination of the usual pregame symptoms of dry mouth, abdominal cramps, leg cramps, nervous defecation, and nausea.

Under ordinary conditions it usually takes approximately 4 hours for a full meal to pass through the stomach and the small intestine. Pregame emotional tension often delays the emptying of the stomach; therefore the undigested food mass remains in the stomach and upper bowel for a prolonged time, even up to or through the actual period of competition, and frequently causes nausea, vomiting, and cramps. This unabsorbed food mass is of no value to the athlete. According to team physicians who have experimented with the liquid food supplements, one of their major advantages is that they clear both the stomach and the upper bowel before game time, thus making available the caloric energy that would otherwise still be in an unassimilated state. There is merit in the use of such food supplements for pregame meals.

## Eating Fast Foods

Eating fast food is a way of life in American society. Athletes, especially young athletes, have for the most part grown up as fast-food junkies. Furthermore, travel budgets and tight schedules dictate that fast food is a frequent choice for coaches on road trips. Aside from occasional problems with food flavor, the biggest concern in consuming fast foods is that 40 to 50 percent of the calories consumed are from fats. To compound this problem, fast food is typically sold in large portions maximizing fat, salt, and calories in a single sitting.

On the positive side, fast-food restaurants have broadened their menus to include whole wheat breads and rolls, salad bars, and low-fat milk products. Many of the larger fast-food restaurants provide nutritional information for consumers upon request or from well-stocked racks. Focus Box 5-2: "Tips for Selecting Fast Foods" provides suggestions for eating more healthfully at fast-food restaurants.

**Tips for Selecting Fast Foods**

- Limit deep-fried foods such as fish and chicken sandwiches and chicken nuggets, which are often higher in fat than plain burgers are. If you are having fried chicken, remove some of the breading before eating.

- Order roast beef, turkey, or grilled chicken, where available, for a lower fat alternative to most burgers.

- Choose a small order of fries with your meal rather than a large one, and request no salt. Add a small amount of salt yourself if desired. If you are ordering a deep-fat-fried sandwich or one that is made with cheese and sauce, skip the fries altogether and try a plain baked potato (add butter and salt sparingly) or a dinner roll instead of a biscuit; or, try a side salad to accompany your meal instead.

- Choose regular sandwiches instead of "double," "jumbo," "deluxe," or "ultimate." And order plain types rather than those with the works, such as cheese, bacon, mayonnaise, and special sauce. Pickles, mustard, ketchup, and other condiments are high in sodium. Choose lettuce, tomatoes, and onions.

- At the salad bar, load up on fresh greens, fruits, and vegetables. Be careful of salad dressings, added toppings, and creamy salads (potato salad, macaroni salad, coleslaw). These can quickly push calories and fat to the level of other menu items or higher.

- Many fast-food items contain large amounts of sodium from salt and other ingredients. Try to balance the rest of your day's sodium choices after a fast-food meal.

- Alternate water, low-fat milk, or skim milk with a soda or a shake.

- For dessert, or a sweet-on-the-run, choose low-fat frozen yogurt where available.

- Remember to balance your fast-food choices with your food selections for the whole day.

## Low-Carbohydrate Diets

For many years it was recommended that fat intake be limited as a means of controlling weight. Recently the recommendation has been to severely limit the intake of carbohydrates in the diet. There are many different versions of a low-carbohydrate diet, all of which recommend a strict reduction in the consumption of carbohydrates. Most "low-carb" diets replace carbohydrates with a high-fat and moderate protein diet. The low-calorie and low-fat diets that have been recommended for years have failed to realize that dietary fat is not necessarily converted into body fat. However carbohydrates are readily converted into fat. When eating a high-carbohydrate meal, the increased blood glucose stimulates insulin production by the pancreas. Insulin allows blood glucose to be used by the cells, but it also causes fat to be deposited, and it stimulates the brain to produce hunger signals. So there is a tendency to eat more carbohydrates, and the cycle repeats. It has been shown that most overweight people became overweight due to a condition called *hyperinsulinemia*— elevated insulin levels in the blood. Restricting carbohydrate intake halts this cycle by decreasing insulin levels. Carbohydrate restriction also increases the levels of glucagon, which is a hormone that causes body fat to be burned and aids in removing cholesterol deposits in the arteries. Severely restricting carbohydrate intake puts the body into a state of ketosis in which blood glucose levels stabilize, insulin level drops, and because the body is burning fat, fairly rapid weight loss occurs.[37]

## GLYCOGEN SUPERCOMPENSATION (LOADING)

For endurance events, maximizing the amount of glycogen that can be stored, especially in muscles, may make the difference between finishing first or at the "end of the pack." Glycogen supplies in muscle and the liver can be increased by reducing the training program a few days before competing and by significantly increasing carbohydrate intake during the week before the event. Reducing training for at least 48 hours before the competition allows the body to eliminate any metabolic waste products that may hinder performance. The high-carbohydrate diet restores glycogen levels in muscle and the liver. This practice is called **glycogen supercompensation.** (In the past this practice has been called glycogen loading.) The basis for this practice is that the quantity of glycogen stored in muscle directly affects the endurance of that muscle.

> **glycogen supercompensation** High-carbohydrate diet.

Glycogen supercompensation is accomplished over a 6-day period divided into three phases. In phase 1 (days 1 to 2), training should be very hard and dietary intake of carbohydrates fairly normal, accounting for about 60 percent of total calorie intake. During phase 2 (days 3 to 5), training is cut back and the individual eats at least 70 percent or more of the diet in carbohydrates. Studies have indicated that glycogen stores may be increased from 50 to 100 percent, theoretically enhancing endurance during a long-term event. Phase 3 (day 6) is the day of the event, during which a normal diet must be consumed.

The effect of glycogen supercompensation in improving performance during endurance activities has not yet been clearly demonstrated. Glycogen supercompensation should not be done more than two to three times during the course of a year. *Glycogen loading is only of value in long-duration events that produce glycogen depletion, such as a marathon or triathlon.*

### Fat Loading

Some endurance athletes have tried fat loading in place of carbohydrate loading. Their intent was to have a better source of energy at their disposal. *The deleterious effects of this procedure outweigh any benefits that may be derived.* Fat loading can lead to cardiac protein and potassium depletion, causing arrhythmias and increased levels of serum cholesterol as a result of the ingestion of butter, cheese, cream, and marbled beef.

## WEIGHT CONTROL AND BODY COMPOSITION

The need for gain or loss of weight in an athlete often poses a problem because the individual's ingrained eating habits are difficult to change. An intelligent and conscientious approach to weight control requires

---

**body composition**
Percent body fat plus lean
body weight.

---

some knowledge of what is involved on the part of the athlete. Such understanding allows athletes to better discipline themselves as to the quantity and kinds of foods they should eat.

## Body Composition

**Body composition** refers to both the fat and nonfat components of the body. That portion of total body weight that is composed of fat tissue is referred to as the percent body fat. That portion of the total body weight that is composed of nonfat or lean tissue, which includes muscles, tendons, bones, connective tissue, and so on, is referred to as lean body weight. Body composition measurements are the most accurate way to determine precisely how much weight an athlete may gain or lose.[7]

In the average college-age female, between 20 and 25 percent of total body weight is made up of fat. The average college-age male has between 12 and 15 percent body fat. Male endurance athletes may get their fat percentage as low as 8 to 12 percent, and female endurance athletes may reach 10 to 18 percent. The recommendation is that body fat percentage not go below 5 percent in males and 12 percent in females, because below these percentages the internal organs tend to lose their protective padding of essential fat, potentially subjecting them to injury.[7]

### Assessing Body Composition

Measuring the thickness of skin folds is based on the fact that about 50 percent of the fat in the body is contained in the subcutaneous fat layers and is closely related to total fat. The remainder of the fat in the body is found around organs and vessels and serves a shock-absorptive function. The skin-fold technique involves measurement of the thickness of the subcutaneous fat layer with a skin-fold caliper.[7]

A second technique for assessing body composition involves measuring bioelectrial impedence. This technique predicts the percentage of body fat by assessing the amount of resistance to the flow of electrical current through the body between selected points. Despite their relative expense, these measurement devices are becoming more and more widely used.

### Assessing Caloric Balance

Positive caloric balance =
weight gain

Negative caloric balance =
weight loss

Changes in body weight are almost entirely the result of changes in caloric balance.

*Caloric balance = Number of Calories Consumed − Number of Calories Expended*

Calories may be expended by three different processes: (1) basal metabolism; (2) work (work may be defined as any activity that requires more energy than sleeping); and (3) excretion. If more calories are consumed than expended, the positive caloric balance results in weight gain. Conversely, weight loss results from a negative caloric balance in which more calories are expended than are consumed.

Caloric balance is determined by the number of calories consumed regardless of whether the calories are contained in fat, carbohydrate, or protein. There are differences in the caloric content of these three foodstuffs:

Carbohydrate = 4 calories per gram

Protein = 4 calories per gram

Fat = 9 calories per gram

Alcohol = 7 calories per gram

(Alcohol should not be considered a macronutrient.)

Estimations of caloric intake for college athletes range between 2,000 and 5,000 calories per day. Estimations of caloric expenditure range between 2,200 and 4,400 calories on the average. Energy demands are considerably higher in endurance athletes, who may require as many as 7,000 calories.

## Methods of Weight Loss

There are several ways to lose weight: (1) dieting (here dieting refers to caloric restriction), (2) increasing the amount of physical exercise, or (3) a combination of diet and exercise.

Weight loss through dieting alone is difficult, and in most cases, dieting is an ineffective means of weight control.[19] Long-term weight control through dieting alone is successful only 20 percent of the time.[5] Through dieting, 35 to 45 percent of the weight decrease results from a loss of lean tissue. The minimum caloric intake for a female should not go below 1,000 to 1,200 calories per day, and for a male, not below 1,200 to 1,400 calories per day.[5]

Weight loss through exercise involves an 80 to 90 percent loss of fat tissue with almost no loss of lean tissue. Weight loss through exercise alone is almost as difficult as losing weight through dieting. However, exercise will not only result in weight reduction but may also enhance cardiorespiratory endurance, improve strength, and increase flexibility.[6] For this reason, exercise has some distinct advantages over dieting in any weight-loss program.

**The most efficient method of decreasing body fat is through some combination of diet and exercise.**[5] A moderate caloric restriction combined with a moderate increase in caloric expenditure will result in a negative caloric balance. This method is relatively fast and easy compared with either of the other methods because habits are moderately changed.

In any weight-loss program, the goal should be to lose 1½ to 2 pounds per week. Weight loss of more than 4 to 5 pounds during a week's time may be attributed to dehydration as opposed to a loss of body fat. The American College of Sports Medicine has established specific guidelines for losing weight, which are listed in Focus Box 5-3.[29]

**Guidelines for Weight Loss**

The American College of Sports Medicine has made the following statements and recommendations regarding weight loss:[29]

- Prolonged fasting and diet programs that severely restrict caloric intake are scientifically undesirable and can be medically dangerous.
- Fasting and diet programs that severely restrict caloric intake result in the loss of large amounts of water, electrolytes, minerals, glycogen stores, and other fat-free tissue (including proteins within fat-free tissues), with minimal amounts of fat loss.
- Mild calorie restriction (500 to 1,000 calories less than the usual daily intake) results in a smaller loss of water, electrolytes, minerals, and other fat-free tissue and is less likely to cause malnutrition.
- Dynamic exercise of large muscles helps to maintain fat-free tissue, including muscle mass and bone density, and results in losses of body weight. Weight loss resulting from an increase in energy expenditure is primarily in the form of fat weight.
- A nutritionally sound diet resulting in mild calorie restriction coupled with an endurance exercise program, along with behavioral modification of existing eating habits, is recommended for weight reduction. The rate of sustained weight loss should not exceed 1 kilogram (2 pounds) per week.
- To maintain proper weight control and optimal body fat levels, a lifetime commitment to proper eating habits and regular physical activity is required.

## Methods of Weight Gain

The aim of a weight-gaining program should be to increase lean body mass, that is, increase muscle as opposed to body fat. Muscle mass should be increased only by muscle work combined with an appropriate increase in dietary intake. It cannot be increased by the intake of any special food or vitamin.[25]

The recommended rate of weight gain is approximately 1 to 2 pounds per week. Each pound of lean body mass gained represents a positive caloric balance, which is an intake in excess of an expenditure of approximately 2,500 calories. One pound of fat represents the equivalent of 3,500 calories; lean body tissue contains less fat, more protein, and more water and represents approximately 2,500 calories. To gain 1 pound of muscle, an excess of approximately 2,500 calories is needed; to lose one pound of fat, approximately 3,500 calories must be expended in activities in excess of intake.[25] Adding 500 to 1,000 calories daily to the usual diet will provide the energy needs of gaining 1 to 2 pounds per week and fuel the increased energy expenditure of the weight-training program. Weight training must be part of the program. Otherwise, the excess intake of energy will be converted to fat.

## DISORDERED EATING

There is an epidemic in this society, especially in sports. This problem is the inordinate concern with being overweight. Out of this obsession has emerged the eating disorders bulimia nervosa, anorexia nervosa,

**5-3 *Critical Thinking***
Exercise

An ice hockey attackman is at an excellent level of fitness and has superb skating ability and stick work. He is convinced that the only thing keeping him from moving to the next level is his body weight. In recent years he has engaged more in weight-training activities to improve his endurance and, to a lesser extent, to increase strength.

? What recommendations should be made for him to be successful in his weight-gaining efforts?

5-4 ▷ *Focus Box*

**Recognizing the Individual with Disordered Eating**

Look for these signs:

- Social isolation and withdrawal from friends and family
- A lack of confidence in athletic abilities
- Ritualistic eating behavior (e.g., organizing food on plate)
- An obsession with counting calories
- An obsession with constantly exercising, especially just before a meal
- An obsession with weighing self
- A constant overestimation of body size
- Patterns of leaving the table directly after eating to go into the restroom
- Problems related to eating disorders (e.g., malnutrition, menstrual irregularities, or chronic fatigue)
- Family history of disordered eating

anorexia athletica, and female athlete triad syndrome. Each of these disorders is increasingly seen in athletes.[4] Focus Box 5-4 provides tips for identifying athletes with disordered eating.

## Bulimia Nervosa

The bulimic individual typically gorges herself with thousands of calories after a period of starvation and then purges herself through induced vomiting and further fasting or through the use of laxatives or diuretics. This secretive binge-eating and purging cycle may go on for years.

The bulimic person is commonly female, ranging in age from adolescence to middle age. One out of every 200 American girls ages 12 to 18 years (1 to 2 percent of the population) will develop patterns of bulimia and/or anorexia nervosa.[3]

Typically the bulimic athlete is white and belongs to a middle-class or upper-middle-class family. She is perfectionistic, obedient, overcompliant, highly motivated, very successful academically, well-liked by her peers, and a good athlete.[13] She most commonly participates in gymnastics, track, and dance. Male wrestlers and gymnasts may also develop bulimia. The formal definition of bulimia is as follows: recurrent episodes of rapid, uncontrollable ingestion of large amounts of food in a short time, usually followed by purging, by either forced vomiting and/or abuse of laxatives or diuretics.

Binge-purge patterns of eating can cause stomach rupture, disrupt heart rhythm, and cause liver damage. Stomach acids brought up by vomiting cause tooth decay and chronically inflame the mucous lining of the mouth and throat.[39]

## Anorexia Nervosa

Thirty to 50 percent of all individuals diagnosed as having anorexia nervosa also develop some symptoms of bulimia. Anorexia nervosa is characterized by a distorted body image and a major concern about weight gain. As with bulimia, anorexia nervosa affects mostly females. It usually begins in adolescence and can be mild without major consequences or can become life threatening. As many as 15 to 21 percent of those individuals diagnosed as anorexic will ultimately die from this disorder. Despite being extremely thin, the athlete sees herself as too fat. These individuals deny hunger and are hyperactive, engaging in abnormal amounts of exercise such as aerobics or distance running.[4] In general, the anorexic individual is highly secretive. Early intervention is essential. Any athlete with signs of bulimia or anorexia nervosa must be confronted in a kind, sympathetic manner. When detected, individuals with eating disorders must be referred for psychological or psychiatric treatment. Unfortunately, simply referring an anorexic person to a health education clinic for help is not usually effective. The key to treatment of anorexia seems to be getting the patient to realize that a problem exists and that he or she could benefit from outside professional help. The individual must voluntarily accept such help if treatment is to be successful.[4]

## Anorexia Athletica

Anorexia athletica is a condition specific to athletes that is characterized by several of the features common to anorexia nervosa, but without the self-starvation practices. Athletes with anorexia athletica may exhibit a variety of signs including disturbance of body image, a weight loss greater than 5 percent of body weight, gastrointestinal complaints, primary amenorrhea, menstrual dysfunction, absence of medical illness explaining the weight reduction, excessive fear of becoming obese, binging or purging, compulsive eating, and/or restriction of caloric intake.

## Female Athlete Triad Syndrome

Female athlete triad syndrome is a potentially fatal problem that involves a combination of disordered eating (either bulimia or anorexia), amenorrhea, and osteoporosis (diminished bone density). New research suggests that an individual may not necessarily have all three conditions and some differences in the extent of each of these three exists in different individuals.[30] Female athlete triad syndrome occurs primarily in female athletes. The incidence of this syndrome is uncertain; however, some studies have suggested that eating disorders in female athletes may be as high as 62 percent in certain sports, with amenorrhea being common in at least 60 percent. However, the major risk of this syndrome is that the bone lost in osteoporosis may not be regained.[4]

## Athletic Injury Management Checklist

This checklist should be considered to ensure the athlete is consuming a nutritious diet.

☐ Generally, does the athlete consume a reasonably well-balanced diet?

☐ Is it necessary for the athlete to take a daily vitamin supplement?

☐ Does the athlete need to take a mineral supplement because of some dietary deficiency?

☐ Is the athlete consuming a sufficient amount of water to stay hydrated?

☐ Are athletes using sports drinks to replace lost fluids and electrolytes?

☐ Is the athlete consuming excess caffeine, sugar, or protein in an effort to enhance performance?

☐ Does the athlete take herbs or consume other types of health foods?

☐ What does the athlete eat for the preevent meal?

☐ Does the athlete appear to be able to balance his or her intake of food with energy expenditure to maintain weight and body composition at an appropriate level?

☐ Is there anything the athlete is doing to make you suspect that the athlete may have an eating disorder?

## SUMMARY

- The classes of nutrients are carbohydrates, fats, proteins, vitamins, minerals, and water.

- Carbohydrates, fats, and proteins provide the energy required for muscular work and also play a role in the function and maintenance of body tissues.

- Protein supplementation is not necessary.

- Vitamins are substances found in foods, which have no caloric value but are necessary to regulate body processes.

- Antioxidants are nutrients that protect the body against various destructive agents.

- Minerals are also involved in regulation of bodily functions and are used to form important body structures.

- Water is the most essential nutrient and should be used with sports drinks in fluid replacement.

- A nutritious diet consists of eating a variety of foods in the amounts recommended on the food pyramid. An athlete whose diet meets those recommendations may not need nutrient supplements.

- Some people need extra iron and calcium.

- The preevent meal should be (1) higher in carbohydrates, (2) easily digested, (3) eaten 2 to 4 hours before an event, and (4) acceptable to the athlete.

- Glycogen supercompensation involves maximizing the stores of carbohydrate in muscle and liver before a competitive event.

- Body composition analysis indicates the percentage of total body weight composed of fat tissue versus the percentage composed of lean tissue.

- Changes in body weight are caused almost entirely by a change in caloric balance, which is a function of the number of calories taken in and the number of calories expended.

- Weight can be lost by increasing caloric expenditure through exercise, by decreasing caloric intake through reducing food intake, or, most effectively, by using a combination of moderate caloric restriction and a moderate increase in physical exercise during the course of each day.

- Bulimia is an eating disorder that involves periodic binging and subsequent purging.

- Anorexia nervosa is a form of mental illness in which a person reduces food intake and increases energy expenditure to the extent that the loss of body fat threatens health and life.

---

### *Solutions to Critical Thinking* Exercises

---

**5-1** In terms of weight control, the important consideration is the total number of calories that this athlete consumes relative to the total number of calories she expends. It makes no difference whether the calories consumed are CHO, fat, or protein. Because fat contains more than twice the number of calories as either CHO or protein, this athlete can eat significantly more food and still have about the same calorie intake if the diet is high in CHO. The necessity of consuming at least some fat in the diet, which is necessary for the production of certain enzymes and hormones, should also be stressed.

**5-2** If this athlete is truly consuming anything close to a well-balanced diet, vitamin supplementation is generally not necessary. However if taking a one-a-day vitamin supplement makes her feel better, no harm is done. The fact that she feels tired could be related to a number of medical conditions (e.g., mononucleosis). An iron deficiency anemia may be detected through a laboratory blood test. The athlete should be referred to a physician for blood work.

**5-3** This athlete must understand the importance of adding lean tissue muscle mass rather than increasing his percent body fat. It is true that caloric intake must be increased so that he is in a positive caloric balance of about 500 calories per day. Additional calorie intake should consist primarily of CHO. Additional supplementation with protein is not necessary. It is absolutely essential that this athlete incorporate a weight-training program using heavy weights that will overload the muscle, forcing it to hypertrophy over time.

**5-4** Treating eating disorders is difficult even for health care professionals specifically trained to counsel these individuals. The athlete should be approached by a support person who shows concern about her weight loss and expresses a desire to help her secure appropriate counseling, not with accusation. Remember that the athlete must first be willing to admit that she has an eating disorder before treatment and counseling will be effective. Eliciting the support of close friends and family can help with treatment.

## REVIEW QUESTIONS AND CLASS ACTIVITIES

1. What is the value of good nutrition in terms of an athlete's performance and injury prevention?
2. Ask coaches of different sports about the type of diet they recommend for their athletes and their rationale for doing so.
3. Have a nutritionist talk to the class about food myths and fallacies.
4. Have each member of the class prepare a week's food diary; then compare it with other class members' diaries.
5. What are the daily dietary requirements according to the food pyramid? Should the requirements of the typical athlete's diet differ from those on the food pyramid? If so, in what ways?
6. Have the class debate the value of vitamin and mineral supplements.
7. Describe the advantages and disadvantages of supplementing iron and calcium.
8. Is there some advantage to preevent nutrition?
9. Are there advantages and/or disadvantages in the vegetarian diet for the athlete?
10. Discuss the importance of having an athlete monitor body composition.
11. Explain the most effective technique for losing weight.
12. Contrast the signs and symptoms of bulimia and anorexia nervosa. If a coach is aware of an athlete who may have an eating disorder, what should he or she do?

## REFERENCES

1. American College of Sports Medicine: 1991. Position stand on exercise and fluid replacement, *Med Sci Sports Exerc* 28:1.
2. Antonio, J: 2001. *Sports supplements,* Philadelphia, PA, Lippincott Williams & Wilkins.
3. Balch, P: 2006. *Prescription for nutritional healing: a practical A-to-Z reference to drug-free remedies using vitamins, minerals, herbs and food supplements,* New York, Penguin Group.
4. Beals, K: 2004. *Disordered eating among athletes: a comprehensive guide for health professionals,* Champaign, IL, Human Kinetics.
5. Brownell, K, Horgen, K: 2003. *Food fight; the inside story of America's obesity crisis—and what we can do about it,* New York, McGraw-Hill.
6. Brukner, Po. Khan, K, Inge, K, Crawford, S: 2002. Maximizing performance: nutrition. In Brukner, P. (ed.), *Clinical sports medicine,* 2nd rev. ed, Sydney, McGraw-Hill.

7. Brzycki, M: 2004. What's the most accurate way to measure body composition? *Fitness management* 20(2):45.

8. Burke, L (ed.): 2006. *Clinical sports nutrition*. 3rd ed, Sydney, McGraw-Hill.

9. Casa D, Armstrong L, Hillman S: 2000. National Athletic Trainers Association position statement: fluid replacement for athletes, *Journal of Athlete Training* 35(2):212.

10. Clark, N: 2007. Organic foods. *American Fitness* 25(5):34.

11. Clark, N: 2008. *Nancy Clark's sports nutrition guidebook*. Champaign, IL, Human Kinetics.

12. Clark, N: 2008. Organic foods for athletes? ACSM Fit Society Page, p. 6.

13. Claude-Pierre P: 1999. *The secret language of eating disorders*, New York, Vintage Books.

14. Coleman, E: 2001. Carbohydrate during stop-and-go sports, *Sports medicine digest* 23(12):142–143.

15. Coleman, E: 2001. Nutrition update: position stand on nutrition and athletic performance, *Sports medicine digest* 23(5):54–55.

16. Daniels, D: 2000. *Exercises for osteoporosis*. New York, Hatherleigh Press.

17. Dubnov, G, Constantini, NW: 2004. Prevalence of iron depletion and anemia in top-level basketball players, *International journal of sport nutrition and exercise metabolism* 14(1):30–37.

18. Froiland, K, Koszewski, W, Hingst, J: 2004. Nutritional supplement use among college athletes and their sources of information, *International journal of sport nutrition and exercise metabolism* 14(1):104–120.

19. Herriot, A, Thomas, D, Hart, K: 2008. A qualitative investigation of individuals' experiences and expectations before and after completing a trial of commercial weight loss programs. *Journal of Human Nutrition & Dietetics* 21(1):72.

20. Is organic food really more nutritious? 2007. Tufts University Health & Nutrition 25(7):8.

21. Izquierdo, M, Ibanez, J, Gonzalez-Badillo, JI, Gorostiaga, EM: 2002. Effects of creatine supplementation on muscle power, endurance, and sprint performance, *Medicine and science in sports and exercise* 4(2):332–343.

22. Kleiner, SM: 2001. The scoop on protein supplements, *Athletic therapy today* 6(1):52–53.

23. Kleiner, SM, Greenwood-Robinson, M: 2001. Performance herbs. In Kleiner, SM (ed), *Power eating*, 2nd ed, Champaign, IL, Human Kinetics.

24. Johnson, KD: 2001. Ephedra and ma huang consumption: do the benefits outweigh the risks? *Strength and conditioning journal* 23(5):32–37.

25. Litt, A: 2004. Tactics for gaining weight, In Litt, A. *Fuel for young athletes*, Champaign, IL, Human Kinetics.

26. Maughn, R: 2004. Dietary supplements, *Journal of sport sciences*, 22(1):95–113.

27. Maughn, R: 2002. *Sports nutrition*, Malden, MA, Blackwell Scientific.

28. Maughan, R, Murray, R: 2001. *Sports Drinks: Basic Science and Practical Aspects*, Boca Raton, FL.

29. McArdle, W, Katch, F, Katch, V: 2005. *Sports and exercise nutrition*, Philadelphia, Lippincott, Williams and Wilkins.

30. Nattiv A, Loucks AB, Manore M: 2007. American College of Sports Medicine position stand. The female athlete triad. *Med Sci Sports Exerc* 39(10):1867–82.

31. Powers, S, DeRuisseau, K: 2004. Dietary antioxidants and exercise, *Journal of sport sciences* 22(1):81–94.

32. Sanborn CF et al.: 2000. Disordered eating and the female athlete triad, *Clin Sports Med* 19(2):199.

33. Sawyer, T. H. (ed.), 2003. *A guide to sport nutrition: for student-athletes, coaches, athletic trainers, and parents,* Champaign, Ill., Sagamore Publishing.

34. Sen, CK: 2001. Antioxidants in exercise nutrition. *Sports medicine* 31(13): 891–908.

35. Sforzo, GA: 2002. Sports supplements. (Review) *Medicine and science in sports and exercise* 34(1):183.

36. Sharkey, B: 2002. Nutrition and health: In Sharkey, B (ed), *Fitness & Health,* 5th ed, Champaign, IL, Human Kinetics.

37. Spriet, L, Gibala, M: 2004. Nutritional strategies to influence adaptations to training, *Journal of sport sciences,* 22(1):127–141.

38. Stevenson, SW, Dydley, GA: 2001. Creatine loading, resistance exercise performance and muscle mechanics. *Journal of conditioning research* 15(4):413–419.

39. Sundgot-Borgen J: 2000. Eating disorders in athletes. In Sundgot-Borgen J, editor, *Nutrition in sport,* Oxford, Blackwell.

40. US Department of Agriculture. *Dietary Guidelines for Americans 2005,* Washington DC, US Government Printing Office.

41. Wardlaw GM, Smith A: 2005. *Contemporary nutrition,* Boston, McGraw-Hill.

42. Williams M: 2004. *Nutrition for health, fitness, and sport,* St Louis, McGraw-Hill.

## ANNOTATED BIBLIOGRAPHY

Bernadot, D: 2005. *Advanced sports nutrition,* Champaign, IL, Human Kinetics.

   *This text presents cutting-edge nutritional concepts tailored for application by athletes in any sport.*

Clark N: 2003. *Nancy Clark's sports nutrition guidebook,* Champaign, IL, Human Kinetics.

   *Complete guide to eating for the vigorous person. Provides the basics of sports nutrition and includes over 100 fast recipes for meals that enhance physical performance.*

Fink, H, Burgoon, L, Mikesky, A: 2009. *Practical applications in sports nutrition,* Sudbury, MN, Jones and Bartlett.

   *Provides an introduction to sports nutrition including general nutrition concepts and a thorough explanation of athletic performance and consultation skills.*

Wardlaw, G: 2005. *Contemporary nutrition.* New York, McGraw-Hill.

   *This text presents cutting-edge nutritional concepts tailored for application by athletes in any sport.*

Williams M: 2004. *Nutrition for health fitness and sport,* Boston, McGraw-Hill.

   *Provides the reader with thorough coverage of the role nutrition plays in enhancing health, fitness, and sport performance. Current research and practical activities are incorporated throughout.*

## WEB SITES

The American Dietetic Association: www.eatright.org
   *This site includes access to the journal published by the American Dietetic Association and provides informative nutritional tips and a section entitled "gateway to nutrition."*

Eating Disorders: www.something-fishy.org/

Organizing and Establishing
an Effective Athletic Health
Care System

*Eating disorder information can be found here, including information about anorexia, bulimia, and overeating as well as information about how to access support groups.*

Food and Nutrition Information
Center: www.nalusda.gov/fnic
*Part of the information centers at the National Agricultural Library, this site provides access to information on healthy eating habits, food composition, and many additional resources.*

Gatorade Sports Science Institute
www.gssiweb.com/
*This Web site provides information for coaches, athletic trainers, physicians,*

*nutritionists, and others in the field of sports medicine, sports nutrition, and exercise science.*

Healthy Biz 2000
www.healthybiz2000.com/
trainer.html
*Information about sports nutrition and nutritional supplements for fitness and weight loss.*

Yahoo Health and Nutrition
Information:
www.yahoo.com/Health/Nutrition
*Includes diet analysis information, nutritional facts, and links to many informative sites.*

# PART 2

## Techniques for Preventing and Minimizing Sport-Related Injuries

# Selecting and Using Protective Sports Equipment

## CHAPTER 6

*When you finish this chapter you will be able to:*

- Discuss legal concerns related to the use of protective equipment.
- Identify the different types of protective equipment available for various parts of the body.
- Describe the proper technique for fitting a football helmet and shoulder pads.
- Discuss what consideration should be given to shoe selection.
- Discuss the efficacy of knee and ankle braces in reducing injuries.

Because of the nature of sports activity, injuries often occur. A number of factors either singly or collectively can contribute to the incidence of injury. Certainly the selection, fitting, and maintenance of protective equipment are critical in injury prevention.[23] Thus it is essential to have some knowledge about the types of protective equipment available for a particular sport and how that equipment should best be fitted and maintained to reduce the possibility of athletic injury.[3,36]

This protection is particularly important in direct contact and collision sports such as football, hockey, and lacrosse, but it can also be important in indirect contact sports such as basketball and soccer. Selecting and purchasing protective sports equipment makes a major commitment to safeguard athletes' health and welfare.[28]

## SAFETY STANDARDS FOR SPORTS EQUIPMENT AND FACILITIES

There is serious concern about the standards for protective sports equipment, particularly material durability standards—concerns that include who should set these standards, mass production of equipment, equipment testing methods, and requirements for wearing protective equipment.

Standards are also needed for protective equipment maintenance, both to keep it in good repair and to determine when to throw it away. Too often, old, worn-out, and ill-fitting equipment is passed down from the varsity players to the younger and often less-experienced players, compounding their risk of injury.[26] Those purchasing equipment must learn to be less concerned with the color, look, and style of a piece of equipment and more concerned with its ability to prevent injury.[10] Many national organizations are addressing these issues. Engineering, chemistry, biomechanics, anatomy, physiology, physics, computer science, and other

> Old, worn-out, ill-fitting equipment should never be passed down to younger, less-experienced players; it compounds their risk of injury.

**Equipment Regulatory Agencies**

American National Standards Institute
1819 L Street NW
Washington, DC 20036
(202) 293-8020
http://www.ansi.org

American Society for Testing Materials
100 Barr Harbor Drive
West Conshohocken, PA 19428-2959
(610) 832-9585
http://www.astm.org

Athletic Equipment Manufacturers Association
Dorothy Cutting
Cornell University Athletic Department
P.O. Box 729
Ithaca, NY 14851
(607) 255-4115
http://www.wisc.edu/ath/aema/

Hockey Equipment Certification Council
18103 TransCanada Highway
Kirkland, QC H9J 324
Canada
(514) 697-9900
http://www.hecc.net

National Athletic Trainers Association
2952 Stemmons Freeway
Dallas, TX 75247-6196
(214) 637-6282
http://www.nata.org

National Collegiate Athletic Association
700 W. Washington Street
P.O. Box 6222
Indianapolis, IN 46206-6222
http://www.ncaa.org

National Association of Intercollegiate Athletics
6120 S. Yale Avenue
Suite 1450
Tulsa, OK 74136
(918) 494-8828
http://www.naia.org

National Federation of State High School
Athletic Associations
P.O. Box 690
Indianapolis, IN 46200
(317) 972-6900
http://www.nfhs.org

National Operating Committee on Standards
for Athletic Equipment
P.O. Box 12290
Overland, KS 66282-2290
http://www.nocsae.org

Sporting Goods Manufacturers Association
200 Castlewood Drive
North Palm Beach, FL 33418
(561) 842-4100
http://sgma@ix.netcom.com

U.S. Consumer Product Safety Commission
4330 East-West Highway
Bethesda, MD 20814-4408
(301) 504-0990
http://www.cpsc.gov

related disciplines are being utilized to solve problems inherent in safety standardization of sports equipment and facilities. Focus Box 6-1 lists regulatory agencies.

### Equipment Reconditioning and Recertification

The National Operating Committee on Standards for Athletic Equipment (NOCSAE) has established voluntary test standards that have been developed to reduce head injuries by identifying minimum safety requirements for football helmets/face masks, baseball/softball batting helmets, baseballs and softballs, and lacrosse helmets/face masks. These standards have been adopted by various regulatory bodies for sports, including the

NCAA and the National Federation of State High School Associations. Factors such as the type of helmet and the amount and intensity of usage will determine the condition of each helmet over a period of time. The NOCSAE helmet standard is not a warranty, but simply a statement that a particular helmet model met the requirements of performance tests when it was manufactured or reconditioned. NOCSAE does recommend that the consumer adhere to a program of periodically having used helmets reconditioned and recertified. Because of the difference in the amount and intensity of usage on each helmet, the consumer should use discretion regarding the frequency with which certain helmets are to be reconditioned and recertified. Helmets that regularly undergo the reconditioning and recertification process can meet standard performance requirements for many seasons, depending on the model and usage. Keeping equipment (such as helmets and pads) as well as clothing clean can help the equipment last longer. In addition, various skin conditions and infections can occur unnecessarily if equipment and clothing are not kept clean (see Chapter 23). Focus Box 6-2 provides guidelines for purchasing and reconditioning helmets.

---

( 6-2 )    *Focus Box*

---

**Guidelines for Purchasing and Reconditioning Helmets**

- Purchase only NOCSAE approved helmets.
- Purchase helmets for appropriate skill level (example: Do not purchase youth helmets for high school football).
- Assign a code number to each helmet purchased and record the date of purchase for each helmet.
- Fit helmets according to manufacturer's recommendations.
- Recheck helmets for proper fit during the season.
- Review written warranty information and comply with manufacturer's requirement(s) for cleaning/reconditioning/recertification.
- Replace or repair broken or damaged helmets before returning to service.
- Develop a written accounting of player use, inspections, reconditioning, recertification, and disposal of each helmet.
- Clean helmets according to manufacturer's recommendations on a regular schedule during the season and at the end of the season prior to off-season storage.
- Recertify/recondition each football helmet according to manufacturer's warranty.
- Recertify/recondition helmets every two years using a certified NOCSAE approved vendor if no warranty exists or after the warranty expires.
- Make certain equipment is kept clean to avoid skin infections.

## LEGAL CONCERNS IN USING PROTECTIVE EQUIPMENT

As with other aspects of sports participation there is increasing litigation related to the use of protective equipment. Both manufacturers and those who purchase sports equipment must foresee all possible uses and misuses of the equipment and must warn the user of any potential risks inherent in using or misusing that equipment.

If an injury occurs as the result of an athlete using a piece of equipment and if that piece of equipment is determined to be defective or inadequate for its intended purpose, the manufacturer is considered liable. If a piece of protective equipment is modified in any way either by the athlete or by any other individual (e.g., removing some pads from inside a football helmet) the liability on the part of the manufacturer is voided, and thus the individual who modified the equipment becomes liable.

If a piece of equipment is modified and an athlete wearing that equipment is injured, it is likely that any lawsuit would involve both the individual who modified the piece of equipment individually and the employing institution. This becomes a case of tort (described in Chapter 3) in which the injured athlete must show that an individual was negligent in his or her decision to alter a piece of equipment and that the negligence resulted in injury. That person would then be legally liable for that action.

## USING OFF-THE-SHELF VERSUS CUSTOM PROTECTIVE EQUIPMENT

Protective equipment can be purchased from a variety of manufacturers and suppliers including athletic equipment manufacturers and medical equipment suppliers. "Off-the-shelf" equipment is premade and packaged by the manufacturer and when taken out of the package may be used immediately without modification. Examples of off-the-shelf equipment are neoprene sleeves, sorbethane shoe inserts, and protective ankle braces. Customized equipment is constructed according to the individual characteristics of the athlete. Using off-the-shelf items may cause problems with sizing and exact fit. In contrast, a custom-made piece of equipment can be specifically sized and made to fit the protective and support needs of the individual.

## HEAD PROTECTION

Direct-collision sports such as football and hockey require special protective equipment, especially for the head. Football involves more body contact than does hockey, but hockey players generally move faster and therefore create greater impact forces. Besides direct head contact stemming from hitting the boards, hockey has the added injury elements of swinging sticks and fast-moving pucks. Other sports using fast-moving projectiles are baseball, with its pitched ball and swinging bat, and track and field, with the javelin, discus, and heavy shot, which can also produce serious head injuries.[27,28]

**6-1 Critical Thinking**
Exercise

Junior varsity high school football players are issued their equipment. These athletes and their parents know very little about the equipment's potential for preventing injury.

? What is the responsibility of the institution in educating the team and their parents about equipment safety limits?

## Football Helmets

The National Operating Committee on Standards for Athletic Equipment (NOCSAE) has developed standards for football helmet certification.[16] An approved helmet must protect against concussive forces that may injure the brain.[18]

Schools must provide the athlete with quality equipment, especially the football helmet. **All helmets must have a NOCSAE certification.** The fact that a helmet is certified does not mean that it is completely failsafe. Athletes and their parents must be apprised of the dangers that are inherent in any sport, particularly football. To make this point especially clear, NOCSAE has adopted the following recommended warning to be placed on all football helmets:

> *Warning: Do not strike an opponent with any part of this helmet or face mask. This is a violation of football rules and may cause you to suffer severe brain or neck injury: including paralysis or death. Severe brain or neck injury may also occur accidentally while playing football.* NO HELMET CAN PREVENT ALL SUCH INJURIES. USE THIS HELMET AT YOUR OWN RISK.

Each player's helmet must have a visible exterior warning label ensuring that players have been made aware of the risks involved in the game of American football. The label must be attached to each helmet by both the manufacturer and the reconditioner.[18]

Each player must read this warning, after which it is read aloud by the coach or equipment manager. The athlete then signs a statement agreeing that he or she understands this warning.

A variety of football helmets are available, although only a few companies manufacture helmets (Figure 6-1).

Football helmets must withstand repeated blows that are of high mass and low velocity.

**6-2 Critical Thinking**
Exercise

The potential risks involved in wearing a football helmet must be explained to the football players.

? What are the most critical points to stress?

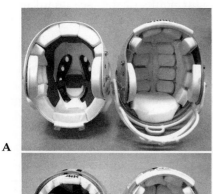

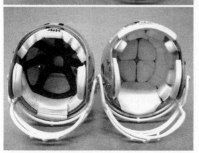

A

B

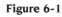

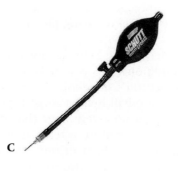

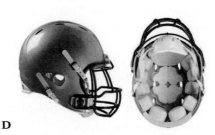

C

D

**Figure 6-1**

**Football Helmets:**
(A) Fluid-filled helmet.
(B) Air-filled helmet.
(C) Pump for inflating air/helmets.
(D) Revolution helmet.

**Proper Football Helmet Fit**

To properly fit a football helmet:

- The helmet should fit snugly around all parts of the player's head (front, sides, and crown), and there should be no gaps between the pads and the head or face.
- The cheek pads should fit snugly against the sides of the face.
- It should cover the base of the skull. The pads placed at the back of the neck should be snug but not to the extent of discomfort.
- It should not come down over the eyes. It should sit (front edge) ¼ inch (1.91 cm) above the player's eyebrows.
- The ear holes should be aligned with the external opening in the ear canal.
- The face mask should be attached securely to the helmet, allowing a complete field of vision.
- It should not shift when manual pressure is applied.
- It should not recoil on impact.
- The chin strap should be an equal distance from the center of the helmet.
- Straps must keep the helmet from moving up and down or side to side.

Football helmets generally use either fluid-filled or air-filled pockets to absorb the forces of impact (Figure 6-1A, B, and C). The lightweight Revolution helmet from Riddell marks the first significant structural change in football helmet design in nearly 25 years (Figure 6-1D). The protective shell has been computer designed and extends to the jaw area to provide protection to the side of the head and the jaw as well as improved front-to-back fit and stability. The distance between the helmet shell and the head has been increased. The padding inflates to provide a custom fit to every player's head shape. The face guard system is designed to isolate the attachment points of the face guard from the shell, thus reducing jarring to the player from low-level impacts to the face guard.

When fitting helmets, always wet the player's hair to simulate playing conditions; this will make the initial fitting easier. Closely follow the manufacturer's directions for a proper fit (see Focus Box 6-3).

The football helmet must be routinely checked for proper fit, especially in the first few days that it is worn (Figure 6-2). If air bladder helmets are used by a team that travels to a different altitude and air pressure, the helmet fit must be routinely rechecked.

Chin straps are also important in maintaining the proper head and helmet relationship. Two basic types of chin straps are in use today—a two-snap and a four-snap strap. Many players prefer the four-snap chin strap because it keeps the helmet from tilting forward and backward.

Jaw pads are also essential to keep the helmet from rocking laterally. They should rest snugly against the player's cheekbones. Even if a helmet's ability to withstand the forces of the game is certified, it is of no avail if the helmet is not properly fitted or maintained.

Even high-quality helmets are of no use if not properly fitted or maintained.

Ice hockey helmets must withstand the high-velocity impact of a stick or puck and the low-velocity forces of falling or hitting a board.

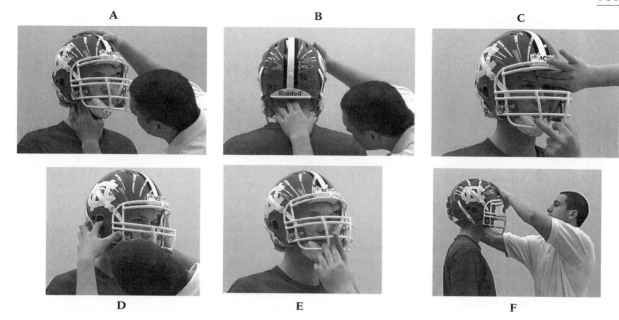

A          B          C

D          E          F

## Ice Hockey Helmets

As with football helmets, there has been a concerted effort to upgrade and standardize ice hockey helmets[22] (Figure 6-3). In contrast to football, blows to the head in ice hockey are usually singular rather than multiple. An ice hockey helmet must withstand both high-velocity impacts (e.g., being hit with a stick or a puck, which produces a force that has low mass and high velocity) and the high mass–low velocity forces produced by running into the boards or falling on the ice. In each instance, the hockey helmet, like the football helmet, must be able to spread the impact over a large surface area through a firm exterior shell and at the same time be able to decelerate forces that act on the head through a proper energy-absorbing liner. All hockey players must wear protective helmets that carry the stamp of approval from the Canadian Standards Association (CSA).

## Baseball/Softball Batting Helmets

Like ice hockey helmets, the baseball/softball helmet must withstand high-velocity impacts. Unlike football and ice hockey, baseball and softball

**Figure 6-2**

Fitting a football helmet: (A) Check fit under all pads: should be sung, (B) should cover base of skull, (C) should be 2 finger widths above eyebrow, (D) ear holes should align with center of ear, (E) Face mask should sit 3 finger widths from mouth, (F) Helmet should not shift when manual pressure is applied in all directions.

**Figure 6-3**

**Ice hockey helmets**

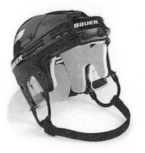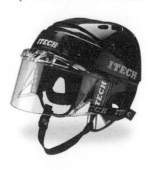

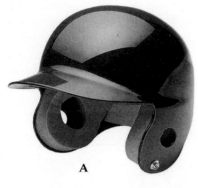
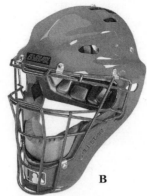
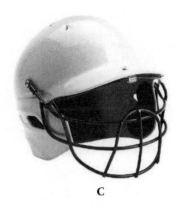

A
B
C

**Figure 6-4**

There is some question about how well baseball batting helmets protect against high-velocity impacts. (A) Batter's helmet. (B) Catcher's helmet and mask. (C) Batter's helmet with face mask and face shield.

have not produced a great deal of data on batting helmets.[23] It has been suggested, however, that baseball/softball helmets do not adequately dissipate the energy of the ball during impact (Figure 6-4). A possible answer is to add external padding or to improve the helmet's suspension. The use of a helmet with an ear flap can afford some additional protection to the batter. Each on-deck batter and runner is required to wear a baseball/softball head protector that carries a NOCSAE stamp similar to that on football helmets. From youth league through high school, catchers must wear a one-piece mask and helmet (Figure 6-4B).

## Cycling Helmets

Unlike other helmets discussed, cycling helmets are designed to protect the head during one single impact. Football, hockey, and baseball helmets are more durable and can survive repeated impact. Many states require the use of cycling helmets, especially for adolescents (Figure 6-5).

## Lacrosse Helmets

Helmets are required equipment for all male lacrosse players. Women's lacrosse requires only a protective eyeguard. Lacrosse helmets are made of a hard plastic with a wire mesh cage, or face mask, to protect the front of the face (Figure 6-6). The face mask must have a center bar running from the top to the bottom. The helmet is designed to absorb

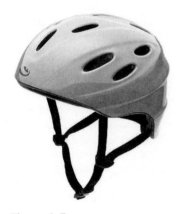

**Figure 6-5**

**Cycling helmet**

**Figure 6-6**

(A) Men's lacrosse helmet. (B) Inside padding. (C) Goalie's helmet with throat protector.

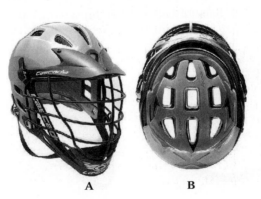

A
B
C

repeated impact from a hard, high-velocity projectile. Helmets come in a variety of sizes and are usually measured in inches. Lacrosse helmets use a four-point buckling system both to ensure that they stay on and to allow for a better fit. Goalie helmets add a throat protector.

## FACE PROTECTION

Devices that provide face protection fall into four categories: full face guards, mouth guards, ear guards, and eye protection devices.

### Face Guards

Face guards are used in a variety of sports to protect the face from carried or flying objects during a collision with another player (Figure 6-7). Since the adoption of face guards and mouth guards for use in football, mouth injuries have been reduced more than 50 percent (Figure 6-8A). The catcher in baseball, hockey players, lacrosse players, and football players should all be adequately protected against facial injuries, particularly lacerations and fractures (Figure 6-8B).

In sports, the face may be protected by:
- face guards
- mouth guards
- ear guards
- eye protection devices

A variety of face masks and bars are available to the player, depending on the position played and the protection needed. In football no face protection should have fewer than two bars. Proper mounting of the face mask and bars is imperative for maximum safety. All mountings should be made in such a way that the bar attachments are flush with the helmet. A 3-inch (7.62 cm) space should exist between the top of the face guard and the lower edge of the helmet. No helmet should be drilled more than one time on each side, and this drilling must be done by a factory-authorized reconditioner. Attachment of a bar or face mask not specifically designed for the helmet can invalidate the manufacturer's warranty.

Ice hockey face masks have been shown to reduce the incidence of facial injuries. In high school, face masks are required for all players,

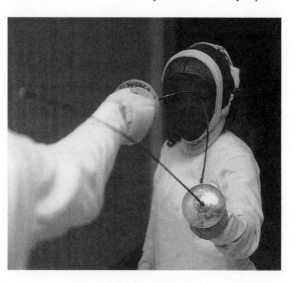

**Figure 6-7**

Sports such as fencing require complete face protection.

**Figure 6-8**

(A) Football face mask
(B) Baseball catcher's face mask
(C) Ice hockey face mask
(D) Lacrosse face mask

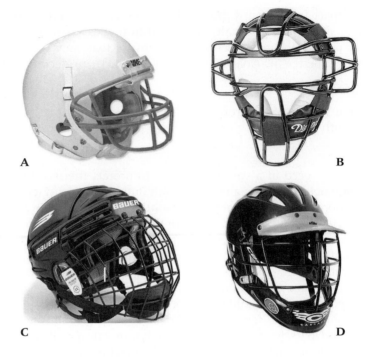

A

B

C

D

not just the goalkeeper. Helmets should be equipped with commercial plastic-coated wire-mesh guards that must meet standards set by the Hockey Equipment Certification Council (HECC) and the American Society for Testing Materials (ASTM) (Figure 6-8C). The openings in the guard must be small enough to prevent a hockey stick from penetrating. Plastic guards such as polycarbonate face shields have been approved by the HECC/ASTM and by the CSA Committee on Hockey Protective Equipment. In addition to face protectors, goalkeepers should wear commercial throat protectors.

## Laryngotracheal (Throat) Protection

A laryngotracheal injury, though relatively uncommon, can be fatal. Baseball catchers, lacrosse goalies, and ice hockey goalies are most at risk. Throat protection should be mandatory for these position players (Figure 6-9).[28]

## Mouth Guards

The majority of dental traumas can be prevented if the athlete wears a customized intraoral mouth guard[17] (Figure 6-10). In addition to protecting the teeth, the intraoral mouth guard absorbs the shock of chin blows and helps reduce the chance of cerebral concussion. Mouth guards serve also to minimize lacerations to the lips and cheeks and fractures to the lower jaw.[4]

The mouth guard should provide a tight fit, comfort, unrestricted breathing, and unimpeded speech during competition.[2] The athlete's air

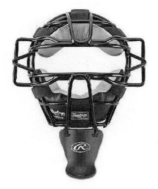
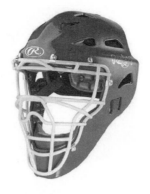

**Figure 6-9**

A throat protector can be attached to the face mask.

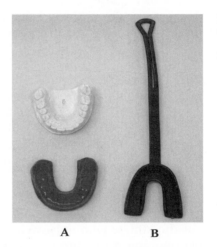

**Fıgure 6-10**

(A) Customized and (B) moldable mouth protectors.

**A**      **B**

passages should not be obstructed in any way by the mouthpiece. It is best when the mouthpiece is retained on the upper jaw and projects backward only as far as the last molar, thus permitting speech.

Cutting down mouth guards to cover only the front four teeth should never be condoned. It invalidates the manufacturer's warranty against dental injuries, and a cut-down mouth guard can easily become dislodged and lead to an obstructed airway, which poses a serious life-threatening situation for the athlete. Maximum protection is afforded when the mouth guard is composed of a flexible, resilient material and is form fitted to the teeth and upper jaw.[4]

Three types of mouth guards generally used in sports include the ready-made stock variety, a commercial mouth guard formed after submersion in boiling water, and the custom-fabricated type, which is formed over a mold made from an impression of the athlete's maxillary arch.

Many high schools and colleges now require that mouth guards be worn at all times (particularly in football) during competition and must be visible to the officials.

A properly fitted mouth guard protects the teeth, absorbs blows to the chin, and can help prevent concussion.

**Figure 6-11**

Ear protection: (A) Wrestler's ear guard. (B) Water polo player's ear protection.

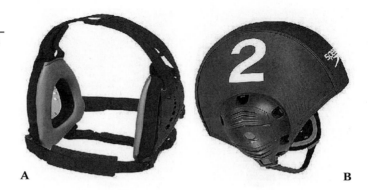

A                                                                                    B

Mouth guards tend to wear down during the course of a season. Coaches should routinely inspect each athlete's mouth guard to determine if replacement is necessary.

## Ear Guards

With the exception of boxing and wrestling, most contact sports do not make a special practice of protecting the ears. Both boxing and wrestling can cause irritation of the ears to the point that permanent deformity can result (see Figure 22-13). To avoid this problem special ear guards should be routinely worn. Recently a very effective ear protector has been developed for the water polo player (Figure 6-11).

## Eye Protection Devices

### Glasses

For the athlete who must wear corrective lenses, glasses can be both a blessing and a nuisance. They may slip on sweat, get bent when hit, fog from perspiration, detract from peripheral vision, and be difficult to wear with protective headgear. Even with all these disadvantages, properly fitted and designed glasses can provide adequate protection and withstand the rigors of the sport. Athletes should wear polycarbonate lenses, which are virtually unbreakable. These are the newest type of lenses available, and they are certainly the safest. If the athlete has glass lenses, they must be case-hardened to prevent them from splintering on impact. When a case-hardened lens breaks, it crumbles, eliminating the sharp edges that may penetrate the eye. The cost of this process is relatively low. The only disadvantages are that the glasses are heavier than average and they may be scratched more easily than regular glasses.[16]

Photochromic lenses can also offer a possible sports advantage. These glass lenses become color tinted when exposed to ultraviolet rays from the sun and then return to a clear state when removed from the sun's rays. Plastic lenses for glasses are popular with athletes. They are much lighter in weight than glass lenses and they can be made scratch resistant with a special coating.

## Contact Lenses

The athlete who is able to wear contact lenses without discomfort can avoid many of the inconveniences of glasses.[13] The greatest advantage to contact lenses is that they "become a part of the eye" and move with it.

Contact lenses come mainly in two types: the corneal type, a hard plastic lens that covers just the iris of the eye, and the scleral type, a soft plastic lens that is a little larger. Peripheral vision, astigmatism, and corneal waviness are improved through the use of contact lenses. Unlike regular glasses, contact lenses do not normally cloud during temperature changes. They also can be tinted to reduce glare. For example, yellow lenses can be used against ice glare and blue ones against glare from snow. Generally, athletes prefer the soft, hydrophilic lenses to the hard type. The soft lenses require a shorter adjustment time than the hard lenses do, they can be more easily replaced, and they are more adaptable to the sports environment. Athletes who wear contact lenses should have an extra pair available if needed along with a small mirror and saline solution.

## Eye and Glasses Guards

It is essential that athletes take special precautions to protect their eyes, especially in sports that use fast-moving projectiles and implements (Figure 6-12). Besides the more obvious sports of ice hockey, lacrosse, and baseball, the racquet sports also cause serious eye injury. Athletes not wearing glasses should wear closed eye guards to protect the orbital cavity. Athletes who normally wear glasses with plastic or case-hardened lenses are to some degree already protected against eye injury from an

**Figure 6-12**

(A & B) Athletes playing sports that involve small, fast projectiles should wear closed eye guards. (C) Polycarbonate shield for a football helmet. (D) Shield for an ice hockey face make. (E) Lacrosse/field hockey goggle. (F) Lacrosse goggle.

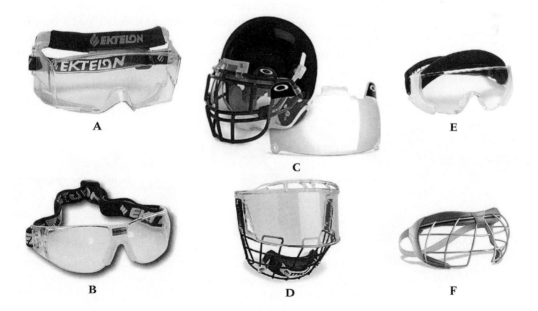

A

C

E

B

D

F

Techniques for Preventing
and Minimizing Sport-
Related Injuries

Eye protection must be worn
by all athletes who play
sports that use fast-moving
projectiles.

implement or projectile; however, greater safety is afforded if the athlete wears a polycarbonate frame that surrounds and fits over the athlete's glasses. The protection that the guard offers is excellent, but it does hinder vision in some planes.[16]

Polycarbonate eye shields can be attached to football face masks, hockey helmets, and baseball/softball helmets (Figure 6-12C).

## TRUNK AND THORAX PROTECTION

Trunk and thorax protection is essential in many contact and collision sports. Sports such as football, ice hockey, baseball, and lacrosse use extensive body protection. Areas that are most exposed to impact forces must be properly covered with some material that offers protection against soft-tissue compression. Of particular concern are the external genitalia and the exposed bony protuberances of the body that have insufficient soft tissue for protection, such as shoulders, ribs, and spine (Figure 6-13).

As discussed earlier, the problem that arises in wearing protective equipment is that, although it is armor against injury to the athlete wearing it, it can also serve as a weapon against all opponents. Standards must become more stringent in determining what equipment is absolutely necessary for body protection and at the same time is not itself a source of trauma. Proper fit and proper maintenance of equipment are essential.

### Football Shoulder Pads

There are two general types of pads, flat and cantilevered.[20] The player who uses the shoulder a great deal in blocking and tackling requires the bulkier cantilevered type, whereas the quarterback and ball receiver use the flat type (Figure 6-14). Over the years the shoulder pad's front and rear panels have been extended along with the cantilever. Focus Box 6-4 lists rules for fitting the football shoulder pad (Figure 6-15).[28]

**Figure 6-13**

Chest and thorax protectors. (A) Baseball catcher's chest protector. (B) Lacrosse goalie chest protector. (C) Ice hockey thorax protector and shoulder pads.

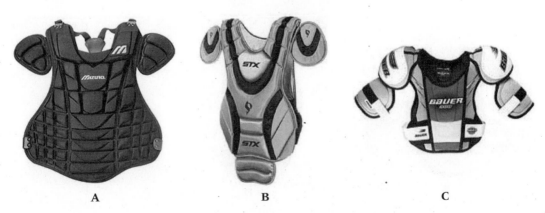

A                                        B                                        C

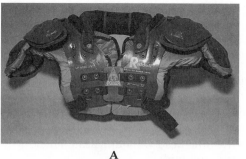

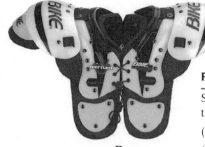

A

B

**Figure 6-14**

Shoulder pads protect both the shoulder and the thorax.

(A) Non-cantilever.

(B) Cantilever.

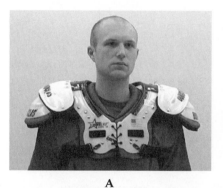

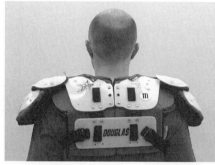

A

B

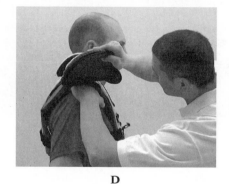

C

D

**Figure 6-15**

Football shoulder pads should be made to protect the player against direct force to the entire shoulder complex. (A) anterior fit, (B) posterior fit, (C) lateral fit, (D) space should be one hand width above shoulder.

A combination of football and ice hockey shoulder pads can be used to prevent injuries high on the upper arm and shoulder. A pair of supplemental shoulder pads is placed under the regular football pads. The deltoid cap of the hockey pad is connected to the main body of the hockey pad by an adjustable lace (Figure 6-16A). The distal end of the deltoid cap is held in place by a Velcro strap. The chest pad is adjustable to ensure proper fit for any size athlete. The football shoulder pads are placed over the hockey pads. The pads should be inspected for a proper fit. Larger football pads may be needed. A neck collar can also be added to the shoulder pads to minimize neck movement (Figure 6-16B).

**6-4** *Focus Box*

**Rules for Fitting Football Shoulder Pads**

- The width of the shoulder is measured to determine the proper size of pad.
- The inside shoulder pad should cover the tip of the shoulder in a direct line with the lateral aspect of the shoulder.
- The epaulets and cups should cover the deltoid muscle and allow movements required by the athlete's specific position.
- The neck opening must allow the athlete to raise the arm over the head without placing undue pressure on the neck yet must not allow the pad to slide back and forth.
- If a split-clavicle shoulder pad is used, the channel for the top of the shoulder must be in the proper position.
- Straps underneath the arm must hold the pads firmly in place, but not so they constrict soft tissue. A collar and drop-down pads may be added to provide additional protection.
- After fitting, have the athlete put the jersey on and make sure pads don't shift.

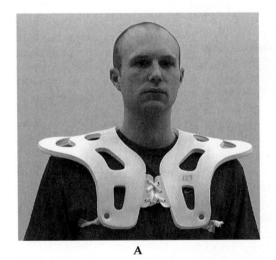

A

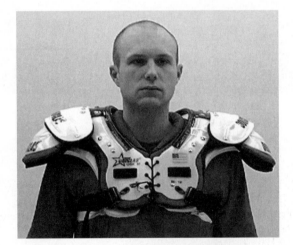

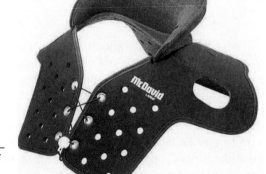

B

**Figure 6-16**

(A) Customized foam is placed on the underside of the shoulder pad to provide additional protection.

(B) Cowboy collar can be attached to the shoulder pad.

## Sports Bras

Manufacturers have made significant efforts to develop athletic support bras for women who participate in all types of physical activity.[8] In the past, the primary concern was for breast protection against external forces that could cause bruising. Most sports bras are now designed to minimize excessive vertical and horizontal movements of the breasts that occur with running and jumping.[22] Several styles of sports bras are now available.[31]

1. For women with smaller breasts it is not as critical to provide compression or support and thus a less elastic *lightweight* bra is sufficient (Figure 6-17A).

2. A *compressive bra* is perhaps the most common and is recommended for women with medium size breasts. Compressive bras function like wide elastic bandages, binding the breasts to the chest wall (Figure 6-17B).

3. *Support bras* are a bit more heavy duty and provide good upward support with elastic material. They tend to have wide bands under the breasts with wide shoulder straps in the back. They are designed for women with larger breasts (Figure 6-17C).

In contact sports additional padding may be placed inside the cup if needed. Women competing in ice hockey, for example, wear protective plastic chest pieces that attach to their shoulder pads to protect the breast tissue from contusions (Figure 6-17D).

## Rib Protection

Several manufacturers provide off-the-shelf pads for rib protection. Many of the rib protectors and rib belts can be modified, replacing stock

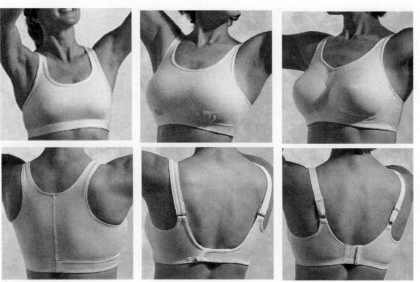
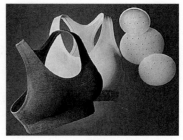

**Figure 6-17**

Sports bras. (A) Lightweight pullover bra. (B) Compressive bra. (C) Support bra with underwire. (D) Protective sports bra with cup inserts.

A          B          C          D

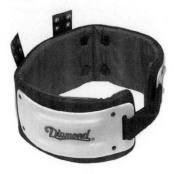

**Figure 6-18**

**Protective rib belt**

pads with customized thermomoldable plastic protective devices[17] (Figure 6-18). Recently many lightweight pads have been developed to protect the athlete against external forces. A jacket for the protection of a rib injury incorporates a pad composed of air-inflated, interconnected cylinders that protect against severe external forces. This same principle has been used in the development of other protective pads. Chest protection should be worn by baseball batters in the preadolescent age group.

### Hips and Buttocks

Pads in the region of the hips and buttocks are often needed by athletes in collision and high-velocity sports such as hockey and football. Other athletes needing protection in this region are amateur boxers, snow skiers, equestrians, jockeys, and water skiers. Two popular commercial pads are the girdle and belt types (Figure 6-19).

### Groin and Genitalia

Sports involving high-velocity projectiles (e.g., hockey, lacrosse, and baseball) require cup protection for male participants. The cup comes as a stock item that fits into place in a jockstrap or athletic supporter (Figure 6-20).

**Figure 6-19**

**Girdle-style hip and coccygeal pads**

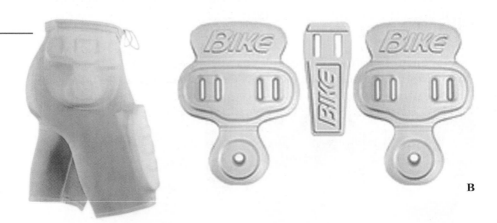

A

B

**Figure 6-20**

A cup, held in place by an athletic supporter, used for protecting the genitals against high-velocity projectiles.

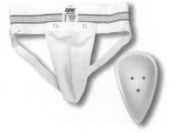

# LOWER EXTREMITY PROTECTIVE EQUIPMENT

## Footwear

It is essential that the coach and equipment personnel make every effort to select and fit their athletes with proper shoes and socks (Figure 6-21).

### Socks

Poorly fitted socks can create a variety of problems for the foot. For example, socks that are too short apply excessive pressure to the fourth and fifth toes. Socks that are too long can cause skin irritation because of wrinkles. All socks should be clean, dry, and without holes to avoid irritations. Manufacturers provide double-knit tubular socks without heels that decrease friction considerably within the shoe. The heelless tubular sock is especially good for the basketball player. The sock's material also should be considered. Cotton socks can be too bulky; a combination of materials such as cotton and some lightweight synthetic material is less bulky and dries faster.

All athletic socks should be clean and dry and without holes. Socks of the wrong size can irritate the skin.

### Shoe Selection

The athletic and fitness shoe manufacturing industry has become extremely sophisticated and offers a number of options when it comes to purchasing shoes for different activities.[14,15,33,34] Figure 6-21 shows the

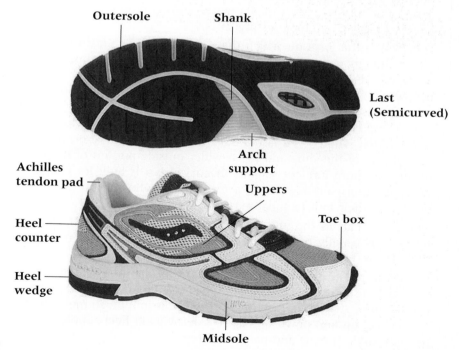

**Figure 6-21**

**Parts of a well-designed sports shoe**

major parts of a shoe. The following guidelines can help in selecting the
most appropriate shoe:[12]

- *Toe box.* There should be plenty of room for the toes in the fitness
  shoe. Most experts recommend a ½- to ¾-inch distance between the
  longest toe and the front of the shoe. A few fitness shoes are made
  in varying widths. If an athlete has a very wide or narrow foot,
  most shoe salespersons can recommend a specific shoe for that foot.
  The best way to make sure there is adequate room in the toe box is
  to have the foot measured and then try on the shoe.

- *Sole.* The sole should possess two qualities. First, it must provide a
  shock absorptive function; second, it must be durable. Most shoes
  have three layers on the sole: a thick spongy layer, which absorbs
  the force of the foot strike under the heel; a midsole, which
  cushions the midfoot and toes; and a hard rubber layer, which
  comes in contact with the ground. The average runner's feet strike
  the ground between 1,500 and 1,700 times per mile. Thus it is
  essential that the force of the heel strike be absorbed by the
  spongy layer to prevent overuse injuries from occurring in the
  ankles and knees. "Heel wedges" are sometimes inserted on either
  the inside or outside surface of the sole underneath the heel
  counter to accommodate and correct for various structural
  deformities of the foot that may alter normal biomechanics of the
  running gait. A flared heel may be appropriate for running shoes
  but is not recommended in aerobic or court shoes. The sole must
  provide good traction and must be made of a tough material that
  is resistant to wear. Most of the better-known brands of shoes
  have well-designed, long-lasting soles.

- *Last.* This is the form on which the shoe is built. The last may be
  either straight, semicurved, or curved. A straight lasted shoe is filled
  in on the inside/medial side of the shoe to increase stability for
  people who have a flat arch or run on the inside of their foot
  (pronators). A semicurved last is designed for the average or normal
  foot. There is a small curve on the medial side of the foot to fit a
  normal arch. The curved last is built with a larger curve on the
  medial side of the shoe and has a wider outside portion of the shoe
  to provide more forefoot stability. A curved last is built for people
  with an abnormally high arch or for runners who run on the
  outside of their foot (supinators).

- *Shank.* The part of the sole between the heel and the metatarsal
  heads. It is usually reinforced with material of sufficient density to
  support the weight of the wearer.

- *Heel counters.* The heel counter is the portion of the shoe that
  prevents the foot from rolling from side to side at heel strike. The
  heel counter should be firm but well fitted to minimize movement
  of the heel up and down or side to side. A good heel counter may
  prevent ankle sprains and painful blisters.

- *Shoe uppers.* The upper part of the shoe is made of some combination of nylon and leather. The uppers should be lightweight, quick drying, and well ventilated. The uppers should have some type of extra support in the saddle area, and there should be some extra padding in the area of the Achilles tendon just above the heel counter.

- *Arch support.* The arch support should be made of some durable yet soft supportive material and should smoothly join with the insole. The support should not have any rough seams or ridges inside the shoe, which may cause blisters.

**Shoe fitting** Fitting sports footgear is always difficult, mainly because the individual's left foot varies in size and shape from the right foot. Therefore measuring both feet is imperative. To fit the sports shoe properly, the athlete should approximate the conditions under which he or she will perform, such as wearing athletic socks, jumping up and down, and running. It is also desirable to fit the athlete's shoes at the end of the day to accommodate the gradual increase in size that occurs from the time of awakening. The athlete must carefully consider this choice because he or she will be spending countless hours in those shoes (Table 6-1).[1]

During performance conditions the new shoe should feel snug but not too tight.[11] The sports shoe should be long enough that all toes can be fully extended without being cramped. Its width should permit full movement of the toes, including flexion, extension, and some spreading. A good point to remember is that the wide part of the shoe should match the wide part of the foot to allow the shoe to crease evenly when the athlete is on the balls of the feet. The shoe should bend (or "break") at its widest part generally at the metatarsal head (ball) of the foot;

*A properly fitted shoe will bend where the foot bends.*

---

**TABLE 6-1** Shoe comparisons

|  | Tennis | Aerobic | Running |
|---|---|---|---|
| Flexibility | Firm sole, more rigid than running shoe | Sole between running and tennis shoe | Flexible ball of foot |
| Uppers | Leather or leather with nylon | Leather or leather with nylon | Nylon or nylon mesh |
| Heel flare | None | Very little | Flared for stability |
| Cushioning | Less than a running shoe | Between running and tennis shoe | Heel and sole well padded |
| Soles (Last) | Polyurethane | Rubber or polyurethane | Carbon-based material for greater durability |
| Tread | Flattened | Flat or pivot dot | Deep grooves for grip |

when the break of the shoe and the ball joint coincide, the fit is correct. However, if the break of the shoe is in back or in front of the normal bend of the foot (metatarsophalangeal joint), the shoe and the foot will be opposing one another, causing abnormal skin and structural stresses to occur. Two measurements must be considered when fitting shoes: (1) the distance from the heel to the bend in the foot and (2) the distance from the heel to the end of the longest toe. An individual's feet may be equal in length from the heels to the balls of the feet but different between heels and toes. Shoes, therefore, should be selected for the longer of the two measurements. Other factors to consider when buying the sports shoe are the stiffness of the sole and the width of the shank, or narrowest part of the sole. A shoe with a too rigid, nonyielding sole places a great deal of extra strain on the foot tendons. A shoe with too narrow a shank also causes extra strain because it fails to adequately support the athlete's inner, longitudinal arches. Two other shoe features to consider are innersoles to reduce friction and built-in arch supports.[11]

**Price** Unfortunately, in many instances price is the primary consideration in buying athletic shoes. When buying athletic shoes, remember that in many activities shoes are important for performance and prevention of injury. Thus it is worth a little extra investment to buy a quality pair of shoes.

**The specialty soled shoe** The cleated or specialty soled sports shoe presents some additional problems in selection. For example, American football shoes use the multi-short-and-cleated polyurethane sole and often use a five-in-front-and-two-in-back cleat arrangement that is common with the soccer-type sole. Both football and soccer shoes have cleats no longer than ½ inch (1.27 cm) (Figure 6-22). Special-soled shoes are also worn when playing on a synthetic surface. If cleated shoes are used, no matter what the sport, the cleats must be properly positioned under the two major weight-bearing joints and must not be felt through the soles of the shoes.

### Using Orthotics

An orthotic is a device for correcting biomechanical problems that exist in the foot that can potentially cause an injury.[30] The orthotic is a plastic, thermoplastic, rubber, sorbethane, or leather support that is placed in the shoe as a replacement for the existing insole.[21] Ready-made orthotics can be purchased in sporting goods or shoe stores. Some athletes need orthotics that are custom made by a physician, podiatrist, athletic trainer, or physical therapist. These are more expensive but can be well worth the expense if the athlete's feet cause pain and discomfort, especially when exercising (Figure 6-23).

### Heel Cups

Heel cups should be used for a variety of conditions including plantar fasciitis, a heel spur, Achilles tendonitis, and heel bursitis (Figure 6-24).

**6-3 Critical Thinking**
Exercise

A high school basketball player is given advice on purchasing a pair of basketball shoes.

? What fitting factors must be taken into consideration when purchasing basketball shoes?

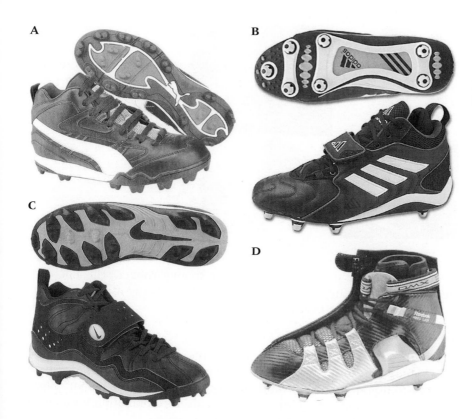

**Figure 6-22**

Variations in cleated shoes—the longer the cleat, the higher the incidence of injury.

A

B

C

D

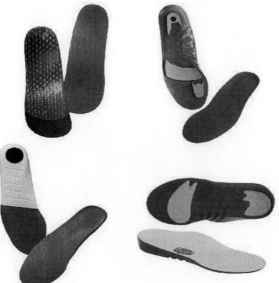

**Figure 6-23**

**Commercially manufactured orthotic devices**

**Figure 6-24**

**Different styles of heel cups.**

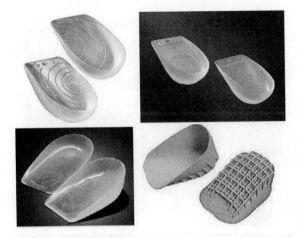

Heel cups may be either hard plastic or spongy rubber. The heel cup helps to compress the fat pad under the heel, providing more heel cushioning during weight-bearing activities.

## Commercial Ankle Supports

Currently, semirigid ankle braces such as the Air Stirrup are being used successfully to restrain ankle motion. Compared with ankle taping, these devices do not loosen significantly during exercise (Figure 6-25).[6] Commercial ankle stabilizers, used either alone or in combination with ankle taping, are becoming increasingly popular in sports.[13,19]

## Shin and Lower Leg Protection

The shin is commonly neglected in contact and collision sports. Commercially marketed hard-shelled, molded shin guards are used in field hockey and soccer (Figure 6-26). Some shin guards can now be customized by placing the guard in hot water and molding it to the shin. Athletes should not try to cut the shin guards down to make them smaller.

**Figure 6-25**

Commercial ankle supports for an injured ankle. (A) Lace-up brace. (B) Lace-up with straps brace. (C) Rigid support brace.

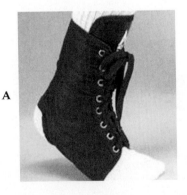

A

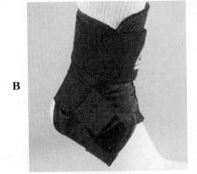

B

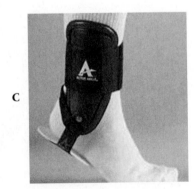

C

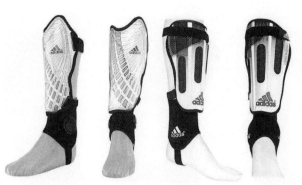

**Figure 6-26**

**Soccer shin guards**

## Thigh and Upper Leg Protection

Thigh and upper leg protection is necessary in collision sports such as football, soccer, and hockey. Generally, pads slip into ready-made pockets in the uniform (Figure 6-27). In some instances customized pads should be constructed and held in place with tape or an elastic wrap. Neoprene sleeves can be used for support following strain to the quadriceps, hamstrings, or groin muscles (Figure 6-28).[5]

## Knee Braces

Because of the high incidence of injury to the knee joint, manufacturers have designed a host of different knee braces for a variety of purposes. *Protective knee braces* are used prophylactically to prevent injuries to the medial collateral ligament in contact sports such as football (Figure 6-29A).[25,32] Although these protective braces have been widely used in the past, the American Orthopedic Society for Sports

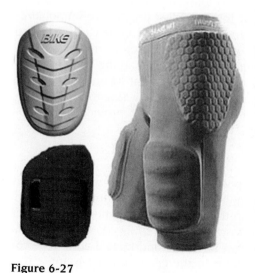

**Figure 6-27**

**Protective thigh pads**

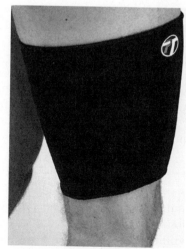

**Figure 6-28**

**Neoprene thigh sleeve for muscle strains**

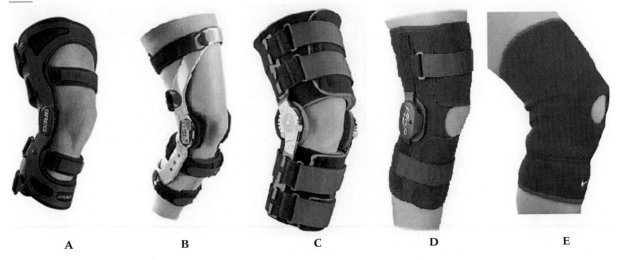

| A | B | C | D | E |

**Figure 6-29**

Knee braces. (A) Prophylactic knee brace. (B) Functional brace. (C) Rehabilitative brace. (D) Neoprene with medial support-brace. (E) Neoprene brace.

Medicine has expressed concern about their efficacy in reducing injuries to the collateral ligaments. Several studies have actually shown an increase in the incidence of injuries to the medial collateral ligament in athletes wearing these braces.[25]

*Functional knee braces* may be worn both during and following the rehabilitative period to provide support during functional activities (Figure 6-29B).[9,29] Functional braces can be purchased ready made or can be custom made. Some physicians strongly recommend that their patients consistently wear these braces during physical activity whereas others do not feel that they are necessary.[7,35]

*Rehabilitative braces* are widely used following surgical repair or reconstruction of the knee joint to allow for controlled progressive immobilization (Figure 6-29C). These braces have hinges that can be easily adjusted to allow range of motion to be progressively increased over time.

*Neoprene braces with medial and lateral supports* may be used by individuals who have sustained injury to the collateral ligaments and feel that they need extra support medially and laterally (Figure 6-29D).

A variety of *neoprene sleeves* may also be used to provide some support for patellofemoral conditions (Figure 6-29E).[5]

## ELBOW, WRIST, AND HAND PROTECTION

As with the lower extremity, the upper extremity requires protection from injury and prevention of further injury after trauma. Although the elbow joint is less commonly injured than the ankle, knee, or shoulder, it is still vulnerable to instability, contusion, and muscle strain. A variety of off-the-shelf protective neoprene sleeves and pads and hinged adjustable rehabilitative braces can offer protection to the elbow (Figure 6-30).

In sports medicine, injuries to the wrist, hand, and fingers are often trivialized and considered insignificant. But injuries to the distal aspect of the upper extremity can be functionally disabling, especially in those

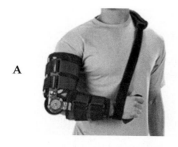

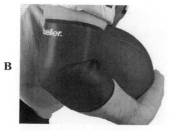

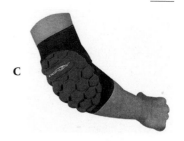

**Figure 6-30**

Elbow braces and supports. (A) Rehabilitation elbow brace. (B) Neoprene elbow sleeve. (C) Elbow pad.

sports that involve throwing and catching. In both contact and non-contact sport activities the wrist, hand, and particularly the fingers are susceptible to fracture, dislocation, ligament sprains, and muscle strains. Protective gloves are essential in preventing injuries in sports like lacrosse and ice hockey (Figure 6-31). It is also common to use both off-the-shelf and custom-molded splints both for support and to immobilize an injury (Figure 6-32).

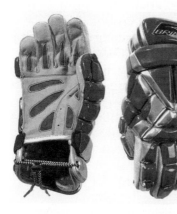

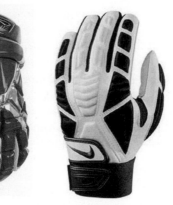

**Figure 6-31**

Hand protection is essential in lacrosse and ice hockey.

**Figure 6-32**

Wrist supports. (A) Off-the-shelf neoprene wrist support. (B) and (C) Custom molded wrist and thumb splints.

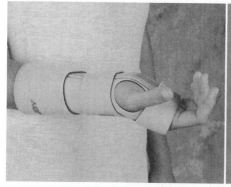

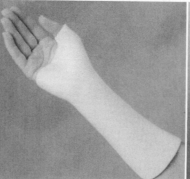

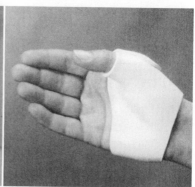

A

B

C

## Athletic Injury Management Checklist

The following checklist contains factors that must be considered when selecting, purchasing, and fitting athletic equipment to help minimize liability.

- ☐ Buy sports equipment from reputable manufacturers.
- ☐ Buy the safest equipment that resources will permit.
- ☐ Make sure that all equipment is assembled correctly.
- ☐ Ensure that the person who assembles equipment is competent to do so and follows the manufacturer's instructions to the letter.
- ☐ Maintain all equipment properly, according to the manufacturer's guidelines.
- ☐ Use equipment only for the purpose for which it was designed.
- ☐ If an athlete is wearing some type of immobilization device (i.e., cast, brace), make certain that this does not violate the rules of that sport.[20]
- ☐ Warn athletes who use the equipment about all possible risks that using the equipment could entail.
- ☐ Use great caution in the construction or customizing of any piece of equipment.
- ☐ Use no defective equipment.
- ☐ Routinely inspect all equipment for defects, and render all defective equipment unusable.

## SUMMARY

- The proper selection and fitting of sports equipment are essential in the prevention of many sports injuries.
- Because of the current number of lawsuits, both durability of material and fit and wear requirements must meet sports equipment standards.
- Manufacturers must foresee all the possible uses and misuses of their equipment and warn the user of any potential risks.
- Head protection in many collision and contact sports is of particular concern: The helmet must be used as intended and not as a weapon; proper fit is also a requirement.
- A warning label on the outside of the helmet must indicate that it is not fail-safe, and the helmet must be used as intended.
- Face protection is of major importance in sports that have fast-moving projectiles, that use implements that come in close proximity to other athletes, and that are characterized by body collisions.
- The customized mouth guard, fitted to individual requirements, provides the best protection for the teeth and also helps protect against concussions.

- Eyes must be protected against projectiles and sports implements.
- The safest eye guard for the athlete not wearing glasses is the closed type that completely protects the orbital cavity.
- Many sports require protection of various parts of the athlete's body. American football players, ice hockey players, and baseball/softball catchers are examples of players who require body protection.
- Socks must be clean, without holes, and made of appropriate materials.
- Shoes must be suited to the sport and must be fitted to the larger foot; the wide part of the foot must match the wide part of the shoe; if the shoe has cleats, they must be positioned at the metatarsophalangeal joints.
- The hand, wrist, and elbow are also vulnerable to sports trauma and require special protective devices.

### *Solutions to Critical Thinking* Exercises

**6-1** The following steps should be taken:

1. A team meeting is called in which the risks entailed in the use and fitting of the equipment are fully explained.
2. A defective piece of equipment must be immediately reported and repaired.
3. A letter is sent out to each parent or guardian explaining equipment limitations. This letter is signed and returned to the athletic trainer.
4. A meeting of parents, team members, and coaches is called to further explain equipment limitations.

**6-2** It must be explained that the helmet cannot prevent serious neck injuries. Striking an opponent with any part of the helmet or face mask can place abnormal stress on cervical structures. Most severe neck injuries occur from striking an opponent with the top of the helmet; this action is known as axial loading.

**6-3** The following points should be emphasized.

- Purchase shoes to fit the large foot.
- Fit shoes wearing athletic socks.
- Purchase shoes at the end of the day.
- Each foot is measured from the heel to the end of the largest toe.
- Shoes feel snug but comfortable when jumping up and down and performing cutting motions.
- Shoe length and width allow full toe function.
- Wide part of foot matches the wide part of the shoe.
- Shoe bends at widest part of shoe.

## REVIEW QUESTIONS AND CLASS ACTIVITIES

1. What are the legal responsibilities in terms of protective equipment?
2. Invite an attorney to class to discuss product liability.
3. What are the various sports with high-risk factors that require protective equipment?
4. How can safety equipment be selected and used to decrease the possibility of sports injuries and litigation?
5. Why is continual inspection and/or replacement of used equipment important?

6. What are the standards for fitting football helmets? Are there standards for any other helmets?
7. Invite your school equipment manager to class to demonstrate all the protective equipment and how to fit it to the athlete.
8. Why are mouth guards important, and what are the advantages of custom-made mouth guards over the stock type?
9. What are the advantages and disadvantages of glasses and contact lenses in athletic competition?
10. How do you fit shoulder pads for different-sized players and their positions?
11. Why is breast protection necessary? Which types of sport bras are available and what should the athlete look for when purchasing one?
12. How do you properly fit shoes? What type of shoes should you use for various sports and different floor and field surfaces?
13. What types of knee braces are on the market today? Do they provide adequate support and protection from injury?

## REFERENCES

1. AAPSM running shoes recommendations: 2005. *American Academy of Podiatric Sports Medicine newsletter* (Rockville, Md.), March p. 4.
2. Amis T et al.: 2000. Influence of intraoral maxillary sports mouthguards on the airflow dynamics of oral breathing, *Med Sci Sports Exerc* 32(2):284.
3. Athletic equipment, *Athletic business* (Madison, Wis), Feb 2003:27 (2). P. 206;211–222.
4. Banky J: 1999. Mouthguards and dental injury: an update, *Sports Coach* 22(3):30.
5. Birmingham TB, Inglis JT, Kramer JF: 2000. Effect of a neoprene sleeve on knee joint kinesthesis: influence of different testing procedures, *Med Sci Sports Exerc* 32(2):304.
6. Bot SDM, van Mechelen W: 1999. The effect of ankle bracing on athletic performance, *Sports Med* 27(3): 171.
7. Brownstein B: 1998. Migration and design characteristics of functional knee braces, *J Sport Rehab* 7(1):33.
8. Breast support for female athletes. 2002. *Sport research review/NIKE sport research review* 1:1–14.
9. Chew, K T, Lew, H: 2007. Current evidence and clinical applications of therapeutic knee braces. American journal of physical medicine & rehabilitation 86(8):678–686.
10. Collins, K: 2007. Equipping the high school football player. *Hughston health alert* 19(4):1.
11. Cuddy S: 1998. The right running shoe: the first step in avoiding running injuries, *Sports Med Update* 13(3): 8.
12. Denton, J: 2008. Ch-ch-changes: the evolution of running shoes. *Running times* 360(1):82.
13. Fiolkowski P: 1998. Considerations in the use of ankle braces, *Ath Ther Today* 3(4):38.
14. Hamilton, A: 2008. Running shoe choice and foot loading during running. *Peak performance* 259(1):11.
15. How to buy athletic shoes: 2003. *Sports Medicine Australia: a resource book for the professional enthusiast*, (1):47–49.
16. International Federation of Medicine: 1999. Position statement: eye injuries and eye protection in sports, *Ath Ther Today* 4(5):6.
17. Labella, CR, Smith, BW, Sigurdsson, A: 2002. Effect of mouthguards

on dental injuries and concussions in college basketball, *Medicine and science in sports and exercise* 34(1): 41–44.

18. Mazzola G: 1998. At your service: reconditioning your football helmets, *Coach Ath Dir* 68(4):40.

19. Mogolov, R: 2007. Ankle brace improvements pay off for athletes. *Training & conditioning* 17(7):48.

20. Newell, K: 2004. Well equipped: innovation that every football program needs, *Coach and athletic director* (Jefferson City, Mo.), March 73 (8):60–62.

21. Nigg BM, Nurse MA, Stefanyshyn DJ: 1999. Shoe inserts and orthotics for sport and physical activities, *Med Sci Sports Exerc* 31(7 suppl):S421.

22. Page KA, Steele JR: 1999. Breast motion and sports brassiere design: implications for future research, *Sports Med* 27(4):205.

23. Peterson, L, Renstrom, P: 2001. Sports and protective equipment. In Peterson, L (ed), *Sports injuries: their prevention and treatment*, 3rd ed, Champaign, IL, Human Kinetics, pp. 79–89.

24. Rules and equipment: 2001. In *Coaching youth football*, 3rd ed, Champaign, IL, Human Kinetics, 63–90.

25. Sauers EL, Harter RA: 1998. Efficacy of prophylactic knee braces: current research perspectives, *Ath Ther Today* 3(4):14, 1998.

26. Steinbach, P: 2002. Armor for all. With player safety paramount, the purchasing of football equipment must ensure adequate supply and proper fit of helmets, shoes and everything in between. *Athletic business* 26(8): 96–98; 100; 102.

27. Steinbach, P: Head and shoulders: injury prevention, *Athletic business* 28(3):10, 2004.

28. Street S, Runkle D: 1999. *Athletic protective equipment: care, selection, and fitting*, Boston, McGraw-Hill.

29. Styf J: 1999. The effects of functional knee bracing on muscle function and performance, *Sports Med* 28(2):77.

30. Swanik CB: 2000. Orthotics in sports medicine, *Ath Ther Today* 5(1):5.

31. The best new sports bras: 2008. *Shape* 27(7):124.

32. Walters, R: 2007. The evolution of prophylactic knee bracing in sports, *Coach & Athletic Director* 76(10):66.

33. Werd, M: 2002. Shoe recommendation listing, *American Academy of Podiatric Sports Medicine newsletter*, Spring 9.

34. Wischnia B, Carrozza P: 2000. Spring 2000 shoe buyer's guide, *Runner's World* 35(3):37.

35. Wojtys, EM, Huston, LJ: 2000. Functional knee braces—the 25-year controversy. In Chan, KM (ed), *Controversies in orthopedic sports medicine*, Champaign, IL, Human Kinetics, 106–118.

36. Yang, J, Bowling, M: 2005. Use of discretionary protective equipment in high school athletes: prevalence and determinants. *American journal of public health* 95 (11):1996.

## ANNOTATED BIBLIOGRAPHY

Street S, Runkle D: 1999 *Athletic protective equipment: care, selection, and fitting*, Boston, McGraw-Hill.

*This reference book provides an overview of available athletic equipment and its usage. The text is a resource for athletic trainers, coaches, and physical education teachers.*

Techniques for Preventing
and Minimizing Sport-
Related Injuries

## WEB SITES

Riddell: http://riddell.com
*Riddell is an equipment manufacturing company, and this site gives information about the safety of the products they sell and the necessary standards for safety equipment.*

The Training Room:
www.thetrainingroom.com
*Sports orthopedic braces, orthotics, protective sports equipment, and athletic injury treatment.*

National Operating Committee on Standards for Athletic Equipment:
www.nocsae.org
*Provides detailed information and recommendations on the appropriate use and maintenance of different types of athletic equipment.*

Road Runner Sports:
www.roadrunnersports.com
*Provides good information for fitting shoes, sports bras, and running apparel.*

Douglas Protective Equipment:
www.douglaspads.com
*Manufacturer and distributor of football, hockey, and baseball protective padding. Custom fitting players at all levels for over 12 years.*

Protective Eyewear for Young Athletes
www.kidsource.com/kidsource/content/eyewear.html
*A joint statement of the American Academy of Pediatrics and American Academy of Ophthalmology.*

# Handling Emergency Situations and Injury Assessment

## CHAPTER 7

*When you finish this chapter you will be able to:*

- Establish a plan for handling emergency situations at your institution.
- Explain the importance of knowing cardiopulmonary resuscitation (CPR) and how to manage an obstructed airway.
- Describe techniques for control of hemorrhage.
- Assess the types of shock and their management.
- Describe the various phases of injury assessment.
- Explain the importance of controlling swelling during initial injury management.
- Describe techniques for moving and transporting the injured athlete.

Most sports injuries do not result in life-or-death emergency situations, but when such situations do arise, prompt care is essential.[6] Time becomes the critical factor, and assistance to the injured athlete must be based on knowledge of what to do and how to do it—how to perform effective first aid immediately.[22] There is no room for uncertainty, indecision, or error. A mistake in the initial management of injury can prolong the time required for rehabilitation and can potentially create a life-threatening situation for the athlete.[7] Therefore it is critical to be well prepared to handle whatever emergency situation may arise.[23]

It must be reemphasized that **all fitness professionals, coaches, and others in areas related to exercise and sport science should be trained and certified in cardiopulmonary resuscitation (CPR), the use of an automatic external defibrillator (AED), and first aid.** However, these individuals are limited beyond providing initial CPR/AED and first aid. The extent of what they can and cannot do legally is determined by the laws and statutes of different states. Much of the information contained in this chapter is intended for informational purposes only and is in no way meant to encourage individuals to act outside of the scope of their responsibilities.[13]

*Time becomes critical in an emergency situation.*

## THE EMERGENCY ACTION PLAN

The prime concern of emergency aid is to maintain cardiovascular function and, indirectly, central nervous system function, because failure of any of these systems may lead to death.[7] The key to emergency aid in

Techniques for Preventing
and Minimizing Sport-
Related Injuries

the sports setting is the initial evaluation of the injured athlete. Time is of the essence, so this evaluation must be done rapidly and accurately so that proper aid can be rendered without delay. In some instances these first steps not only will be lifesaving but also may determine the degree and extent of permanent disability.

As discussed in Chapter 1, the sports medicine team—the coach, the athletic trainer, and the team physician—must at all times act reasonably and prudently. This behavior is especially important during emergencies.

All sports programs must have a prearranged emergency action plan (EAP) that can be implemented immediately when necessary.[4,26] (See Focus Box 2-5 on page 29.) The following issues must be addressed when developing the emergency action plan:

All sports programs must
have an emergency action
plan.

1. Develop separate emergency action plans for each sport's field, courts, or gymnasiums[12] (see Focus Box 2-5: "Sample Emergency Action Plan").
   a. Determine the personnel who will be on the field during practices and competitions (e.g., athletic trainers, athletic training students, physicians, emergency medical technicians, rescue squad). Each person should understand exactly what his or her role and responsibility is if an emergency occurs. It is also recommended that the sports medicine team practice the use and operation of emergency equipment, such as stretchers and automatic external defibrillators (AED).[14] Everyone involved should know the location of the nearest AED.
   b. Decide what emergency equipment should be available for each sport. The emergency equipment needs for football will likely be different from those of the cross-country team.
2. Establish specific procedures and policies regarding the removal of protective equipment, particularly the helmet and shoulder pads. These procedures will be discussed later in this chapter.[22]
3. Make sure phones are readily accessible. Cellular or digital phones are recommended. However, a land line should also be readily available in case cell phone service is not available. If cellular phones are not available, all staff personnel and athletes should know the location of the telephone; phones should be clearly marked. Use 911 if available, but realize that in some areas all service is not accessible by cellular phones and thus land lines should be used to access the emergency medical system. Occasionally, calls made on cell phones may be redirected out of the local area. Thus it is critical to ask what area the local 911 call has been directed to.

4. All staff should be familiar with the community-based emergency health care delivery plan, including existing communication and transportation policies.[12] It is also critical to be familiar with emergency care facility admission and treatment policies, particularly when rendering emergency care to a minor. Someone should specifically be designated to make an emergency phone call. Most emergency medical systems can be accessed by dialing 911, which connects the caller to a dispatcher who has access to rescue squad, police, and fire personnel. The person making the emergency phone call must provide the following information:
   a. Type of emergency situation
   b. Type of suspected injury
   c. Present condition of the athlete
   d. Current assistance being given (e.g., cardiopulmonary resuscitation)
   e. Location of telephone being used
   f. Exact location of emergency (give names of streets and cross streets) and how to enter facility

5. Make sure keys to gates or padlocks are easily accessible. Staff members should have the appropriate keys.

6. Inform all staff and maintenance personnel of the emergency plan at a meeting held annually before the beginning of the school year. Each individual must know his or her responsibilities should an emergency occur.

7. Assign someone to accompany the injured athlete to the hospital.

8. Carry contact information for all athletes, coaches, and other personnel at all times, particularly when traveling. For minors, consent forms should also be available when traveling.

9. In certain situations at both high schools and colleges, staff members may be called upon to provide emergency services not only to athletes but also to coaches, referees, and in some cases parents and other spectators who may develop an emergent condition during the course of an athletic event. The emergency action plan should include plans for managing these situations with the help of emergency medical services and other local health care providers.[26]

## Cooperation between Emergency Care Providers

Individuals providing emergency care to the injured athlete must cooperate and act professionally. Too often, the rescue squad personnel, a physician, an athletic trainer, or a coach disagree over exactly how the injured athlete should be handled and transported. The coach or athletic trainer is usually the first individual to deal with the emergency situation. The athletic trainer has generally had more training and experience in moving and transporting an injured athlete than the physician has. **If an athletic trainer or physician is not available, the rescue squad should be called to handle an emergency situation.** If the rescue squad is called and responds, the emergency medical technicians (EMTs) should have the final say on how the athlete is to be transported.

To alleviate potential conflicts, it is a good idea to establish procedures and guidelines and to arrange practice sessions at least once a year with all parties concerned for handling the injured athlete. The rescue squad may not be experienced in dealing with someone who is wearing a helmet or other protective equipment. Before an incident occurs the EMTs should understand how athletes wearing various types of athletic equipment should be managed. When dealing with the injured athlete, all egos should be put aside. Certainly the most important consideration is what is the best for the athlete.

### Parent Notification

According to HIPAA regulations discussed in Chapter 2, if the injured athlete is a minor, it is essential that actual consent to treat the athlete be obtained from the parent. **Actual consent may be given in writing either before or during an emergency.** Actual consent is notification that the parent has been informed about what medical personnel thinks is wrong and what that person intends to do, and parental permission is granted to give treatment for a specific incident. If the athlete's parents cannot be contacted, then the predetermined wishes of the parent given at the beginning of a season or school year can be acted upon. If there is no informed consent, then implied consent on the part of the athlete to save his or her life takes precedence. Focus Box 7-1 provides an example of a parental consent form for medical treatment of a minor.

### PRINCIPLES OF ON-THE-FIELD INJURY ASSESSMENT

Appropriate medical care cannot be delivered to the injured athlete until some systematic assessment of the situation has been made. This assessment (Figure 7-1) helps to determine the nature of the injury and

---

**7-1** ❯ *Focus Box*

**Consent Form for Medical Treatment of a Minor**

By this signature, I hereby consent to allow the physician(s) and other health care provider(s) selected by myself or the school to perform a preparticipation examination on my child and to provide treatment for any injury or condition resulting from participating in athletics and activities for his or her school during the school year covered by this form. I further consent to allow said physician(s) or health care provider(s) to share appropriate information concerning my child that is relevant to participation in athletics and activities with coaches and other school personnel as deemed necessary.

_____          _____
Parent or Guardian                                              Date

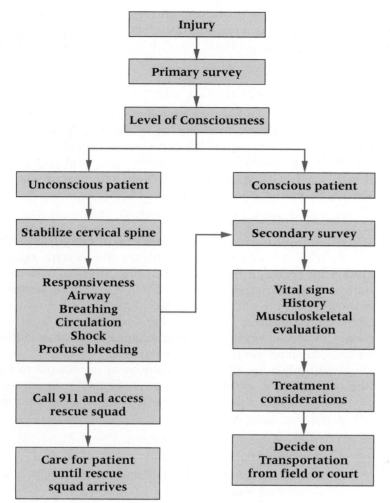

**Figure 7-1**

**Flowchart showing the appropriate emergency procedures for the injured patient**

provides direction in the decision-making process concerning the emergency care that must be rendered.[8] The ***primary survey*** refers to assessment of potentially life-threatening problems including airway, breathing, circulation, severe bleeding, or shock. It takes precedence over all other aspects of victim assessment and should be used to correct life-threatening situations.[24] Once the condition of the victim is stabilized, the ***secondary survey*** is used to take a closer look at the injury sustained by the athlete. The secondary survey gathers specific information about the injury from the athlete, systematically assesses vital signs and symptoms, and allows for a more detailed evaluation of the injury. The secondary survey is done to uncover additional problems in other parts of the body not necessarily associated with the injury, which do not pose an immediate threat to life but which may do so if they remain uncorrected.[24]

An injured athlete who is conscious and stable does not require a primary survey. However, the unconscious athlete must be monitored for life-threatening problems throughout the assessment process.

## PRIMARY SURVEY

### Treatment of Life-Threatening Injuries

Life-threatening injuries take precedence over all other injuries sustained by the athlete. Situations that are considered life threatening include those that require CPR (i.e., obstruction of the airway, no breathing, no circulation), profuse bleeding, and shock. **Whenever there is a life-threatening situation, the rescue squad should always be called by dialing 911.**

### The Unconscious Athlete

The state of unconsciousness provides one of the greatest dilemmas in sports. **With an unconscious athlete, the rescue squad should always be accessed by dialing 911, regardless of whether the situation is life threatening.** Unconsciousness may be defined as a state of insensibility in which there is a lack of conscious awareness. This condition can be brought about by a blow to either the head or the solar plexus, or it may result from general shock. It is often difficult to determine the exact cause of unconsciousness.

The unconscious athlete must always be considered to have a life-threatening injury, which requires an immediate primary survey. Here are guidelines that should be followed when dealing with the unconscious athlete:

1. The body position should be noted immediately and the level of consciousness and responsiveness determined.
2. Airway, breathing, and circulation should routinely be established immediately.
3. Injury to the neck and spine is always a possibility in the unconscious athlete.
4. If the athlete is wearing a helmet, it should never be removed until neck and spine injury have been unequivocally ruled out. However, the face mask must be immediately cut away and removed to allow for CPR.
5. If the athlete is supine and not breathing, establish airway, breathing, and circulation (ABC) immediately.
6. If the athlete is supine and breathing, do nothing until consciousness returns.
7. If the athlete is prone and not breathing, logroll him or her carefully to supine position and begin CPR immediately.
8. If the athlete is prone and breathing, do nothing until consciousness returns, and wait for the rescue squad.
9. Monitor and maintain life support for the unconscious athlete until emergency medical personnel arrive.

## Overview of Emergency Cardiopulmonary Resuscitation (CPR)

It is essential that a careful evaluation of the injured athlete be made to determine whether CPR should be conducted. **(The following is an overview of CPR and is intended only for those individuals who are certified in CPR.)** It should also be noted that, because of the serious nature of CPR, updates should routinely be studied through courses offered by the American Red Cross, the American Heart Association, or the National Safety Council. The techniques presented are recommended for both an adult and a child (ages 1–12) (Figure 7-2). The sequence of both adult and child CPR is the same. However, there are minor differences in the specific techniques, which will be identified throughout the following section.

Anyone providing care in an emergency situation that will require CPR should be aware that the Good Samaritan laws were enacted to give legal protection to individuals who willingly provide emergency care to an injured victim. It is recommended that a first aid care provider obtain consent from the victim before rendering first aid. However in the case of an unconscious individual who requires CPR, consent would be implied, meaning that they would give consent if they could.[3]

The rescuer should follow the emergency action steps: **Check-Call-Care.**[3] *Check* the scene to find out what happened and to identify other individuals who might help and then check the victim for consciousness. *Call* 911 to access the rescue squad and then initiate *care* for the victim.

In 2008, the American Heart Association, proposed changes that simplifies CPR techniques for those people who have *not* been certified in CPR. This technique, referred to as "hands-only CPR," only requires a rescuer to call 911, then to perform uninterrupted chest compressions—100 a minute—until paramedics take over or an automated external defibrillator is available to restore a normal heart rhythm. This action should be taken only for adults who unexpectedly collapse, stop breathing, and are unresponsive.[1]

### Equipment Considerations

Protective equipment worn by an athlete may complicate life-saving CPR procedures. A great deal of controversy exists as to whether equipment should be removed or left in place. The presence of a football, ice hockey, or lacrosse helmet with a face mask and various types of shoulder pads associated with each sport obviously makes CPR more difficult if not impossible.[11,17]

Removing the face mask should be the first step.[27] The face mask does not hinder the evaluation of the airway but it may hinder treatment. A number of techniques using various instruments have been recommended to remove the face mask, including electric screwdrivers (Figure 7-3D), which work well as long as the screws are not rusted; or wire cutters, bolt cutters, scissors, or scalpels, none of which work very well.[15] Three devices, the Anvil Pruner, the Trainer's Angel, and the

194

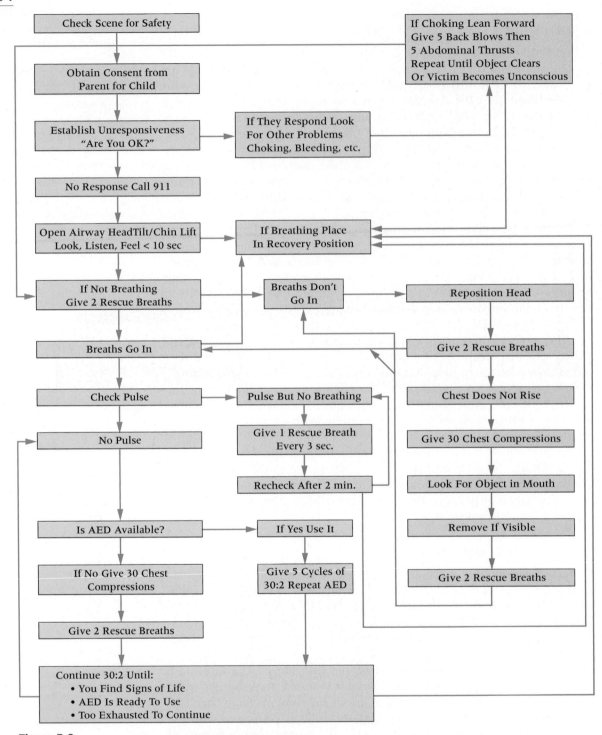

**Figure 7-2**

**Flowchart for Adult and Child CPR**

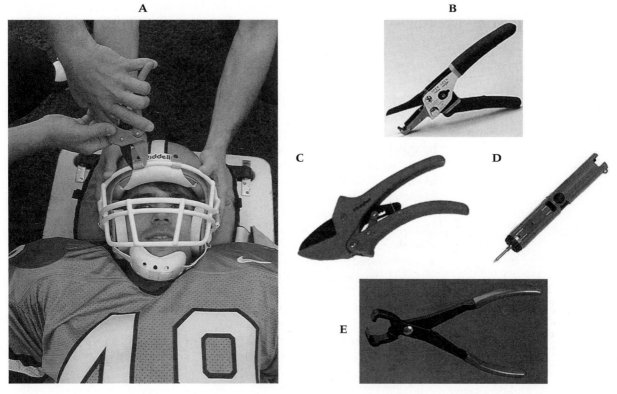

A

B

C

D

E

**Figure 7-3**

(A) A number of different tools can be used to cut or remove the plastic grommets that hold the face mask, including (B) FM Extractor (C) Anvil Prune (D) Electric cordless screwdriver (E) Trainer's Angel.

FM Extractor, have been effective in quickly cutting the plastic clips (Figure 7-3).[15] Most recently the recommended technique has been to use a combination of both an electric screwdriver and one of the three cutting devices.[10]

In 1992, the Occupational Safety and Health Administration (OSHA) mandated the use of barrier devices to protect the rescuer from transmission of bloodborne pathogens during CPR (Figure 7-4). It is possible

**Figure 7-4**

A barrier mask protects the rescuer from potential exposure to bloodborne pathogens.

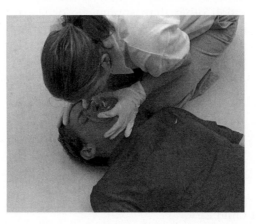

to slip the barrier mask under the face mask, attach the one-way mouthpiece or valve through the bars of the face mask, and begin CPR within 5 to 10 seconds without removing the face mask.[16]

Decisions to remove a helmet and shoulder pads before initiating CPR should be based on the potential of injury to the cervical spine. **The helmet should not be removed from an athlete with a suspected cervical spine injury.** The exception to this rule is if the airway is compromised. If it is reasonably certain that no injury has occurred to the cervical spine, both the helmet and shoulder pads can be quickly removed before initiating CPR. If there is ANY possibility of injury to the cervical spine, care must be taken to minimize movement of the head and neck while permitting CPR to be performed. The face mask should be dealt with as recommended earlier, and the jersey and shoulder pad strings and/or straps should be cut and the shoulder pads spread apart so that the chest may be compressed according to CPR guidelines. Although removal of the helmet and shoulder pads has been recommended by some, it seems that no matter how much care is taken, removal creates unnecessary movement of the cervical spine and delays initiation of CPR, neither of which is best for the injured athlete.[28]

If cervical neck injury is suspected yet the athlete is conscious and breathing and does not require CPR, the athlete should be transported with the helmet, chin strap, and shoulder pads in place. The face mask should be removed in case CPR becomes necessary.

### Establish Unresponsiveness

First, establish unresponsiveness of the athlete by tapping or gently shaking his or her shoulder and shouting, "Are you okay?" Note that shaking should be avoided if the athlete has a possible neck injury. If the athlete is unresponsive, the emergency medical system (EMS) should be activated immediately by dialing 911. Someone should be specifically instructed to dial 911. That person should also be instructed to get an automatic external defibrillator (AED) if available (AEDs are discussed in detail on page 199). If the athlete is not breathing, carefully position the athlete in the supine position. If the athlete is in a position other than supine, he or she must be carefully rolled over as a unit, avoiding any twisting of the body, because CPR can be administered only with the athlete lying flat on the back with knees straight or slightly flexed. In cases of suspected cervical spine injury, care must be taken to minimize cervical movement during logrolling. Then proceed with CPR.[20]

### Opening the Airway

Open the airway by using the head tilt–chin lift method (Figure 7-5).[3] Lift under the chin with one hand while pushing down on the victim's forehead with the other, avoiding the use of excessive force. The tongue is the most common cause of airway obstruction; the forward lift of the jaw raises the tongue away from the back of the throat, thus clearing

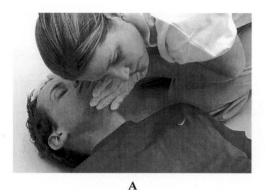
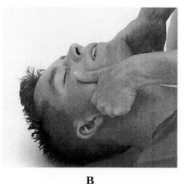

A                    B

**Figure 7-5**

(A) Head-tilt/chin-lift technique for establishing an airway (B) Alternative jaw thrust technique.

the airway.[2] In cases where cervical injury is suspected, the rescuer should use the jaw-thrust techniques to open the airway. In this alternative technique, the rescuer hooks the index finger under the curve of the jaw pulling forward. This pulls the tongue away from the back of the throat.

### Establishing Breathing

1. To determine if the victim is breathing, maintain the open airway, place your ear over the victim's mouth, observe the chest, and look, listen, and feel for breath sounds for 5–10 seconds (Figure 7-5).

2. With the hand that is on the athlete's forehead, pinch the nose shut, keeping the heel of the hand in place to hold the head back (if there is no neck injury). OSHA has mandated the use of barrier shields (and disposable gloves if available) by individuals to minimize the risk of transmitting bloodborne pathogens (Figure 7-4). These shields have a plastic or silicone sheet that spreads over the face and separates the individual from the athlete. Some models have a tubelike mouthpiece, which may help in situations in which the athlete is wearing a face mask. If a barrier shield is not available, taking a normal breath, place your mouth over the athlete's mouth to provide an airtight seal and give two slow, full breaths at a rate of one breath per second. Observe the chest rise and fall. Remove your mouth, and listen for the air to escape through passive exhalation. If the airway is obstructed, reposition the victim's head and try again to ventilate. If still obstructed, give thirty chest compressions. Then look for an object in the mouth and perform a finger sweep with the index finger to clear visible objects from the mouth (Figure 7-6).[16] Be careful not to push the object further into the throat. Continue to repeat this sequence until ventilation occurs.

**Figure 7-6**

Finger sweeping of the mouth is essential in attempting to remove a foreign object from a choking victim.

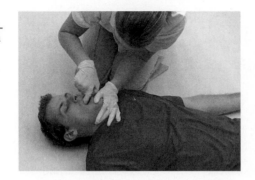

### Establishing Circulation

1. In the adult and child, feel for a pulse at the carotid artery. Place two fingers on the center of the neck and slide them toward you into the groove on the side of the neck. Monitor for 5 to 10 seconds.

2. If there is no pulse and an AED is available, the AED should be used as soon as possible (see page 199). Deliver 1 shock followed immediately by chest compressions.[2]

3. If no AED is available and there are no evident signs of circulation (i.e., breathing, coughing, or movement) chest compressions should begin immediately after giving two rescue breaths.[2]

4. Maintain an open airway. Position yourself close to the side of the athlete's chest.

5. Next, the heel of one hand is positioned on the sternum between the nipples (Figure 7-7). The other hand is placed on top of the hand on the sternum so that the heels of both hands are parallel and the fingers are directed straight away from the athletic trainer (Figure 7-7). Fingers can be extended or interlaced, but they must be kept off the chest wall.

6. Elbows are kept in a locked position with arms straight and shoulders positioned over the hands, enabling the thrust to be straight down.

**Figure 7-7**

Establish circulation:
(A) Pulse is checked at the carotid artery.
(B) Compressions are done with the heel of the hands on the middle of the sternum between the nipples.

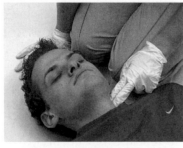

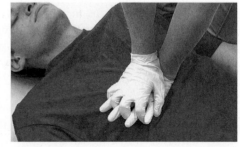

A

B

7. In a normal-sized adult, enough force must be applied to depress the sternum 1½ to 2 inches (4 to 5 cm). In a child, the sternum should be compressed 1 to 1½ inches. After depression, there must be complete release of the sternum to allow the heart to refill. The time of release should equal the time of compression. For one rescuer, compression must be given at the rate of 100 times per minute, maintaining a ratio of thirty chest compressions to two full breaths (30:2) for all victims from infants to adults.[2]

8. After five cycles of thirty compressions and two breaths (30:2), or about 2 minutes, recheck the pulse at the carotid artery (allow 5 seconds) while maintaining head tilt. If no pulse is found, continue the 30:2 cycle beginning with chest compressions.

**Using an automatic external defibrillator** An automatic external defibrillator (AED) is a device that evaluates the heart rhythm of a victim of sudden cardiac arrest.[20] It is capable of delivering an electrical charge to the heart, and does not require the expertise of a medical professional.[20] To prevent human error, all machines now have computers that evaluate heart rhythm and decide if deployment is appropriate. AEDs have become an essential tool in the treatment of out-of-hospital cardiac arrest.[14] The American Heart Association estimates that 100,000 deaths could be prevented each year with rapid defibrillation. Over the years, the devices have become safer, more reliable, and more maintenance free. The new technologies used in these devices make them suitable for use by anyone who has had basic training.[3]

AEDs are extremely easy to use; anyone trained to use cardiopulmonary resuscitation (CPR) should be trained to use an AED. Most AEDs are designed to be used by people without medical backgrounds, such as police, firefighters, flight attendants, security guards, fitness professionals, coaches, and lay rescuers, as long as the procedure is coordinated with existing EMS systems and the person administering the procedure has received proper training. Public places where AEDs might be located include police cars, theaters, sports arenas, public buildings, business offices, and airports. An increasing number of commercial airplanes are now equipped with AEDs and enhanced medical kits. Formal training programs, such as those offered by the American Heart Association's Heart-saver AED course, can be taught in as little as 4 hours. However, operating an AED is so simple that it can be done successfully even without formal training. Training is recommended for as many people as possible. Local and state regulations determine the training requirements for public access defibrillator (PAD) programs.

The legal requirements that allow the lay public to use AEDs are determined on a state-by-state basis. In some states there is true public access defibrillation, meaning that anyone with knowledge of an AED can use one anytime it is available. For example, a traveler in an airport may retrieve and use an AED mounted in a public location. In other states, use of AEDs is more restricted. Some states require a formal training program, the direct involvement of an authorizing doctor, or that the AED rescuer be part of a formal in-house response team. In most states, any individual using an AED in a good faith attempt to save the life of a cardiac arrest victim will be covered by some form of a Good Samaritan statute.

The broad deployment of a new generation of portable defibrillators for use by trained lay rescuers can help save countless lives.

Anyone can be certified to use an AED in most states and can learn to use an AED in about an hour.[14] AED users also need yearly training not only on the use of the device but also on CPR. Maintenance is minimal on AEDs. The devices are equipped with long-life batteries and have features that notify the users when the battery needs replacement.

To use an AED the rescuer simply applies the two electrodes to the right apex and the left base of the chest (Figure 7-8). To operate most devices, push the "on" button and listen for a voice on the machine to direct you whether or not to push the defibrillator button. If the pulse resumes, place the victim into the recovery position (see Figure 7-11) until the rescue squad arrives. If the pulse does not resume, the rescuer should continue external compressions at a 30 (compressions): 2 (breaths) ratio. **All staff personnel should be certified in CPR/AED and should take a refresher examination at least once a year.**

### Obstructed Airway Management

Choking is a possibility in many sports activities; for example, an athlete may choke on a mouth guard, a broken piece of dental work, chewing gum, or even a chew of tobacco. When such emergencies arise, early

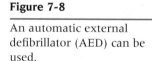

**Figure 7-8**

An automatic external defibrillator (AED) can be used.

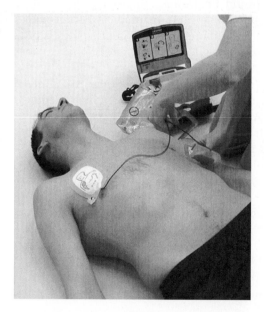

recognition and prompt, knowledgeable action are necessary to avert a tragedy. An unconscious athlete can have an obstructed airway when the tongue falls back in the throat, thus blocking the upper airway. Blood clots resulting from head, facial, or dental injuries may impede normal breathing, as may vomiting. When complete airway obstruction occurs, the individual is unable to speak, cough, or breathe.

### Conscious Victim

If the athlete is conscious, he or she makes is a tremendous effort to breathe, the head is forced back, and the face initially is flushed and then becomes cyanotic as oxygen deprivation occurs. If partial airway obstruction is causing the choking, some air passage can be detected, but during a complete obstruction no air movement is discernible.

For the victim who is conscious and has an airway obstruction, the standing abdominal thrust technique is performed until he or she is relieved.[2]

First, if the victim cannot cough, speak, or breathe, have someone call 911. The rescuer should obtain consent from the victim before proceeding. Lean the victim forward supporting the chest with one hand and deliver five back blows between the scapulae with the other (Figure 7-9). Then, stand behind and to one side of the athlete. Place both arms around the waist just above the belt line, and permit the athlete's head, arms, and upper trunk to hang forward (Figure 7-10). Grasp one of your fists with the other, placing the thumb side of the grasped fist immediately below the xiphoid process of the sternum, clear of the rib cage. Now sharply and forcefully thrust the fists into the abdomen, inward, and upward. This "hug" pushes up on the diaphragm, compressing the air in the lungs, creating forceful pressure against the blockage, and thus usually causing the obstruction to be promptly expelled. Repeat the maneuver until the athlete is relieved or becomes unconscious.

### Unconscious Victim

If a conscious victim with an obstructed airway eventually loses consciousness, the rescuers should help the victim get to the ground without falling. The victim must be on his or her back. If the athlete loses consciousness, open the airway,[2] and try to ventilate with two rescue breaths. If the airway is still obstructed, reposition the head and try again. Look to see if an object is visible in the mouth and only then perform a finger sweep. Then give thirty chest compressions. Repeat this sequence as long as necessary. Victims who begin breathing on their own should be placed on their side in the recovery position (Figure 7-11).[3]

**Finger sweeping**  If a foreign object such as a mouth guard is lodged in the mouth or the throat and is visible, it may be possible to remove or release it with the fingers (see Figure 7-6).[3] Care must be taken that the probing does not drive the object deeper into the throat. Once the object is removed, if the athlete is not already breathing, attempt to ventilate.[3]

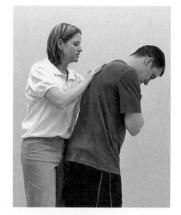

**Figure 7-9**

**Obstructed airway back blows**

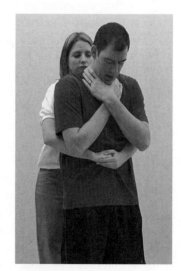

**Figure 7-10**

**Standing abdominal thrusts for a conscious victim with an obstructed airway**

**Figure 7-11**

**Recovery position**

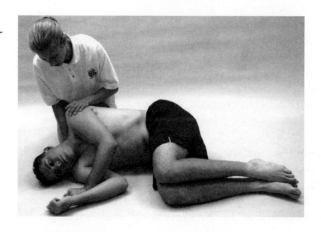

Infant CPR

While the sequence for infant (under 1 year) CPR is similar to adult and child CPR, there are some differences in technique.[3] The procedures for providing CPR to an infant are summarized in Focus Box 7-2.

## 7-2 *Focus Box*

**CPR Procedures for an Infant**

- Analyze the scene.
- Place the infant on his or her back on a firm, flat surface.
- Check the infant for responsiveness. If no response, have someone else dial 911.
- Check for breathing and/or movement for less than 10 seconds.
- If not moving or breathing, tilt the infant's head to a neutral position.
- Using a resuscitation mask give two rescue breaths by blowing puffs of air into the infant.
- Check for a pulse at the brachial artery on the inside of the upper arm for no more than 10 seconds.
- Scan the infant for severe bleeding.
- If there is no pulse movement or breathing,
  — Keep one hand on the infant's forehead to maintain an open airway.
  — Place two or three fingers on the center of the chest just below the nipple line.
- Give thirty chest compressions.
  — Compress the chest about ½ to 1 inch at 100 compressions per minute.
  — Take pressure off the chest between compressions.
- Replace the resuscitation mask and give two rescue breaths.
- Repeat cycles of thirty chest compressions and two rescue breaths.
- Continue CPR until
  — Another trained rescuer arrives and takes over.
  — You are too exhausted to continue.
  — The scene becomes unsafe.
  — You notice an obvious sign of life.

## Controlling Bleeding

An abnormal external or internal discharge of blood is called a *hemorrhage*. The hemorrhage may be venous, capillary, or arterial and may be external or internal. Venous blood is characteristically dark red with a continuous flow, capillary bleeding exudes from tissue and is a reddish color, and arterial bleeding flows in spurts and is bright red. NOTE: The coach or fitness professional must always be concerned with exposure to bloodborne pathogens and other diseases when coming in contact with someone's blood or other body fluids. It is essential to take *universal precautions* to minimize this risk. Disposable nonlatex gloves should be used routinely whenever the coach comes in contact with blood or other body fluids. This topic is discussed in detail in Chapter 8.

### Controlling External Bleeding

External bleeding stems from open skin wounds such as abrasions, incisions, lacerations, punctures, or avulsions. The control of external bleeding is most effectively accomplished by use of direct pressure. Elevation and pressure points may also help to control bleeding.

**Direct pressure** Pressure applied directly over a wound with the hand over a sterile gauze pad is now recommended as the primary technique for controlling bleeding. The pressure is applied firmly against the resistance of a bone (Figure 7-12). As a gauze pad becomes soaked, additional pads should be placed on top of those already in place to facilitate the clotting process. Pressure may also be applied with a compression bandage holding sterile gauze in place over the wound.

**Elevation** Elevation provides an additional means for the reduction of external hemorrhage. Elevating a hemorrhaging part against gravity reduces hydrostatic blood pressure and facilitates venous and lymphatic drainage; consequently, elevating slows bleeding.[16]

**Pressure points** When direct pressure combined with elevation fails to slow hemorrhage, the use of pressure points may be the method of choice. Eleven points on each side of the body have been identified for controlling external bleeding; the two most commonly used are the brachial artery in the upper limb and the femoral artery in the lower

External bleeding can usually be managed by using direct pressure, elevation, or pressure points.

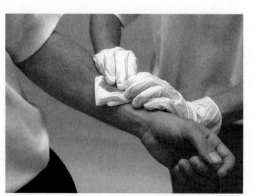

**Figure 7-12**

Direct pressure for the control of bleeding is applied with the hand over a sterile gauze pad.

**Figure 7-13**

The two most common sites for direct pressure are the (A) brachial artery and (B) the femoral artery.

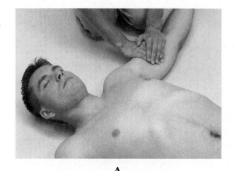
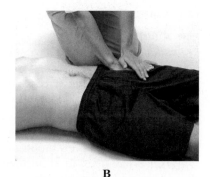

A                                        B

limb. The brachial artery is compressed against the medial aspect of the humerus, and the femoral artery is compressed as it is detected within the femoral triangle (Figure 7-13).

### Internal Hemorrhage

Internal hemorrhage is invisible to the eye unless manifested through some body opening or identified through x-ray studies or other diagnostic techniques. Its danger lies in the difficulty of diagnosis. When internal hemorrhaging occurs, either subcutaneously such as in a bruise or contusion, intramuscularly, or in joints, the athlete may be moved without danger in most instances. However, the detection of bleeding within a body cavity such as the skull, thorax, or abdomen is of the utmost importance because it could mean the difference between life and death. Because the symptoms are obscure, internal hemorrhage is difficult to diagnose properly. As a result of this difficulty, **athletes with internal injuries require hospitalization under complete and constant observation by a medical staff to determine the nature and extent of the injuries.** All severe hemorrhaging eventually results in shock and should therefore be treated on this premise. Even if there is no outward indication of shock, the athlete should be kept quiet and body heat should be maintained at a constant and suitable temperature (see the section on shock for the preferred body position).[20]

### Managing Shock

With any injury shock is a possibility. But when severe bleeding, fractures, or internal injuries are present, the potential for shock increases. Shock occurs when a diminished amount of blood is available to the circulatory system. As a result, not enough oxygen-carrying blood cells are available to the tissues, particularly those of the nervous system. When shock occurs, a quantity of plasma is lost from the blood vessels to the tissue spaces of the body, leaving the blood cells within the vessels, thus causing stagnation and slowing the blood flow. This general collapse of the vascular system causes widespread tissue death, which eventually causes the death of the individual unless treatment is given.

Certain conditions such as extreme fatigue, exposure to extreme heat or cold, extreme dehydration and mineral loss, or illness predispose an athlete to shock. In a situation with potential for a shock condition, the athletic trainer or coach should use other signs to assess the possibility of the athlete's lapsing into a state of shock as an aftermath of the injury. The most important clue to potential shock is the recognition of a severe injury. It may happen that none of the usual signs of shock is present.

### Symptoms and Signs

The major signs of shock are moist, pale, cool, clammy skin; weak and rapid pulse; increased and shallow respiratory rate; decreased blood pressure; and in severe situations urinary retention and fecal incontinence. If conscious, the athlete may display a disinterest in his or her surroundings or may display irritability, restlessness, or excitement. There may also be extreme thirst.[16]

### Management

Depending on the causative factor for the shock, the following emergency care should be given:

1. Dial 911 to access emergency care.
2. Maintain body temperature as close to normal as possible.
3. Elevate the feet and legs 8 to 12 inches for most situations. However, shock positioning varies according to the type of injury.[2] For example, for a neck injury, the athlete should be immobilized as found; for a head injury, his or her head and shoulders should be elevated; and for a leg fracture, his or her leg should be kept level and should be raised after splinting.

Shock can also be compounded or initially produced by the psychological reaction of the athlete to an injury situation. Fear or the sudden realization that a serious situation has occurred can result in shock. In the case of a psychological reaction to an injury, the athlete should be instructed to lie down and avoid viewing the injury. This athlete should be handled with patience and gentleness, but firmness as well. Spectators should be kept away from the injured athlete. Reassurance is of vital concern to the injured individual. The person should be made comfortable by loosening his or her clothing. Nothing should be given by mouth until a physician has determined that no surgical procedures are indicated.

## CONDUCTING A SECONDARY ASSESSMENT

If the athlete has no life-threatening injuries, a secondary assessment should be conducted to survey the entire body for injury.

Signs of shock:
- Blood pressure is low.
- Systolic pressure is usually below 90 mm Hg.
- Pulse is rapid and very weak.
- Athlete may be drowsy and appear sluggish.
- Respiration is shallow and extremely rapid.
- The athlete's skin is pale, cool, clammy.

Secondary assessment consists of:
- history
- observation
- physical examination
- special tests

Vital signs to observe:
- pulse
- respiration
- blood pressure
- temperature
- skin color
- pupils
- state of consciousness
- weakness of movement
- sensory changes

## Recognizing Vital Signs

Anyone providing emergency care has to be able to evaluate the existing physiological signs and symptoms of injury. Among these *vital signs* are heart rate, breathing rate, blood pressure, temperature, skin color, pupils of the eye, movement, the presence of pain, and level of consciousness. **It is important to be able to recognize when one or more of the vital signs does not appear to be normal.** Table 7-1 provides a list of what is considered to be normal with each of these vital signs. An individual with any abnormal vital sign should be referred to a physician.

## On-Field Injury Inspection

Two phases of injury assessment take place during the secondary evaluation. The first involves the initial on-field injury inspection during which early decisions are made relative to (1) the seriousness of the injury and (2) how the injured athlete should be transported from the

**TABLE 7-1** Vital Signs

| Sign | Description |
|---|---|
| Pulse | Normal pulse rate per minute for adults ranges between 60 and 80 beats and in children from 80 to 100 beats. Trained athletes usually have slower pulses. Pulse rate is measured at the carotid artery in the neck or the radial artery in the wrist (Figure 7-14). |
| Respiration | Normal breathing rate per minute is approximately 12 breaths in adults and 20 to 25 breaths in children. Breathing may be shallow (indicating shock), irregular, or gasping (indicating cardiac involvement). |
| Blood pressure | Normal systolic pressure for 15- to 20-year-old males ranges from 100 to 140 mm Hg. The diastolic pressure, on the other hand, usually ranges from 60 to 90 mm Hg. The normal blood pressure of females is usually 8 to 10 mm Hg lower than in males for both systolic and diastolic pressures. Blood pressure can only be measured using a blood pressure cuff (Figure 7-15). |
| Temperature | Normal body temperature is 98.6° F (37° C). Core temperature is most accurately measured in the rectum or at the tympanic membrane in the ear (Figure 7-16). |
| Skin color | Red skin may indicate heatstroke, high blood pressure, or elevated temperature. Pale, ashen, or white skin can mean insufficient circulation, shock, fright, hemorrhage, heat exhaustion, or insulin shock. Blue skin (cyanotic), primarily noted in lips and fingernails, usually means an airway obstruction or respiratory insufficiency. |
| Pupils | Pupils should be of equal size. Pupil should respond to light, resulting in constriction or dilation. Response is more critical than pupil size. |
| State of consciousness | Normally the athlete is alert, is aware of the environment, and responds quickly to vocal stimulation. |
| Weakness of movement | Weakness of one side of the body compared to the other is not normal and may indicate nerve damage. |
| Sensory changes | Numbness, tingling, or complete loss of sensation is not normal. |

playing field. Quite often this on-field inspection must be done by the coach when an athletic trainer is not available. The more thorough off-field assessment is usually done by an athletic trainer or physician, if necessary.

A logical process must be used to evaluate accurately the extent of a musculoskeletal injury.[19] It is critical to be aware of the major signs that reveal the site, nature, and above all, severity of the injury. Detection of these signs can be facilitated, as is true with all trauma, by understanding the mechanism or traumatic sequence and by methodically inspecting the injury. Knowledge of the mechanism of an injury is extremely important in determining which area of the body is most affected.

In an attempt to understand the mechanism of injury, a brief history of the complaint must be taken. The athlete is asked, if possible, about the events leading up to the injury and how it occurred. The athlete is further asked what was heard or felt when the injury took place. Such sounds as a snap, crack, or pop at the moment of injury often indicate bone fracture or injury to ligaments or tendons. A visual observation of the injured site is made, comparing it to the uninjured body part. The initial visual examination can disclose obvious deformity, swelling, and skin discoloration.

Finally, the region of the injury is gently palpated. Feeling, or palpating, a part can, in conjunction with visual and audible signs, indicate the nature of the injury. Palpation is started away from the injury and gradually moved toward it. The extent of point tenderness, the extent of irritation (whether it is confined to soft tissue alone or extends to the bony tissue), and deformities that may not be detected by visual examination alone can be determined through palpation.

After the brief on-field injury inspection, the following decisions should be made:

1. The seriousness of the injury.
2. The type of first aid and immobilization necessary.

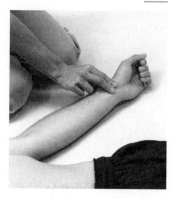

**Figure 7-14**

Pulse rate can be taken at the radial artery.

Some athletes normally have irregular and unequal pupils.

**7-2 Critical Thinking**
Exercise

A recreational tennis player complains of pain in his shoulder that he has had for about a week. He indicates that he first hurt the shoulder when lifting weights but did not think it was a bad injury. During the past week he has not been able to lift because of pain. He has, however, continued to play but his shoulder seems to be getting worse instead of better.

? What is the process for evaluating this injury?

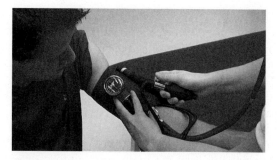

**Figure 7-15**

Blood pressure is measured using a sphygmomanometer and a stethoscope.

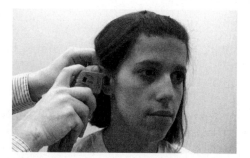

**Figure 7-16**

Thermometer for measuring tympanic membrane temperature.

Decisions that can be made from the secondary survey:
- seriousness of injury
- type of first aid required
- whether injury warrants referral to a physician
- type of transportation needed

3. Whether the injury warrants immediate referral to a physician for further assessment.
4. The manner of athlete transportation from the injury site to the sidelines, training room, or hospital.

**It is important to document in written form the findings of the on-the-field exam.** This should be done as soon after evaluating the injury as practical to ensure accuracy in reporting what was found during the evaluation and the course of action taken.

## OFF-FIELD ASSESSMENT

A more thorough off-field evaluation is performed by either an athletic trainer, physical therapist, or physician once the athlete has been removed from the site of initial injury to a place of comfort and safety. This detailed assessment may be performed on the sidelines, in an emergency room, in the athletic health care facility, or in a sports medicine clinic. The evaluation scheme is divided into four broad categories: history, observation, physical examination (palpation) and special tests[8] (HOPS). Numerous special tests can provide additional information about the extent of injuries.[19] The following discussion provides a brief overview of some of the steps and techniques that can be used in an off-field assessment.

### History

Obtaining as much information as possible about the injury is of major importance. Understanding how the injury occurred and listening to the complaints of the athlete and how key questions are answered can provide important clues to the exact nature of the injury. The examiner becomes a detective in pursuit of as much accurate information as possible, which will lead to a determination of the true nature of the injury. From the history the examiner develops strategies for further examination and possible immediate and follow-up management.

### Observation

Along with gaining knowledge and understanding of the athlete's major complaint from a history, general observation is also performed, often at the same time the history is taken. What is observed is usually affected by the athlete's major complaints.

### Palpation

The two areas of palpation are bony and soft tissue. As with all examination procedures, palpation must be performed systematically, starting with very light pressure followed by gradually deeper pressure and usually beginning away from the site of complaint, then gradually moving toward it.

### Special Tests

Special tests have been designed for almost every body region as means for detecting specific pathologies. They are often used to substantiate what has been learned from other testing. For example, special tests are commonly used to determine ligament stability, impingement signs, tightness of specific structures, muscle imbalance, and body alignment discrepancies. Special tests for various joints are discussed in Chapters 14 through 22.

## IMMEDIATE TREATMENT FOLLOWING ACUTE MUSCULOSKELETAL INJURY

Musculoskeletal injuries are extremely common in sports. Appropriate first aid must be provided immediately to control hemorrhage and associated swelling. **Every initial first-aid effort should be directed toward one primary goal—reducing the amount of swelling resulting from the injury.** If swelling can be controlled initially, the amount of time required for injury rehabilitation will be significantly reduced. Initial management of musculoskeletal injuries should include protection, rest, ice, compression, and elevation (PRICE). Focus Box 7-3 summarizes the specific technique for initial management of acute injuries (Figure 7-17).

### Protection

Protection from further injury should occur immediately following injury. If there is a fracture or some joint instability, the injured structure should be immobilized with some type of splint or brace. Choosing an appropriate method of transporting the injured athlete from the field can also help to protect an injury from further damage.

PRICE (protection, rest, ice, compression, elevation) are essential in the emergency care of musculoskeletal injuries.

### Rest

Rest after any type of injury is an extremely important component of any treatment program. Once a body part is injured, it immediately begins the healing process. If the injured part is not rested and is subjected to

---

**7-3** ⟩ **Focus Box**

**Initial Management of Acute Injuries**

The appropriate technique for initial management of the acute musculoskeletal injury, regardless of where it occurs, is the following:

1. Apply a compression wrap directly over the injury. Wrapping should start distally and continue proximally. Tension should be firm and consistent. It may be helpful to wet the elastic wrap to facilitate the passage of cold from ice packs. A dry compression wrap should be left in place for at least 72 hours or until there is little chance of continued swelling.

2. Surround the injured area entirely with ice packs or bags and secure them in place. The ice should be left on for 20 minutes initially and then 1 hour off and 30 minutes on as much as possible over the next 24 hours. During the following 48-hour period, ice should again be applied as often as possible.

3. The injured part should be elevated for most of the initial 72-hour period after injury. It is particularly important to keep the injury elevated while sleeping. This elevation also allows the damaged part to rest after the injury. The initial management of an injury is extremely important to reduce the length of time required for rehabilitation. The end of the mattress can be elevated by placing pillows or a rolled up blanket underneath.

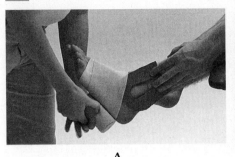 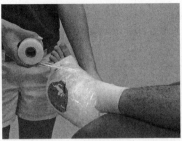 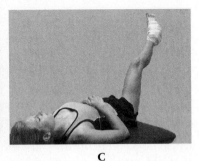

A        B        C

**Figure 7-17**

PRICE technique: (A) A wet compression wrap should be applied over the horseshoe pad; (B) ice bags should be secured in place by a dry compression wrap or plastic wrap; and (C) the leg should be elevated during the initial treatment period.

external stresses and strains, the healing process never gets a chance to do what it is supposed to do. Consequently the injured part does not heal, and the time required for rehabilitation is markedly increased. The number of days necessary for resting varies with the severity of the injury. Parts of the body that have experienced minor injury should be rested for approximately 48 to 72 hours before a rehabilitation program is begun.

### Ice (Cold Application)

The initial treatment of acute injuries should use cold.[18] Therefore ice is used for most conditions involving strains, sprains, and contusions. Ice is most commonly used immediately after injury to decrease pain and promote local constriction of the vessels (vasoconstriction), thus controlling hemorrhage and edema. Cold applied to an acute injury lowers metabolism and the tissue demands for oxygen, and reduces hypoxia. With ice treatments, the athlete usually reports an uncomfortable sensation of cold, followed by burning, then an aching sensation, and finally complete numbness.

Because subcutaneous (under the skin) fat conducts cold slowly, applications of cold for short periods are ineffective in cooling deeper tissues. For this reason, treatments of at least 20 minutes are recommended. Prolonged application of cold, however, can cause tissue damage.[18]

Ice packs should be applied to the area for at least 72 hours after an acute injury. With many injuries, regular ice treatments may be continued for several weeks.

For best results, ice packs (crushed ice and towel) should be applied over a compression wrap. Frozen gel packs should not be used directly against the skin, because they reach much lower temperatures than ice packs. A good rule of thumb is to apply a cold pack to a recent injury for a 20-minute period and repeat every 1 to 1½ hours throughout the waking day. Depending on the severity and site of the injury, cold may be applied intermittently for 1 to 72 hours. For example, a mild strain will probably require 1 day of 20-minute periods of cold application, whereas a severe knee or ankle sprain might need 3 to 7 days of intermittent cold. If in doubt about the severity of an injury, it is best to extend the time that ice is applied.[18]

## Compression

**Immediate compression of an acute injury is perhaps more important than ice in controlling swelling.** Placing external pressure on an injury assists in decreasing hemorrhage and hematoma formation by mechanically reducing the space available for swelling to accumulate. Fluid seepage into interstitial spaces is retarded by compression, and absorption is facilitated. However, application of compression to an anterior compartment syndrome or to certain injuries involving the head and neck is contraindicated (see Chapter 15).

Many types of compression are available. An elastic wrap that has been soaked in water and frozen in a refrigerator can provide both compression and cold when applied to a recent injury. Pads can be cut from felt or foam rubber to fit difficult-to-compress body areas. A horseshoe-shaped pad, for example, placed around the malleolus in combination with an elastic wrap and tape provides an excellent way to prevent or reduce ankle edema. Although cold is applied intermittently, compression should be maintained throughout the day and, if possible, throughout the night. Pressure buildup in the tissues may make it painful to leave a compression wrap in place for a long time. However, the wrap must be left in place even though there may be significant discomfort because compression is so important in the control of swelling. The compression wrap should be left in place for at least 72 hours after an acute injury. In many chronic overuse problems, such as tendonitis, tenosynovitis, and particularly bursitis, the compression wrap should be worn until swelling is almost entirely gone.

## Elevation

Along with cold and compression, elevation reduces internal bleeding. The injured part, particularly an extremity, should be elevated to eliminate the effects of gravity on blood pooling in the extremities. Elevation assists the veins, which drain blood and other fluids from the injured area and return them to the central circulatory system. The greater the degree of elevation, the more effective the reduction in swelling. For example, in an ankle sprain the leg should be placed so that the ankle is virtually straight up in the air. The injured part should be elevated as much as possible during the first 72 hours.

## EMERGENCY SPLINTING

**If an athlete appears to have a fracture, dial 911 and access the rescue squad immediately. Any suspected fracture should be splinted before the athlete is moved.** Transporting a person with a fracture without proper immobilization can result in increased tissue damage, hemorrhage, and shock. The application of splints should be a simple process through the use of commercial emergency splints.[16]

Regardless of the type of splint used, the principles of good splinting remain the same. Two major concepts of splinting are (1) to splint

A suspected fracture must be splinted before the athlete is moved.

**Figure 7-18**

(A) Rapid form vacuum immobilizer. (B) Air splint.

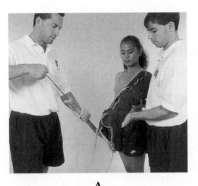

A

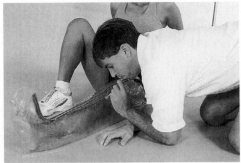

B

from one joint above the fracture to one joint below the fracture and (2) to splint the injury in the position it is found. If at all possible, do not move the athlete until he or she has been splinted.

## Rapid Form Vacuum Immobilizers

The rapid form vacuum immobilizer is a new type of splint that is widely used by both EMTs and athletic trainers. It consists of styrofoam chips contained inside an airtight cloth sleeve that is pliable. It can be molded to the shape of any joint or angulated fracture using Velcro straps. A handheld pump sucks the air out of the sleeve, giving it a cardboard-like rigidity. This splint is most useful for injuries that are angulated and must be splinted in the position in which they are found (Figure 7-18A).

## Air Splints

An air splint is a clear plastic splint that is inflated with air around the affected part; it can be used for extremity splinting, but its use requires some special training. This splint provides support and moderate pressure to the body part and affords a clear view of the site for x-ray examination. The inflatable splint should not be used if it will alter a fracture deformity (Figure 7-18B).

## Splinting of Lower-Limb Fractures

Fractures of the ankle or leg require immobilization of the foot and knee. Any fracture involving the knee, thigh, or hip needs splinting of all the lower-limb joints and one side of the trunk.

## Splinting of Upper-Limb Fractures

Fractures around the shoulder complex are immobilized by a shoulder sling, with the upper limb bound to the body securely. Upper-arm and elbow fractures must be splinted in the position they are found. Lower-arm and wrist fractures should be splinted in a position of forearm flexion and should be supported by a sling. Hand and finger dislocations and fractures should be splinted with tongue depressors, gauze rolls, or aluminum splints.

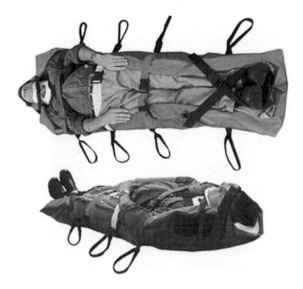

**Figure 7-19**

**Rapid form total body immobilizer**

### Splinting of the Spine and Pelvis

Injuries involving a possible spine or pelvic fracture are best splinted and moved using a spine board. Recently, a total body rapid form vacuum immobilizer has been developed for dealing with spinal injuries (Figure 7-19). The effectiveness of this piece of equipment as an immobilization device has yet to be determined.

## MOVING AND TRANSPORTING THE INJURED ATHLETE

Moving, lifting, and transporting the injured athlete must be executed using techniques that prevent further injury. Moving or transporting the athlete improperly may cause more additional injuries than any other emergency procedure.[2] There is no excuse for poor handling of the injured athlete. Planning should take into consideration all the possible transportation methods and the necessary equipment to execute them. Capable and well-trained personnel, spine boards, stretchers, and a rescue vehicle may be needed to transport the injured athlete.

Great caution must be taken when transporting the injured athlete.

### Suspected Spinal Injury

**When spinal injuries are suspected, immediately dial 911 and access the EMS and wait until the rescue squad arrives before attempting to move the athlete.** The only exception is in cases in which the athlete is not breathing and logrolling the athlete onto the back is required for CPR.

A suspected spinal injury requires extremely careful handling and is best left to properly trained paramedics, EMTs, or athletic trainers who are more skilled and have the proper equipment for such transport.[28] If such personnel are not available, moving should be done under the express direction of a physician, and a spine board should be used. One danger inherent in moving an athlete with a suspected spinal injury, in particular a cervical injury, is the tendency of the neck and head to turn because of the victim's inability to control his or her movements. Torque so induced creates a possibility of spinal cord or root damage when small fractures are present. The most important principle in transporting an individual on a spine board is to keep the head and neck in alignment with the long axis of the body. In such cases it is best to have one individual whose sole responsibility is to ensure and maintain proper positioning of the head and neck until the head is secured to a spine board.[5]

### Placing the Athlete on a Spine Board

Once an injury to the neck has been recognized as severe, a physician and rescue squad should be summoned immediately. After the rescue squad has been called, the coach should assume the responsibility for providing primary emergency care that involves maintaining normal breathing, treating for shock, and keeping the athlete quiet and in the position found until medical assistance arrives. Ideally, transportation should not be attempted until the physician has examined the athlete and has given permission to move him or her. Once the rescue squad arrives, they assume responsibility for positioning the athlete on the spine board and carrying the athlete on the spine board to the rescue vehicle. The athlete should be transported while lying on his or her back with the curve of the neck supported by a rolled-up towel or pad or encased in a stabilization collar. Neck stabilization must be maintained throughout transportation, first to the emergency vehicle, then to the hospital, and throughout the hospital procedure.[9] If stabilization is not continued, additional spinal cord damage and paralysis may ensue (Figure 7-20).

### Stretcher Carrying

**Figure 7-20**

The athlete should be placed on the spine board with the head securely stabilized.

Whenever a serious injury other than a spinal injury is suspected, the best and safest mode of transportation for a short distance is by stretcher. With each segment of the body supported, the athlete is gently lifted and placed on the stretcher, which is carried adequately by four

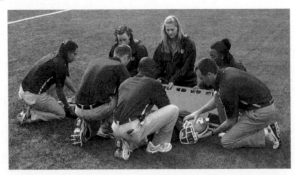
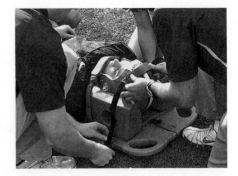

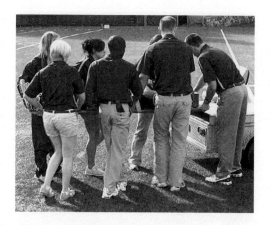

**Figure 7-21**

Whenever a serious injury is suspected, a stretcher is the safest method for transporting the athlete.

assistants, two supporting the ends of the stretcher and two supporting either side (Figure 7-21). Any person with an injury serious enough to require the use of a stretcher must be carefully examined before being moved.

When transporting a person with a limb injury, be certain the injury is splinted properly before transport. Athletes with shoulder injuries are more comfortably moved in a semi-sitting position, unless other injuries preclude such positioning. If injury to the upper extremity is such that flexion of the elbow is not possible, the individual should be transported on a stretcher with the limb properly splinted and carried at the side and with adequate padding placed between the arm and the body.

### Ambulatory Aid

Ambulatory aid (Figure 7-22) is support or assistance given to an injured athlete who is able to walk. Before the athlete is allowed to walk, he or she should be carefully scrutinized to make sure that the injuries are minor. Whenever serious injuries are suspected, walking should be prohibited. Complete support should be given on both sides of the athlete by two individuals who are approximately the same height. The athlete's arms are draped over the assistants' shoulders, and their arms encircle his or her back.

### Manual Conveyance

Manual conveyance (Figure 7-23) may be used to move a mildly injured individual a greater distance than can be walked with ease. As with the use of ambulatory aid, any decision to carry the athlete must be made only after a complete examination to determine the existence of potentially serious conditions. The most convenient carry is performed by two assistants.

### Fitting and Using the Crutch or Cane

When an athlete has a lower-limb injury, weight bearing may be contraindicated. Situations of this type call for the use of crutches or a cane.

Properly fitting a crutch or cane is essential to avoid placing abnormal stresses on the body.

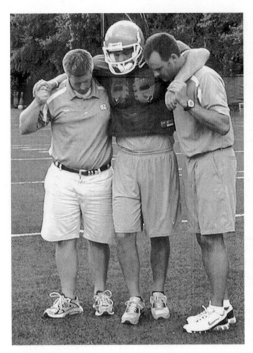

**Figure 7-22**

**The ambulatory aid method of transporting a mildly injured athlete**

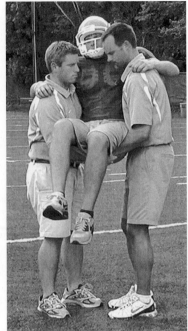

**Figure 7-23**

**Manual conveyance method for transporting a mildly injured athlete**

Very often, the athlete is assigned one of these aids without proper fitting or instruction in its use. Improper fit and usage can place abnormal stresses on various body parts. Constant pressure of the body weight on the crutch's axillary pads can cause crutch palsy. This pressure on the axillary or radial nerves and blood vessels can lead to temporary or even permanent numbness in the hands. Faulty mechanics in the use of crutches or canes can produce chronic low back and/or hip strain.

### Fitting the Athlete

The adjustable crutch is well suited to the athlete (Figure 7-24). For a correct fit the athlete should wear low-heeled shoes and stand with good posture and the feet close together. The crutch length is determined first by placing the tip 6 inches (15 cm) from the outer margin of the shoe and 2 inches (5 cm) in front of the shoe. The underarm crutch brace is positioned 1 inch (2.5 cm) below the anterior fold of the axilla. Next, the hand brace is adjusted so that it is even with the athlete's hand and the elbow is flexed at approximately a 30-degree angle. Fitting a cane to the athlete is relatively easy. Measurement is taken from the superior aspect of the greater trochanter of the femur to the floor while the athlete is wearing street shoes.

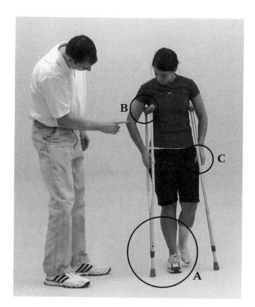

**Figure 7-24**

The crutch must be properly fitted to the athlete. (A) The crutch tips are placed 6 inches [15 cm] from the outer margin of the shoe and 2 inches [5 cm] in front of the shoe. (B) The underarm crutch brace is positioned 1 inch [2.5 cm] below the anterior fold of the axilla. (C) The hand brace is placed even with the athlete's hand, with the elbow flexed approximately 30 degrees.

### Walking with Crutches or Cane

Many elements of crutch walking correspond with walking. The technique commonly used in sports injuries is the tripod method. In this method, the athlete swings through the crutches without making any surface contact with the injured limb or by partially bearing weight with the injured limb. The following sequence is performed:

1. The athlete stands on one foot with the affected foot completely elevated or partially bearing weight.

2. Placing the crutch tips 12 to 15 inches (30 to 37.5 cm) ahead of the feet, the athlete leans forward, straightens the elbows, pulls the upper crosspiece firmly against the side of the chest, and swings or steps between the stationary crutches (Figure 7-25). The athlete should avoid placing the major support in the axilla.

3. After moving through, the athlete recovers the crutches and again places the tips forward.

An alternate method is the four-point crutch gait. In this method, the athlete stands on both feet. One crutch is moved forward and the opposite foot is stepped forward. The crutch on the same side as the foot that moved forward moves just ahead of the foot. The opposite foot steps forward, followed by the crutch on the same side, and so on.

Once the athlete is able to move effectively on a level surface, negotiating stairs should be taught. As with level crutch walking, a tripod is maintained on stairs. In going upstairs, the unaffected support leg moves up one step while the body weight is supported by the hands. The full weight of the body is transferred to the support leg, followed by moving the crutch tips and affected leg to the step. In going down-

**Figure 7-25**

Crutch gait. (A) Tripod
method. (B) Four point gait.

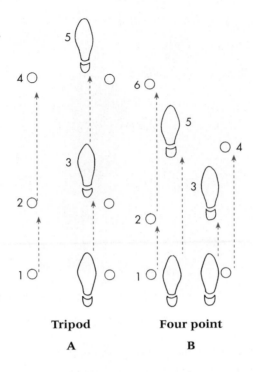

**Tripod**

**A**

**Four point**

**B**

stairs, the crutch tips and the affected leg move down one step followed by the support leg. If a handrail is available, both crutches are held by the outside hand, and a similar pattern is followed as with the crutch on each side. The phrase "up with the good—down with the bad" may help the athlete remember the correct sequence.

When the injured athlete needs to be partially weight bearing, a cane or perhaps a single crutch can be used to help with balance. In this case the athlete should hold the cane or crutch in the hand on the uninjured side and move the cane forward simultaneously with the injured leg. The athlete should avoid leaning too heavily on the cane or crutch. If this is a problem then the athlete should use two crutches.

**Athletic Injury Management Checklist**

The following checklist includes steps that should be taken in initial management and assessment of injury.

☐ Have an established emergency action plan in place.
☐ Conduct annual training for all staff to practice executing the emergency action plan.
☐ Determine if the athlete is conscious or unconscious.
☐ If the athlete is unconscious, dial 911 and access the emergency medical system.

☐ Conduct primary survey looking for life-threatening injuries (loss of breathing, bleeding, shock).

☐ Take appropriate measures to manage loss of breathing, bleeding, or shock until the rescue squad arrives. The rescue squad takes over injury management.

☐ If there is no loss of consciousness and no life-threatening injury conduct a secondary survey.

☐ Immobilize the injury if necessary.

☐ Determine how the athlete should be transported from the field.

☐ Notify the parents of injury if the athlete is a minor.

☐ Manage the injury using appropriate first aid measures (PRICE).

☐ Fit the athlete with a crutch or cane if necessary.

☐ Refer the athlete to the team or family physician.

## SUMMARY

• An emergency is defined as "an unforeseen combination of circumstances and the resulting state that calls for immediate action." The prime concern of emergency aid is to maintain cardiovascular function and, indirectly, central nervous system function. All sports programs should have an emergency action plan that is activated anytime an athlete is seriously injured.

• A systematic assessment of the injured athlete should be made to determine appropriate emergency care. A primary survey assesses and deals with life-threatening situations. Once stabilized, the secondary survey makes a more detailed assessment of the injury.

• All staff personnel should be certified in CPR/AED. To relieve an obstructed airway, abdominal thrusts or chest compressions and/or a finger sweep of the throat should be performed. An AED can be critical in restoring normal heart rhythm.

• Hemorrhage can occur externally and internally. External bleeding can be controlled by direct pressure, applying pressure at pressure points, and by elevation. Internal hemorrhage can occur subcutaneously, intramuscularly, or within a body cavity.

• Secondary assessment consists of four major areas: history, general observation, physical examination, and special tests. Special tests depend on the body site.

• Protection, rest, ice, compression, and elevation (PRICE) should be used for the immediate care of a musculoskeletal injury. Ice should be applied for at least 20 minutes every 1 to 1½ hours, and compression and elevation should be continuous for at least 72 hours following injury.

- Any suspected fracture should be splinted before the athlete is moved. Commercial rapid form vacuum immobilizers and air splints are most often used in an athletic training setting.

- Great care must be taken in moving the seriously injured athlete. The unconscious athlete must be handled as though he or she has a cervical fracture. Moving an athlete with a suspected serious neck injury must be performed only by persons specifically trained to do so. A spine board should be used, avoiding any movement of the cervical region.

- The proper fitting and instruction in the use of crutches or a cane by an athlete with an injury to the lower extremity is essential.

*Solutions to Critical Thinking* Exercises

**7-1** Because of the mechanism of injury, it should be suspected that the athlete has a cervical neck injury. The head should be stabilized throughout. If the athlete is prone and breathing, do nothing until consciousness returns. An on-field exam should establish the athlete's unresponsiveness. Then the athlete should be carefully logrolled onto a spine board because CPR could be necessary at any time. The face mask should be removed in case CPR is required. The helmet and shoulder pads should be left in place. The athlete should then be transported to the emergency facility. Remember, in this situation the worst mistake that can be made is not exercising enough caution.

**7-2** First a subjective history should be taken from the injured athlete, followed by an objective examination that includes observation, palpation, special tests, tests for joint stability, and a functional performance evaluation.

**7-3** The ankle should be wrapped with a wet elastic compression wrap. Ice should be applied to both sides of the joint over the compression wrap and secured. The ankle should be elevated such that the leg is above 45 degrees at a minimum. The compression wrap, ice, and elevation should be maintained initially for at least 30 minutes but not longer than an hour. Some determination should be made as to whether a fracture is suspected. Make the appropriate referral to a physician.

## REVIEW QUESTIONS AND CLASS ACTIVITIES

1. What considerations are important in a well-planned system for handling emergency situations?
2. Discuss the rules for managing and moving an unconscious athlete.
3. What are the life-threatening conditions that should be evaluated in the primary survey?
4. What are the ABCs of life support?
5. Identify the major steps in giving CPR and managing an obstructed airway. When may these procedures be used in a sports setting?
6. List the basic steps in assessing a musculoskeletal injury.
7. What techniques should be used to stop external hemorrhage?
8. What are the signs and symptoms of shock and how do you treat it?

9. What first-aid procedures are used to decrease hemorrhage, inflammation, and pain from a musculoskeletal injury?
10. Discuss the process for assessing an injury.
11. Describe the basic concepts of emergency splinting.
12. How should an athlete with a suspected spinal injury be transported?
13. What techniques can be used when transporting an athlete with a suspected musculoskeletal injury?
14. Explain how to properly fit crutches.

## REFERENCES

1. AHA clarifies CPR guidelines, recommends "hands-only" CPR for bystanders: 2008. *PT: Magazine of physical therapy* 16(6):16.
2. American Heart Association: 2005. Highlights of the 2005 American Heart Association guidelines for cardiopulmonary resuscitation and emergency cardiovascular care, *Currents in emergency cardiovascular care* 16(4):1–8.
3. American Red Cross: 2006. *CPR/AED for the professional rescuer.* Yardley, PA, American Red Cross.
4. Andersen, JC, Courson, RW, Kleiner, DM, McLoda, TA: 2002. National Athletic Trainers' Association position statement: emergency planning in athletics, *Journal of athletic training* 37(1):99–104.
5. Broglio, S, Dillon, M: 2005. Emergency management of head and cervical-spine injuries, *Athletic therapy today* 10(2):24.
6. Brukner, P, Khan, K, Hunte, G: 2002. Sporting emergencies. In Brukner, P (ed), *Clinical sports medicine,* 2nd ed, Sydney, McGraw-Hill.
7. Courson, R. 2007. Preventing sudden death on the athletic field: the emergency action plan, *Current sports medicine reports* 6(2):93.
8. Delforge, G: 2002. Sports injury assessment and problem identification. In Delforge, G. (ed), *Musculoskeletal trauma: implications for sports injury management.* Champaign, IL, Human Kinetics.
9. Del Rossi, G, Horodyski, M: 2008. The 6-plus–person lift transfer technique compared with other methods of spine boarding, *Journal of athletic training* 43(1):6.
10. Gale, S, Decoster, L. 2008. The combined tool approach for face mask removal during on-field conditions, *Journal of athletic training* 43(1):14.
11. Helmet removal guidelines: 2001. In Shultz, SJ et al. (ed), *Sports medicine handbook,* Indianapolis, Ind., National Federation of State High School Associations.
12. Herbert, D: 2007. Emergency preparedness recommendations for high school and college athletic programs, *Exercise standards & malpractice reporter* 21(4):58.
13. Herbert, DL: 2004. Planning for an emergency response: in the absence of an AED, facility operators can ensure their members are safe and their facilities are protected from legal claim by adhering to strict standards of care, *Fitness management* 20(3):46–47.
14. Herbert, D.L.: 2004. Update on AEDs in health and fitness facilities, *Sports medicine standards and malpractice reporter* (16)(3):41–42.
15. Jenkins, HL, Valovich, TC, Arnold, BL, Gansneder, BM: 2001. Removal tools are faster and produce less force and torque on the helmet than cutting tools during face-mask retraction, *Journal of athletic training* 37(3):246–251.
16. Karren KJ, Limmer, D: 2007. *First aid for colleges and universities,* Upper Saddle River, NJ, Pearson.

17. Kleiner, DM: 2001. 10 questions about football-helmet and face-mask removal: a review of the recent literature, *Athletic therapy today,* 6(3): 29–35.
18. Knight K: 1995. *Cryotherapy in sport injury management,* Champaign, IL, Human Kinetics.
19. Magee DL: 2007. *Orthopedic physical assessment,* Philadelphia, WB Saunders.
20. National Safety Council: 2004. *First aid CPR and AED Essentials,* Boston, Jones & Bartlett.
21. Ransone J, Dunn-Bennett LR: 1999. Assessment of first-aid knowledge and decision making of high school athletic coaches, *Journal of athletic training* 34(3): 267.
22. Rubin, A: 2004. *Sports injuries and emergencies: a quick response manual,* New York, McGraw-Hill.
23. Shores, A: 2001. Raising the safety standard. New program provides emergency training for volunteer coaches, *Sports medicine update* 16(1):40–41.

24. Starkey C, Ryan J: 2002. *Evaluation of orthopedic and athletic injuries,* Philadelphia, FA Davis.
25. Steinbach, P.: Emergency situation: countless young athletes are taking the field without a trained care provider on the sideline, but new efforts to equip coaches with basic first-aid knowledge are coming to the rescue, *Athletic business* 27(11): 62–64; 66; 68, 2003.
26. Sturgill, G, Martin, R: 2006. Being prepared for a medical emergency, *Journal of physical education & recreation* 12(1):58–62.
27. Swartz, E: 2007. Efficient football helmet face mask removal, *Athletic therapy today* 12(2):21.
28. Walsh, K: 2001. Thinking proactively: the emergency action plan, *Athletic therapy today* 6(5):57–62.
29. Waninger KN: 1998. On-field management of potential cervical spine injury in helmeted football players: leave the helmet on, *Clin J Sportmed* 8(2):124.

**ANNOTATED BIBLIOGRAPHY**

American College of Emergency Physicians: 2009. *Sports first aid and injury prevention,* Boston, Jones and Bartlett.
*This text teaches coaches how to administer basic first aid to sick and injured athletes.*
Karren KJ, Limmer, D: 2007. *First aid for colleges and universities,* Upper Saddle River, NJ, Pearson.
*A well-illustrated, simple approach to the treatment of emergency illness and injury.*
Leikin JB, Feldman BJ: 2000. *American Medical Association handbook of first aid and emergency care,* Philadelphia, Random House.
*Covering urgent emergency situations and the common injuries and ailments that occur in every family, this AMA guide takes the reader step-by-step through basic first-aid techniques, the* medical symptoms to recognize before an emergency occurs, and what to do when one does.
Magee DJ: 2007. *Orthopedic physical assessment,* Philadelphia, WB Saunders.
*An extremely well-illustrated book, with excellent depth of coverage. Its strength lies in its coverage of injuries commonly found during athletic training.*
Thygerson A: 2004. National Safety Council: *First aid CPR and AED Essentials,* Boston, Jones and Bartlett.
*A complete and widely used first aid text that addresses all aspects of first aid CPR and AED use*
Starkey C, Ryan J: 2003. *Orthopedic and athletic injuries, Evaluation Handbook,* Philadelphia, 2003, FA Davis.
*A detailed, well-illustrated text that addresses all aspects of injury assessment for the athletic trainer.*

**WEB SITES**

American Red Cross:
www.redcross.org
*The American Red Cross offers many emergency services and training. This site describes those services and introduces information about various training opportunities.*

American Heart Association:
www.amhrt.org

National Safety Council:
www.nsc.org/
*The National Safety Council is a membership organization with resources on safety, health, and environmental topics, training, products, publications, news, and more.*

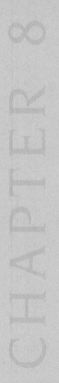

## CHAPTER 8

# Bloodborne Pathogens, Universal Precautions, and Wound Care

*When you finish this chapter you will be able to:*

- Explain what bloodborne pathogens are and how they can infect fitness professionals and athletes.
- Describe the transmission, symptoms and signs, and treatment of hepatitis B (HBV).
- Describe the transmission, signs and symptoms, management, and treatment of hepatitis C (HCV).
- Describe the transmission, symptoms, and signs of human immunodeficiency virus (HIV) infection.
- Describe how HIV is most often transmitted.
- List the pros and cons of sports participation of athletes with an HBV or HIV infection.
- Identify universal precautions as mandated by the Occupational Safety and Health Administration and how they apply to the coach.
- Discuss the various types of skin wounds.

I t has always been important for any health care provider to be concerned with maintaining an environment that is as clean and sterile as possible.[1,7] In our twenty-first century society, it has become critical for everyone in the population to take measures to prevent the spread of infectious diseases.[25] Failure to do so may expose any individual to potentially life-threatening situations.[24]

**Because of the close physical contact that occurs through athletic participation, the potential for spread of infectious disease among fitness professionals, coaches, athletes, and sports medicine personnel is of major concern. Everyone must be aware of the potential dangers of exposure to blood or other infectious materials and take whatever measures are necessary to prevent contamination** (Figure 8-1).[25]

## WHAT ARE BLOODBORNE PATHOGENS?

*Bloodborne pathogens* are pathogenic microorganisms that can potentially cause disease. They may be present in human blood and other bodily fluids including semen, vaginal secretions, cerebrospinal fluid, synovial fluid, and any other fluid contaminated with blood.[23] The three most significant bloodborne pathogens include the hepatitis B virus (HBV), hepatitis C virus (HCV), and the human immunodeficiency virus (HIV).[29] A number of

**Bloodborne pathogens:**
- hepatitis B (HBV)
- hepatitis C (HCV)
- human immunodeficiency virus (HIV)

**Mode of transmission:**
- human blood
- semen
- vaginal secretions
- cerebrospinal fluid
- synovial fluid

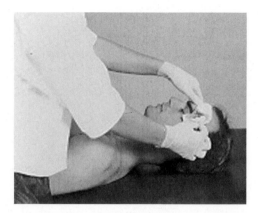

**Figure 8-1**

Precautions must be taken to prevent exposure and transmission of bloodborne pathogens.

other bloodborne diseases exist, including hepatitis A, hepatitis D, hepatitis E, and syphilis. Although HIV has been more widely addressed in the media, HBV and HCV have a higher possibility for spread.[18] HBV is stronger and more durable than HIV.[7] HBV can be spread more easily via sharp objects, open wounds, or bodily fluids when compared to HIV.

## Hepatitis B Virus

HBV is a major cause of viral infection that results in swelling, soreness, and loss of normal function in the liver. The number of cases of HBV has risen dramatically during the last 10 years.[28]

### Signs of HBV

The signs in a person infected with HBV include flulike symptoms such as fatigue, weakness, nausea, abdominal pain, headache, fever, and possibly jaundice. It is possible that an individual infected with HBV will exhibit no signs or symptoms and may go undetected. In these individuals, the HBV antigen will always be present and thus the disease may be unknowingly transmitted to others through exposure to blood or other bodily fluids or by intimate contact.

An infected person's blood may test positive for the HBV antigen within 2 to 6 weeks after the symptoms develop. Approximately 85 percent of those infected recover within 6 to 8 weeks.

### Prevention

Good personal hygiene and avoiding high-risk activities are the best ways to avoid HBV.[7] HBV can survive for at least a week in dried blood or on contaminated surfaces and may be transmitted through contact with these surfaces. Caution must be taken to avoid contact with any blood or other fluid that potentially contains a bloodborne pathogen.

### Management

A vaccine is now available that can prevent contraction of HBV. The vaccine requires a series of three inoculations spread over a 6-month period.

In 1991 the Occupational Safety and Health Administration (OSHA) mandated that vaccination against HBV must be made available by an employer at no cost to any individual who may be exposed to blood or other bodily fluids and may thus be at risk of contracting hepatitis B.[11] **Any individual working in an allied health care profession who may potentially come in contact with blood should receive HBV immunization.**

### Hepatitis C

Originally referred to as non-A, non-B hepatitis, hepatitis C is both an acute and chronic form of liver disease caused by the hepatitis C virus (HCV). HCV is the most common chronic bloodborne infection in the United States. At least 85 percent of those infected acutely with HCV become chronically infected, and 67 percent develop chronic liver disease. It is the leading indication for liver transplant. Three percent of those with chronic liver disease die from cirrhosis or liver cancer. It is estimated that 3.9 million Americans have been infected with HCV, of whom 2.7 million are chronically infected.[16]

#### Symptoms and Signs

Eighty percent of those infected with HCV have no signs or symptoms. Those who are symptomatic may be jaundiced and/or have mild abdominal pain, particularly in the upper right quadrant; loss of appetite; nausea; fatigue; muscle or joint pain; and/or dark urine.

#### Prevention

HCV is not spread by sneezing, hugging, coughing, food or water, sharing eating utensils or drinking glasses, or casual contact. It is rarely spread through sexual contact. It is spread by contact with the blood of an infected person.[16] It is most commonly transmitted by sharing needles or syringes. Therefore, it is a significant risk of getting a tattoo or body piercing. However it can also be transmitted by sharing personal care items that might have blood on them (razors, toothbrushes). Athletic trainers should always follow routine barrier precautions and safely handle needles and other sharp objects.

#### Management

Unlike HBV, presently there is no vaccine for preventing HCV transmission. Several blood tests can be done to determine if a person has been infected with HCV. A physician may order just one or a combination of these tests. It is possible to find HCV within one to two weeks after being infected with the virus. A single positive test indicates infection with HCV. However a single negative test does not prove that a person is not infected. When hepatitis C is suspected, even though an initial test is negative, the test should be repeated.[16]

HCV-positive persons should be evaluated by their doctor for liver disease. Interferon and ribavirin are two drugs used in combination that appear to be the most effective for the treatment of persons with chronic hepatitis C. Drinking alcohol can make liver disease worse.

## Human Immunodeficiency Virus

HIV infection is caused by a family of complex viruses that invade normal healthy cells, thus decreasing the effectiveness of the host cell in preventing disease. HIV is a viral infection that has the potential to eventually destroy the immune system. The rapid increase in the number of known individuals who are HIV positive is alarming. The World Health Organization has estimated that worldwide 42 million people were living with HIV/AIDS as of the year 2004.[37]

### Symptoms and Signs of HIV

As with HBV, HIV is transmitted by exposure to infected blood or other bodily fluids or by intimate sexual contact. Symptoms of HIV include fatigue, weight loss, muscle or joint pain, painful or swollen glands, night sweats, and fever. HIV antibodies can be detected in a blood test within a year following exposure. Like people with HBV, people with HIV may be unaware that they have contracted the virus and may go as long as 8 to 10 years before developing any signs or symptoms. Unfortunately most individuals who test positive for HIV have a high probability of eventually developing acquired immunodeficiency syndrome (AIDS). Table 8-1 summarizes information on HBV, HCV, and HIV.

AIDS: Acquired
immunodeficiency syndrome

### Acquired Immunodeficiency Syndrome

AIDS is an acronym for acquired immunodeficiency syndrome. A syndrome is a collection of signs and symptoms that are recognized as the effects of an

**TABLE 8-1** Transmission of Hepatitis B and C Viruses and Human Immunodeficiency Virus

| Disease | Symptoms and Signs | Mode of Transmission | Infectious Materials |
|---|---|---|---|
| Hepatitis B virus | Flulike symptoms, jaundice | Direct and indirect contact | Blood, saliva, semen, feces, food, water, and other products |
| Hepatitis C virus | Jaundice, upper right quadrant pain, loss of appetite, nausea, fatigue, dark urine | Direct and indirect contact with blood | Blood |
| Human immuno-deficiency virus/ acquired immuno-deficiency syndrome | Fever, night sweats, weight loss, diarrhea, severe fatigue, swollen lymph nodes, lesions | Direct and indirect contact | Blood, semen, vaginal fluid |

Techniques for Preventing
and Minimizing Sport-
Related Injuries

infection. A person who has AIDS has no protection against even the simplest infections and thus is extremely vulnerable to developing a variety of illnesses, opportunistic infections, and/or cancers that cannot be stopped.[3] A positive HIV test cannot predict when the individual might show the symptoms of AIDS. Those individuals who develop AIDS generally die within 2 years after the symptoms appear.

### Management

Unlike HBV, there is no vaccine for HIV. Much research is being done to find a preventive vaccine and an effective treatment. Presently, it appears that certain combinations of various antiviral drugs, which have been labeled "cocktails," can slow replication of the virus and improve prospects for survival.

### Prevention

HIV is most often transmitted through intimate sexual contact.

The use of latex condoms can reduce the chances of contracting HIV.

The best means for prevention is through education.[16] Athletes should be educated about HIV. Athletes must be made to understand that their greatest risk for contracting HIV is through intimate sexual contact with an infected partner and not through contact that occurs during athletic participation. Practicing safe sex is of major importance. (See Focus Box 8-1.) The athlete must choose nonpromiscuous sex partners and use condoms for vaginal or anal intercourse. Latex condoms provide a barrier against both HBV and HIV. Male condoms should have reservoir tips to reduce the chance of ejaculate being released from the sides of the condom. Condoms that are prelubricated are less likely to tear. Water-based, greaseless spermicides or lubricants should be avoided. If the condom tears, a vaginal spermicide should be used immediately. The condom should carefully be removed and discarded.[9]

---

**8-1**    *Focus Box*

**HIV Risk Reduction**

- Avoid contact with others' bodily fluids, feces, and semen.
- Avoid sharing needles (e.g., injecting anabolic steroids or human growth hormones).
- Choose nonpromiscuous sex partners.
- Limit sex partners.
- Consistently use condoms.
- Avoid drugs that alter good judgment.
- Avoid sex with known HIV carriers.
- Get regular tests for sexually transmitted diseases (STDs).
- Practice good hygiene before and after sex.

# DEALING WITH BLOODBORNE PATHOGENS IN ATHLETICS

In general the chances of transmitting HIV among athletes is low. There is minimal risk of on-field transmission of HIV from one player to another in sports.[30] One study involving professional football estimated that the risk of transmission from player to player was less than one per 1 million games. In fact, at this writing there have been no validated reports of HIV transmission in sports.[9]

Sports that have a potentially higher risk for transmission are those that involve close physical contact and possible direct contact with the blood of another person.[38] Sports such as the martial arts, wrestling, and boxing have more theoretical potential for transmission.[9] (See Focus Box 8-2.)

## Policy Regulation

Athletes participating in organized sports are subject to procedures and policies relative to transmission of bloodborne pathogens.[21] The United States Olympic Committee (USOC), the National Collegiate Athletic Association (NCAA), the National Federation of State High School Athletic Associations, the National Basketball Association, the National Hockey League, the National Football League, and Major League Baseball have established policies to help prevent the transmission of bloodborne pathogens. They have also initiated programs to help educate athletes under their control.

All institutions should take the responsibility for educating their student-athletes about how bloodborne pathogens are transmitted.[33] Efforts should also be made to educate the parents of high-school athletes.[4] Professional, collegiate, and high-school athletes should be made to understand that the real risk of contracting HBV or HIV is through their off-the-field activities, which may include unsafe sexual practices and sharing needles, particularly in the use of steroids.[33] Athletes, perhaps more than other individuals in the population, tend to think that they are immune and that infection will always happen to someone else.

> **8-1 Critical Thinking**
> Exercise
>
> A wrestler is concerned about the possibility of contracting HIV from wrestling with a sweaty partner.
>
> ? What can this athlete be told to help him ease his fear?

---

**8-2** **Focus Box**

**Risk Categories for Sports[11]**

- Greatest risk: Boxing, tae kwon do, wrestling, rugby
- Moderate risk: Basketball, field hockey, football, ice hockey, judo, soccer, team handball
- Lowest risk: Archery, badminton, baseball, bowling, canoeing/kayaking, cycling, diving, equestrian sports, fencing, figure skating, gymnastics, modern pentathalon, raquetball, rhythmic gymnastics, roller skating, rowing, shooting, softball, speed skating, skiing, swimming, synchronized swimming, table tennis, volleyball, water polo, weightlifting, yachting

For additional information on
HIV and AIDS care, contact
the Centers for Disease
Control and Prevention
(CDC) National AIDS Hotline:
1-800-342-2437.

Each institution should implement policies and procedures concerning bloodborne pathogens.[31] A recent survey of NCAA institutions found that a large number of health care providers at many colleges and universities demonstrated significant deficits in following the universal guidelines mandated by OSHA. In a sports medicine or other health care setting, following these universal precautions protects the athlete, the coach, and the health care providers.[27]

### HIV and Athletic Participation

There is no definitive answer as to whether asymptomatic HIV carriers should participate in sports.[6,35] Bodily fluid contact should obviously be avoided, and the participant should also avoid engaging in exhaustive exercise that may lead to an increased susceptibility to infection.[18]

The Americans with Disabilities Act of 1991 states that athletes infected with HIV cannot be discriminated against and may be excluded from participation only on a medically sound basis. Exclusion must be based on objective medical evidence that takes into consideration the risk of infection to others and of potential harm to the athlete and what means can be taken to reduce these risks.[3]

### Testing Athletes for HIV

HIV testing should not be used as a screening tool to determine if an athlete can participate in sports. Mandatory testing for HIV may not be allowed for legal reasons related to the Americans with Disabilities Act. In terms of importance, mandatory testing should be secondary to education to prevent transmission of HIV. Neither the NCAA nor the Centers for Disease Control and Prevention (CDC) recommends mandatory HIV testing for athletes.[31]

Athletes who engage in high-risk activities should be encouraged to seek voluntary anonymous testing for HIV. A blood test may detect the presence of the HIV virus within 3 months to 1 year following exposure. Testing therefore should occur at 6 weeks, at 3 months, and at 1 year after exposure.[9]

Many states have enacted laws that protect the confidentiality of the HIV-infected person. For example, you cannot ask anyone if they are HIV positive on a medical history form. Coaches should be familiar with the laws of their state and make every effort to guard the confidentiality and anonymity of HIV testing for their athletes.[36]

## UNIVERSAL PRECAUTIONS IN AN ATHLETIC ENVIRONMENT

The guidelines instituted by OSHA were developed to protect the health care provider and the patient against bloodborne pathogens.[28] It is essential that every sports program develop and carry out a bloodborne pathogen exposure control plan.[15] This plan should include counseling, education, volunteer testing, and the management of bodily fluids.[31]

Throughout the remainder of this text, wherever there is a discussion of an injury or a technique of care that requires universal precautions the following icon will appear in the margin.

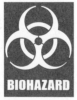
BIOHAZARD

OSHA's guidelines should be followed by anyone coming in contact with blood or other bodily fluids. Following are considerations specific to the sports arena.

### Preparing the Athlete

Before an athlete participates in practice or competition, all open skin wounds or lesions must be covered with a dressing that is fixed in place and does not allow for transmission to or from an athlete.[10] An occlusive dressing lessens the chances of cross-contamination and also reduces chances of the wound reopening by keeping it moist and pliable.

### When Bleeding Occurs

As mandated by the NCAA and the USOC, open wounds or other skin lesions considered a risk for disease transmission should be treated aggressively.[32] This means that athletes with active bleeding must be removed from participation as soon as possible and only returned when it is deemed safe by the medical staff.[5] Uniforms containing blood must be evaluated for infectivity. A uniform that is saturated with blood must be removed and changed before the athlete can return to competition.[8] All personnel managing potential infective wound exposures must follow universal precautions.[28]

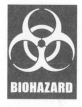

**BIOHAZARD**

### Personal Precautions

Health care personnel working directly with bodily fluids on the field must make use of the appropriate protective equipment in all cases in which there is potential contact with bloodborne pathogens. Protective equipment includes disposable nonlatex gloves, gowns, or aprons; masks and shields; eye protection; nonabsorbant gowns; and disposable mouthpieces for resuscitation devices.[28] **One-time use nonlatex gloves should be used in treating the athlete.** The choice of glove type should be appropriate to the situation. The ideal prophylactic glove is made of latex. Unfortunately, many people have allergies to latex. Thus, one should consider wearing nonlatex gloves such as those made of vinyl or synthetic rubber. These gloves may be used when the superior barrier protection of latex is not needed such as when there is minimal prospect for long-term exposure to blood or body fluids.[13] Double gloving is suggested when there is heavy bleeding or when sharp instruments are used. Gloves are always carefully removed following their use (see Focus Box 8-3). In cases of emergency, heavy toweling may be used until gloves can be obtained.[1]

Hands and all skin surfaces that come in contact with blood or other bodily fluids should be washed immediately with soap and water or other antigermicidal agents.

First-aid kits must have protection for hands, face, and eyes and resuscitation mouthpieces. Kits should also make towelettes available for cleaning skin surfaces.[2]

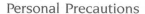

**8-2 Critical Thinking**
Exercise

A soccer player jumps to win a head ball and an opponent's head smashes the right eyebrow, creating a significant laceration. The athlete is conscious but is bleeding profusely from the wound.

? What techniques are most effective to control the bleeding, and what should be done to close the wound?

Nonlatex gloves should be worn when dealing with blood or bodily fluids.

Techniques for Preventing
and Minimizing Sport-
Related Injuries

### Glove Removal and Use (Figure 8-2)

1. Avoid touching personal items when wearing contaminated gloves.
2. Remove first glove by using the other gloved hand and turn inside out, beginning at the wrist and peeling off without touching skin.
3. Remove second glove while trapping the other glove inside making sure not to touch ungloved hand to soiled surfaces.
4. Discard gloves that have been used, discolored, torn, or punctured in white biohazard bags.
5. Wash hands immediately after glove removal.

## Availability of Supplies and Equipment

In keeping with universal precautions, the sports program must have available chlorine bleach, antiseptics, proper receptacles for soiled equipment and uniforms, wound care bandages, and a designated container for disposal of sharps such as needles, syringes, or scalpels.[21]

Universal precautions
minimize the risk of exposure
and transmission.

Biohazard warning labels should be fixed to regulated wastes, refrigerators containing blood, and other containers used to store or ship potentially infectious materials (Figure 8-3). The labels are fluorescent orange or red and should be affixed to containers. White bags should be used for disposal of potentially infected materials such as contaminated gloves and bandages. Sealed white bags can be placed in regular trash containers for disposal.

### 8-3 *Critical Thinking*
Exercise

All institutions sponsoring athletic programs must initiate and carry out a bloodborne pathogen exposure control plan.

? What is the policy on universal precautions in an athletic environment as proposed by OSHA?

### Disinfectants

All contaminated surfaces, such as the field or court, should be cleaned immediately with a solution consisting of one part bleach to ten parts water (1:10) or with a disinfectant approved by the Environmental Protection Agency.[48] Disinfectants should inactivate the virus. Towels or other linens that have been contaminated should be bagged and separated from other

**Figure 8-2**

Technique for removing
nonlatex gloves

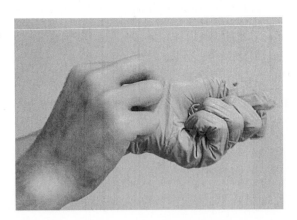

laundry. Soiled linen is to be transported in red or orange containers or bags that prevent soaking or leaking and are labeled with the biohazard warning labels (refer to Figure 8-3). Contaminated laundry should be washed in hot water (71°C for 25 minutes) using a detergent that deactivates the virus. Laundry done outside the institution should be taken to a facility that follows OSHA standards. Gloves must be worn during bagging and cleaning of contaminated laundry.[15]

### Sharps

*Sharps* refers to sharp objects such as needles, razor blades, and scalpels. Extreme care should be taken when handling and disposing of sharps to minimize risk of puncturing or cutting the skin. OSHA mandates that sharps be disposed of in a leakproof and puncture-resistant container.[4,11] The container should be red or orange and labeled as a biohazard (Figure 8-4).

## Protecting the Caregiver

It must be pointed out that OSHA guidelines for bloodborne pathogens are intended to protect staff personnel and other employees and not the athlete.[11] Staff other than sports medicine personnel and occasionally coaches do not normally come in contact with blood or other bodily fluids from an injured athlete, so their risk is considerably reduced. It is the responsibility of the high school, college, professional team, or

Contaminated surfaces should be cleaned with a 10 percent bleach solution.

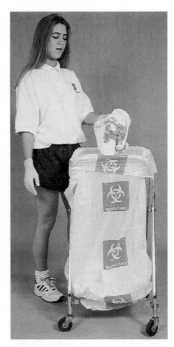

**Figure 8-3**

Soiled linens should be placed in a leakproof bag marked as a biohazard.

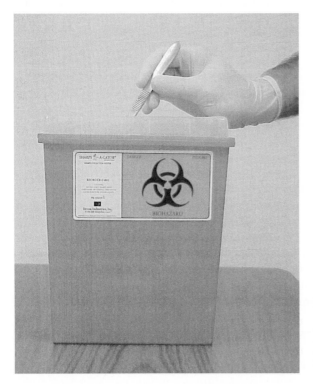

**Figure 8-4**

Sharps should be disposed of in a red, puncture-resistant, plastic container marked as a biohazard.

clinic to ensure the safety of all staff members as potential health care providers by instituting and annually updating policies for education on the prevention of transmission of bloodborne pathogens through contact with athletes. The institution must provide the necessary supplies and equipment to carry out these recommendations. All staff members have the personal responsibility of adhering to these policies and guidelines and enforcing them.

### Protecting the Athlete from Exposure

Several additional recommendations may further help protect the athlete. The USOC supports the required use of mouthpieces in those high-risk sports listed in Focus Box 8-2. All athletes should shower immediately after practice or competition. Athletes who may be exposed to HIV or HBV should be evaluated for immunization against HBV.

### Postexposure Procedures

Following a report of an exposure incident, the exposed individual should have a confidential medical evaluation that includes documentation of the exposure route, identification of the source individual, a blood test, counseling, and an evaluation of reported illness. Again, the laws that pertain to reporting and notification of the test results relative to confidentiality vary from state to state.[11]

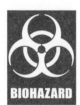

## CARING FOR SKIN WOUNDS

Skin wounds are extremely common in sports. A wound is defined as trauma to tissues that causes a break in the continuity of that tissue.[11] The skin consists of two layers, the epidermis and the dermis. Because of the soft, pliable nature of skin, it can be easily traumatized. Numerous mechanical forces can injure soft tissue. These forces produce friction or rubbing, scraping, compression or pressure, tearing, cutting, and penetration, each of which can adversely affect the skin's integrity.[24] Wounds are classified according to the mechanical force that caused them.

### Types of Wounds

Various types of wounds may be classified as follows (Figure 8-5):

*Abrasions* are common conditions in which the skin is scraped against a rough surface such as grass, artificial playing surface, floor, or mat. The top layer of skin wears away, exposing numerous blood capillaries. This exposure, with dirt and foreign materials scraping and penetrating the skin, increases the probability of infection unless the wound is properly debrided and cleansed.[5]

*Lacerations*, also common in sports, occur when a sharp or pointed object tears the tissues, giving a wound the appearance of a jagged-edge cavity. As with abrasions, lacerations present an environment conductive to infections. The same mechanism that causes a laceration also can lead to a skin avulsion, in which a piece of skin is ripped off.[14]

*Puncture wounds* can easily occur during physical activities and can be fatal. Direct penetration of tissues by a pointed object such as a track shoe spike can introduce the tetanus bacillus into the bloodstream, possibly making the athlete a victim of lockjaw. All puncture wounds and severe lacerations should be referred immediately to a physician.

*Avulsion wounds* occur when skin is torn from the body and are frequently associated with major bleeding. If the torn tissue may possibly be reattached, the avulsed tissue should be placed on moist gauze, preferably saturated with saline solution. It is then put into a plastic bag, immersed in cold water, and taken along with the athlete to the hospital for reattachment.[11]

*Incisions* are wounds with smooth edges that often appear where a blow has been delivered over a sharp bone or a bone that is poorly padded. They are not as serious as the other types of exposed wounds.

## Immediate Care

It is of the utmost importance to the well-being of the athlete that open wounds be cared for immediately.[17] All wounds, even those that are relatively superficial, must be considered to be contaminated by microorganisms and therefore must be cleaned, medicated (when called for), and dressed.[19] To minimize the chances of infection, it is critical that the wound be cleaned as thoroughly as possible.[30] It is recommended that the wound initially be cleaned using copious amounts of soap and water or sterile saline. Neither bacterial solutions nor hydrogen peroxide should be used to clean the wound initially. Dressing wounds requires a sterile environment to prevent infections.[17]

## Dressings

Sterile dressings should be applied to keep a fresh wound clean. Sterile dressings come in various sizes from simple gauze pads to adhesive bandages. Occlusive dressings appear to be extremely effective in minimizing scarring.[26] If a wound is discharging fluid (serum), the dressing should be changed often to minimize bacterial growth. After drainage has stopped, there is no need for a dressing. Antibacterial ointments may be applied to limit surface bacterial growth and prevent the dressing from sticking to the wound. Topical antibiotics are recommended. Wounds may be cleansed with hydrogen peroxide several times daily over the next several days before the reapplication of ointment. Good wound care will minimize the inflammatory response, speed healing, and minimize scarring.

## Are Sutures Necessary?

Deeper lacerations, incisions, or occasionally puncture wounds may require some sort of manual closure using sutures. If an athlete has a wound that appears to be severe the athlete should be sent to the physician, who will make a decision as to whether it is necessary to use sutures to close the wound. Sutures should be put in as soon as possible but

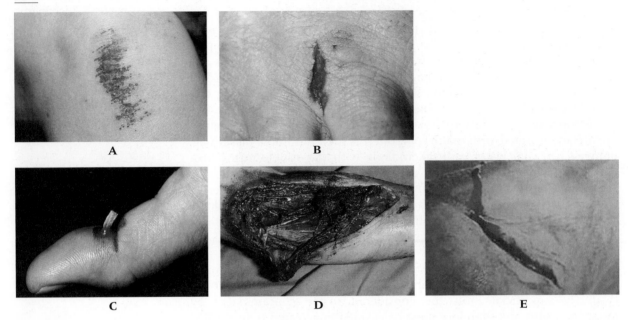

**Figure 8-5**

Wounds: (A) Abrasion of shoulder. (B) Laceration of hand. (C) Puncture of thumb. (D) Avulsion of forearm. (E) Incision on sole of foot.

certainly within a maximum of 12 hours following injury. In relatively simple wounds, the edges may be brought in close approximation by the use of sutures to minimize scar formation. Before closing a wound with a suture, the doctor will usually anesthetize the local area with a short acting medication. Fine suture material and minimal tightening limit any additional tissue damage, inflammation, and scarring. Wounds in areas that heal slower (areas that are less vascularized) or are in high stress areas require larger suture material and that the stitches be left in longer. Sometimes sutures may be removed after only a few days to minimize scarring.

The physician may decide that the wound does not require sutures and that the torn tissues may be approximated using steri-strips or butterfly bandages.

## Signs of Wound Infection

The classic signs of infection are the same as those for inflammation, including pain, heat, redness, swelling, and disordered function. In addition pus may form due to an accumulation of white blood cells, and a fever may occur as the immune system fights the bacterial infection.[26] Most wound infections can be treated with antibiotic drugs. However, in recent years some strains of a bacterium found on the skin called *staphylococcus aureus* have become resistant to some antibiotics. The bacteria are referred to as methicillin-resistant staphylococcus aureus (MRSA). MRSA strains are much more difficult to treat because many antibiotics do not work. Therefore, infections tend to become more severe than they may otherwise have been if the cause of the infection is not diagnosed early, and antibiotics that do not work are

**TABLE 8-2** Care of skin wounds

| Type of Wound | Action of Coach | Initial Care | Follow-up Care |
|---|---|---|---|
| Abrasion | 1. Provide initial care.<br><br>2. Wound seldom requires medical attention unless infected. | 1. Cleanse abraded area with soap and water; debride with brush.<br>2. Apply an antibiotic ointment to keep abraded surface moist. In sports it is not desirable for abrasions to acquire a scab. Place either an occlusive dressing or a nonadherent sterile pad (Telfa pad) over the ointment. | 1. Change dressing daily and look for signs of infection. |
| Laceration | 1. Cleanse around the wound. Avoid wiping more contaminating agents into the area.<br>2. Apply dry, sterile compress pad and refer to physician. | 1. Complete cleansing and suturing are accomplished by a physician; injections of tetanus vaccine may be required. | 1. Change dressing daily and look for signs of infection. |
| Puncture | 1. Cleanse around the wound. Avoid wiping more contaminating agents into the area.<br>2. Apply dry, sterile compress pad and refer to physician. | 1. Complete cleansing and injections of tetanus vaccine, if needed, are managed by a physician. | 1. Change dressing daily and look for signs of infection. |
| Avulsion | 1. Clean around wound; save avulsed tissue.<br>2. Apply dry, sterile compress pad to control bleeding and refer to physician. | 1. Wound is cleansed thoroughly; avulsed skin is replaced and sutured by a physician; tetanus vaccine injection may be required. | 1. Change dressing daily and look for signs of infection. |
| Incision | 1. Clean around wound.<br>2. Apply dry, sterile compress pad to control bleeding and refer to physician. | 1. Cleanse wound.<br>2. Suturing and injections of tetanus vaccine are managed by a physician, if needed. | 1. Change dressing daily and look for signs of infection. |

given at first. Infections that start in the skin may spread to cause more serious infections.[24] MRSA is discussed in detail in Chapter 23.

### Tetanus

Tetanus is a bacterial infection that causes fever and convulsions. A tetanus infection occurs most often with a puncture wound. Tonic spasm of skeletal muscles is always a possibility for any nonimmunized athlete. The tetanus bacillus enters a wound as a spore and, depending

**Suggested Practices in Wound Care**

The following are suggested procedures to reduce the possibility of
wound infections.

1. Make sure all instruments used, such as scissors, tweezers, and swabs,
   are sterilized.
2. Wash hands thoroughly and put on nonlatex gloves.
3. Clean a skin lesion using soap and water.
4. Place a nonmedicated dressing on a lesion if the athlete is to be sent
   for medical attention.
5. Avoid touching any parts of a sterile dressing that will come in contact
   with a wound.
6. Place medication on a pad rather than directly on a lesion.
7. Secure the dressing with tape or a wrap.
8. If necessary, follow the procedures described in this chapter for control
   of bleeding.

on individual susceptibility, acts on the motor end plate of the central
nervous system. After initial childhood immunization with a tetanus
vaccine, boosters should be given every 10 years.[11] An athlete not im-
munized should receive an injection of tetanus immune globulin
(Hyper-Tet) immediately after sustaining a skin wound. Focus Box 8-4
describes how to help reduce wound infections and Table 8-2 details the
care of wounds.

**Athletic Injury Management Checklist**

The following is a checklist for practicing universal precautions
in dealing with bloodborne pathogens.

☐ Wash hands frequently throughout the day.
☐ Make sure all open wounds or skin lesions are covered before
   practice or competition.
☐ Routinely use nonlatex gloves when dealing with bleeding or
   wound care.
☐ Remove athletes with active bleeding from competition.
☐ Ensure that a uniform saturated with blood is removed and
   changed.
☐ Clean up blood spills with a disinfecting solution.
☐ Use the appropriate technique when removing gloves.
☐ Dispose of all soiled materials in a biohazard bag.
☐ Dispose of sharps in a biohazard container.
☐ Wash hands thoroughly after taking universal precautions.
☐ Report all exposure incidents.

## SUMMARY

- Bloodborne pathogens are microorganisms that can potentially cause disease and are present in human blood and other bodily fluids, including semen, vaginal secretions, synovial fluid, and any other fluid contaminated with blood. Hepatitis B virus (HBV), hepatitis C virus (HCV), and human immunodeficiency virus (HIV) are bloodborne pathogens.

- A vaccine is available to prevent HBV. Currently no effective vaccine exists for treating HIV.

- An individual infected with HIV may develop acquired immuno-deficiency syndrome (AIDS), which is fatal.

- The risks of contracting HBV, HCV, or HIV may be minimized by avoiding exposure to blood and other bodily fluids and by practicing safe sex.

- The risk of an athlete being exposed to bloodborne pathogens on the field is minimal. Off-the-field activities involving risky sexual behaviors pose the greatest threat for transmission.

- Various national medical and sports organizations have established policies and procedures for dealing with bloodborne pathogens in the athletic population.

- The Occupational Safety and Health Administration (OSHA) has established rules and regulations that protect the health care employee.

- Universal precautions must be taken to avoid bloodborne pathogen exposure. All sports programs must carry out a plan for counseling, education, volunteer testing, and the management of exposure.

---

*Solutions to Critical Thinking* Exercises

**8-1** Athletes must be made to understand that their greatest risk for contracting HIV is through intimate sexual contact with an infected partner and not through contact that occurs during athletic participation. It is highly unlikely that sweat carries HIV. However, this athlete should become concerned if his opponent begins bleeding; he should wait until the bleeding has been controlled and the wound securely covered before resuming physical contact.

**8-2** The first step is to take precautions to protect against the transmission of bloodborne pathogens. The wound should be cleaned with soap and water. Direct pressure should be applied to the wound over several layers of sterile gauze, which hopefully will absorb the bleeding. Ice may also be applied to help minimize the bleeding. The athlete, if not dizzy, should remain in a sitting position and should be referred to a physician for suturing. Sterile strips or a butterfly bandage may also be applied, although sutures generally leave a smaller scar. All blood-contaminated supplies should be disposed of in a clearly marked biohazard bag.

**8-3** Universal precautions should be practiced by anyone coming in contact with blood or other body fluids. This plan must include counseling, education, voluntary testing, and management of bodily fluids.

## REVIEW QUESTIONS AND CLASS ACTIVITIES

1. Define and identify the bloodborne pathogens.
2. Discuss HBV transmission, symptoms and signs, prevention, and treatment.
3. Discuss the pros and cons of allowing the participation of an athlete who is an HBV carrier.
4. Discuss HIV transmission, symptoms and signs, prevention, and treatment.
5. How is HIV transmitted and why is it eventually fatal at this time?
6. Should an athlete who tests positive for HBV or HIV be allowed to participate in sports?
7. How can an athlete avoid the risk of HIV infection?
8. Define OSHA and discuss its universal precautions for preventing exposure to bloodborne pathogens.
9. What precautions should a coach take when caring for a bleeding athlete on the field?
10. What are the different kinds of wounds that can occur and how should they be managed?

## REFERENCES

1. American Academy of Pediatrics: 1991. Human immunodeficiency virus [acquired immunodeficiency syndrome (AIDS) virus] in athletic settings, *Pediatrics* 88:640.
2. American Medical Association Department of HIV, Division of Health Science: 1993. *Digest of HIV/AIDS policy,* Chicago, American Medical Association.
3. American Medical Society for Sports Medicine and the American Academy for Sports Medicine: 1995. Human immunodeficiency virus (HIV) and bloodborne pathogens in sport, joint position statement, *Am J Sports Med* 23: 510.
4. Arnold BL: 1995. A review of selected blood-borne pathogen position statements and federal regulations, *J Ath Train* 30(2):171.
5. Basler, RSW, Garcia, MA, Gooding, KS: 2001. Immediate steps for treating abrasions, *Physician and sportsmedicine* 29(4):69–70.
6. Brown L, Dortman P: 1993. What is the risk of HIV infection in athletic competition? International Conference on AIDS 19939:PO-C21-3102.
7. Buxton BP et al: 1994. Prevention of hepatitis B virus in athletic training, *J Ath Train* 29(2):107.

8. Clark, G, Lorenzi, D: 2008. Blood on the gym floor: application of universal precautions, *Strategies* 21(3):15.
9. Clem, K, Borchers, J: 2007. HIV and the athlete. *Clinics in sports medicine* 26(3):413.
10. Deere, R, Stopka, C, Curran, K, Bolger, C: 2001. Universal precautions for blood borne pathogens: a checklist for your program, *Strategies* 14(6):18–19.
11. Farb, D, Gordon, B: 2004. OSHA *Bloodborne pathogens*, Library Edition, The University of Health Care.
12. Fincher LA: 1999. Wound care management, *Ath Ther Today* 4(1):11.
13. First national guideline on latex allergy: 2007. *Occupational Health* 60(6):37.
14. Glazer, JL: 2002. Laceration care, *Physician and sportsmedicine* 30(7):50.
15. Guidelines on handling contests: 2007. *Interscholastic athletic administration* 34(2):18.
16. Hamann B: 2006. *Disease: identification, prevention, and control,* New York, McGraw-Hill.
17. Honshik, K, Romeo, M: 2007. Sideline skin and wound care for acute injuries. *Current sports medicine reports* 6(3):147.

18. Howe WB: 2004. The athlete with chronic illness. In Birrer RB, editor: *Sports medicine for the primary care physician,* ed 3, Boca Raton, Fla, CRC Press.

19. Irion, G: 2002. *Comprehensive wound management* (1st ed.), Thorofare, N.J., Slack, Inc.

20. Karon, JM, Fleming, PL, Steketee, RW, De Cock, KM: 2001. HIV in the United States at the turn of the century: an epidemic in transition, *American journal of public health* 91(7):1060–1068.

21. Klossner, D, (ed.): 2007. *NCAA 2007–2008 sports medicine handbook,* Indianapolis, IN, NCAA.

22. Lindsey, J, Krohmer, J: 2008. *Bloodborne pathogens,* Boston, Jones and Bartlett.

23. Lindsey, J, Krohmer, J: 2008. *Bloodborne pathogens,* Boston, Jones and Bartlett.

24. Knight, KL: 2001. Acute care of injuries and illnesses. In Knight, KL: (ed), *Assessing clinical proficiencies in athletic training: a modular approach,* 3rd ed, Champaign, IL, Human Kinetics.

25. Luke, A, D'Hemecourt, P: 2007. Prevention of infectious diseases in athletes. *Clinics in sports medicine* 26(3):321.

26. McCulloch, JM, Kloth, LC: 2002. *Wound healing: alternatives in management,* 3rd ed, Philadelphia, FA Davis.

27. McGraw C, Dick R, Schneidewind K: 1993. Survey of NCAA institutions concerning HIV/AIDS policies and universal precautions, *Med Sci Sport Exer* 25:917.

28. National Safety Council: 2009. *Bloodborne pathogens,* New York, McGraw-Hill.

29. Pirozzolo, J, LeMay, D: 2007. Blood-borne infections, *Clinics in sports medicine* 26(3):425.

30. Rabenberg, VS, Ingersoll, CD, Sandrey, MA, Johnson, MT: 2002. The bactericidal and cytotoxic effects of antimicrobial wound cleansers, *Journal of athletic training* 37(1): 51–54.

31. Rogers KJ: 1995. Human immunodeficiency virus in sports. In Torg JS, Shephard RJ, editors: *Current therapy in sports medicine,* St. Louis, Mosby.

32. Sankaran G, editor: 1999. *HIV/AIDS in sport: impact, issues, and challenges,* Champaign, IL, Human Kinetics.

33. Shultz, SJ: 2001. Preventing transmission of blood-borne pathogens. In Shultz, SJ et al, (ed), *Sports medicine handbook,* Indianapolis, IN, National Federation of State High School Associations.

34. Stockard, A: 2005. Methicillin-resistant staphylococcal(sic) aureas (MRSA) skin infection in athletes, *Texas coach* 49(7):42–44.

35. Stringer WW: 1999. HIV and aerobic exercise: current recommendations, *Sports med* 28(6):389.

36. Thomas CE: 1996. The HIV athlete: 1996 policy, obligations, and attitudes, *Sport Sci Rev* 5(2):12.

37. United States Department of Health and Human Services, AIDS/HIV Statistics, http://www.niaid.nih.gov/factsheets/aidsstat.htm

38. Zeigler T: 1997. *Management of bloodborne infections in sport,* Champaign, IL, Human Kinetics.

## ANNOTATED BIBLIOGRAPHY

Klossner, D, editor: 2007. *National Collegiate Athletic Association 2007–2008 sports medicine handbook,* Indianapolis, NCAA.

*A complete discussion of bloodborne pathogens and intercollegiate athletic policies and administration.*

National Safety Council, editors: 2009. *Bloodborne pathogens,* New York, McGraw-Hill.

*A manual that presents OSHA's regulations specific to bloodborne pathogens.*

Techniques for Preventing
and Minimizing Sport-
Related Injuries

Hamann B: 2006. *Disease: identification, prevention, and control,* New York, McGraw-Hill.

*Designed for health educators; detailed coverage of AIDS and hepatitis.*

Occupational Safety and Health Administration: 1992. *As it should be done: workplace precautions against bloodborne pathogens,* Washington, DC, US Department of Labor.

*This 24-minute video explains how workers can protect themselves against occupational exposure to bloodborne pathogens, such as Hepatitis B Virus (HBV) and the Human Immunodeficiency Virus (HIV). This program is targeted primarily to health care workers and related professionals.*

## WEB SITES

Occupational Safety and Health Administration (OSHA): www.osha.gov

Department of Health and Human Services: www.os.dhhs.gov

HIV/AIDS Prevention: www.cdc.gov/hiv

Centers for Disease Control and Prevention: www.cdc.gov

National Institute of Health: www.nih.gov

Bloodborne pathogens self-study module: www2.umdnj.edu/eohssweb/publications/biosafetytraining.htm

*A self-study module that details work practice controls and current knowledge of HBV, HIV, and other bloodborne pathogens.*

# Understanding the Potential Dangers of Adverse Environmental Conditions

*When you finish this chapter you will be able to:*

- Describe the physiology of hyperthermia and the clinical signs of heat stress and how they can be prevented.
- Identify the causes of hypothermia and the major cold disorders and how they may be prevented.
- Explain how an athlete should be protected from exposure to the sun.
- Describe precautions that should be taken in an electrical storm.

O ne of the primary responsibilities of a coach or any other fitness professional in preventing injuries is to make certain that the practice and playing environment is as safe as it can possibly be. Certainly no one has control over the weather. However, **the potential dangers of having athletes engage in practices or competitions when adverse weather or environmental conditions exist cannot be ignored. Ignoring or minimizing the potential threat to the health and well-being of athletes who are forced to practice or compete under adverse environmental conditions can have serious legal consequences should a situation arise that results in injury to an athlete.** The adverse environmental conditions that tend to pose the greatest potential for injury in the athletic population are hot, humid, sunny conditions that cause **hyperthermia;** cold and windy conditions that cause **hypothermia**; lightning and thunderstorms; and overexposure to the sun.

**hyperthermia**
Increased body temperature.

## HYPERTHERMIA

An ever-present concern of practicing or competing in a hot humid environment is the problem of hyperthermia. Hyperthermia refers to an increase in body temperature. In recent years, particularly among football players and wrestlers, a number of deaths have been caused by hyperthermia.[3] It is vitally important to understand when environmental heat and humidity are at a dangerous level and to act accordingly. Remember that an individual does not have to be in the south to experience heat-related illnesses. Heat and humidity occur in every geographic region of the United States, and anyone who supervises athletes that practice and compete in these environmental conditions must be able to recognize the clinical signs of heat stress and manage them properly.

**hypothermia**
Decrease of body temperature.

## CHAPTER 9

Heat can be gained or lost
through:
- metabolic heat production
- conductive heat exchange
- convective heat exchange
- radiant heat exchange
- evaporative heat loss

## Heat Stress

Regardless of the level of physical conditioning, extreme caution must be taken when exercising, particularly in hot, humid weather. Prolonged exposure to extreme heat can result in heat illness.[16,22] Heat stress is certainly preventable, but each year many athletes suffer illness and, occasionally, death from some heat-related cause.[36] Athletes who exercise in hot, humid environments are particularly vulnerable to heat stress. The physiological processes in the body can continue to function only as long as body temperature is maintained within a normal range.[35] Maintenance of normal temperature in a hot environment depends on the ability of the body to dissipate heat. Heat can be dissipated from the body through four mechanisms: conduction (direct contact with a cooler object); convection (contact with a cooler air or water mass); radiation (heat generated from metabolism); and evaporation (sweat evaporating from the skin surface). It must be added that the body can also gain heat through conduction, convection, and radiation if the surrounding environment is hotter than the body temperature or if the body is exposed to direct sunlight. By far most of the heat that is dissipated from the body is through the process of evaporation.

Sweat glands in the skin allow water to be transported to the surface where it evaporates, taking large quantities of heat with it. When the temperature and radiant heat of the environment become higher than body temperature, loss of body heat becomes highly dependent on the process of sweat evaporation. The sweat must evaporate for heat to be dissipated. But the air must be relatively free of water for evaporation to occur. Heat loss through evaporation is severely impaired when the relative humidity reaches 65 percent and virtually stops when the humidity reaches 75 percent. The heat index takes both ambient air temperature and relative humidity into account and attempts to determine how hot it actually feels to the human body (Figure 9-1).

It must be emphasized that, while heat illness is most likely to occur in a hot, humid environment, it is possible that heat illnesses can also occur in colder environments when the athlete allows himself or herself to become dehydrated and the body cannot dissipate heat through sweating.

## Monitoring the Heat Index

Common sense must be exercised when overseeing the health care of athletes training or competing in the heat. Obviously, when the combination of heat, humidity, and bright sunshine is present, extra caution is warranted.[9] The universal *wet bulb globe temperature (WBGT) index* provides an objective means for determining necessary precautions for practice and competition in hot weather.[28] The index incorporates readings from several different thermometers. The dry bulb temperature (DBT) is recorded from a standard mercury thermometer. The wet bulb temperature (WBT) uses a wet wick or piece of gauze wrapped around the

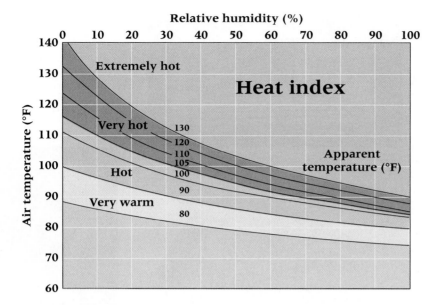

**Figure 9-1**

The heat index takes both air temperature and relative humidity into account.

end of a thermometer that is swung around in the air. Globe temperature (GT) measures the sun's radiation and uses a black metal casing around the end of the thermometer.[9]

The DBT and WBT can easily be measured using a *psychrometer*. It consists of two identical thermometers—the wet bulb thermometer, so called because its bulb is covered with a jacket of tight-fitting muslin cloth that can be saturated with distilled water, and the dry bulb thermometer. When the cloth is soaked and the thermometers are properly ventilated, the wet bulb temperature will be lower than the dry bulb temperature (actual air temperature) because of cooling due to the evaporation of water from the cloth. The drier the air is, the greater the evaporation, and thus the more wet bulb temperature is depressed. Ventilation is provided by a suction fan (aspiration psychrometer) (Figure 9-2A) or by whirling the thermometers at the end of a handle (sling psychrometer) (Figure 9-2B). Newer psychrometers use special digital sensors (Figure 9-2C). Recording the temperature requires about 90 seconds. Either instrument is relatively inexpensive and easy to use, although it appears that the old sling psychrometer may have the greatest accuracy.[32] The WBGT index is easily calculated using charts that are provided with the psychrometer. The digital psychrometer calculates the heat index automatically. Once the WBGT index has been calculated, Table 9-1 can be used to make recommendations relative to fluid replacement and the length of work and rest periods.

## Heat Illnesses

It should be obvious that heat-related problems have the greatest chance of occurring on days when the sun is bright and the temperature and

**Figure 9-2**

(A) A physiodyne, or
(B) a sling psychrometer, or
(C) a digital psychrometer
    may be used to determine
    the WBGT heat index.

**A**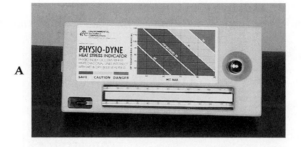

**B**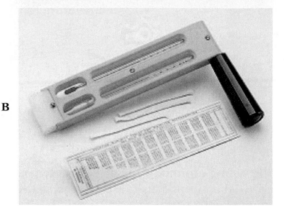

**C**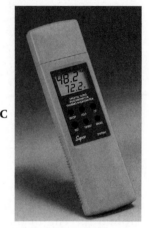

---

**TABLE 9-1** WBGT index and recommendations for fluid replacement and work/rest periods

| Heat Category | WBGT °F | Easy Work Work/Rest* | Easy Work Water Per Hour | Moderate Work Work/Rest* | Moderate Work Water Per Hour | Hard Work Work/Rest* | Hard Work Water Per Hour |
|---|---|---|---|---|---|---|---|
| 1 | 78–81.9 | No limit | ½ qt. | No limit | ¾ qt. | 40/20 min | ¾ qt. |
| 2 | 82–84.9 | No limit | ½ qt. | 50/10 min | ¾ qt. | 30/30 min | 1 qt. |
| 3 | 85–87.9 | No limit | ¾ qt. | 40/20 min | ¾ qt. | 30/30 min | 1 qt. |
| 4 | 88–89.9 | No limit | ¾ qt. | 30/30 min | ¾ qt. | 20/40 min | 1 qt. |
| 5 | >90 | 50/10 min | 1 qt. | 20/40 min | 1 qt. | 10/50 min | 1 qt. |

*Rest means minimal physical activity (sitting or standing) and should be accomplished in the shade if possible.

relative humidity are high. But it is certainly true that various forms of heat illness, including heat syncope and exertional heat cramps, heat exhaustion, heatstroke, or hyponatremia can occur whenever the body's ability to dissipate heat is impaired.[26]

### Heat Syncope

Heat syncope, or heat collapse, is associated with rapid physical fatigue during overexposure to heat. It is usually caused by standing in heat for long periods or by not being accustomed to exercising in the heat. It is caused by peripheral vasodilation of superficial vessels, hypotension, or a pooling of blood in the extremities, which results in dizziness, fainting, and nausea. Heat syncope is quickly relieved by laying the athlete down in a cool environment and replacing fluids.[30]

### Exertional Heat Cramps

Heat cramps are extremely painful muscle spasms that occur most commonly in the calf and abdomen, although any muscle can be involved (Table 9-2). *The occurrence of heat cramps is related primarily to excessive loss of water and loss of electrolytes, particularly sodium. Electrolytes* are ions (sodium, chloride, potassium, magnesium, and calcium) that are essential elements in muscle contraction.[20]

Heat cramps occur because of some imbalance between water and electrolytes.

Profuse sweating involves losses of large amounts of water as well as electrolytes, thus destroying the balance in concentration of these elements within the body. This imbalance ultimately results in painful muscle contractions and cramps. The person most likely to get heat cramps is one who is in fairly good condition who simply overexerts in the heat.

**Treatment** Heat cramps may be prevented by adequate replacement of fluids and increased intake of sodium.[4] The immediate treatment for heat cramps is ingestion of large quantities of fluid and sodium, and mild stretching with ice massage of the muscle in spasm.[29] An athlete who experiences heat cramps will generally not be able to return to practice or competition for the remainder of the day because cramping is likely to reoccur.

### Exertional Heat Exhaustion

Heat exhaustion results from inadequate replacement of fluids lost through sweating (Table 9-2). Clinically, the victim of heat exhaustion collapses and manifests profuse sweating, pale skin, mildly elevated temperature (102° F), dizziness, hyperventilation, and rapid pulse.

Heat exhaustion results from dehydration.

It is sometimes possible to spot athletes who are having problems with heat exhaustion. They may begin to develop heat cramps. They may become disoriented and light-headed, and their physical performance will not be up to their usual standards when fluid replacement has not been adequate. In general, persons in poor physical condition who attempt to exercise in the heat are most likely to get heat exhaustion.

**Treatment** Immediate treatment of heat exhaustion requires ingestion and eventually intravenous replacement of large quantities of fluids. It is essential to obtain an accurate core temperature. Temperature can be measured in the ear with a tympanic membrane thermometer. However, a rectal temperature is the most accurate indicator of core temperature to differentiate heat exhaustion from heatstroke. In heat exhaustion the core temperature will be around 102° F. If possible, the athlete should be placed in a cool environment, although it is more critical to replace fluids.[27]

**TABLE 9-2** Heat Disorders: Treatment and Prevention

| Disorder | Cause | Clinical Features and Diagnosis | Treatment | Prevention |
|---|---|---|---|---|
| Heat syncope (fainting) | Rapid physical fatigue in heat and blood pooling in extremities | Dizziness, nausea, fainting | Lay athlete down in a cool environment, replace fluids | Acclimatize athlete and make sure they are appropriately hydrated |
| Exertional heat cramps | Hard work in heat; sweating heavily; imbalance between water and electrolytes | Muscle twitching and cramps, usually after midday; spasms in arms, legs, abdomen | Ingesting large amounts of water and sodium, mild stretching, and ice massage of affected muscle | Acclimatize athlete properly; provide large quantities of water; increase intake of sodium, calcium, and potassium |
| Exertional heat exhaustion | Prolonged sweating; inadequate replacement of body fluid losses; diarrhea; intestinal infection | Excessive thirst, dry tongue and mouth; weight loss; fatigue; weakness; incoordination; mental dullness; small urine volume; slightly elevated body temperature; high serum protein and sodium; reduced swelling | Bed rest in cool room, immediate oral fluid replacement, increase fluid intake to 6 to 8 l/day; sponge with cool water; keep record of body weight; keep fluid balance record; provide semiliquid food until salination is normal, IV fluids if drinking is impaired | Supply adequate water and other liquids<br><br>Provide adequate rest and opportunity for cooling |
| Exertional heatstroke | Thermoregulatory failure of sudden onset | Abrupt onset, preceded by headache, vertigo, and fatigue, flushed skin; relatively less sweating than seen with heat exhaustion; pulse rate increases rapidly and may reach 160 to 180; respiration increases; blood pressure seldom rises; temperature rises rapidly to 104° F; athlete feels as if he or she is burning up; diarrhea, vomiting; circulatory collapse may produce death; can lead to permanent brain damage | Emergency measures to reduce temperature must be taken immediately (e.g., immerse the athlete in a tub of ice water, or sponge cool water and air fan over body, massage limbs); transport to hospital as soon as possible | Ensure proper acclimatization, proper hydration<br><br>Educate those supervising activities conducted in the heat<br><br>Adapt activities to environment<br><br>Screen participants with past history of heat illness for malignant hyperthermia |
| Exertional hyponatremia | Fluid/electrolyte disorder resulting in low concentration of sodium in the blood | Progressively worsening headache, nausea and vomiting, swelling in hands and feet, lethargy or apathy, low blood sodium, compromised CNS | Do not try to rehydrate; transport to medical facility; sodium levels must be increased and fluid levels decreased | Hydrate with sports drinks; increase sodium intake; make sure fluid intake equals fluid loss |

## Exertional Heatstroke

Unlike heat cramps and heat exhaustion, heatstroke is a serious, life-threatening emergency (Table 9-2). The specific cause of heatstroke is unknown; however, it is clinically characterized by sudden collapse with loss of consciousness; flushed, hot skin; less sweating than is seen with heat exhaustion; shallow breathing; a rapid, strong pulse; and, most important, a core temperature of 104° F or higher.[12] Basically heatstroke is a breakdown of the thermoregulatory mechanism caused by excessively high body temperature; the body loses the ability to dissipate heat through sweating.[34]

Heatstroke can occur suddenly and without warning. *The athlete may or may not show signs of heat cramps or heat exhaustion.* **The possibility of death from heatstroke can be significantly reduced if body temperature is lowered to normal within 45 minutes.** The longer the body temperature is elevated to 104° F or higher, the higher the mortality rate.[21]

**Treatment** *It is imperative that the victim be transported to a hospital as quickly as possible.* Every first-aid effort should be directed to lowering body temperature. Get the athlete into a cool environment. Strip all clothing off the athlete. **It is most effective to immerse the athlete in ice water.**[13,14,42] Alternatives would be to place ice bags in the ampits, groin, and neck, or sponge him or her down with cold water, and fan with a towel. The replacement of fluid is not critical in initial first aid.

*Heatstroke is a life-threatening emergency.*

*Managing heatstroke requires a heroic effort to lower body temperature.*

## Exertional Hyponatremia

Hyponatremia is a condition involving a fluid/electrolyte disorder that results in an abnormally low concentration of sodium in the blood.[2] It is most often caused by ingesting so much fluid before, during, and after exercise that the concentration of sodium is decreased. It also can occur due to too little sodium in the diet or in ingested fluids over a period of prolonged exercise. An individual with a high rate of sweating and a significant loss of sodium, who continues to ingest large quantities of fluid over a several hour period of exercise (as in a marathon or triathlon), is particularly vulnerable to developing hyponatremia. Hyponatremia can be avoided completely by making certain that fluid intake during exercise does not exceed fluid loss and that sodium intake is adequate.[11]

*Hyponatremia results from a low concentration of sodium and too much fluid.*

The signs and symptoms of exertional hyponatremia may include a progressively worsening headache; nausea and vomiting; swelling of the hands and feet; lethargy, apathy, or agitation; and low blood sodium. Ultimately, a very low concentration of sodium can compromise the central nervous system creating a life-threatening situation.[2]

**Treatment** If hyponatremia is suspected and blood sodium levels cannot be determined onsite, measures to rehydrate the athlete should be delayed and the athlete should be transported immediately to a medical facility.[2] At the medical facility the delivery of sodium, certain diuretics,

The prevention of
hyperthermia involves
• unrestricted fluid
  replacement
• gradual acclimatization
• identification of susceptible
  individuals
• lightweight uniforms
• routine weight record
  keeping

**9-1 Critical Thinking**
Exercise

A high school athletic director in
southern Louisiana is concerned
about the likelihood that several
of the football players will suffer
heat-related illness during preseason practice the first 2 weeks
of August.

? What intervention strategies
can be implemented to help
the athletes avoid heat-related
illnesses?

or intravenous solutions may be necessary. A physician should clear the athlete before he or she is allowed to return to play.

### Preventing Heat Illness

**It is essential to understand that heat illness is preventable.** Exercising common sense and caution will keep heat illnesses from occurring.[35] The following suggestions should be considered when planning a practice or competitive program during hot weather.

#### Fluid Replacement

**The single most important step that can be taken to minimize the chance of heat illness is to make absolutely certain that athletes are appropriately hydrated.** Regardless of whether the athlete is practicing or competing in a hot humid environment or a cold damp environment the athlete needs to continually rehydrate by replacing fluids lost through evaporation of sweat[5] (Figure 9-3). Unfortunately dehydration occurs frequently during physical activity because athletes do not ingest enough fluid to match sweat loss even though unlimited fluids are readily available.[35] In fact, seldom is more than 50 percent of this fluid loss replaced. **Ideally, fluid replacement should match sweat loss.** Fluid is most effectively replaced at regular intervals of about 15 minutes.

The problem in fluid replacement is how rapidly the fluid can be eliminated from the stomach into the intestine, from which it can enter the bloodstream. Water is absorbed rapidly from the intestine. Beverages containing 6 percent carbohydrate (glucose) are absorbed at about the same rate as water as long as there is normal hydration.[33] Cold drinks (45° to 55° F [7.2° to 12.8° C]) tend to empty more rapidly from the stomach than do warmer drinks; they are not more likely to induce cramps, nor do they offer any particular threat to a normal heart.[31] Drinks that contain alcohol and caffeine act as diuretics and act to promote dehydration.

**Figure 9-3**

Athletes must have unlimited
access to water or sports
drinks, especially in hot
weather.

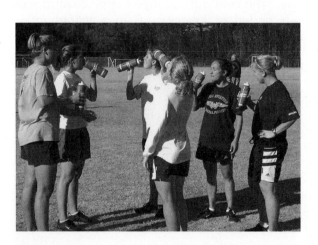

Athletes can tell if they are appropriately hydrated by paying attention to the color and volume of their urine. Within 60 minutes of exercise, a nearly clear urine of normal to above-normal output indicates that the athlete is appropriately hydrated.

### Using Sports Drinks

It has been shown that replacing lost fluids with a sports drink is more effective than using water alone.[31] Research has shown that because of the flavor of the sports drinks an athlete is likely to drink more than plain water. In addition, sports drinks replace both fluids and electrolytes that are lost in sweat and also provide energy to the working muscles.

Water is a good thirst quencher but it is not a good rehydrator because water "turns off" your thirst before you're completely rehydrated. Water also "turns on" the kidneys prematurely so you lose fluid in the form of urine much more quickly than when drinking a sports drink. The small amount of sodium in sports drinks allows the body to hold onto the fluid consumed rather than losing it through urine.[12,27]

Not all sports drinks are the same. How a sports drink is formulated dictates how well it works in providing rapid rehydration and energy. The optimal level of carbohydrate is 14 grams per 8 ounces of water for quickest absorption and energy.[35] Thus sports drinks should be used without diluting. Research has shown that full-strength sports drinks are absorbed just as fast as water. Most contain no carbonation or artificial preservatives, making them satisfying during exercise and causing no stomach bloating. Also most sports drinks contain a minimal number of calories. It has been shown that sports drinks are effective in improving performance during both endurance activities and short-term high-intensity activities such as soccer, basketball, and tennis that last from 30 minutes to an hour.[15] Focus Box 9-1 provides recommendations for fluid replacement.

### Gradual Acclimatization

Gradual acclimatization is a critical consideration in avoiding heat stress. Acclimatization should involve not only becoming accustomed to heat but also becoming acclimatized to exercising in hot temperatures.[14] A good preseason conditioning program—started well before the advent of the competitive season and carefully graded as to intensity—is recommended. During the first 5 or 6 days, an 80 percent acclimatization can be achieved on the basis of a 2-hour practice period in the morning and a 2-hour practice period in the afternoon. Complete acclimatization may take a minimum of 10 to 14 days.[6]

### Identifying Susceptible Individuals

Athletes with a large muscle mass are particularly prone to heat illness.[22] Body build must be considered when determining individual susceptibility to heat stress. Overweight individuals may have as much as 18 percent greater heat production than underweight individuals

9-1 > *Focus Box*

**Recommendations for Fluid Replacement***

- Athletes should begin all exercise sessions well hydrated.
- To ensure proper hydration the athlete should consume 17 to 20 ounces of water or a sports drink 2 to 3 hours before exercise and then 7 to 10 ounces 20 minutes before exercise.
- Fluid replacement beverages should be easily accessible during activity and should be consumed at a minimal rate of 7 to 10 ounces every 10 to 20 minutes.
- During activity the athlete should consume the maximal amount of fluid that can be tolerated.
- A cool, flavored beverage at 50 to 59° F is recommended.
- Addition of proper amounts of carbohydrates and electrolytes to a fluid replacement solution is recommended for exercise events that last longer than 1 hour.
- A 6 percent carbohydrate solution appears to be optimal.
- For exercise lasting less than 1 hour the addition of carbohydrates and electrolytes does not seem to enhance physical performance.

*Based on recommendations from ACSM[3] and NATA.[12,27]*

because metabolic heat is produced proportionately to surface area. It has been found that heat illness victims tend to be overweight. Death from heatstroke increases at a ratio of approximately four to one as body weight increases.[22]

Women are apparently more physiologically efficient in body temperature regulation than are men. Although women possess as many heat-activated sweat glands as men do, they sweat less and manifest a higher heart rate when working in heat. Although slight differences exist, the same precautionary measures apply to both genders.

Other individuals who are susceptible to heat stress include children and older adults, those with relatively poor fitness levels, those with a history of heat illness, and anyone with a febrile condition.

### Keeping Weight Records

Careful weight records of all players must be kept. Weights should be measured both before and after practice for at least the first 2 weeks of practice. If a sudden increase in temperature and/or humidity occurs during the season, weight should be recorded again for a time. A loss of 3 to 5 percent of body weight reduces blood volume and could lead to a health threat.[22] A rule should be established that the athlete should be held out of practice until normal body weight has been regained.

### Uniforms

Uniforms should be selected on the basis of temperature and humidity. Initial practices should be conducted in light-colored, short-sleeved

**9-2**    *Focus Box*

Recommendations for preventing heat illness*

- Ensure that appropriate medical care is available.
- Conduct a thorough physician-supervised preparticipation exam to identify susceptible individuals.
- Acclimatize athletes over ten to fourteen days.
- Educate athletes and coaches regarding prevention, recognition, and treatment of heat illnesses.
- Educate athletes to balance fluid intake with sweat and urine losses to maintain adequate hydration.
- Encourage athletes to sleep six to eight hours per night in a cool environment.
- Monitor environmental conditions and develop guidelines for altering practice sessions based on those conditions.
- Provide an adequate supply of water or sports drinks to maintain hydration.
- Weigh high-risk athletes before and after practice to make certain they are not dehydrated.
- Minimize the amount of equipment and clothing worn in hot humid conditions.
- Minimize warm-up time in hot humid conditions.
- Allow athletes to practice in shaded areas and use cooling fans when possible.
- Have appropriate emergency equipment available (e.g., fluids, ice, immersion tank, rectal thermometer, telephone or two-way radio).

*From NATA Position Statement on Exertional Heat Illnesses, 2002.[6]

T-shirts, shorts, and socks, moving gradually into short-sleeved net jerseys, lightweight pants, and socks as acclimatization proceeds. All early-season practices and games should be conducted in lightweight uniforms. Because of the specialized equipment worn by the players, football requires particular consideration. In hot, humid environments, the helmet should be removed as often as possible.

Focus Box 9-2 provides recommendations for preventing heat illness.

## HYPOTHERMIA

Cold weather is a frequent adjunct to many outdoor sports in which the sport itself does not require heavy protective clothing; consequently, the weather becomes a pertinent factor in injury susceptibility.[7] In most instances, the activity itself enables the athlete to increase the metabolic rate sufficiently for normal physiological functioning and to dissipate the resulting heat and perspiration through the usual physiological mechanisms.[1] An athlete may fail to warm up sufficiently or may become chilled because of relative inactivity for varying periods demanded by

Many sports played in cold weather do not require heavy protective clothing; thus, weather becomes a factor in injury susceptibility.

**Temperature (°F)**

| Calm | 40 | 35 | 30 | 25 | 20 | 15 | 10 | 5 | 0 | −5 | −10 | −15 | −20 | −25 | −30 | −35 | −40 | −45 |
|------|----|----|----|----|----|----|----|----|----|----|----|----|----|----|----|----|----|----|
| 5 | 36 | 31 | 25 | 19 | 13 | 7 | 1 | −5 | −11 | −16 | −22 | −28 | −34 | −40 | −46 | −52 | −57 | −63 |
| 10 | 34 | 27 | 21 | 15 | 9 | 3 | −4 | −10 | −16 | −22 | −28 | −35 | −41 | −47 | −53 | −59 | −66 | −72 |
| 15 | 32 | 25 | 19 | 13 | 6 | 0 | −7 | −13 | −19 | −26 | −32 | −39 | −45 | −51 | −58 | −64 | −71 | −77 |
| 20 | 30 | 24 | 17 | 11 | 4 | −2 | −9 | −15 | −22 | −29 | −35 | −42 | −48 | −55 | −61 | −68 | −74 | −81 |
| 25 | 29 | 23 | 16 | 9 | 3 | −4 | −11 | −17 | −24 | −31 | −37 | −44 | −51 | −58 | −64 | −71 | −78 | −84 |
| 30 | 28 | 22 | 15 | 8 | 1 | −5 | −12 | −19 | −26 | −33 | −39 | −46 | −53 | −60 | −67 | −73 | −80 | −87 |
| 35 | 28 | 21 | 14 | 7 | 0 | −7 | −14 | −21 | −27 | −34 | −41 | −48 | −55 | −62 | −69 | −76 | −82 | −89 |
| 40 | 27 | 20 | 13 | 6 | −1 | −8 | −15 | −22 | −29 | −36 | −43 | −50 | −57 | −64 | −71 | −78 | −84 | −91 |
| 45 | 26 | 19 | 12 | 5 | −2 | −9 | −16 | −23 | −30 | −37 | −44 | −51 | −58 | −65 | −72 | −79 | −86 | −93 |
| 50 | 26 | 19 | 12 | 4 | −3 | −10 | −17 | −24 | −31 | −38 | −45 | −52 | −60 | −67 | −74 | −81 | −88 | −95 |
| 55 | 25 | 18 | 11 | 4 | −3 | −11 | −18 | −25 | −32 | −39 | −46 | −54 | −61 | −68 | −75 | −82 | −89 | −97 |
| 60 | 25 | 17 | 10 | 3 | −4 | −11 | −19 | −26 | −33 | −40 | −48 | −55 | −62 | −69 | −76 | −84 | −91 | −98 |

Wind (mph)

Frostbite times ☐ 30 minutes ☐ 10 minutes ■ 5 minutes

**Figure 9-4**

### Wind Chill Factor

Low temperatures can pose serious problems for the athlete, but wind chill could be a critical factor.

Low temperatures accentuated by wind and dampness can pose major problems for athletes.

the particular sport, during either competition or training. Consequently, the athlete is predisposed to hypothermia or a lowered body temperature.[24]

Low temperatures alone can pose some problems, but when such temperatures are further accentuated by wind, the chill factor becomes critical (Figure 9-4).[39] A third factor, dampness or wetness, further increases the risk of hypothermia. Air at a temperature of 50° F is relatively comfortable, but water at the same temperature is intolerable. Certainly the combination of cold, wind, and dampness creates an environment that easily predisposes the athlete to hypothermia.

As muscular fatigue builds up during strenuous physical activity in cold weather, the rate of exercise begins to drop and may reach a level at which the body heat loss to the environment exceeds the metabolic heat protection, resulting in definite impairment of neuromuscular responses and exhaustion. A relatively small drop in body core temperature can induce shivering sufficient to materially affect the athlete's neuromuscular coordination. Shivering ceases below a body temperature of 85° to 90° F (29.4° to 32.2° C). Death is imminent if the core temperature rises to 107° F (41.6° C) or drops to between 77° and 85° F (25° to 29° C).[8]

### Cold Disorders

Cold injuries in sports include:
• frostnip
• frostbite

Athletes need to replace fluids when working out in a cold environment as much as they do in a hot environment.[17] Because dehydration reduces blood volume, less fluid is available for warming the tissues. Athletes performing in a cold environment should be weighed before and after practice, especially in the first 2 weeks of the season.[7] Severe overexposure to a cold climate occurs less often than hyperthermia does in a warm climate; however, it is still a major risk of winter sports, long-distance running in cold weather, and swimming in cold water.[28]

### Frostnip

Frostnip involves ears, nose, cheeks, chin, fingers, and toes. It commonly occurs during a high wind, severe cold, or both. The skin initially appears very firm, with cold, painless areas that may peel or blister in 24 to 72 hours. Affected areas can be treated early by firm, sustained pressure of the hand (without rubbing), by blowing hot breath on the spot, or if the injury is to the fingertips, by placing them in the armpits.

### Frostbite

Superficial frostbite involves only the skin and subcutaneous tissue. The skin appears pale, hard, cold, and waxy. Palpating the injured area reveals a sense of hardness but with yielding of the underlying deeper tissue structures. When rewarming, the superficial frostbite at first feels numb, then stings and burns. Later the area may produce blisters and be painful for a number of weeks.[28]

Deep frostbite is a serious injury indicating that tissues are frozen. This medical emergency requires immediate hospitalization. As with frostnip and superficial frostbite, the tissue is initially cold, hard, pale or white, and numb. Rapid rewarming is required, including hot drinks, heating pads, or hot water bottles that are 100° to 110° F (38° to 43° C).[28] During rewarming the tissue becomes blotchy, red, swollen, and extremely painful. Later the injury may become gangrenous, causing a loss of tissue.

### Prevention

Apparel for competitors must be geared to the weather. The clothing should not restrict movement, should be as lightweight as possible, and should consist of material that permits the free passage of body heat and sweat that otherwise accumulates on the skin or the clothing and provides a chilling effect when activity ceases.[25] **The athlete should routinely dress in thin layers of clothing that can easily be added or removed to prevent sweating as the temperature decreases or increases.**[10] To prevent chilling, warm-up suits should be worn before exercise, during activity breaks or rest periods, and at the termination of exercise.[7]

## OVEREXPOSURE TO SUN

Athletes, along with coaches, athletic trainers, and other support staff, frequently spend a great deal of time outdoors in direct sunlight. Applying sunscreens to protect these individuals from overexposure to ultraviolet radiation (UVR) is seldom done.

### Long-Term Effects on Skin

The most serious effects of long-term UVR exposure are premature aging of the skin and skin cancer.[19] Lightly pigmented individuals are more susceptible. Premature aging of the skin is characterized by dryness,

SPF stands for sun protection factor

cracking, and a decrease in the elasticity of the skin. Skin cancer is the most common malignant tumor found in humans and has been epidemiologically and clinically associated with exposure to UVR. Fortunately the rate of cure exceeds 95 percent with early detection and treatment.[18]

### Using Sunscreens

Sunscreens applied to the skin can help prevent many of the damaging effects of UVR.[19] A sunscreen's effectiveness in absorbing the sunburn-inducing radiation is expressed as the sun protection factor (SPF). An SPF of 6 indicates that an athlete can be exposed to UVR six times longer than without a sunscreen before the skin will begin to turn red. Higher numbers provide greater protection. However, athletes who have a family or personal history of skin cancer may experience significant damage to the skin even when wearing an SPF 15 sunscreen. Therefore, these individuals should wear an SPF 30 sunscreen.[37]

Sunscreen should be worn regularly by athletes, coaches, and athletic trainers who spend time outside. This caution is particularly relevant for individuals with fair complexions, light hair, or blue eyes or those whose skin burns easily. People with dark complexions should also wear sunscreens to prevent sun damage.

Sunscreens are needed most between the months of March and November but should be used year-round. Sunscreens are needed most between 10 A.M. and 4 P.M. and should be applied 15 to 30 minutes before sun exposure.[37] Although clothing and hats provide some protection from the sun, they are not a substitute for sunscreens (a typical white cotton T-shirt provides an SPF of only 5). Reflected sunlight from water, sand, and snow may effectively increase sun exposure and risk of burning.

### SAFETY IN LIGHTNING AND THUNDERSTORMS

Research indicates that lightning is the number two cause of death by weather phenomena, accounting for 110 deaths per year.[41] As a result of the inherent danger associated with electrical storms to athletes and staff who practice and compete outdoors, the NATA has established a position statement with specific guidelines for athlete trainers.[41] Each institution should develop a specific emergency action plan to be implemented in case of a lightning storm that includes establishing a chain of command to determine who should monitor both the weather forecast and changing weather of a threatening nature, and to determine who makes the decision both to remove from and ultimately to return a team to the practice field based on specific preestablished criteria.[41] If you hear thunder or see lightning, you are in immediate danger and should seek a protective shelter in an indoor facility at once. An indoor facility is recommended as the safest protective shelter. However, if an

**9-2 Critical Thinking**
Exercise

A triathlete is competing in a triathlon. She is extremely concerned about getting sunburned and has liberally applied sunscreen with an SPF of 30 during the early morning. It is a very hot, sunny day and she is sweating heavily. She is worried that her sunscreen has worn off and asks her workout partner for more sunscreen. She hands her sunscreen with an SPF of 15, and the triathlete complains that it is not strong enough to protect her.

? Will she be well protected by the sunscreen she has been given?

indoor facility is not available, an automobile is a relatively safe alternative. If neither of these is available, the following guidelines are recommended. Avoid standing near large trees, flagpoles, or light poles. Choose an area that is not on a hill. As a last alternative, find a ditch, ravine, or valley. At times, the only natural forewarning that might precede a strike is feeling your hair stand on end and your skin tingle. At this point, you are in imminent danger of being struck by lightning and should drop to the ground, assuming a crouched position immediately. Do not lie flat. Should a ground strike occur near you, lying flat increases the body's surface area that is exposed to the current traveling through the ground.[36] Avoid standing water (pools), showers, telephones, and metal objects at all times (metal bleachers, umbrellas, etc.).[41]

The most dangerous storms give little or no warning; thunder and lightning are not heard or seen. Lightning is always accompanied by thunder, although 20 percent to 40 percent of thunder cannot be heard because of atmospheric disturbances. The **flash-to-bang method** provides an estimation of how far away lightning is occurring.[41] From the time lightning is sighted, count the number of seconds until the bang occurs and divide by 5 to calculate the number of miles away the lightning is occurring.[38] When the flash-to-bang count is at 30 (6 miles) there is inherent danger, and conditions should be closely monitored. When the count is 15 (3 miles) everyone should leave the field immediately and seek safe shelter.[38]

The NATA, the NCAA, and the National Severe Storms Service recommend that 30 minutes should pass after the last sound of thunder is heard or lightning strike is seen before resuming play.[38] This is enough time to allow the storm to pass and move out of lightning strike range. The perilous misconception that it is possible to see lightning coming and have time to act before it strikes could prove to be fatal. In reality, the lightning that we see flashing is actually the return stroke flashing upward from the ground to the cloud, not downward. When you see the lightning strike, it already has hit.[41]

### Lightning Detectors

A lightning detector is a hand-held instrument with an electronic system to detect the presence and the distance of lightning/thunderstorm activity occurring within a 40-mile distance (Figure 9-5).[38] It allows you to know the level of activity of the storm and it determines if it is moving toward, away from, or parallel to your position. When the lightning detector detects a lightning stroke, it emits an audible warning tone and lights the range indicator allowing you to see the distance to the last, closest detected lightning strike. Lightning detectors are under $200 and are thus an inexpensive alternative to contracting with a weather service to provide information on potentially dangerous weather conditions over a pager system.

**flash-to-bang method**
Estimates how far away lightning is occurring; determined by the number of seconds from the lightning flash until the sound of thunder divided by 5.

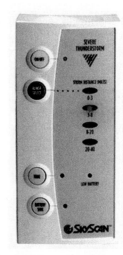

**Figure 9-5**

Portable hand-held lightning detector

## Athletic Injury Management Checklist

The following checklist includes basic guidelines that should be followed during an electrical storm.

☐ In situations in which thunder or lightning may be present and you feel your hair stand on end and skin tingle, immediately assume a crouched position: Drop to your knees, place your hands and arms on your legs, and lower your head. Do not lie flat.

☐ If thunder and/or lightning can be heard or seen, stop activity and seek protective shelter immediately. An indoor facility is recommended as the safest protective shelter. However, if an indoor facility is not available, an automobile is a relatively safe alternative. If neither of these options is available, you should avoid standing under large trees and telephone poles. If the only alternative is a tree, choose a small tree in a wooded area that is not on a hill. As a last alternative, find a ravine or valley. In all instances outdoors, assume the aforementioned crouched position.

☐ Avoid standing water and metal objects at all times (e.g., metal bleachers, metal cleats, umbrellas, etc.).

☐ Allow 30 minutes to pass after the last sound of thunder or lightning strike before resuming play.

---

### ◐ 9-3 *Critical Thinking*
Exercise

A lacrosse team is practicing on a remote field with no indoor facility in close proximity. The weather is rapidly worsening, with the sky becoming dark and the wind blowing harder. Twenty minutes are left in the practice session and suddenly, there is a bolt of lightning and an immediate burst of thunder.

? How should this extremely dangerous situation be handled?

## SUMMARY

- Environmental stress can adversely affect an athlete's performance and pose a serious health problem.

- Regardless of the athletes' level of physical conditioning, use extreme caution when conducting exercises in hot, humid weather. Prolonged exposure to extreme heat can result in heat cramps, heat exhaustion, heatstroke, or hyponatremia.

- Heat illness is preventable. Exercising common sense and caution will keep heat illnesses from occurring. Coaches can prevent heat illness by encouraging adequate fluid replacement, acclimatizing athletes gradually, identifying susceptible individuals, keeping weight records, and selecting appropriate uniforms.

- Hypothermia is most likely to occur in a cool, damp, windy environment. Extreme cold exposure can cause conditions such as frostnip and frostbite.

- Athletes, coaches, and athletic trainers should be protected from overexposure to ultraviolet radiation (UVR) by the routine application of sunscreens.

- Thirty minutes should be allowed to pass after the last sound of thunder is heard or last lightning strike is seen before play is resumed.

---

*Solutions to Critical Thinking* Exercises .

**9-1** It is essential to understand that heat-related illnesses are preventable. The athletes should come into preseason practice at least partially acclimatized to working in a hot, humid environment and during the first week of practice should become fully acclimatized. Temperature and humidity readings should be monitored and practice should be modified according to conditions. Practice uniforms should maximize evaporation and minimize heat absorption to the greatest extent possible. Weight records should be maintained to identify individuals who are becoming dehydrated. Most important, the athletes must keep themselves hydrated by constantly drinking large quantities of water both during and between practice sessions.

**9-2** The sun protection factor (SPF) indicates the sunscreen's effectiveness in absorbing the sunburn-inducing radiation. An SPF of 15 indicates that an athlete can be exposed to UVR fifteen times longer than without a sunscreen before the skin begins to turn red. Therefore the athlete needs to understand that a higher SPF doesn't indicate a greater degree of protection. She must simply apply the SPF 15 sunscreen twice as often as necessary with an SPF 30 sunscreen.

**9-3** As soon as lightning is observed, practice should end immediately and the athletes should seek shelter. If an indoor facility is not available, an automobile is a relatively safe alternative. The athletes should avoid standing under large trees or telephone poles. As a last alternative, athletes should assume a crouched position in a ditch or ravine. Athletes should avoid any standing water or metal objects around the fields.

## REVIEW QUESTIONS AND CLASS ACTIVITIES

1. How do temperature and humidity cause heat illnesses?
2. Describe the symptoms and signs of the most common heat disorders.
3. What steps should be taken to avoid heat illnesses?
4. How is heat lost from the body to produce hypothermia?
5. Identify the physiological basis for the body's susceptibility to a cold disorder.
6. What should athletes do to prevent heat loss?
7. How should athletes protect themselves from the effects of ultraviolet radiation?
8. What precautions can be taken to minimize injury during an electrical storm?

## REFERENCES

1. ACSM: 2006. Position stand: prevention of cold injuries during exercise, *Medicine & science in sports & exercise* 38(11):2012–2029.

2. Armstrong, LE: 2004. Exertional hyponatraemia, *Journal of sports sciences* 22(1)144–145.

3. Armstrong LE, Epstein Y, Green-leaf JE: 1997. ACSM position stand: heat and cold illnesses during distance running, *Med Sci Sports Exerc* 28(12): i–x.

4. Bergeron, MF: 2002. Averting heat cramps, *Physician and sportsmedicine* 30(11):14.

5. Berning, JR: 2002. 10 essentials for avoiding dehydration, *Strategies* 16(1):18.

6. Binkley, H, Beckett, J, Casa, D, Kleiner, D, Plummer, P: 2002. National Athletic Trainers Association position statement: exertional heat illnesses, *Journal of Athletic Training* 37(3):329–342.

7. Bodine KL: 2000. Avoiding hypothermia: caution, forethought, and preparation, *Sports Med Alert* 6(1):6.

8. Brukner, P: 2002. Exercise in the cold. In Brukner, P. (ed.), *Clinical sports medicine*, 2nd rev. ed, Sydney, McGraw-Hill.

9. Budd, G: 2008. Wet-bulb globe temperature (WBGT)—its history and its limitations. *Journal of science & medicine in sport* 11(1):20.

10. Campbell, J, Sebastianelli, W: 2007. Athletics in extreme cold: do's and don't's. *Sports Medicine Update*: 2–6

11. Carter III, R: 2008. Exertional heat illness and hyponatremia: an epidemiological perspective. *Current sports medicine reports* 7(4):S20.

12. Casa, D, Armstrong, L, Hillman, S, Mountain, S, Reiff, R: 2000. National Athletic Trainers Association position statement: fluid replacement for athletes, *Journal of Athletic Training* 35(2):212–224.

13. Casa, D, Mcdermott, B: 2007. Cold water immersion: the gold standard for exertional heatstroke treatment, *Exercise & Sport Sciences Reviews* 35(3):141.

14. Clements, J, Casa, D J, Knight, C: 2002. Ice-water immersion and cold-water immersion provide similar cooling rates in runners with exercise induced hyperthermia, *Journal of athletic training*, 37(2): 146–150.

15. Coombes, JS, Hamilton, KL: 2000. The effectiveness of commercially available sports drinks, *Sports medicine* 29(3):181–209.

16. Coris, EE, Ramirez, AM, Van Durme, DJ: 2004. Heat illness in athletes: the dangerous combination of heat, humidity and exercise, *Sports medicine* 34(1):9–16.

17. Dabinett J: 1998. Preparing for competition in hot and humid environments, *Sports Exerc Injury* 4(1):10.

18. Davis, JL: 2000. Sun and active patients: preventing acute and cumulative skin damage, *Physician and sportsmedicine* 28(7):79–85.

19. Davis M: 2003. Ultraviolet therapy. In Prentice W, editor: *Therapeutic modalities in sports medicine and athletic training* New York, McGraw-Hill.

20. Eichner ER: 1999. Heat cramps: salt is simplest, most effective antidote, *Sports Med Digest* 21(8):88.

21. Eichner, ER: 2002. Heat stroke in sports: causes, prevention, and treatment, *Sports science exchange* 15(3):1–4.

22. Graver, D, Armstrong, LE: 2003. *Exertional heat illnesses,* Champaign, Ill., Human Kinetics.

23. Heat illness symptoms and treatments: 2003. *The journal of physical education, recreation & dance* 74(7): 12–13.

24. Hinch, Moroz, DE, Radomski, MW: 2003. Exercise in the cold, *Wellness-Options* 4(11)43–44.

25. Hoffman, J: 2002. Exercise in the cold. In Hoffman, J (ed), *Physiological aspects of sport training and performance*, Champaign, IL, Human Kinetics.

26. Howe, A, Boden, B: 2007. Heat-related illness in athletes, *American journal of sports medicine* 35(8): 1384–1395.

27. Inter-Association Task Force on Exertional Heat Illnesses Consensus Statement: 2003. *NATA news* 6:24–29.

28. Kanzenbach TL, Dexter WW: 1999. Cold injuries: protecting your patients from the dangers of hypothermia and frostbite, *Postgrad Med* 105(1):72.

29. Kay D, Marino FE: 2000. Fluid ingestion and exercise hyperthermia: implications for performance, thermoregulation, metabolism and the development of fatigue, *J Sports Sci* 18(2):71.

30. Kleiner, DM: 2002. A new exertional heat illness scale, *Athletic therapy today* 7(6), Nov, 65–70.

31. Maughan, RJ, Murray, R: 2000. *Sports drinks: basic science and practical aspects*, Boca Raton, Florida, CRC Press.

32. McCann DJ, Adams WC: 1997. Wet bulb globe temperature index and performance in competitive distance runners, *Med Sci Sports Exerc* 29(7): 955.

33. Montain SJ, Maughan RJ, Sawka MN: 1996. Fluid replacement strategies for exercise in hot weather, *Ath Ther Today* 1(4):24.

34. Moss, RI: 2002. Another look at sudden death and exertional hyperthermia, *Athletic therapy today* 7(3): 44–45.

35. Murray R: 1996. Dehydration, hyperthermia, and athletes: science and practice, *J Ath Train* 31(3):248.

36. *NCAA sports medicine handbook,* Indianapolis, IN, 2007–2008: 2007. National Collegiate Athletic Association.

37. Peterson, J: 2008. 10 nice-to-know facts about being in the sun, *ACSM's health & fitness journal* 12(4):48.

38. Polanshek, K: 2001. When lightning strikes, *Athletics administration* 36(1):36.

39. Sallis R, Chassay CM: 1999. Recognizing and treating common cold-induced injury in outdoor sports, *Med Sci Sports Exerc* 31(10):1367.

40. Sparling PB, Millard-Stafford M: 1999. Keeping sports participants safe in hot weather, *Physician Sportsmed* 27(7):27.

41. Walsh, K, Bennett, B, Cooper, M, Holle, R: 2000. National Athletic Trainers Association position statement: lightning safety for athletics and recreation, *Journal of Athletic Training* 35(4):471–477.

42. What is the optimum water temperature for cooling athletes with exertional heat illness? 2003. *Sports medicine digest* 25(7):78.

## ANNOTATED BIBLIOGRAPHY

Grarer, D, Armstrong, L: 2003. *Exertional heat illness*, Champaign, IL, Human Kinetics.

*This book takes a look at the science behind the various types of heat illnesses and the basis for treatment.*

Klossner D(ed): 2007. *NCAA sports medicine handbook 2007–2008*, Indianapolis, IN, National Collegiate Athletic Association.

*Contains guidelines and recommendations for preventing heat illness, hypohydration, and cold stress, and for lightning safety.*

Strauss RH, editor: 1996. *Sports medicine*, Philadelphia, WB Saunders.

*Provides four pertinent chapters on the subject of environmental disorders that can affect the athlete.*

WEB SITES

National Athletic Trainers Association: www.nata.org

*Site contains detailed position papers on heat illness, fluid replacement, and lightning safety.*

National Lightning Safety Institute (NLSI): www.lightningsafety.com/

*National Lightning Safety Institute provides consulting, education, training, and expert witness relating to lightning hazard mitigation.*

FEMA: Extreme Heat Fact Sheet: www.fema.gov/hazard/heat/index.shtm

*Fact Sheet: Extreme Heat. Doing too much on a hot day, spending too much time in the sun, or staying too long in an overheated place can cause heat-related illnesses.*

WebMDHealth: Heat Illness (Heat Exhaustion, Heatstroke, Heat Cramps): www.webmd.com/a-to-z-guides/heat-exhaustion

*Prolonged or intense exposure to hot temperatures can cause heat-related illnesses, such as heat exhaustion, heat cramps, and heatstroke (also known as sunstroke).*

A Hypothermia Treatment Technology WebSite: www.hypothermia-ca.com

OA Guide to Hypothermia & Cold Weather Injuries: www.princeton.edu/~oa/safety/hypocold.shtml

The Gatorade Sports Science Institute: www.gssiweb.com

*This Web site provides the most up-to-date recommendations for fluid replacement and preventing heat illness.*

# Bandaging and Taping Techniques

*When you finish this chapter you will be able to:*

- Explain the need for and demonstrate the application of elastic bandages.
- Demonstrate site preparation for taping.
- Know the various types of tape that can be used.
- Understand what you are trying to accomplish by the application of a specific taping technique.
- Demonstrate basic skills in the use of taping for a variety of body parts.

Bandaging and taping techniques are used routinely to accomplish a variety of specific objectives including:

- Providing compression to minimize swelling in the initial management of injury.
- Reducing the chances of injury by applying tape prophylactically (for prevention) before an injury occurs.
- Providing additional support to an injured structure.

Correctly and effectively applying a bandage or a "tape job" to a specific body part is a skill anyone can master to accomplish the objectives listed.[12]

There are advantages and disadvantages to using bandaging and taping techniques. Certainly bandaging and taping skills are not difficult. They can be mastered by anyone willing to spend time practicing and learning what works best in a given situation.[14] Of course certain taping and bandaging techniques are more advanced and should be used only by those with some advanced experience. As a "taper" gains more experience, it becomes evident that there are many nuances to taping and there are certainly variations to taping techniques presented in this text. Individual athletes may like slight modifications in taping techniques. Techniques that work well on one athlete may not work as well on others. Each athlete is a bit different anatomically and adjustments may be necessary to accommodate these anatomic variations. However, there are some very basic techniques that can be easily applied with only a little training. Tape should not be applied by coaches or other fitness professionals who do not have at least some understanding of the type of injury that exists and the reasons that an athlete needs to be taped in the first place.

Anyone can master taping and bandaging with practice.

## CHAPTER 10

On the negative side, tape is expensive and some schools simply don't have the budget to purchase large quantities of elastic and nonelastic tape. Applying tape is also time consuming.[3]

Moreover, the effectiveness of taping in preventing or at least minimizing the chances of injury is controversial.[7,13] The amount of support and motion limitation that tape provides has also been questioned.[5,10] Several research studies have indicated that the use of commercially manufactured braces may be equally effective if not more effective than taping for limiting movement and preventing injury.[9,12,18]

**Taping and bandaging techniques should never be used as a substitute for a sound rehabilitation program designed to correct problems of weakness and instability that in many cases create the need for taping and bandaging.**

## ELASTIC BANDAGES

Elastic bandages can be applied for a variety of purposes. They are most often used for compression of an acute injury to limit the amount of swelling that occurs (Figure 10-1). They may also be used to secure a dressing for a wound or to hold a pad or an ice bag in place. An elastic bandage is also useful in providing support to injured soft tissue structures. Elastic wraps are active bandages; they let the athlete move without restriction.

Elastic bandages are generally made of two-ply cotton yarns, reinforced with heat-resistant elastic rubber threads that are often made of latex. (Athletes that may have allergies to latex should be warned.) The bandages come in a variety of widths and lengths and should be selected according to the body part to be bandaged. The sizes most frequently used are the 2-, 3-, 4-, and 6-inch widths by either 5- or 6-yard length. The 4- and 6-inch bandages are usually also available in double lengths of 10 yards.

### Application

The elastic bandage must be applied in a specific manner to maximize its effectiveness. When an elastic bandage is to be placed on a body part,

Elastic bandages
- apply firm even pressure
- wrap distal to proximal

**Figure 10-1**

Technique for using an elastic wrap

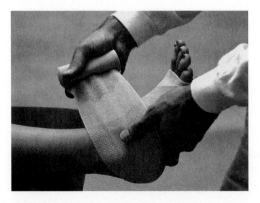

the roll should be held in the preferred hand with the loose end extending from the bottom of the roll. The back surface of the loose end is placed on the part and held in position by the other hand. The bandage will stay in place and not loosen and migrate as much if a corner edge of the first anchor is "dog eared," that is, angled such that it sticks out 2 to 3 inches and then is folded down over the bandage as it wraps over the initial anchor. The bandage is then unrolled and passed around the injured area. As the hand pulls the material from the roll, it also standardizes the bandage pressure and guides the bandage in the proper direction. To anchor and stabilize the bandage, a number of turns, one on top of the other, are made. Circling a body part requires the operator to alternate the bandage roll from one hand to the other and back again.

For maximum benefit from an elastic bandage, it should be applied uniformly and firmly but not too tightly. Excessive or unequal pressure can hinder the normal blood flow within the body part. The following points should be considered when using the elastic bandage:

- Wrapping should always begin distally and move proximally (i.e., start at the toes and wrap up the leg).
- A body part should be wrapped in the position of maximum muscle contraction to ensure unhampered movement and circulation.
- It is better to use a large number of turns with moderate tension than a limited number of turns applied too tightly.
- Each turn of the bandage should be overlapped by at least one half of the overlying wrap to prevent the separation of the material while engaged in activity. Separation of the bandage turns tends to pinch and irritate the skin.

When limbs are wrapped, fingers and toes should be checked often for signs of circulation impairment. Abnormally cold or cyanotic (bluish) fingers or toes are signs of excessive bandage pressure.

## Elastic Bandaging Techniques

### Ankle and Foot Spica

The ankle and foot **spica** bandage (Figure 10-2) is used in sports for the compression of new injuries, for holding wound dressings in place, and to stabilize or secure smaller body part on a larger one.

**Materials needed**   Depending on the size of the ankle and foot, a 2- or 3-inch (5 to 7.5 cm) wrap is used.

**Position of the athlete**   The athlete sits with ankle and foot extended over a table.

**Procedure**

1. An anchor is placed around the foot near the metatarsal arch.
2. The elastic bandage is brought across the instep and around the heel and returned to the starting point. Make sure to completely cover the heel leaving no spaces.

Check circulation after applying an elastic wrap.

> spica (spy ka)
> A figure-eight bandage, with one of the two loops being larger.

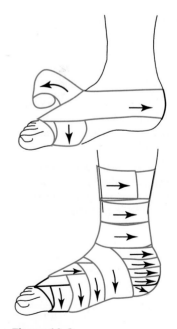

**Figure 10-2**

Ankle and foot spica

**Figure 10-3**

Spiral bandage

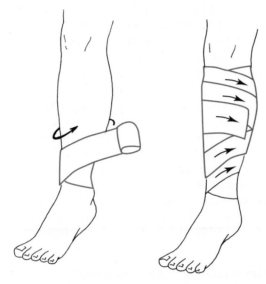

3. The procedure is repeated several times, with each succeeding revolution progressing upward on the foot and the ankle.

4. Each spica overlaps approximately one-half of the preceding layer.

Lower Leg Spiral Bandage

The spiral bandage (Figure 10-3) is widely used in sports for covering a large area of a cylindrical part.

**Materials needed**   Depending on the size of the area, a 3- or 4-inch (7.5 to 10 cm) wrap is required.

**Position of the athlete**   If the wrap is for the lower limb, the athlete bears weight on the opposite leg.

**Procedure**

1. The elastic bandage is anchored at the smallest circumference of the limb and is wrapped upward in a spiral against gravity.

2. To prevent the bandage from slipping down on a moving extremity, two pieces of tape should be folded lengthwise and placed on the bandage at either side of the limb or tape adherent can be sprayed on the part.

3. After the bandage is anchored, it is carried upward in consecutive spiral turns, each overlapping the other by at least ½ inch.

4. The bandage is terminated by locking it with circular turns, which are then firmly secured by tape.

Groin Support

The following procedure is used to support a groin strain and hip adductor strains (Figure 10-4).

**Materials needed**   One roll of extra-long 6-inch (15 cm) elastic bandage, a roll of 1½-inch (3.8 cm) adhesive tape, and nonsterile cotton.

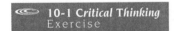
**10-1 *Critical Thinking***
Exercise

A baseball player strains his right groin while running the bases.

? Describe the elastic wrap technique that should be applied when the athlete returns to his sport and why.

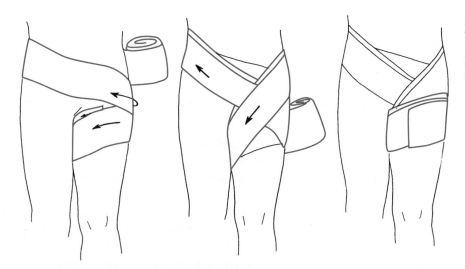

**Figure 10-4**

Elastic groin support

Leg should be internally rotated.

**Position of the athlete**   The athlete stands on a table with weight placed on the uninjured leg. The affected limb is relaxed and internally rotated.

**Procedure**

1. A piece of nonsterile cotton or a felt pad may be placed over the injured site to provide additional compression and support.
2. The end of the elastic bandage is started at the upper part of the inner aspect of the thigh and is carried posteriorly around the thigh. Then it is brought across the lower abdomen and over the crest of the ilium on the opposite side of the body.
3. The wrap is continued around the back, repeating the same pattern and securing the wrap end with 1½-inch (3.8 cm) adhesive tape.

**Note**   Variations of this method can be seen in Figure 10-5, used to support injured hip flexors.

**10-2 Critical Thinking**
*Exercise*

A wrestler sustains a blow to the left shoulder resulting in injury.

**?** A sponge rubber doughnut is applied to protect the shoulder from further injury. How is the doughnut held in place?

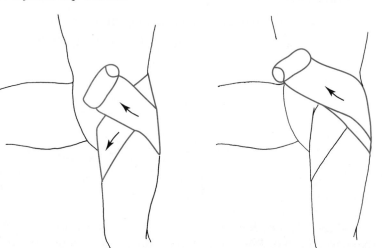

**Figure 10-5**

Hip spica for hip flexors

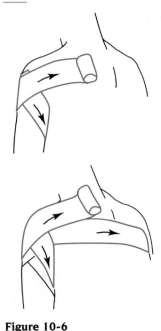

**Figure 10-6**

Elastic shoulder spica

### Shoulder Spica

The shoulder spica (Figure 10-6) is used mainly for the retention of wound dressings and for moderate muscular support.

**Materials needed**   One roll of extra-long 4- to 6-inch (10 to 15 cm) elastic wrap, 1½-inch adhesive tape, and padding for axilla (armpit).

**Position of the athlete**   Athlete stands with side toward the operator.

**Procedure**

1. The axilla must be well padded to prevent skin irritation and constriction of blood vessels.
2. The bandage is anchored by one turn around the affected upper arm.
3. After anchoring the bandage around the arm on the injured side, the wrap is carried around the back under the unaffected arm and across the chest to the injured shoulder.
4. The affected arm is again encircled by the bandage, which continues around the back. Every figure-eight pattern moves progressively upward with an overlap of at least half of the previous underlying wrap.
5. For sprains of the acromioclavicular joint, the wrap should cross directly over the top of the joint.

### Elbow Figure Eight

The elbow figure-eight bandage (Figure 10-7) can be used to secure a dressing in the antecubital fossa or to restrain full extension in hyper-extension injuries. When it is reversed, it can be used on the posterior aspect of the elbow.

**Materials needed**   One 3-inch elastic roll and 1½-inch adhesive tape.

**Position of the athlete**   Athlete flexes elbow between 45 degrees and 90 degrees, depending on the restriction of movement required.

**Procedure**

1. Anchor the bandage by encircling the lower arm.
2. Bring the roll obliquely upward over the posterior aspect of the elbow.

**Figure 10-7**

Elastic elbow figure-eight bandage

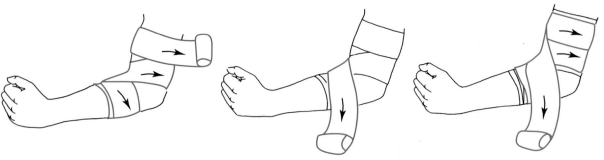

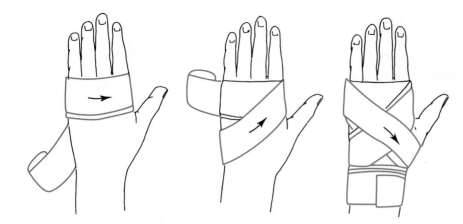

**Figure 10-8**

Hand and wrist figure eight

3. Carry the roll obliquely upward, crossing the antecubital fossa; then pass once again completely around the upper arm and return to the beginning position by again crossing the antecubital fossa.

4. Continue the procedure as described, but for every new sequence move upward toward the elbow one half the width of the underlying wrap.

### Hand and Wrist Figure Eight

A figure-eight bandage (Figure 10-8) can be used for mild wrist and hand support and for holding dressings in place.

**Materials needed**   One 2-inch bandage.

**Position of the athlete**   Athlete positions elbow at a 45-degree angle.

**Procedure**

1. The anchor is executed with one or two turns around the palm of the hand.

2. The roll is carried obliquely across the anterior or posterior portion of the hand, depending on the position of the wound, to the wrist, which it circles once, then it is returned to the primary anchor.

3. As many figures as needed are applied.

## NONELASTIC AND ELASTIC ADHESIVE TAPING

### Nonelastic White Adhesive Tape

Nonelastic white adhesive tape has great adaptability for use in sports because of its uniform adhering qualities, lightness, and the relative strength of the backing materials.[15] All of these qualities are of value both in securing wound dressings in place and in providing support and protection to injured areas.[6] This tape comes in a variety of sizes; 1-, 1½, and 2-inch widths are commonly used in sports medicine. When nonelastic white adhesive tape is purchased, factors such as cost, grade of backing, quality of adhesive, and properties of unwinding should be considered.

Techniques for Preventing
and Minimizing Sport-
Related Injuries

When purchasing white
adhesive tape, consider
• grade of backing
• quality of adhesive
• winding tension

### Tape Grade

Nonelastic white adhesive tape is most often graded according to the number of longitudinal and vertical fibers per inch of backing material. The heavier and more costly tape contains eighty-five or more longitudinal fibers and sixty-five vertical fibers per square inch. The lighter, less expensive grade has sixty-five or fewer longitudinal fibers and forty-five vertical fibers.[2]

### Adhesive Properties

The tape should adhere readily when applied and should maintain this adherence in the presence of profuse perspiration and activity. Besides sticking well, the adhesive must contain as few skin irritants as possible and must be easily removed without leaving a residue or pulling away the superficial skin.[4]

### Winding Tension

The winding tension of a tape roll is important to the operator. If tape is to be applied for protection and support, there must be even and constant unwinding tension. In most cases a proper wind needs little additional tension to provide sufficient tightness.

## Elastic Adhesive Tape

Elastic adhesive tape is often used in sports medicine. Because of its conforming qualities, stretch tape is used for small, angular body parts, such as the feet, wrist, hands, and fingers. Elastic adhesive tape also allows for expansion of body parts such as a muscle that is contracting or the foot, which expands during weight bearing. As with nonelastic white adhesive tape, elastic adhesive tape comes in a variety of widths; 1-, 2-, 3-, and 4-inch widths are typical.

## Waterproof Tape

Store tape in a cool place,
and stack it flat.

Occasionally a swimmer, diver, or waterpolo player might require an application of adhesive tape. It is recommended that special waterproof tape be used in these instances. If waterproof tape is not available duct tape is an effective substitute.

## Storing Adhesive Tape

When storing tape, take the following steps:
■ Store in a cool place.
■ Stack so that the tape rests on its flat top or bottom to avoid distortion.

## Preparation for Taping

Skin surface should be
cleansed and hair should be
shaved before applying tape.

Special attention must be given when applying tape directly to the skin.[13] Focus Box 10-1 gives a list of supplies needed for proper taping. Perspiration, oil, and dirt prevent tape from adhering to the skin. Whenever tape is used, the skin surface should be cleaned with soap and

---

**10-1** ) **Focus Box**

**Taping Supplies**

Effective taping requires the availability of numerous supplies:

1. Razor for hair removal.
2. Soap for cleaning skin.
3. Alcohol for removal of oil from skin.
4. Adhesive spray for tape adherent.
5. Prewrap material for skin protection.
6. Heel and lace pads.
7. White adhesive tape (linen-backed tape) (½-inch, 1-inch, 1½-inch, and 2-inch).
8. Adhesive and stretch tape (1-inch, 2-inch, 3-inch, and 4-inch).
9. Felt and foam padding material.
10. Tape scissors.
11. Tape cutters.
12. Elastic bandages (2-inch, 3-inch, 4-inch, and 6-inch).

---

water to remove all dirt and oil. Also, hair should be shaved to prevent additional irritation when the tape is removed (Figure 10-9A). Tape should not be applied if the skin is hot or cold. A quick-drying tape adherent spray can be used to help the tape adhere to the skin although it is not absolutely necessary (Figure 10-9B). Also, at certain points such as over bony prominences the tape can produce friction blisters. Extra foam or gauze pads (heel and lace pads) with a small amount of lubricant can help to minimize the occurrence of blisters (Figure 10-9C).

Taping directly on skin provides maximum support. However, applying tape day after day can lead to skin irritation. A roll of foam that is thin, porous, extremely lightweight, and resilient called "underwrap" or "prewrap" easily conforms to the contours of the part to be taped and protects the skin to some degree. Underwrap material should be overlapped by ½ the thickness, molding it no thicker than 2 layers (Figure 10-9D).[13]

## Proper Taping Technique

The correct tape width depends on the area to be covered. The more acute the angles, the narrower the tape must be to fit the many contours. For example, the fingers and toes usually require ½- or 1-inch (1.25 or 2.5 cm) tape; the ankles require 1½-inch (3.75 cm) tape; and the larger skin areas such as thighs and back can accommodate 2- to 3-inch (5 to 7.5 cm) tape with ease.[16]

## Tearing Tape

With some practice nonelastic white adhesive tape can be easily torn by hand. Tearing elastic tape is more difficult and it is usually necessary to

*10-3 Critical Thinking*
Exercise

A freshman football player has a chronically weak ankle that he has sprained several times. He wants to have the ankle taped before games and practices but has never had it taped before.

**?** What can be done to minimize the occurrence of blisters and ensure that the tape provides support?

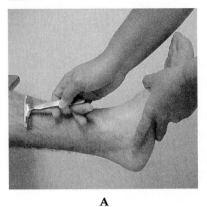 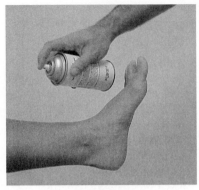 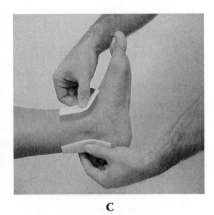

A    B    C

**Figure 10-9**

Taping preparation:
(A) Shaving. (B) Applying
tape adherent spray.
(C) Placing heel and lace
pads. (D) Applying one layer
of underwrap. (E) Applying
anchor strips.

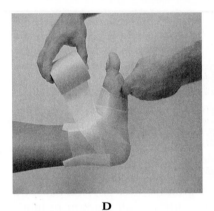 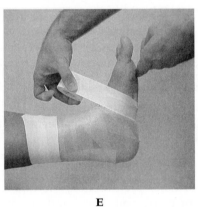

D    E

cut it with scissors. Various techniques can be used in tearing tape
(Figure 10-10).[17] The following is a suggested procedure:

1. Hold the tape roll in the preferred hand with the index finger
   hooked through the center of the tape roll and the thumb
   pressing its outer edge.

**Figure 10-10**

Technique for tearing
adhesive tape

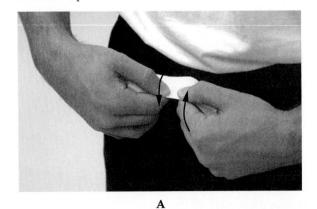 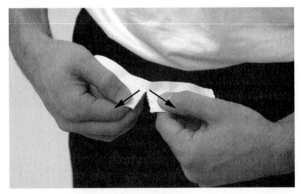

A    B

2. With the other hand, grasp the loose end between the thumb and index finger.

3. With both hands in place, pull both ends of the tape so that it is tight. Next, make a quick, scissorslike move to tear the tape. In tearing tape the movement of one hand is away from the body and the other hand toward the body. Remember, do not try to bend or twist the tape to tear it.

When tearing is properly executed, the torn edges of the nonelastic white adhesive tape are relatively straight, without curves, twists, or loose threads sticking out. Once the first thread is torn, the rest of the tape tears easily. Learning to tear tape effectively from many different positions is essential for speed and efficiency.[11]

## Removing Adhesive Tape

Tape usually can be removed from the skin by hand, by tape scissors or tape cutters, or by chemical solvents.[1]

### Manual Removal

When pulling tape from the body, be careful not to tear or irritate the skin. Tape must not be wrenched in an outward direction from the skin but should be pulled in a direct line with the body (Figure 10-11). Remember to remove the skin carefully from the tape and not to peel the tape from the skin. One hand gently pulls the tape in one direction, and the opposite hand gently presses the skin away from the tape.

### Use of Tape Scissors or Cutters

The characteristic tape scissors or cutters have a blunt nose that slips underneath the tape smoothly without gouging the skin. Take care to avoid cutting the tape too near the site of the injury, lest the scissors aggravate the condition. If possible cut on the uninjured side.

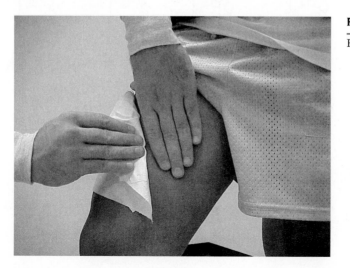

**Figure 10-11**

Removing adhesive tape

### Using "Tape Remover"

Tape remover is an alcohol-based liquid that is useful for removing adherent residue from the skin. It works best when scrubbing the area with a towel or cloth. Some individuals have a skin sensitivity to this chemical that produces a reaction. Everyone should wash the tape remover off using soap and water.

## COMMON TAPING TECHNIQUES

### Arch

Taping the arch supports the entire plantar aspect of the foot (Figure 10-12). Arch taping may be used in cases of plantar fasciitis, arch sprain (see Chapter 14), or shin splints (see Chapter 15).

**Materials needed**   One roll of 1-inch (2.5 cm) and one roll of 1½-inch (3.8 cm) white adhesive tape and tape adherent.

**Position of the athlete**   The athlete sits on a taping table with the foot to be taped extending approximately 6 inches (15 cm) over the edge of the table. The foot should be relaxed.

**Procedure**

1. Place an anchor strip around the ball of the foot (1). If the injury is acute, the anchor strip should be placed around the metatarsal heads to minimize swelling of the toes.
2. Starting at the third metatarsal head, take the tape around the heel from the lateral side and meet the strip where it began (2 and 3).
3. The next strip starts near the second metatarsal head and finishes on the fourth metatarsal head (4).

**Figure 10-12**

Arch taping technique

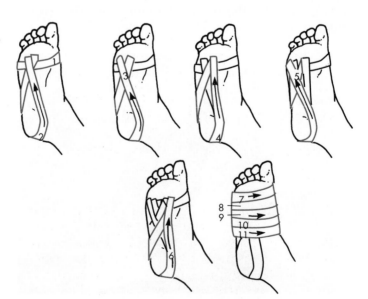

4. The last strip begins on the fourth metatarsal head and finishes on the fifth (5). The technique, when completed, forms a fanshaped pattern covering the metatarsal region (6).

5. Lock strips (7 through 11) using 1½-inch (3.8 cm) tape and encircling the complete arch.

### Great Toe

This procedure is used for taping a sprained great toe (Figure 10-13).

**Materials needed** One roll of 1-inch (2.5 cm) white adhesive tape and tape adherent.

**Position of the athlete** The athlete assumes a sitting position.

**Procedure**

1. The greatest support is given to the joint by a half-figure-eight taping (1 through 3). Start the series at an acute angle on the top of the foot and swing down between the great and first toes, first encircling the great toe and then coming up, over, and across the starting point. Repeat this process, starting each series separately. Precut strips can be applied to the appropriate surface of the great toe to prevent it from moving into a position that causes pain, prior to application of the half-figure-eight strips.

2. After the required number of half-figure-eight strips are in position, place one lock piece around the ball of the foot (4).

### Toes

**Materials needed** One roll of ½- to 1-inch (1.25 to 2.5 cm) tape, ⅛-inch (0.3 cm) sponge rubber, and tape adherent.

**Position of the athlete** The athlete assumes a sitting position.

**Procedure**

1. Cut a ⅛-inch (0.3 cm) sponge rubber wedge and place it between the affected toe and a healthy one.

2. Wrap two or three strips of tape around the toes (Figure 10-14). This technique splints a fractured toe with a nonfractured one.

### Ankle

Ankle taping applied directly to the athlete's skin affords the greatest support; however, when applied and removed daily, skin irritation occurs.[8] To avoid this problem, apply an underwrap material. Before taping, follow these procedures:[1]

1. Shave all the hair off the foot and ankle.

2. Apply a coating of tape adherent to protect the skin and offer an adhering base. NOTE: It may be advisable to avoid the use of a tape adherent, especially if the athlete has a history of developing tape blisters. In cases of skin sensitivity, the ankle surface should be thoroughly cleansed of dirt and oil and an underwrap material applied; or tape directly to the skin.

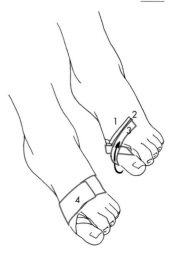

**Figure 10-13**

Taping for a sprained great toe

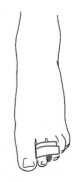

**Figure 10-14**

Taping for fracture of a toe

If the athlete has sensitive
skin, thoroughly clean the
area to be wrapped.

3. Apply a gauze pad coated with friction-proofing material such
   as grease over the instep and to the back of the heel.
4. If underwrap is used, apply a single layer. The tape anchors
   extend beyond the underwrap and adhere directly to the skin.
5. Do not apply tape if skin is cold or hot from a therapeutic
   treatment.

The closed basket weave technique (Figure 10-15) offers strong tape
support and is primarily used in athletic training for newly sprained or
chronically weak ankles.[5]

**Materials needed**   One roll of 1½-inch (3.8 cm) white adhesive
tape and tape adherent.

**Position of the athlete**   The athlete sits on a table with the leg extended and the foot held at a 90-degree angle.

**Procedure**

1. Place an anchor around the ankle approximately 5 or 6 inches
   (12.5 to 15 cm) above the malleolus, just below the belly of
   the gastrocnemius muscle, and a second anchor around the
   instep just proximal to the styloid process of the fifth
   metatarsal (1 and 2).
2. Apply the first strip posteriorly to the malleolus and attach it
   to the anchor strips (3). NOTE: When applying strips, pull the

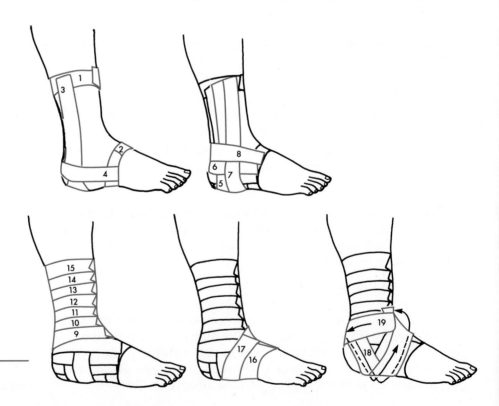

**Figure 10-15**

Closed basket weave
ankle taping

foot into eversion for an inversion strain and into a neutral
position for an eversion strain.

3. Start the first horizontal strip of the basket weave directly
   under the malleolus and attach it to the foot anchor (4).

4. In an alternating series, place three vertical strips and three
   horizontal strips on the ankle with each piece of tape
   overlapping at least half of the preceding strip (5 through 8).
   These strips and the anchors should not put pressure on the
   5th metatarsal.

5. After applying the basket weave series, continue the horizontal
   strips up the ankle, thus giving circular support (9 through 15).

6. For arch support, apply two or three circular strips lateral to
   medial (16 and 17).

7. After completing the conventional basket weave, apply two or
   three heel locks to ensure maximum stability (18 and 19).
   Start the heel lock on the dorsum (top) of the foot at the
   ankle joint. Angle the tape around the back and above the
   calcaneous, then, under the heel, then back up over the top of
   the ankle. Repeat this same pattern on the other side of the
   ankle joint moving in the opposite direction. For individuals
   with lateral (inversion) ankle sprains, the ankle should be
   pulled outward by applying more tension on the tape in a
   lateral direction. For medial (eversion) sprains, the ankle
   should be pulled inward by applying more tension on the tape
   in a medial direction. For extra support, two figure-eights
   could be added.

### Achilles Tendon

Achilles tendon taping (Figure 10-16) is designed to prevent the Achilles
tendon from overstretching.

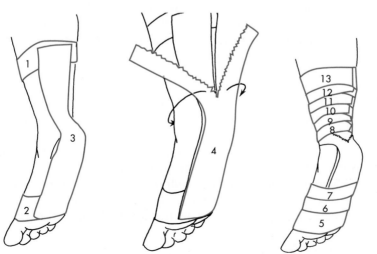

**Figure 10-16**

Achilles tendon taping

Techniques for Preventing
and Minimizing Sport-
Related Injuries

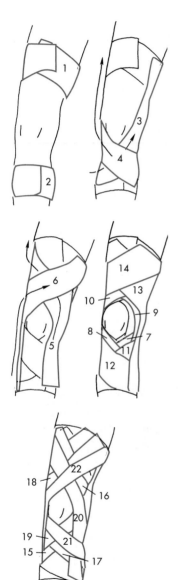

**Figure 10-17**

Taping for injuries to the
ligaments of the knee

**Materials needed**  One roll of 3-inch (7.5 cm) elastic tape, one roll
of 1½-inch (3.8 cm) white adhesive tape, heel and lace pad (placed on
the Achilles tendon just above the calcaneus), and tape adherent.

**Position of the athlete**  The athlete kneels or lies face down, with
the affected foot hanging relaxed over the edge of the table.

**Procedure**

1. Apply two anchors with 1½-inch (3.8 cm) tape, one circling
   the leg loosely approximately 7 to 9 inches (17.5 to 22.5 cm)
   above the malleoli and the other encircling the ball of the foot
   (1 and 2).

2. Cut two strips of 3-inch (7.5 cm) elastic tape approximately
   8 to 10 inches (20 to 25 cm) long. Moderately stretch the first
   strip from the ball of the athlete's foot along its plantar aspect
   up to the leg anchor (3). The second elastic strip (4) follows
   the course of the first, but cut it and split it down the middle
   lengthwise. Wrap the cut ends around the lower leg to form a
   lock. CAUTION: Keep the wrapped ends above the level of the
   strain.

3. Complete the series by placing two or three lock strips of
   elastic tape (5 through 7) loosely around the arch and five or
   six strips (8 through 13) around the athlete's lower leg.

**Notes**

1. Locking too tightly around the lower leg and foot tends to
   restrict the normal action of the Achilles tendon and create
   more tissue irritation.

2. A variation to this method is to use three 2-inch-wide (5 cm)
   elastic strips in place of strips 3 and 4. Apply the first strip at
   the plantar surface of the first metatarsal head and end it on
   the lateral side of the leg anchor. Apply the second strip at the
   plantar surface of the fifth metatarsal head and end it on the
   medial side of the leg anchor. Center the third strip between
   the other two strips and end it at the posterior aspect of the
   calf. Wrap strips of 3-inch (7.5 cm) elastic tape around the
   forefoot and lower calf to close them off.

### Knee

Athletes with unstable knees, like those with ankle instabilities, should
never use tape and bracing as a replacement for proper exercise rehabilitation. If properly applied, taping can help protect the knee and aid
in the rehabilitation process (Figure 10-17).

**Materials needed**  One roll of 2-inch (5 cm) white adhesive tape,
one roll of 3-inch (7.5 cm) elastic tape, a 1-inch (2.5 cm) heel lift,
heel and lace pads (placed in the crease behind the knee), and skin
adherent.

**Position of the athlete**   The athlete stands on a 3-foot (90 cm) table with the injured knee held in a moderately relaxed position by a 1-inch (2.5 cm) heel lift. The hair is completely removed from an area 6 inches (15 cm) above to 6 inches (15 cm) below the patella.

**Procedure**

1. Lightly encircle the thigh and leg at the hairline with a 3-inch (7.5 cm) elastic anchor strip (1 and 2).

2. Precut 12 elastic tape strips, each approximately 9 inches (22.5 cm) long. Stretching them to their utmost, apply them to the knee as indicated in Figure 10-17 (3 through 14).

3. Apply a series of three strips of 2-inch (5 cm) white adhesive tape (15 through 22). Some individuals find it advantageous to complete a knee taping by wrapping loosely with an elastic wrap, thus providing an added precaution against the tape's coming loose from perspiration.

**Caution**   Tape must not constrict patella.

Elbow

Tape the elbow as follows to prevent hyperextension (Figure 10-18).

**Materials needed**   One roll of 1½-inch (3.8 cm) white adhesive tape, heel and lace pad (placed in the crease of the elbow), tape adherent, and 2-inch (5 cm) elastic bandage.

**Position of the athlete**   The athlete stands with the affected elbow flexed at 90 degrees.

**Procedure**

1. Apply 3 anchor strips loosely around the forearm (1 through 3). Apply three anchor strips loosely around the upper arm, approximately 2 inches (25 cm) to above the curve of the elbow (antecubital fossa) (4 through 6).

2. Construct a checkrein by cutting a 10-inch (25 cm) and a 4-inch (10 cm) strip of tape and laying the 4-inch (10 cm) strip against the center of the 10-inch (25 cm) strip, blanking out that portion. Next place the checkrein so that it spans the two anchor strips with the blanked-out side facing downward. Leave checkrein extended 1 to 2 inches past anchor strips on both ends. This allows anchoring of the checkreins with circular strips to secure against slippage (7).

3. Place five additional 10-inch (25 cm) strips of tape over the basic checkrein.

4. Finish the procedure by securing the checkrein with three lock strips on each end (8 through 13). A figure-eight elastic wrap applied over the taping will prevent the tape from slipping because of perspiration.

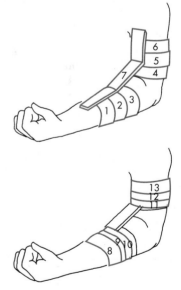

**Figure 10-18**

Taping to restrict elbow motion

**Figure 10-19**

Wrist taping technique

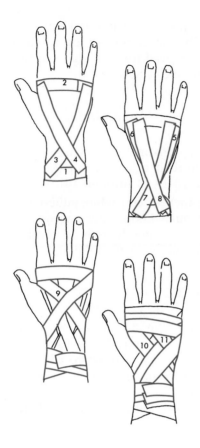

### Wrist

Wrist taping (Figure 10-19) stabilizes and protects badly injured wrists.

**Materials needed** One roll of 1-inch (2.5 cm) white adhesive tape and tape adherent.

**Position of the athlete** The athlete stands with the affected hand flexed toward the injured direction and the fingers moderately spread to increase the breadth of the wrist for the protection of nerves and blood vessels.

**Procedure**

1. Apply one anchor strip around the wrist approximately 3 inches (7.5 cm) from the hand (1); wrap another anchor strip around the spread hand (2).

2. With the wrist bent toward the side of the injury, run a strip of tape from the anchor strip near the little finger obliquely across the wrist joint to the wrist anchor strip. Run another strip from the anchor strip on the index finger side across the wrist joint to the wrist anchor. This forms a crisscross over the wrist joint (3 and 4). Apply a series of four or five crisscrosses, depending on the extent of splinting needed (5 through 8).

3. Apply two or three series of figure-eight tapings over the crisscross taping (9 through 11). Start by encircling the wrist once, carry a strip over the back of the hand obliquely, encircling the hand twice, and then carry another strip obliquely upward across the back of the hand to where the figure-eight started. Repeat this procedure to ensure a strong, stabilizing taping.

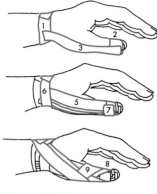

### Thumb

Sprained thumb taping (Figure 10-20) is designed to give both protection for the muscle and joint and support to the thumb.

**Materials needed**   One roll of 1-inch (2.5 cm) white adhesive tape and tape adherent.

**Position of the athlete**   The athlete should hold the injured thumb in a relaxed neutral position.

**Figure 10-20**

Taping for a sprained thumb

**Procedure**

1. Place an anchor strip loosely around the wrist and another around the distal end of the thumb (1 and 2).

2. From the anchor at the tip of the thumb to the anchor around the wrist, apply four splint strips in a series on the side of greater injury (dorsal or palmar side) (3 through 5) and hold them in place with one lock strip around the wrist and one encircling the tip of the thumb (6 and 7).

3. Add three thumb spicas. Start the first spica on the radial side at the base of the thumb and carry it under the thumb, completely encircling it, and then cross the starting point. The strip should continue around the wrist and finish at the starting point. Each of the subsequent spica strips should overlap the preceding strip by at least ⅔ inch (1.7 cm) and move downward on the thumb (8 and 9). The thumb spica with tape provides an excellent means of protection during recovery from an injury.

### Athletic Injury Management Checklist

The following is a checklist for applying adhesive tape to an injured body part.

☐ If the part to be taped is a joint, place it in the position in which it is to be stabilized. If the part is muscle, make the necessary allowance for contraction and expansion.

☐ Overlap the tape at least half the width of the tape below. Unless tape is overlapped sufficiently, the active athlete will separate it, exposing the underlying skin to irritation.

☐ Avoid continuous taping. Tape continuously wrapped around a part may cause constriction. It is suggested that one turn be made at a time and that each encirclement be torn to overlap the starting end by approximately 1 inch. This rule is particularly true of white adhesive tape.

☐ Keep the tape roll in the hand whenever possible. By learning to keep the tape roll in the hand, seldom putting it down, and by learning to tear the tape, an operator can develop taping speed and accuracy.

☐ Smooth and mold the tape as it is laid on the skin. To save additional time, tape strips should be smoothed and molded to the body part as they are put in place; this is done by stroking the top with the fingers, palms, and heels of both hands.

☐ Allow tape to fit the natural contour of the skin. Each strip of tape must be placed with a particular purpose in mind. Linen-backed tape is not sufficiently elastic to bend around acute angles but must be allowed to fall as it may, fitting naturally to the body contours. Failing to allow this fit creates wrinkles and gaps that can result in skin irritations.

☐ Start taping with an anchor piece and finish by applying a lock strip. Commence taping, if possible, by sticking the tape to an anchor piece that encircles the part. This placement affords a good medium for the stabilization of succeeding tape strips so that they will not be affected by the movement of the part.

☐ Where maximum support is desired, tape directly over skin. In cases of sensitive skin, prewrap may be used as a tape base. With prewrap, some movement can be expected between the skin and the base.

☐ Do not apply tape if skin is hot or cold from a therapeutic treatment.

## SUMMARY

- Elastic bandages, when properly applied, can contribute to recovery from sport injuries.

- Elastic bandages must be applied uniformly, firmly but not so tightly as to impede circulation.

- Tape is used in a variety of ways—as a means of holding a wound dressing in place, as support, and as protection against musculoskeletal injuries.

- For supporting and protecting musculoskeletal injuries, two types of tape are currently used—nonelastic white adhesive and elastic adhesive.

- Tape must be stored in a cool place and must be stacked on the flat side of each roll.

- The skin of the athlete must be carefully prepared before tape is applied.

- The skin should first be carefully cleaned; then all hair should be removed.

- An adherent may be applied, followed by an underwrap material, if needed, to help avoid skin irritation.

- Tape must be applied in a manner that provides the least amount of irritation and the maximum support.

- All tape applications require great care that the proper materials are used, that the proper position of the athlete is ensured, and that procedures are carefully followed.

---

*Solutions to Critical Thinking* Exercises

**10-1** A 6-inch (15 cm) elastic wrap as a hip adductor restraint should be applied. This technique is designed to prevent the groin from being overstretched and the hip adductors reinjured.

**10-2** A 4-inch (10 cm) elastic shoulder spica is used to hold the doughnut in place.

**10-3** First the ankle should be shaved. Then a tape adherent spray should be applied. Heel and lace pads with a small amount of lubricant should be applied over bony prominences. One layer of underwrap can be applied. Tape should be applied with even pressure leaving no gaps.

## REVIEW QUESTIONS AND CLASS ACTIVITIES

1. What are elastic bandages used for? How do you apply them?
2. Observe the athletic trainer bandaging and taping in the athletic training room.
3. What types of tape are available? What is the purpose of each type? What qualities should you look for in selecting tape?
4. How should you prepare an area to be taped?
5. How should you tear tape?
6. How should you remove tape from an area? Demonstrate the various methods and cutters that can be used to remove tape.
7. What are some general rules for tape application and why should you follow them?
8. What are some common taping procedures?
9. Bring the different types of tape to class. Discuss their uses and the qualities to look for in purchasing tape. Have the class practice tearing tape and preparing an area for taping.
10. Take each joint or body part and demonstrate the common taping procedures used to give support to that area. Have the students pair up and practice these taping jobs on each other. Discuss the advantages and disadvantages of using tape as a supportive device.

## REFERENCES

1. Alt W, Lohrer H, Gollhofer A: 1999. Functional properties of adhesive ankle taping: neuromuscular and mechanical effects before and after exercise, *Foot Ankle Int* 20(4):238.
2. Austin, K: 1994. *Taping techniques,* Chicago, Mosby-Wolfe.
3. Beam, J: 2006. *Orthopedic taping, wrapping, bracing and padding,* Philadelphia, FA Davis.
4. Bragg, RW, Macmahon, JM, Overom, EK, Yerby, SA, Matheson, GO, Carter, DR, Andriacchi, TP: 2002. Failure and fatigue characteristics of adhesive athletic tape, *Medicine and science in sports and exercise* 34(3):403–410.
5. Briggs, J: 2001. Bandaging, strapping and taping. In Briggs, J: (ed), *Sports therapy: theoretical and practical thoughts and considerations,* Chichester, England, Corpus Publishing Limited.
6. Callaghan MJ: 1997. Role of ankle taping and bracing in the athlete, *Br J Sports Med* 31(2):102.
7. DesRochers, DM, Cox, DE: 2002. Proprioceptive benefit derived from ankle support, *Athletic therapy today* 7(6):44–45.
8. Heit EJ, Lephart SM, Rozzi SL: 1996. The effect of ankle bracing and taping on joint position sense in the stable ankle, *J Sport Rehab* 5(3):206.
9. Hughes, T, Rochester, P: 2008. The effects of proprioceptive exercise and taping on proprioception in subjects with functional ankle instability: A review of the literature. *Physical therapy in sport* 9(3):136.
10. Hunt, E, Short, S: 2006. Collegiate athletes' perceptions of adhesive ankle taping: a qualitative analysis, *Journal of Sport Rehabilitation* 15(4):280.
11. Jones K: 1996. Athletic taping and bracing. In Sallis RE, Massamino F, editors: *Essentials of sport medicine,* St Louis, MO, Mosby–Year Book.
12. Knight, KL: 2001. Taping, wrapping, bracing, and padding. In Knight, KL: (ed), *Assessing clinical proficiencies in athletic training: a modular approach,* 3rd edition, Champaign, IL, Human Kinetics.
13. Manfroy PP, Ashton-Miller JA, Wojtys EM: 1997. The effect of exercise, prewrap, and athletic tape on the maximal active and passive ankle resistance to ankle inversion, *Am J Sports Med* 25(2):156.
14. Perrin DH: 2005. *Athletic taping and bracing,* Champaign, IL, Human Kinetics.
15. Sports Medicine Council of British Columbia: 1995. *Manual of athletic taping,* Philadelphia, FA Davis.
16. *Sports taping basics: lower body:* 1996. Champaign, IL, Human Kinetics.
17. *Sports taping basics: upper body:* 1996. Champaign, IL, Human Kinetics.
18. Wilkerson, GB: 2002. Biomechanical and neuromuscular effects of ankle taping and bracing, *Journal of athletic training,* 37(4):436–445.

## ANNOTATED BIBLIOGRAPHY

Beam, J: 2006. *Orthopedic taping, wrapping, bracing and padding,* Philadelphia, FA Davis.

*This highly illustrated manual is an all-inclusive examination of taping, wrapping, bracing and padding techniques for the prevention, treatment, and rehabilitation of common athletic injuries and conditions.*

MacDonald, R: 2004. *Taping techniques: principles and practice,* Philadelphia, Elsevier.

*Provides an illustrated guide to taping techniques for those involved in the treatment and rehabilitation of sports injuries and other conditions such as muscle imbalances, unstable joints, and neural control. Chapters organized by body part*

give indications and instructions for taping for specific conditions.

Prentice W: 2009. *Arnheim's principles of
athletic training*, New York, McGraw-
Hill.

    *Contains a comprehensive chapter on a
variety of taping and bandaging skills
with complete descriptions of techniques.*

Perrin DH: 2005. *Athletic taping and
bracing*, Champaign, IL, Human
Kinetics.

    *Discusses specific injuries; gives step-
by-step instructions for applying tape,
braces, wraps, and orthotics; and presents
stretching and strengthening exercises
that reduce the chances of reinjury.*

Sports Medicine Council of British
Columbia: 1995. *Manual of athletic
taping*, Philadelphia, FA Davis.

    *Guidelines for taping and wrapping
athletes' joints and limbs to both prevent
and manage injuries. Chapters include
injury recognition; anatomy and taping
techniques for the ankle, foot, knee, wrist,
hand, elbow, and muscles and tendons;
and resources.*

First aider, Gardner, Kan, Cramer Products.

    *Published seven times throughout the
school year, this periodical contains useful
taping and bandaging techniques that
have been submitted by readers.*

*Sports Medicine Guide*, Mueller Sports
Medicine, 1 Quench Dr, Prairie du
Sac, WI, 53578.

    *Published four times a year, this quar-
terly often presents, along with discus-
sions on specific injuries, many innova-
tive taping and bandaging techniques.*

**WEB SITES**

Properties of Athletic Tape:
    www.bloodandbones.com/
    tape.html

Cramer Sports Medicine:
    www.cramersportsmed.com/

Mueller Sports Medicine—Retail Tape
    and Wrap:
    www.muellersportsmed.com/
    Retail_Tape_and_Wrap.htm

Johnson & Johnson: www.jnj.com/

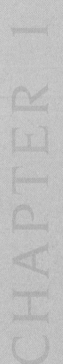

## CHAPTER 11

# Understanding the Basics of Injury Rehabilitation

*When you finish this chapter you will be able to:*

- Explain the philosophy of the rehabilitative process in a sports medicine environment.
- Identify the individual short-term and long-term goals of a rehabilitation program.
- Describe the criteria and the decision-making process for determining when the injured athlete may return to full activity.
- Discuss how a coach might use therapeutic modalities in a rehabilitation program.

## THERAPEUTIC EXERCISE VERSUS CONDITIONING EXERCISE

The basic principles of training and conditioning exercises that were discussed in some detail in Chapter 4 also apply to techniques of therapeutic, rehabilitative, or reconditioning exercises that are specifically concerned with restoring normal body function following injury. The term *therapeutic exercise* is perhaps most widely used to indicate exercises that are used in a rehabilitation program, whereas the term *conditioning exercise* refers to those activities that minimize the possibility of injury while maximizing performance.

The purpose of this chapter is to provide some knowledge and understanding of a basic plan for a typical rehabilitation program that an athletic trainer or a physical therapist would use to deal with the injured athlete. **It is NOT intended to prepare a coach or other fitness professionals to oversee a rehabilitation program for an injured athlete. It must be made absolutely clear that state laws and statutes limit anyone other than health care providers (i.e., athletic trainers, physical therapists, physicians, etc.) in the extent to which he or she can legally be involved in supervising or designing the rehabilitation program.** However, it should also be emphasized that controlling initial swelling and managing the pain associated with acute injury are first aid techniques that everyone may legally perform.

## PHILOSOPHY OF ATHLETIC INJURY REHABILITATION

Although every effort is made to create a safe playing environment and prevent injuries, the nature of athletic participation dictates that injuries will eventually occur. Fortunately, few of the injuries that occur in an athletic setting are life threatening. The majority of the injuries are not serious and lend themselves to rapid rehabilitation. Long-term

The long-term goal is to return the injured athlete to practice or competition as quickly and safely as possible.

The athletic trainer is responsible for design, implementation, and supervision of the rehabilitation program.

rehabilitation programs require the supervision of a highly trained professional to be safe and effective. In an athletic setting, the athletic trainer or perhaps a physical therapist assumes the primary responsibility for design, implementation, and supervision of the rehabilitation program for the injured athlete.[9]

The competitive nature of athletics necessitates an aggressive approach to rehabilitation. Because of the short competitive season in most sports, the injured athlete does not have the luxury of simply sitting around and doing nothing until the injury heals. *The goal for the injured athlete is to return to activity as soon as safely possible.*[9] Consequently, the tendency is to try to push the athlete to return. Unfortunately there is a thin line between not pushing the athlete hard enough or fast enough and being overly aggressive. In either case, a mistake in judgment on the part of the person overseeing the rehabilitation program may hinder the athlete's return to activity. Health care professionals overseeing the rehabilitation program must make decisions about how to progress that program on the limitations of the healing process.

## BASIC COMPONENTS AND GOALS OF A REHABILITATION PROGRAM

Designing an effective rehabilitation program is simple if several basic components are addressed. These basic components may also be considered as the short-term goals of a rehabilitation program and should include (1) providing correct immediate first aid and management following injury to limit or control swelling; (2) reducing or minimizing pain; (3) restoring full range of motion; (4) reestablishing core stability; (5) restoring or increasing muscular strength, endurance, and power; (6) reestablishing neuromuscular control; (7) improving balance; (8) maintaining cardiorespiratory fitness; and (9) incorporating appropriate functional progressions.[9] *The long-term goal is almost invariably to return the injured athlete to practice or competition as quickly and safely as possible.*

### Providing Correct First Aid and Controlling Swelling

As discussed in detail in Chapter 7, the process of rehabilitation begins immediately after injury. Initial first-aid and management techniques are perhaps the most critical part of any rehabilitation program. How the injury is managed initially has a significant impact on the course of the rehabilitative process.[1] Everything that is done in first-aid management of any injury should be directed toward controlling the swelling.[8] To control and significantly limit the amount of swelling, the PRICE principle— protection, rest, ice, compression, and elevation—should be applied (Figure 11-1). Each factor plays a critical role in limiting swelling, and all these elements should be used simultaneously (see Chapter 7).

### Controlling Pain

When an injury occurs, the athlete experiences some degree of pain. The extent of the pain is determined in part by the severity of the injury, by the athlete's individual response to and perception of pain, and

**11-1 Critical Thinking Exercise**

A soccer player has been diagnosed as having a grade 2 sprain of the MCL in her knee. The team physician has referred the athlete to a physical therapist, who is charged with the responsibility of overseeing the rehabilitation program.

? What are the short-term goals of a rehabilitation program, and how can these be best achieved?

Components of a rehabilitation program:
- controlling swelling
- reducing pain
- restoring full range of motion
- reestablishing core stability
- restoring muscle strength, endurance, power
- reestablishing neuromuscular control
- regaining balance
- maintaining cardio-respiratory fitness
- incorporating functional progressions

Controlling swelling:
- protection
- rest
- ice
- compression
- elevation

**Figure 11-1**

The PRICE technique should be used immediately following injury to limit swelling.

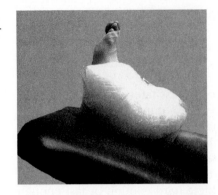

**Figure 11-2**

Stretching techniques are used with tight musculotendinous structures to improve range of motion. (A) Dynamic (ballistic) stretching. (B) Static stretching. (C) PNF stretching. (D) Stretching with exercise ball. (E) Stretching with foam roller.

by the circumstances under which the injury occurred. Acute pain can be effectively controlled by using the PRICE technique immediately after injury.[7] In addition, using appropriate therapeutic modalities such as ice, heat, or electrical stimulating currents can help modulate pain throughout the rehabilitation process.[10]

## Restoring Range of Motion

Injury to a joint is always followed by some associated loss of motion. That loss of movement may be caused by resistance of the muscle and its tendon to stretch, by contracture of the ligaments and capsule around a joint, or by some combination of the two. The athlete should engage in dynamic (ballistic), static, or PNF (see Chapter 4) stretching activities designed to improve flexibility (Figure 11-2).

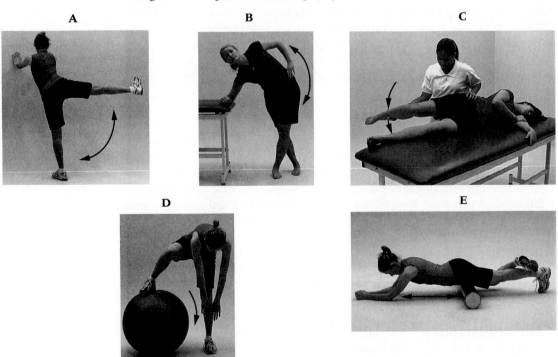

A    B    C

D    E

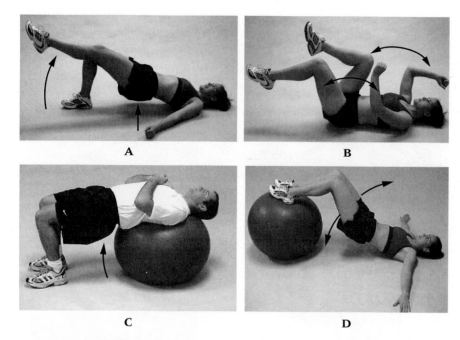

A            B

C            D

**Figure 11-3**

Core stability exercises: (A) Single-leg bridge (B) Dead bug (C) Bridge on ball (D) Hamstring curl on stability ball.

## Reestablishing Core Stability

Core stability is absolutely essential to developing functional strength (Figure 11-3). The core is considered to be the lumbo-pelvic-hip complex, which functions to dynamically stabilize the entire kinetic chain during functional movements. Without proximal or core stability, the distal movers cannot function optimally to efficiently utilize their strength and power. Thus core stability should be addressed prior to engaging in any form of strengthening.

## Restoring Muscular Strength, Endurance, and Power

Muscular strength, endurance, and power are among the most essential factors in restoring the function of a body part to preinjury status. Isometric, progressive resistance (isotonic), isokinetic, and plyometric exercises performed in either an open or closed kinetic chain can benefit rehabilitation (see Chapter 4).[4] A major goal in performing strengthening exercises is to work through a full, pain-free range of motion.

### Isometric Exercise

Isometric exercises are commonly performed in the early phase of rehabilitation when a joint is immobilized for a period of time. They are useful in cases in which using resistance training through a full range of motion may make the injury worse. Isometrics increase static strength and assist in decreasing the amount of atrophy. Isometrics also can lessen swelling by causing a muscle pumping action to remove fluid and edema.

**11-2 *Critical Thinking***
Exercise

A runner complains of anterior knee pain. She has greatly cut back on the distance of her training runs and indicates that she has been taking anti-inflammatory medication to help her continue to train. However, she is frustrated because her knee seems to be getting worse instead of better.

**?** What can be recommended to most effectively help her deal with her knee pain?

**Figure 11-4**

Progressive resistance (isotonic) exercise techniques include (A) free weights, (B) exercise machines, (C) elastic bands or tubing, and (D) manual resistance.

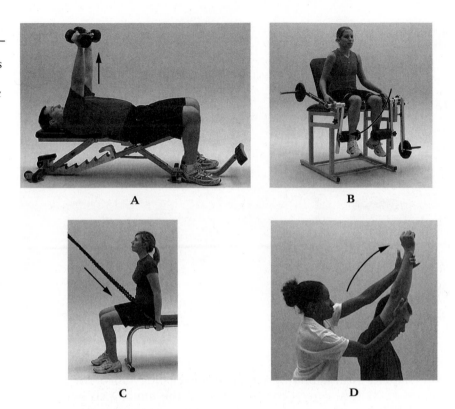

A

B

C

D

### Progressive Resistance Exercise

Progressive resistance exercise (PRE) is the most commonly used strengthening technique in a rehabilitation program. PRE may be done with free weights, exercise machines, or rubber tubing (Figure 11-4). Progressive resistance exercise uses isotonic contractions in which force is generated against resistance while the muscle is changing in length. In a rehabilitation program, both eccentric (shortening) and concentric (lengthening) strengthening exercises should be used.

Limited range of movement = stretching.

Strengthening exercises:
- isometrics
- progressive resistance exercise
- isokinetics
- plyometrics

### Isokinetic Exercise

Isokinetic exercise is occasionally used in the rehabilitative process.[3] It is most often incorporated during the later phases of a rehabilitation program primarily for diagnostic purposes. Isokinetics use a fixed speed with accommodating resistance to provide maximal resistance throughout the range of motion (Figure 11-5). The speed of movement can be altered in isokinetic exercise. Isokinetic measures are commonly used as criteria for return of the athlete to functional activity following injury.

### Plyometric Exercise

Plyometric exercises are most often incorporated into the later stages of a rehabilitation program. Plyometrics use a quick stretch of a muscle to facilitate a subsequent concentric contraction. Plyometric exercises are useful in restoring or developing the athlete's ability to produce dynamic movements associated with muscular power (Figure 11-6). The ability to generate force very rapidly is a key to successful performance in many sport activities. It is critical to address the element of muscular power in rehabilitation programs for the injured athlete.

## Reestablishing Neuromuscular Control

Neuromuscular control is the mind's attempt to teach the body conscious control of a specific movement.[6] Neuromuscular control relies on the central nervous system to interpret and integrate sensory and movement information coming from muscles and joints and then to control those individual muscles and joints to produce coordinated movement.[11] Following injury and subsequent rest and immobilization, the central nervous system "forgets" how to put this information together. Regaining neuromuscular control means regaining the ability to follow some previously established sensory pattern. Strengthening exercises, particularly those that tend to be more functional, are essential for reestablishing neuromuscular control.[11]

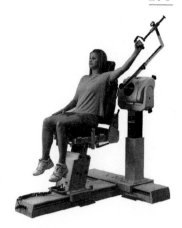

**Figure 11-5**

Isokinetic exercise is most often used in the later stages of rehabilitation.

Neuromuscular control produces coordinated movements.

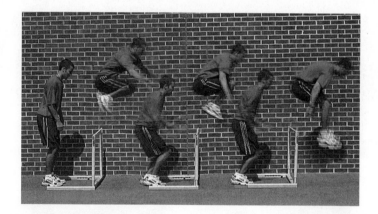

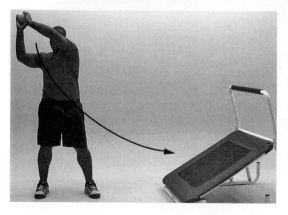
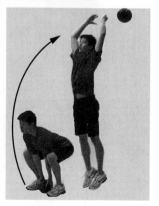

**Figure 11-6**

Plyometric exercise focuses on improving dynamic power movements.

### Regaining Balance

The ability to balance and maintain postural stability is essential to reacquiring athletic skills.[2] A rehabilitation program must include functional exercises that incorporate balance training to prepare the athlete for return to activity (Figure 11-7). Failure to address balance problems may predispose the athlete to reinjury.[3]

### Maintaining Cardiorespiratory Fitness

Maintaining cardiorespiratory fitness is perhaps the single most neglected component of a rehabilitation program. An athlete spends a considerable amount of time preparing the cardiorespiratory system to handle the increased demands made upon it during a competitive season. When injury occurs and the athlete is forced to miss training time, levels of cardiorespiratory fitness may decrease rapidly. Thus substitute alternative activities should be used that allow the athlete to maintain existing levels of cardiorespiratory fitness as early as possible in the rehabilitation period (Figure 11-8).[6]

**Figure 11-7**

Reestablishing neuromuscular control and balance are critical components in regaining functional performance capabilities. (A) Balancing on BAPS board. (B) Dynadisc. (C) Rockerboard.

**A**

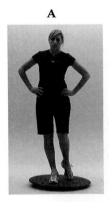

**B**

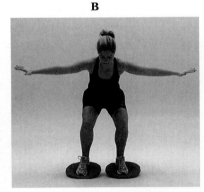

**C**

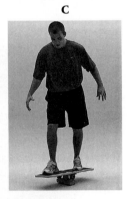

**Figure 11-8**

Every rehabilitation program must include some exercise designed to maintain cardiorespiratory fitness. (A) Upper and lower extremity ergometic. (B) Aquatic exercise.

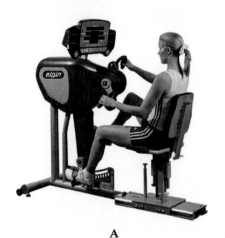

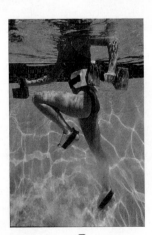

**A**

**B**

---

$\boxed{11\text{-}1}$    *Focus Box*

**Return to Running Following Lower Extremity Injury Functional Progression:**

- Walking
- Jogging on track with walking of curves
- Jogging full track
- Running on track with jogging of curves
- Running full track
- Running for fitness—2 to 3 miles three times per week
- Lunges—90 degree, pivot, 180 degree
- Sprints—"W," triangle, 6 second, 20 yd, 40 yd, 120 yd
- Acceleration/deceleration runs
- Shuffle slides progressing to shuffle run
- Carioca

---

Depending on the nature of the injury, several possible activities can help the athlete maintain fitness levels. A lower extremity injury necessitates non-weight-bearing activities. Pool activities provide an excellent means for injury rehabilitation. Cycling also can positively stress the cardiorespiratory system.

## Functional Progressions

The purpose of any rehabilitation program is to restore normal function following injury. Functional progressions involve a series of gradually progressive activities designed to prepare the individual for return to a specific sport (Focus Box 11-1).[11] Those skills necessary for successful participation in a given sport are broken down into component parts, and the athlete gradually reacquires those skills within the limitations of his or her own individual progress.[12] Every new activity introduced must be carefully monitored to determine the athlete's ability to perform and his or her physical tolerance. If an activity does not produce additional pain or swelling, the level should be advanced; new activities should be introduced as quickly as possible. Ultimately, the rehabilitating athlete should be challenged with position-specific drills and activities.

Functional progressions will gradually assist the injured athlete in achieving normal pain-free range of motion, in restoring adequate strength levels, and in regaining neuromuscular control throughout the rehabilitation program.

## Functional Testing

Functional testing uses functional progression drills for the purpose of assessing the athlete's ability to perform a specific activity (Figure 11-9). Functional testing involves the performance of a single maximal effort

*Functional progressions incorporate sport-specific skills into the rehabilitation program.*

**11-3 *Critical Thinking***
Exercise

Following an ankle sprain, a basketball player is placed in an ankle immobilizer and given crutches with instructions to begin with totally non-weight-bearing movement and progress to full weight-bearing movement without crutches as soon as possible. After 4 days the athlete is out of the immobilizer and can walk without crutches but still has a significant limp.

? What can be done to help the athlete regain a normal gait pattern, and why is it important to do so as soon as possible?

**Figure 11-9**

Performance on functional tests can determine the capability of the athlete to return to full activity.

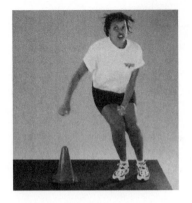 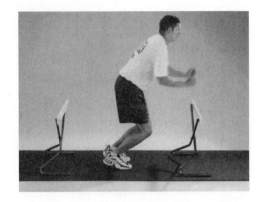

All exercise rehabilitation must be conducted as part of a carefully designed plan.

to give some idea of how close the athlete is to a full return to activity. For years a variety of functional tests have been used to assess the athlete's progress, including agility runs (e.g., figure eights, shuttle runs, cariocas), side stepping, vertical jumps, hopping for time or distance, and co-contraction tests.[11] If preseason testing was done, the performance of the injured athlete on a functional test can be compared with the preseason baseline test to determine if the athlete is functionally ready to return to full activity.

## USING THERAPEUTIC MODALITIES

Most athletic trainers and physical therapists routinely incorporate the use of therapeutic modalities including cold (cryotherapy), heat (thermotherapy), ultrasound, electrotherapy, massage, traction, and intermittent compression into their rehabilitation programs. Athletic trainers and physical therapists have had formal classroom instruction and supervised clinical experience in using various therapeutic modalities and in many states are licensed to do so.[10]

**In the absence of an athletic trainer or physical therapist, simple inexpensive therapeutic modalities such as cold, heat, or perhaps massage might be used to treat an injured athlete; using other modalities is usually beyond the scope of a coach's expertise. It is essential to be aware of and follow the laws of different states that specifically dictate how certain therapeutic modalities can be used.[10]**

### Ice Packs (Bags)

Ice packs are most often used for minimizing swelling and for analgesia immediately following injury. Flaked or crushed ice can be encased in a wet towel and placed on the part to be treated. An ice pack made by placing crushed or chipped ice in a self-sealing plastic bag may also be used. Both types of ice packs can easily mold to the contour of the part. Besides toweling, an elastic wrap should be available and should be used to hold the pack firmly in place. Usually an elastic bandage compression wrap and elevation are used with an ice pack. These packs are safely used for 20 minutes. Ice massage may also be useful to help with analgesia and then repeated after 1 hour.[10]

## Hot Packs

Hot packs are most often used postacutely (after swelling has stopped) to increase blood and lymphatic flow and facilitate reabsorption of the by-products of the injury process into the lymphatic system. Heat may also be used for its analgesic and relaxation effects. Caution should be exercised in using heat too early following injury. Cold should be used for at least 72 hours post injury before using any type of heat.

Commercial moist heat packs, sometimes called *hydrocollator packs,* contain silicate gel in a cotton pad, which is immersed in thermostatically controlled hot water at a temperature of 160° F. Each pad retains water and a relatively constant heat level for a 20- to 30-minute treatment period. A minimum of six layers of toweling or commercial terry cloth are used between the packs and the skin. The athlete should not lie on top of the hot pack. Focus Box 11-2 provides basic indications and contraindications for using heat or ice.

## Massage

Massage is defined as the systematic manipulation of the soft tissues of the body. The movements of gliding, compressing, stretching, percussing, and vibrating are regulated to produce specific responses in the athlete. Massage causes mechanical, physiological, and psychological responses.[10]

Mechanical responses to massage occur as a direct result of the graded pressures and movements of the hand on the body. Such actions encourage venous and lymphatic drainage and mildly stretch superficial

---

( 11-2 )     ***Focus Box***

**Using Ice versus Heat?**

- Use ice immediately after injury to minimize swelling and reduce pain.
- Ice should be used for a minimum of 72 hours following acute injury.
- Heat is used to increase blood flow to the area of injury.
- Using heat too soon increases the chances of additional swelling.
- If you are trying to decide whether to use ice or heat, you will always be safest using ice.
- It is safe to switch from ice to heat when:
  - there is little or no chance of additional swelling.
  - the injury is not tender to touch.
  - any discoloration from the injury is starting to dissipate.

and scar tissue. Connective tissue can be effectively stretched by friction massage, which helps prevent rigidity in scar formation. Massage can increase circulation and, as a result, increase metabolism and aid in the removal of metabolites such as lactic acid. It also helps to remove edema by increasing circulation at and around the injury site, assisting in the normal venous blood return to the heart. Relaxation can be induced by slow, superficial stroking of the skin that is beneficial for tense, anxious athletes who may require gentle hands-on treatment.[10]

**11-3**    *Focus Box*

**Full Return to Activity**

In considering the athlete's return to activity, the following concerns should be addressed:

- *Physiological healing constraints.* Has rehabilitation progressed to the later stages of the healing process?
- *Pain status.* Has pain disappeared, or is the athlete able to play within his or her own levels of pain tolerance?
- *Swelling.* Is there still a chance that swelling may be exacerbated by a return to activity?
- *Range of motion.* Is range of motion adequate to allow the athlete to perform both effectively and with minimized risk of reinjury?
- *Strength.* Is strength, endurance, or power great enough to protect the injured structure from reinjury?
- *Neuromuscular control/proprioception/kinesthesia.* Has the athlete "relearned" how to use the injured body part?
- *Cardiorespiratory fitness.* Has the athlete been able to maintain cardiorespiratory fitness at or near the level necessary for competition?
- *Sport-specific demands.* Are the demands of the sport or a specific position such that the athlete will not be at risk of reinjury?
- *Functional testing.* Does performance on appropriate functional tests indicate that the extent of recovery is sufficient to allow successful performance?
- *Prophylactic taping, bracing, padding.* Are any additional supports necessary for the injured athlete to return to activity?
- *Responsibility of the athlete.* Is the athlete capable of listening to his or her body and of knowing enough not to put himself or herself in a potential reinjury situation?
- *Predisposition to injury.* Is this athlete prone to reinjury or a new injury when not 100 percent?
- *Psychological factors.* Is the athlete capable of returning to activity and competing at a high level without fear of reinjury?
- *Athlete education and preventive maintenance program.* Does the athlete understand the importance of continuing to engage in conditioning exercises that can greatly reduce the chances of reinjury?

## CRITERIA FOR FULL RECOVERY

All exercise rehabilitation plans must determine what is meant by complete recovery from an injury. Often it means that the athlete is fully reconditioned and has achieved full range of movement, strength, neuromuscular control, cardiovascular fitness, and sport-specific functional skills. Besides physical well-being, the athlete must also have regained full confidence to return to his or her sport. Specific criteria for a return to full activity after rehabilitation are determined to a large extent by the nature and severity of the specific injury, but also depend on the philosophy and judgment of both the physician and the coach (Focus Box 11-3).[7]

The decision to release an athlete recovering from injury to a full return to athletic activity is the final stage of the rehabilitation/recovery process. The decision should be carefully considered by each member of the sports medicine team involved in the rehabilitation process. The team physician should be ultimately responsible for deciding that the athlete is ready to return to practice and/or competition. That decision should be based on collective input from the coach, the athletic trainer, and the athlete.

### Athletic Injury Management Checklist

The following is a checklist for those components that should be addressed in designing an injury rehabilitation program.

☐ Provide correct immediate first aid and management following injury to limit or control swelling.
☐ Reduce or minimize pain.
☐ Restore full range of motion.
☐ Reestablish neuromuscular control.
☐ Restore or increase muscular strength, endurance, and power.
☐ Improve balance.
☐ Maintain cardiorespiratory fitness.
☐ Incorporate appropriate functional progressions.

## SUMMARY

- The rehabilitation philosophy in sports medicine is an aggressive one, with the ultimate goal being to return the injured athlete to full activity as quickly and safely as possible.

- Short-term goals of a rehabilitation program are (1) providing correct immediate first aid and management following injury to limit or control swelling; (2) reducing or minimizing pain; (3) restoring full range of motion; (4) restoring or increasing muscular strength, endurance, and power; (5) reestablishing neuromuscular control; (6) improving balance; (7) maintaining cardiorespiratory fitness; and (8) incorporating appropriate functional progressions.

• The athlete should be permitted to fully return to activity when he or she is fully reconditioned and has achieved full range of movement, strength, neuromuscular control, cardiovascular fitness, and sport-specific functional skills. Besides physical well-being, the athlete must also have regained full confidence to return to his or her sport.

---

*Solutions to Critical Thinking* Exercises

---

**11-1** In sports medicine, the short-term goals in any rehabilitation program should include controlling pain, regaining range of motion, regaining strength, reestablishing neuromuscular control, and maintaining levels of cardiorespiratory fitness. The approach to rehabilitation should be aggressive. Decisions as to when and how to alter and progress specific components within a rehabilitation program should be based on, and are limited by, the healing process. The long-term goal is to return the athlete to full activity as soon as safely possible.

**11-2** Anterior knee pain can result from many different causes. However, strengthening the quadriceps can often be quite helpful. If full-range-of-motion strengthening exercises increase pain, the athlete should begin with isometric exercises done at different points in the range and should progress to full-range concentric and eccentric resistance exercise as tolerated.

Exercises such as minisquats, stepping exercises, or leg presses are excellent for strengthening quadriceps and tend to be more functional than exercises done on an exercise machine.

**11-3** Following injury and subsequent rest and immobilization, it is not unusual for the athlete to "forget" how to walk. The athlete must relearn neuromuscular control, which means regaining the ability to follow some previously established motor and sensory pattern by regaining conscious control of a specific movement until that movement becomes automatic. Strengthening exercises, particularly those that tend to be more functional, are essential for reestablishing neuromuscular control. Addressing neuromuscular control is critical throughout the recovery process but may be most critical during the early stages of rehabilitation to avoid reinjury or even overuse injuries to additional structures.

## REVIEW QUESTIONS AND CLASS ACTIVITIES

1. Explain the role of the fitness professionals and coaches in a rehabilitation program.
2. Describe the techniques for controlling swelling following injury.
3. Why it is important to modulate pain during a rehabilitation program?
4. How is range of motion restored after an injury?
5. Compare the use of isometric, progressive resistance, isokinetic, and plyometric exercises in rehabilitation.
6. How is neuromuscular control related to movement?
7. Why must an athlete condition the body generally while an injury heals?
8. How and when should functional progressions be incorporated into the rehabilitation program?
9. Describe how to determine if an athlete is ready to return to activity following injury.
10. What modalities can be used in treating the athlete and for what should they be used?

## REFERENCES

1. Brotzman, S, Wilk, K: 2003. *Clinical orthopedic rehabilitation*, Philadelphia, Elsevier Health Sciences.
2. Dvir, Z: 2003. *Isokinetics: muscle testing, interpretation, and clinical applications*, Philadelphia, Elsevier Health Sciences.
3. Guskiewicz K, Perrin D: 1996. Research and clinical applications of assessing balance, *J Sport Rehab* 5(1):45.
4. Kisner C, Colby A: 2007. *Therapeutic exercise: foundations and techniques*, Philadelphia, FA Davis.
5. Lephart, SM: 2000. *Proprioception and neuromuscular control in joint stability*, Champaign, Ill., Human Kinetics.
6. Magnusson P, McHugh M: 1995. Current concepts on rehabilitation in sports medicine. In Nicholas J, Hirschman E: *The lower extremity and spine in sports medicine*, St Louis, Mosby.
7. Malone T, editor: 1996. *Orthopedic and sports physical therapy*, St Louis, Mosby–Year Book.
8. Prentice W: 2009. *Arnheim's principles of athletic training*, ed 13, New York, McGraw-Hill.
9. Prentice W: 2010. *Rehabilitation techniques for sports medicine and athletic training*, New York, McGraw-Hill.
10. Prentice W: 2009. *Therapeutic modalities for sports medicine and athletic training*, ed. 6, New York, McGraw-Hill.
11. Tippett S, Voight M: 1999. *Functional progressions for sport rehabilitation*, Champaign, IL, Human Kinetics.
12. Zachazewski J, Magee D, Quillen S: 1996. *Athletic injuries and rehabilitation*, Philadelphia, WB Saunders.

## ANNOTATED BIBLIOGRAPHY

Brotzman, S, Wilk, K: 2003. *Clinical orthopedic rehabilitation*, Philadelphia, Elsevier Health Sciences.
*Provides practical guidance on the evaluation, treatment, and rehabilitation of patients with orthopaedic problems.*
Prentice W: 2009. *Rehabilitation techniques for sports medicine and athletic training*, ed 5, New York, McGraw-Hill.
*A comprehensive text dealing with all aspects of rehabilitation used in a sports medicine setting.*
Tippett S, Voight M: 1995. *Functional progressions for sport rehabilitation*, Champaign, IL, Human Kinetics.
*Presents scientific principles and practical applications for using functional exercise to rehabilitate athletic injuries.*

### WEB SITES

National Athletic Trainers' Association: www.nata.org
*Accesses rehabilitation in the athletic training journals.*
The Physician and Sportsmedicine: www.physsportsmed.com
*Search back issues and access the ones specifically geared toward weight training and rehabilitation.*
Archives of Physical Medicine and Rehabilitation: www.archives-pmr.org/
Journal of Sport Rehabilitation: www.humankinetics.com/JSR/journalAbout.cfm

# Helping the Injured Athlete Psychologically

## CHAPTER 12

*When you finish this chapter you will be able to:*

- Discuss how athletes might respond psychologically to an injury.
- Describe the progressive reactions to injury, dependent on length of rehabilitation.
- Discuss predictors of injury and interventions.
- Identify stressors in the athlete's life.
- Discuss the concept of buffers for stress management.
- Discuss the importance of goal setting as a means of making the injured athlete compliant in the rehabilitation program.
- Identify the various considerations in managing the psychological impact of injury.
- Describe the decision-making process for returning the injured athlete to competition.

When the body is injured, it is likely that the mind is also affected. Research indicates that athletes who experience a negative psychological response to injury have a longer and more difficult period of rehabilitation.[8] Therefore, information regarding the effect that injury has on the athlete and the possible psychological care that can be given in the sport setting may facilitate the athlete's return to competition.[11]

Certainly the sports medicine team can have a significant impact on the course of rehabilitation for the injured athlete[3] (Figure 12-1). The manner in which these individuals interact with the injured athlete and how the athlete responds psychologically to injury collectively dictate the course of a rehabilitative program.[15] The goal is to get the mind, as well as the body, ready to return to competition.

Coaches and other fitness professionals who work with competitive or recreational athletes must have an understanding of the athlete's psychological reaction to injury and how different individuals deal with injury. The way a coach or fitness professional chooses to support the injured athlete during the period of rehabilitation can have a significant impact on the course of that process. This chapter addresses the athlete's psychological reaction to injury and suggests what the coach can do to have a positive impact.

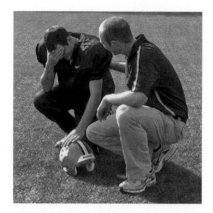

**Figure 12-1**

Sports medicine personnel can have a significant impact on how an athlete deals with an injury psychologically.

## THE ATHLETE'S PSYCHOLOGICAL RESPONSE TO INJURY

Athletes don't all deal with injury in the same manner.[2,17] One athlete may view an injury as disastrous, another may view it as an opportunity to show courage, another athlete may relish the injury to prevent embarrassment over poor performance, to provide an escape from a losing team, or to discourage a domineering parent.[5]

### Injury Severity Classification

Certain factors are commonly seen among athletes going through adjustment to injury and rehabilitation. Severity of injury usually determines length of rehabilitation.[14] Generally injuries may be classified as short term (less than 4 weeks), long term (greater than 4 weeks), chronic (recurring), or terminating (career ending) (Table 12-1).

### Phases of the Injury Process

Regardless of severity of injury and the corresponding length of time required for rehabilitation, the injured athlete has to deal with a variety

**TABLE 12-1** Progressive reactions of injured athletes based on severity of injury and length of rehabilitation

| Length of rehabilitation | Reaction to injury | Reaction to rehabilitation | Reaction to return |
|---|---|---|---|
| Short (< 4 weeks) | shock<br>relief | impatience<br>optimism | eagerness<br>anticipation |
| Long (> 4 weeks) | fear<br>anger | loss of vigor<br>irrational thoughts<br>alienation | acknowledgment |
| Chronic (recurring) | anger<br>frustration | dependence or independence,<br>apprehension | confident or skeptical |
| Termination (career ending) | isolation<br>grief process | loss of athletic identity | closure and renewal |

Techniques for Preventing
and Minimizing Sport-
Related Injuries

Reactive phases:
- reaction to injury
- reaction to rehabilitation
- reaction to return

A volleyball player sprains the medial collateral ligament in her knee during a match.

? What emotional reactions would you expect to see throughout the initial injury, re-habilitation, and return phases of this short-term injury?

Injury-prone athletes are often risk-takers.

of emotions that may occur during three reactive phases of the injury and rehabilitation process.[31] These reactive phases that the injured athlete typically goes through are reaction to injury, reaction to rehabilitation, and reaction to return to competition or career termination.[29] It should be pointed out that all athletes do not necessarily have all reactions nor do all reactions fall precisely into the suggested sequence. Other factors that can influence reactions to injury and rehabilitation are the athlete's coping skills, past history of injury, social support, and personality traits.[29]

With any type of injury, but particularly with those that require lengthy rehabilitation, athletes whose whole lives tend to revolve around a sport may have to make major adjustments in how they perceive themselves and come to terms with how they are perceived within their society.[31] Injuries are a common source of diminished self-esteem. Athletes who have been successful competitively prior to injury frequently continue to have problems after their physical recovery from an injury. While some athletes may have high self-esteem, which encourages them to take added risks, others with low self-esteem may use an injury as a release from the pressure.[9]

## PREDICTORS OF INJURY

### The Injury-Prone Athlete

Some athletes seem to have a pattern of injury, whereas others in exactly the same position with the same physical makeup are injury-free. It has been suggested that some psychological traits at one extreme or the other may predispose the athlete to repeated injury. No one particular personality type has been recognized as injury-prone. However, the individual who likes to take risks seems to represent the injury-prone athlete.[22] Other personality types that seem predisposed to injury are reserved, detached, or tender-minded players and/or apprehensive, overprotective, or easily distracted players.[25] These individuals usually also lack the ability to cope with the stress associated with the risks and its consequences. Other factors may also contribute to the likelihood of injury, such as attempting to reduce anxiety by being more aggressive or continuing to be injured because of fear of failure or guilt over unobtainable or unrealistic goals.[22]

Injury prevention is both psychological and physiological. The athlete who enters a contest while angry, frustrated, or discouraged or while undergoing some other disturbing emotional state is more prone to injury than is the one who is better adjusted emotionally. The angry player, for example, wants to vent that anger in some way and therefore often loses perspective on desirable and approved conduct. In the grip of emotion, skill and coordination are sacrificed, resulting in an injury that otherwise would have been avoided.

### Stress and Risk of Injury

Much has been written about life stress events and the likelihood of illness. Stressors may be positive, such as making all-conference, or negative, such as not making the starting lineup or failing a drug test. Stressors that seem to predispose an athlete to injury are the negative stressors.[30]

Negative stressors lead to lack of attentional focus and muscle tension, which in turn leads to the stress-injury connection. Loss of attentional focus may cause the athlete to miss cues during a play that can set the stage for a possible injury. Muscle tension (bracing or guarding) leads to reduced flexibility, reduced motor coordination, and reduced muscle efficiency, setting the athlete up for a variety of injuries.

Sports are stressors to the athlete.[31] An athlete often walks a fine line between reaching and maintaining peak performance and overtraining. Besides performance concerns, many peripheral stressors can be imposed on the athlete, such as unreasonable expectations by the athlete, the coaches, or the parents. Worries that stem from school, work, and family can also be major causes of emotional stress.

*Stress may be positive or negative.*

### Recognizing and Dealing with Stress

It is important to recognize when an athlete is stressed emotionally. The athlete whose performance is declining and whose personality is changing may need a training program that is less demanding. Conferring with the athlete might reveal emotional and physical problems that need to be dealt with by a counselor, psychologist, or physician.[21]

## Overtraining

Overtraining occurs because of an imbalance between a physical load placed on an athlete and his or her coping capacity.[23] Both physiological and psychological factors underlie overtraining. Overtraining can lead to staleness and eventual burnout.

Overtraining must be recognized early and dealt with immediately. A short interruption of training should be carried out over a three- to five-day period.[26] The athlete should perform a lower amount of work but with the same intensity.[26] When the athlete shows signs of a full recovery, a gradual return to the same workload can be initiated. Competition must be stopped.

### Staleness

Some athletes become "stale" for countless reasons. The athlete could be training too hard and long without proper rest. Staleness is often attributed to emotional problems stemming from daily worries, fears, and anxieties. **Anxiety** is one of the most common mental and emotional stress producers.[23] It is reflected by a vague fear, a sense of apprehension, and restlessness. Typically, the anxious athlete is unable to describe the problem. The athlete feels inadequate in a certain situation but is unable to say why. Heart palpitations, shortness of breath, sweaty palms, constriction in the throat, and headaches may accompany anxiety. Children who are pushed too hard by parents may acquire a number of psychological problems. They may even fail purposely in their sport just to rid themselves of the painful stress of achieving. A parent who acts like

**anxiety**
A feeling of uncertainty or apprehension.

a drill sergeant—one who continually gives negative reinforcements—will likely cause athletes to develop symptoms of overstress.

Staleness is evidenced by a wide variety of symptoms: a deterioration in the usual standard of performance, chronic fatigue, apathy, loss of appetite, indigestion, weight loss, and inability to sleep or rest properly. Stale athletes become irritable and restless, have to force themselves to practice, and exhibit signs of boredom and lassitude about everything connected with the activity.[9]

Athletes who show signs of staleness also increase their potential for both acute and overuse injuries and infections.[26] Stress fractures and tendonitis are typical injuries that can occur during a time of staleness.

### Burnout

Burnout is a syndrome related to physical and emotional exhaustion that leads to a negative self-concept, negative sport attitudes, and loss of concern for the feeling of others.[7] Burnout stems from overwork and can affect both the athlete and the coach.[20]

Burnout can be detrimental to an athlete's general health; it is reflected in frequent headaches, gastrointestinal disturbances, sleeplessness, and chronic fatigue.[7] Athletes suffering from burnout may experience feelings of depersonalization, increased emotional exhaustion, a reduced sense of accomplishment, cynicism, and a depressed mood.

## GOAL SETTING AS A MOTIVATOR TO COMPLIANCE

Establishing progressive attainable goals is essential in rehabilitation.

Goal setting has been shown to be an effective motivator for compliance to rehabilitation of an athletic injury, as well as for reaching goals in a general sport setting.[6,27] Athletes have set goals since their first competition, usually starting at an early age. They set goals to run faster, jump higher, shoot straighter, throw longer, hit harder, and so on. These goals have all had one thing in common: they were not achieved with one burst of effort but came as the result of many short-term goals having been met before the achievement of the long-term goal.[29] Focus Box 12-1 suggests nine factors that should be incorporated into goal setting for the athlete.[13]

In athletic rehabilitation athletes need to know exactly what the goal is and have a sense that it can be met.[4] Telling an athlete that by a certain day the athlete should be partial weight bearing with crutches is neither specific nor measurable. It is more effective to say that by achieving a certain range of motion and strength level the foot can be placed on the ground with weight bearing and that the measurement of success is that the partial weight bearing is without pain. The goal must be a challenge but one that the athlete can reach with reasonable rehabilitation effort.[15] Goals that are easily reached have no reward in success. Goals must be personal and internally satisfying, not a goal imposed on the athlete. The setting of goals needs to be a joint venture between the athlete and the coach to be successful.[6] The athlete has to take responsibility for the progress of the injury and be responsible for doing the necessary rehabilitation.

---

12-1 ⟩ *Focus Box*

**Nine Factors to Incorporate into Goal Setting for the Athlete**

- Set specific and measurable goals
- Use positive versus negative language
- Goals should be challenging but realistic
- Set a reasonable timetable
- Integrate short-, medium-, and long-term goals
- Link outcome to process
- Internalize goals
- Monitor and evaluate goals
- Link sport goals to life goals

---

Goal setting incorporates a multitude of other motivating factors that intuitively appear to increase the odds of compliance by reducing the stress associated with injury rehabilitation.[27] These buffers incorporated within the goal setting paradigm are positive reinforcement when goals are met, time management for incorporating goals into a lifestyle, a feeling of social support when goals are set with the coach, feelings of increased self-efficacy when goals are achieved, and the like. Goals are easily understood by athletes, are concrete concepts, are active events, and have been a natural part of their sport that requires no additional time commitment.[3] Goals can be set daily for a sense of accomplishment, weekly for a sense of progress, and monthly or yearly for long-term achievement.

## PROVIDING SOCIAL SUPPORT TO THE INJURED ATHLETE

The coach is often the first person an athlete interacts with after injury. When athletes are injured they should be shown that the coach cares for the athlete as a person and not just as a part of the team. Their perception of the coach makes a difference in recovery time and effort.[18] First they have to respect the coach as a person before they can trust the coach in the rehabilitative setting. Successful communication between the coach and the athlete is essential for effective rehabilitation.[18] Taking an interest in athletes before injuries have occurred enables the coach to know the athletes' personalities and work with them in helping to build their confidence. Focus Box 12-2 summarizes things that a coach or fitness professional can do to provide social support to an injured athlete throughout a rehabilitation program.

### Be a Good Listener

Active listening is an important skill. Listen to the athlete beyond the complaining. Listen for fear, anger, depression, or anxiety in the athlete's voice. With *fear*, the athlete may be wondering what the pain means in terms of function and if he or she will be accepted by peers. *Anger* is

**12-2 Critical Thinking**
Exercise

A sports psychologist is discussing goals for rehabilitation with an injured soccer player.

? How should goals be set and what can be done to help the athlete feel successful in her rehabilitation program?

12-2 *Focus Box*

Things a coach can do to provide social support for an injured athlete:

■ Be a good listener.
■ Be aware of body language.
■ Project a caring image.
■ Find out exactly what the problem is.
■ Explain the injury to the athlete.
■ Manage the stress of injury.
■ Keep the athlete involved with the team.
■ Help the athlete return to play.

often a feeling of being victimized by the injury and the unfairness of it. In *depression*, the athlete may have an overwhelming feeling of hopelessness or loneliness. With *anxiety*, the athlete wonders how he or she can survive the injury and what will happen if he or she cannot return to full competition.[13]

### Be Aware of Body Language

Body language is important as well. Continuing to work on paperwork while talking to the athlete is sending a noncaring message. Be concerned, and look athletes in the eye with a genuine interest in their problems. This will go a long way toward gaining confidence and respect.

### Project a Caring Image

It is important to consider the athlete as an individual instead of as "the sprained ankle." If the injury is the only consideration, the athlete becomes just an injury and not a person.

The relationship between a care provider and the athlete should be one of person to person. When the athlete is treated as an equal the relationship is improved, and it helps the athlete accept responsibility for his or her own rehabilitation. With injury athletes lose control over their physical efforts. They go from 3 to 4 hours a day of practice or competition to no activity. They are in a temporary lifestyle change. Their feelings affect the success or failure of the rehabilitation process. A care provider must establish rapport and a sense of genuine concern and caring for the athlete, who is not fooled by superficial concern.

Neglecting injured athletes or giving them the perception that they are "outcasts" also can contribute to injury and reinjury. Coaches who foster this attitude are saying to the players that they have no self-worth if they are injured.[15] Some coaches go so far as to prevent team contact until injured players are ready to return or to belittle them in front of their peers, believing that this will make the athlete want to get back to competition quicker. This tactic may work with some players with minor injuries but only causes major adjustment difficulties for athletes who suffer severe injury.

Some coaches refuse to talk to the athlete or tell others that the athlete really doesn't want to play or isn't tough enough. The coach and athlete experience frustration with the injury. During this period either the athletic staff shows its concern for the athlete and in return wins the athlete's loyalty and dedication, or they undermine the athlete's trust, setting up for a let down when the athlete gets in the position of controlling the outcome of a contest and may underperform out of spite.

### Find Out What the Problem Is

During an injury evaluation the athlete should provide as much input about his or her injury as possible. Paraphrasing or restating the information to the athlete is invaluable to the care provider who is unsure of the mechanism of injury or its results. Statements such as "I see" or "Go ahead" or simple silence to allow athletes to fully express themselves are of value. Important information can be gained by asking at the end of gathering subjective information "What have I not asked you or do I need to know about this injury?" Then give the athlete input into the decision of where to go from here.

### Explain the Injury to the Athlete

Either an athletic trainer or a physician should effectively explain the injury to the athlete. Care should be taken to explain the situation to the athlete in understandable terms. In most cases the simplest explanation acceptable to the athlete is the best. Athletes must have injuries explained to them to their satisfaction. Disseminating injury information appropriate to athletes' emotional and intellectual level can be a real challenge. The rate and degree of acceptance are not the same with all athletes. Severity of injury is certainly important, but the athlete's perception of that severity is what matters in the rehabilitation process.[13] Thus the physiological must be interrelated with the psychological.

### Manage the Stress of Injury

The amount of stress associated with playing a sport and the meaning the sport has to the athlete can affect the athlete's compliance to rehabilitation.[30] The athlete has a more successful rehabilitation when engaged fully in the activity of rehabilitation, much as the athlete has a more successful sport career when more interest and involvement are put into the sport. Stress can be a deterrent to engaging in rehabilitation. Several techniques can be used (relaxation, imagery, cognitive restructuring, thought stopping) that may lessen the stressful reaction to injury. Often a change in an athlete's perception concerning injury and rehabilitation can affect outcome.

### Keep the Athlete Involved with the Team

An injured athlete should remain involved with the rest of the team.[22] Following injury, particularly one that requires long-term rehabilitation, athletes may have problems adjusting socially and may feel alienated from

Techniques for Preventing
and Minimizing Sport-
Related Injuries

Injury might mean major
changes in the way an athlete
behaves socially.

the rest of the team. Athletes with an injury that requires weeks or months of rehabilitation before they can return to competition often feel that the coaches have ceased to care, that teammates have no time to spend with them, that friends are no longer around, and that their social life consists of time put into rehabilitation. Occasionally athletes feel that they have received little support from coaches and teammates.

Injured athletes may understand that the coach cares but has no expertise in injury management and must be concerned with getting the team ready without them.[19] Injured athletes may feel unable to maintain or regain normal relationships with teammates. The injured athlete is a reminder that injury can happen, and teammates may pull away from that constant reminder. Friendships based on athletic identification are now compromised because the athletic identification is gone; friends and team members relate to injured athletes only in terms of what they did yesterday or as injured teammates, not as individuals. Injured athletes no longer feel the team camaraderie that provides a sense of belonging or importance. Athletes who can remain involved with the team, however, feel less isolated and less guilty about not being able to help the team (Figure 12-2).

After injury, athletes need the social support to prevent feelings of negative self-worth and loss of identity.[19] As early in the rehabilitation process as possible the athlete should begin sport-specific drills during practice time with his or her athletic team. The athlete then begins to reenter the team culture and is not isolated from the team environment. Thus, the athlete puts more effort into functional, sport-specific situations that are generally less boring. In so doing, the athlete gains a more realistic appreciation of the skills needed to attain preinjury performance levels. The rehabilitation routine is more easily tolerated by athletes if they can see some carryover to their sport.

**Figure 12-2**

It is important to make sure
that the injured athlete stays
involved with the team.

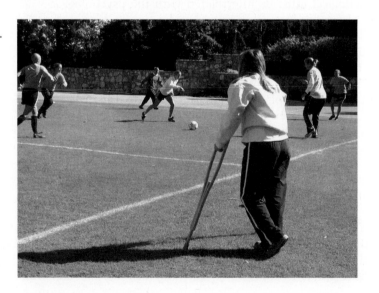

Help the Athlete Return to Play

Often the perception of the athlete who is returning to competition is either that he or she is ready to return and not being allowed to or that he or she is being forced to return before ready. It is important to assist the athlete in making a decision based on the facts and not clouded by emotions.

Occasionally an athlete is unable or unwilling to continue to participate in their sport. Frequently the athlete's identity is intertwined with the sport played.[26] The transition into a completely different culture can be a traumatic experience. It is stressful to enter a culture and not know one's place or identity in that culture. To not know what the game is and what the rules are is frustrating to the injured athlete.

## RETURN TO COMPETITION DECISIONS

Perhaps the most difficult aspect of the rehabilitative process is making a decision as to when it is safe to return to competition. Although physically ready to return to competition, athletes coming back from a traumatic injury may be psychologically compromised by a fear that their return to play may again lead to injury.[28] It is difficult for many athletes to admit to themselves, or a coach, that they are afraid of being hurt again, or that deep down, they even expect it, thus increasing the likelihood of the occurrence. This fear of reinjury must be overcome if the athlete is to restore his or her self-esteem in a positive manner. Certainly the athletic trainer or team physician is well prepared to make such a decision. Unfortunately, untrained personnel, such as fellow teammates, parents, and coaches sometimes assume this responsibility when no athletic trainer is present. **This situation has the potential to result in poor medical care and leaves the coach vulnerable to legal action as a result of negligence.** Courts expect competent medical care to be provided to athletes.

The phrase "you have to play with pain" has been interpreted literally to mean that the athlete has to play through an injury. The difference is that some injuries may be mild and only somewhat painful, resulting in no reinjury in competition, whereas a more severe injury is made worse by continuing to compete. The competitive athlete may be more "body aware" than the general public and therefore more apt to respond to injury with the use of protection, rest, ice, compression, and elevation (PRICE) to promote healing. The general public, on the other hand, is more likely to respond to the pain of injury than to consider the healing process.[16] Therefore the athlete may want to return to competition in spite of pain whereas the nonathlete may want the pain to be treated before any activity is undertaken.

The athlete who continues to play with an unhealed or poorly rehabilitated injury constantly reduces the chances of a healthy life of activity. The athlete has to live past the few years of competition. Most athletes, however, have difficulty seeing past the present season or at best have the goal of participating in their sport until they can no longer compete, regardless of the consequences. The rewards of competition and the admiration of others take sports out of perspective and retard a healthy attitude toward sports. The attitude of some athletes is "Give it up for the sport" because "I'm invincible." Lack of this attitude is viewed by some as weakness or not being a team player. These athletes have difficulty adjusting to an injury, especially a career-ending one.[14]

One research study found that coaches were likely to return players on the basis of status and game situation, whereas the athletic trainer's decisions were more likely to be dictated by the status of the athlete's injury.[13] Athletes who feel that a missed practice or game will relegate them to the bench for the year or those who have been encouraged to play no matter what are candidates for injury and reinjury; thus, they only reinforce the decision of the coach to play someone else. Usually what happens, however, is that athletes with unhealed injuries perform poorly because they are not at full strength.

One method of making an objective decision about the athlete's readiness to return to activity is to collect baseline performance data in the preseason (e.g., 40-yard sprint, vertical jump, shuttle run) and use those scores to compare with scores on those same tests when the athlete seems to be physically and psychologically ready to resume activity. The athlete with 4.5 speed who can run only a 5.0 illustrates to the coach that he or she is not ready for competition. This also illustrates to the athlete that more time and effort are necessary to get ready to return.

The treatment of athletic injury and rehabilitation is more than just physical, emotional, and psychological aspects of the individual. The impact of the environment, the support of the athletic community, and the culture in which the athlete resides at the time of injury combine to influence the course the athlete takes from injury, through rehabilitation, to return to competition.

## REFERRING THE ATHLETE FOR PSYCHOLOGICAL HELP

Although coaches are typically not educated as professional counselors or psychologists, they must nevertheless be concerned with the feelings of the athletes they work with.[21] The coach must have appropriate counseling skills to confront an athlete's fears, frustrations, and daily crises and to refer individuals with serious emotional problems to the proper professionals.[10,17]

The team physician and athletic trainer, like the coach, play an integral part in helping the athlete who is overly stressed.[24] Many psychophysiological responses thought to be emotional are in fact caused by some undetected physical dysfunction. Therefore, referral to a sport psychologist, clinical psychologist, or perhaps a psychiatrist should be routine.[10,17]

**Athletic Injury Management Checklist**

The following is a checklist of things that can be done to address the psychological aspects of dealing with an injured athlete.

☐ Establish a rapport and a sense of genuine concern and caring for the athlete.
☐ Earn the athlete's trust.
☐ Establish good open communication with the athlete.
☐ Take a personal interest in athletes before an injury occurs.
☐ Be a good active listener.
☐ Look the athlete in the eye with genuine interest and use good body language.
☐ Don't neglect or ignore the injured athlete.
☐ Facilitate continuing social support by teammates.
☐ Provide as much information about his or her injury as possible.
☐ Make sure the athlete is included in the decision-making process.

## SUMMARY

- Following injury to the athlete it is essential to pay attention to getting the mind, as well as the body, ready to return to competition.

- Athletes don't all respond to an injury in the same manner.

- Regardless of the severity of injury and the corresponding length of time required for rehabilitation, the injured athlete has to deal with a variety of emotions that may occur during three reactive phases of the injury and rehabilitation process: reaction to injury, reaction to rehabilitation, and reaction to return to competition or career termination.

- No one personality type has been recognized as injury-prone.

- Negative stressors seem to predispose an athlete to injury.

- Setting appropriate goals is an effective motivator for compliance to rehabilitation of an athletic injury.

- The social support provided to the injured athlete, both in what is said and perceived actions, has a major impact on the course of injury rehabilitation.

- Decisions for returning the injured athlete to play should be based on the status of the athlete's injury.

**12-1** Initially the athlete experiences shock and relief, followed by impatience and optimism during the rehabilitation phase, and finally eagerness and anticipation during the return phase.

**12-2** The athlete needs to know exactly what the goal is and have a sense that it can be met. Setting a progressive series of attainable goals is critical so that the athlete does not become frustrated.

## REVIEW QUESTIONS AND CLASS ACTIVITIES

1. How might an athlete possibly respond psychologically to an injury?
2. Identify the sequence of possible emotions associated with the three reactive phases of the injury process for short-term, long-term, chronic, and career-ending injuries.
3. What are some of the personality characteristics of an individual who is likely to be injury-prone?
4. What is the difference between negative and positive stress and which is more likely to cause injury?
5. What are the primary considerations in setting appropriate goals for the injured athlete to achieve during the rehabilitation program?
6. Generate a list of the things that the coach should and should not do in managing the psychological impact of injury on the athlete.
7. What factors should come into consideration in the decision-making process for returning the injured athlete to competition?

## REFERENCES

1. Bone, J, Fry, M: 2006. The influence of injured athletes' perceptions of social support from ATC's on their beliefs about rehabilitation. *Journal of Sport Rehabilitation* 15(2):156.
2. Brewer, B: 2003. Developmental differences in psychological aspects of sport-injury rehabilitation, *Journal of athletic training,* 38(2):152–153.
3. Brewer, BW: 2000. Doing sport psychology in the coaching role. In Andersen, MB (ed), *Doing sport psychology,* Champaign, IL, Human Kinetics.
4. Briggs, J: 2001. The psychology of injury and rehabilitation. In Briggs, J (ed), *Sports therapy: theoretical and practical thoughts and considerations,* Chichester, England, Corpus Publishing Limited.
5. Burton, D, Raedeke, T: 2008. *Sport psychology for coaches,* Champaign, IL, Human Kinetics.
6. Cramer Roh, JL, Perna, FM: 2000. Psychology/counseling: a universal competency in athletic training, *Journal of athletic training* 35(4): 458–465.
7. Cresswell, SL, Eklund, RC: 2004. The athlete burnout syndrome: possible early signs, *Journal of science and medicine in sport:* 7(4): 481–487.
8. Evans, L, Hardy, L: 2002. Injury rehabilitation: a goal-setting intervention study, *Research quarterly for exercise and sport* 73(3): 310–319.
9. Ford IW, Gordon S: 1998. Guidelines for using sport psychology in rehabilitation, *Ath Ther Today* 3(3):41.
10. Green, SL, Weinberg, RS: 2001. Relationships among athletic identity, coping skills, social support, and the psychological impact of injury in recreational participants,

*Journal of applied sport psychology* 13(1): 40–59.

11. Hamson-Utley, J, Jordan, M: 2008. Athletic trainers' and physical therapists' perceptions of the effectiveness of psychological skills within sport injury rehabilitation programs, *Journal of Athletic Training* 43(3):258.

12. Harris, L: 2003. Development of the injured collegiate athlete, *Journal of athletic training,* 38(1):75–82.

13. Hedgpeth E, Gieck, J: 2010. Psychological considerations for rehabilitation of the injured athlete. In Prentice W: *Rehabilitation techniques in sports medicine, and athletic training,* New York, McGraw-Hill.

14. Home, TS: 2008. *Advances in sport psychology,* 2nd ed Champaign, IL, Human Kinetics.

15. Kolt, GS: 2001. Doing sport psychology with injured athletes. In Andersen, MB (ed), *Doing sport psychology,* Champaign, IL, Human Kinetics.

16. Magyar, TM, Duda, JL: 2000. Confidence restoration following athletic injury, *Sport psychologist* 14(4): 372–390.

17. Mensch, J, Miller, G: 2007. *The athletic trainer's guide to psychosocial intervention and referral,* Thoroughfare, NJ, Slack.

18. Mitchell, I, Neil, R, Wadey, R: 2007. Gender differences in athletes' social support during injury rehabilitation. *Journal of Sport & Exercise Psychology* 29:S189.

19. O'Connor, E: 2002. Recognition and referral of psychological issues in sports medicine, *SportEX medicine* (12):7–8.

20. Raedeke, TD: 2004. Coach commitment and burnout: a one-year follow-up, *Journal of applied sport psychology* 16(4):333–349.

21. Robbins, JE, Rosenfeld, LB: 2001. Athletes' perceptions of social support provided by their head coach, assistant coach, and athletic trainer, preinjury and during rehabilitation, *Journal of sport behavior* 24(3):277–297.

22. Rock, JA, Jones, MV: 2002. A preliminary investigation into the use of counseling skills in support of rehabilitation from sport injury, *Journal of sport rehabilitation* 11(4): 284–304.

23. Schwenz, SJ: 2001. Psychology of injury and rehabilitation, *Athletic therapy today* 6(1):44–45.

24. Shelley, GA, Trowbridge, CA, Detling N: 2003. Practical counseling skills for athletic therapists, *Athletic therapy today* 8(2):57–62.

25. Tennenbaum, G, Eklund, R: 2007. *Handbook of sport psychology,* 3rd ed, New York, Wiley.

26. Udry, E: 2002. Staying connected: optimizing social support for injured athletes, *Athletic therapy today* 7(3):42–43.

27. Van Raalte, JL (ed): 2002. *Exploring sport and exercise psychology,* 2nd ed, Washington, American Psychological Association.

28. Weinberg, R, Butt, J, Knight, B: 2001. High school coaches' perceptions of the process of goal setting, *Sport psychologist* 15(1):20–47.

29. Weinberg, R, Gould, D: 2006. *Foundations of sport and exercise psychology,* Champaign, Il, Human Kinetics.

30. Wiese-Bjornstal, D: 2002. To play or not to play? That is the question, *Athletic therapy today* 7(2): 24–26.

31. Weiss, M: 2003. Psychological aspects of sport-injury rehabilitation: A developmental perspective, *Journal of athletic training,* 38(2): 172–175.

32. Williams, JM, Andersen, MB: 1998. Psychosocial antecedents of sport injury: review and critique of the stress and injury model, *Journal of applied sport psychology* 10(1): 5–25.

**ANNOTATED BIBLIOGRAPHY**

Tennenbaum, G, Eklund, R: 2007. *Handbook of sport psychology*, 3rd ed. New York, Wiley.

*A resource for sport psychologists, coaches, and athletes searching for new and effective approaches to pain management, exercise psychology, and building self-confidence. Combines theoretical explanation and practical applications and emphasizes the value of basic and applied research to practice.*

Taylor J, Taylor S: 2004. *Psychological approaches to sports injury rehabilitation*, Gaithersburg, Md, Aspen Publishers.

*This text specifically addresses how to deal with injury rehabilitation from a psychological perspective.*

Van Raalte, JL (ed): 2002. *Exploring sport and exercise psychology*, 2nd ed, Washington, American Psychological Association.

*Provides an overview of the field of sport and exercise psychology, connecting theory and practice, and discussing practical issues.*

Weinberg RS, Gould D: 2005. *Foundations of sport and exercise psychology,* Champaign, IL, Human Kinetics.

*Discusses the techniques that a coach should incorporate for contributing to the success of an athlete.*

## WEB SITES

Association for the Advancement of Applied Sport Psychology: http://aaasponline.org/index.php

*Emphasis on the role of psychological factors in sport and exercise.*

NASPSPA North American Society for Psychology of Sport and Physical Activity: www.naspspa.org/

Sport Psychology Oversite: www.personal.umich.edu/~bing/oversite/sportpsych.html

*A comprehensive list of links to sites that focus on mental training and performance enhancement.*

Mind Games: Applied Sport Psychology for Every Athlete: www.drrelax.com

*A new, Web-based system of individualized psychological training.*

Sport Psychology for Athletes: www.drrelax.com/baseball.htm

*The use of psychological training and preparation.*

# PART 3

## Recognition and Management of Specific Injuries and Conditions

# Recognizing Different Sports Injuries

## CHAPTER 13

*When you finish this chapter you will be able to:*

- Differentiate between acute and chronic injury.
- Briefly describe acute traumatic injuries, including fractures, dislocations and subluxations, contusions, ligament sprains, muscle strains, muscle soreness, and nerve injuries.
- Talk about chronic overuse injuries and differentiate tendinitis, tenosynovitis, bursitis, osteoarthritis, and myofascial trigger points.
- Have at least some understanding of the three phases of the healing process.

No matter how much attention is directed toward the general principles of injury prevention, the nature of physical activity dictates that sooner or later injury will occur. Traditionally, the terms *acute* and *chronic* have been used to describe injuries. Health care professionals have debated the usefulness of these terms in defining injury. The concern has been that at some point all injuries can be considered acute—in other words, every injury has a beginning point. At what point does an acute injury become a chronic injury? Generally, injuries occur either from trauma or from overuse. Acute injuries are caused by trauma; chronic injuries can result from overuse such as the injuries that occur with the repetitive dynamics of running, throwing, or jumping. In this chapter we discuss the more common traumatic and overuse injuries that the coach or fitness professional is likely to see.

The information in this chapter is not meant to encourage fitness professionals, coaches, or others interested in areas related to exercise and sport science to attempt to diagnose injuries that may occur. This should be left to health care professionals, who have considerably more training and expertise. However, being familiar with the various injuries described in this chapter can help in understanding the course of both immediate care and long-term injury management.

Acute injuries = trauma
Chronic injuries = overuse

## ACUTE (TRAUMATIC) INJURIES

### Fractures

**Fractures** (broken bones) occur as a result of extreme stresses and strains placed on bones. Before discussing fractures, a brief discussion of bone anatomy is necessary.[14] The gross structure of the long bones includes the diaphysis, epiphysis, articular cartilage, and periosteum (Figure 13-1). The

Fractures are breaks or cracks in a bone.

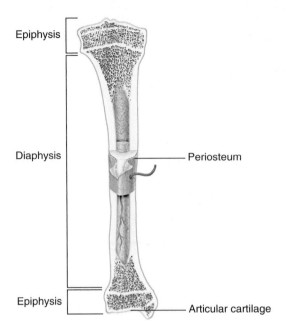

Epiphysis

Diaphysis — Periosteum

Epiphysis — Articular cartilage

**Figure 13-1**

The gross structure of the long bones includes the diaphysis, epiphysis, articular cartilage, and periosteum.

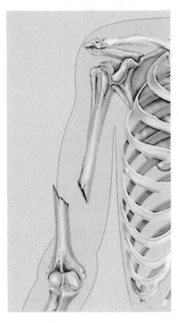

**Figure 13-2**

In an open fracture the end of the fractured bone penetrates the skin.

*diaphysis* is the main shaft of the bone. It is hollow, cylindrical, and covered by compact bone. The *epiphysis* is located at the ends of long bones. It is the growth area of the bone in adolescents. An injury to the epiphysis may affect growth of the long bones in younger athletes (see Chapter 25). The ends of long bones are covered with a layer of *articular cartilage* that covers the joint surfaces of the epiphysis. This cartilage provides protection during movement and cushions jars and blows to the joint. A dense, white, fibrous membrane, the *periosteum,* covers long bones except at joint surfaces. Interlacing with the periosteum are fibers from the muscle tendons. Throughout the periosteum on its inner layer exist countless blood vessels and **osteoblasts** (bone-forming cells). The blood vessels provide nutrition to the bone, and the osteoblasts provide bone growth and repair.

Fractures generally can be classified as either open or closed.[14] In an **open fracture** there is enough displacement of the fractured ends that the bone actually breaks through surrounding tissues, including the skin (Figure 13-2). An open fracture increases the possibility of infection. A **closed fracture** is one in which there is little or no movement or displacement of the broken bones. Both types of fractures can be serious if not managed properly. Signs and symptoms of a fracture include obvious deformity, point tenderness, swelling, and pain on active and

**osteoblasts**
(**os** tee oh blasts)
Bone-forming cells.

**open fracture**
Overlying skin is lacerated by protruding bone fragments.

**closed fracture**
Fracture does not penetrate superficial tissue.

passive movement. There may also be crepitus (popping or a grating sound on movement). The only definitive technique for determining if a fracture exists is to have it x-rayed.

Several different kinds of closed fractures can occur (Figure 13-3). Long bones can be stressed or forced to fail by tension, compression, bending, twisting (torsion), and shear.[10] These forces, either singly or in

Long bones can be stressed by tension, compression, bending, torsion, and shear.

(A) Greenstick

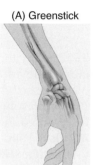

**Greenstick fractures** are incomplete breaks in bones that have not completely ossified. They occur most frequently in the convex bone surface, keeping the concave surface intact. The name is derived from the similarity of such fractures to the break in a green twig taken from a tree.

(D) Comminuted

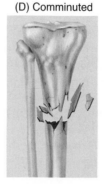

**Comminuted fractures** consist of three or more fragments at the fracture site. They can be caused by a hard blow or a fall in an awkward position. From the physician's point of view, these fractures impose a difficult healing situation because of the displacement of the bone fragments. Soft tissues are often interposed between the fragments, causing incomplete healing. Such cases may need surgical intervention.

(B) Transverse

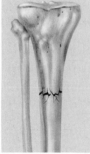

**Transverse fractures** occur in a straight line, more or less at right angles to the bone shaft. A direct outside blow usually causes this injury.

(E) Linear

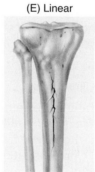

**Linear fractures** are those in which the bone splits along its length. They are often the result of jumping from a height and landing in such a way as to apply force or stress to the long axis.

(C) Spiral

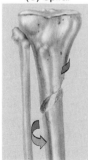

**Spiral fractures** have an S-shaped separation. They are fairly common in football and skiing, in which the foot is firmly planted and the body is suddenly rotated.

(F) Oblique

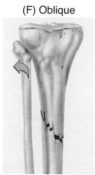

**Oblique fractures** are similar to spiral fractures. They occur when one end receives sudden torsion or twisting and the other end is fixed or stabilized.

**Figure 13-3**

Closed fractures: (A) Greenstick, (B) Transverse, (C) Spiral, (D) Comminuted, (E) Linear, (F) Oblique

combination, can cause a variety of fractures. For example, *spiral fractures* are caused by twisting, whereas *oblique fractures* are caused by the combined forces of axial compression, bending, and torsion. *Transverse fractures* occur because of bending (Figure 13-3). Along with the type of stress, the amount of force must be considered. The more complex the fracture, the more energy is required. External energy can be used to deform and then actually fracture bone. Some energy can be dispersed to soft tissue adjacent to the bone.[13]

### Healing of a Fracture

In most instances the fracture of a bone requires immobilization for some period in a cast. In general, fractures of the long bones of the arm and leg require approximately 6 weeks of casting, and the smaller bones in the hands and feet may require as little as 3 weeks of either casting or splinting. In some instances, immobilization may not be required for healing.[5] For example, breaks of the four small toes are difficult to splint or cast. Of course, complications such as infections may lengthen the time required for both casting and rehabilitation.

Casting time:
Long bones = 6 weeks
Small bones = 3–4 weeks

For a fracture to heal, osteoblasts must lay down extra bone formation, called a **callus**, over the fracture site during the immobilization period. Once the cast is removed, the bone must be subjected to normal stresses and strains so that tensile strength may be regained before the healing process is complete. Cells called **osteoclasts** function to reshape the bone in response to normally applied stresses and strains.[14]

**Callus**
New bone formation over a fracture.

**osteoclasts**
(**os** tee oh klasts)
Cells that absorb and remove osseous tissue.

### Stress Fractures

Perhaps the most common fracture that results from physical activity is a **stress fracture**. Unlike the other types of fractures that have been discussed, the stress fracture results from overuse rather than acute trauma.[18] Common sites for stress fractures include the weight-bearing bones of the leg or foot. In either case, repetitive forces transmitted through the bones produce irritations of the periosteum and fatigue fractures of the underlying bone. The pain usually begins as a dull ache, which becomes progressively painful day after day. Initially, pain is most severe during activity. However, when a stress fracture develops, pain becomes worse after the activity is stopped. Specific causes of stress fractures will be discussed in Chapters 14–15.

**stress fracture**
A fracture at an area of periosteal irritation on the bone.

The biggest problem with a stress fracture is that often it does not show up on an x-ray until the osteoblasts begin laying down bone. At that point, a small white line appears on the x-ray. If a stress fracture is suspected, it is best to stop the activity for a period of at least 14 days and then slowly and gradually allow the athlete to get back into the activity that initially produced the stress fracture.[11] Stress fractures do not usually require casting; however, if they are not handled correctly, they may become true fractures that must be immobilized.

A

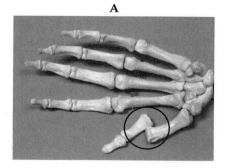

B

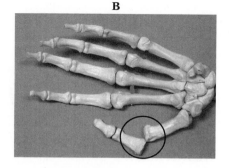

**Figure 13-4**

A joint that is forced beyond its anatomical limits can be (A) dislocated or (B) subluxated.

## Dislocations and Subluxations

A **dislocation** occurs when at least one bone in a joint (articulation) is forced completely out of its normal and proper alignment and must be manually or surgically put back into place or reduced. Dislocations most commonly occur in the shoulder joint, elbow, and fingers, but they can occur wherever two bones articulate (Figure 13-4A). A **subluxation** is like a dislocation except that in this situation a bone comes partially out of its normal articulation but then goes right back into place.[3] Subluxations most commonly occur in the shoulder joint and, in females, in the knee cap (patella) (Figure 13-4B).

In dislocations, deformity is almost always apparent; however, it may be obscured by heavy musculature, making it important for the examiner to routinely palpate, or feel, the injured site to determine the loss of normal contour. Comparison of the injured side with the uninjured side often reveals asymmetry.

Dislocations or subluxations will likely result in a rupture of the stabilizing ligaments and tendons surrounding the joint. Occasionally an avulsion fracture occurs in which an attached tendon or ligament pulls a small piece of bone away from the rest of the bone. In other cases, the force may separate growth plates (epiphysis) or cause a complete fracture of a long bone. These possibilities indicate the importance of administering complete and thorough medical attention to first-time dislocations. It has often been said, "Once a dislocation, always a dislocation." In most cases this statement is true, because once a joint has been either subluxated or completely dislocated, the connective tissues that bind and hold it in its correct alignment are stretched to such an extent that the joint is extremely vulnerable to subsequent dislocations.

A first-time dislocation should always be considered and treated as a possible fracture. Once it has been ascertained that the injury is a dislocation, a physician should be consulted for further evaluation. However, before the athlete is taken to the physician, the injury should be properly splinted and supported to prevent any further damage. **Dislocations should not be reduced immediately, regardless of where they occur.** Ideally the athlete should get an x-ray to rule out fractures or other problems before reduction although a physician

**dislocation**
A bone is forced out of alignment and stays out until surgically or manually replaced or reduced.

**subluxation**
(**sub** lucks ashun)
A bone is forced out of alignment but goes back into place.

**13-1 Critical Thinking**
Exercise

An athlete training for a marathon complains of pain in the lower leg. She consults with her physician, who determines that she has a stress fracture. When she returns to training, she is confused about what a stress fracture is.

? How can the difference between a stress fracture and a trauma-induced fracture be explained, and what is the course of management?

**Figure 13-5**

Structure of a synovial joint

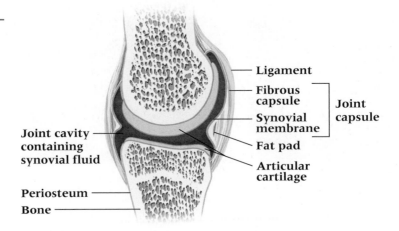

Joint capsule
— Ligament
— Fibrous capsule
— Synovial membrane
— Fat pad
— Articular cartilage

Joint cavity containing synovial fluid

Periosteum

Bone

will often reduce a dislocation without getting an x-ray. Inappropriate techniques of reduction may only exacerbate the problem. Return to activity after dislocation or subluxation is largely dependent on the degree of soft tissue damage.

Ligament Sprains

**sprain**
Injury to a ligament or joint capsule that connects bone to bone.

A **sprain** involves damage to a ligament or joint capsule that provides support to a joint.[4] A ligament is a tough, relatively inelastic band of tissue that connects one bone to another. Before discussing injuries to ligaments, a review of joint structure is necessary (Figure 13-5). All *synovial* joints are composed of two or more bones that articulate with one another to allow motion in one or more planes. The articulating surfaces of the bone are lined with a very thin, smooth, cartilaginous covering called an articular, or *hyaline, cartilage*. All joints are entirely surrounded by a thick, ligamentous *joint capsule*. The inner surface of this joint capsule is lined by a very thin *synovial membrane* that is highly vascularized and innervated. The synovial membrane produces *synovial fluid,* the functions of which include lubrication, shock absorption, and nutrition of the joint.[14]

The articular capsule, ligaments, outer aspects of the synovial membrane, and fat pads of the synovial joint are well supplied with nerves. The inner aspect of the synovial membrane, cartilage, and articular disks, if present, have nerves as well. These nerves, called **mechanoreceptors**, provide information about the relative position of the joint and are found in the fibrous capsule and ligaments.[14]

**mechanoreceptors**
Located in muscles, tendons, ligaments, and joints; provide information on joint position.

Some joints contain a thick fibrocartilage called a *meniscus*. The knee joint, for example, contains two wedge-shaped menisci that deepen the articulation and provide shock absorption in that joint. Finally, the main structural support and joint stability is provided by the ligaments, which may be either thickened portions of a joint capsule or totally separate bands. The anatomical position of the ligaments partly determines what motions a joint is capable of making.[14]

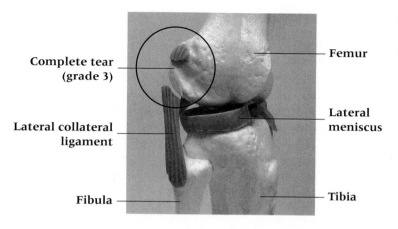

Complete tear
(grade 3)

Femur

Lateral collateral
ligament

Lateral
meniscus

Fibula

Tibia

**Figure 13-6**

A ligament sprain in the knee joint. This would be considered a grade 3 sprain.

If a joint is forced to move beyond normal limits or planes of movement, injury to the ligaments is likely to occur (Figure 13-6). The severity of the damage is subject to many different classifications; however, the most commonly used system involves three grades of sprain.

- *Grade 1 sprain.* There is some stretching and separation of the ligamentous fibers, with minimal instability of the joint. Mild to moderate pain, localized swelling, and joint stiffness should be expected.
- *Grade 2 sprain.* There is some tearing and separation of the ligament fibers, with moderate instability of the joint. Moderate to severe pain, swelling, and joint stiffness should be expected.
- *Grade 3 sprain.* There is total tearing of the ligament, which leads to instability of the joint. A grade 3 sprain can result in a subluxation. Initially, severe pain may be present, followed by little or no pain as a result of total disruption of nerve fibers. Swelling may be great, and the joint tends to become very stiff some hours after the injury. In some cases, a grade 3 sprain with marked instability requires surgical repair. Frequently, the force producing the ligament injury is so great that other ligaments or structures surrounding the joint may also be injured. Rehabilitation of grade 3 sprains involving surgery is a long-term process.

The greatest problem in the rehabilitation of grade 1 and grade 2 sprains is restoring stability to the joint.[14] Once a ligament has been stretched or partially torn, inelastic scar tissue forms, preventing the ligament from regaining its original tension. To restore stability to the joint, the other structures surrounding that joint, primarily muscles and their tendons, must be strengthened. The increased muscle tension provided by strength training can improve stability of the injured joint.

**13-2 *Critical Thinking***
Exercise

A volleyball player has sprained her ankle just 2 days before the beginning of the conference tournament. The athlete, her parents, and her coach are extremely concerned that she is going to miss the tournament and want to know if anything can be done to make her get well more quickly.

? What can this athlete be told about the process of healing?

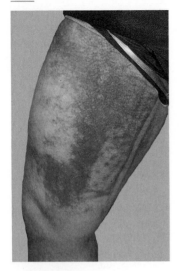

**Figure 13-7**

A contusion occurs when soft tissues are compressed between bone and some external force.

Contusion = Bruise

> **myositis ossificans (my oh sigh** tis ah **sif** ah cans) Calcium deposits that result from repeated trauma.

## Contusions

A **contusion** is another word for a bruise. The mechanism that produces a bruise is familiar. A blow from some external object causes soft tissues (i.e., skin, fat, and muscle) to be compressed against hard bone underneath[12] (Figure 13-7). If the blow is hard enough, capillaries are torn, which allows bleeding into the tissues. Minor bleeding often causes a bluish-purple discoloration of the skin that persists for several days. The contusion may be very sore to the touch, and if damage has occurred to muscle, pain may be experienced on active movement. In most cases the pain ceases within a few days and discoloration disappears usually in a few weeks.[8]

### Myositis Ossificans

The major problem with contusions occurs in an area that is subjected to repeated blows. If the same area, or more specifically, a muscle, is bruised over and over again, small calcium deposits may begin to accumulate in the injured area. These pieces of calcium may be found between several fibers in the muscle belly, or calcium may build up to form a spur, which projects from the underlying bone. These calcium formations may significantly impair movement and are referred to as **myositis ossificans**.[2]

The key to preventing the occurrence of myositis ossificans from repeated contusions is to protect the injured area with padding. If the area is properly protected after the first contusion, myositis may never develop. Protection and rest may allow the calcium to be reabsorbed, eliminating any need for surgery.

The two areas that seem to be the most vulnerable to repeated contusions during physical activity are the quadriceps muscle group on the front of the thigh and the biceps muscle on the front of the upper arm. The formation of myositis ossificans in these or any other areas may be detected by x-rays.

## Muscle Strains

The muscle is composed of separate fibers that are capable of simultaneous contraction when stimulated by the central nervous system. Each muscle is attached to bone at both ends by strong, relatively inelastic tendons that cross over joints.

If a muscle is overstretched or forced to contract against too much resistance, separation or tearing of the muscle fibers occurs. This damage is referred to as a **strain** (Figure 13-8).[2] Muscle strains, like ligament sprains, are subject to various classification systems. The following is a simple system of strain classification:

> **strain**
> A stretch, tear, or rip in the muscle or its tendon.

- *Grade 1 strain.* Some muscle fibers have been stretched or actually torn. There is some tenderness and pain on active motion. Movement is painful, but full range of motion is usually possible.

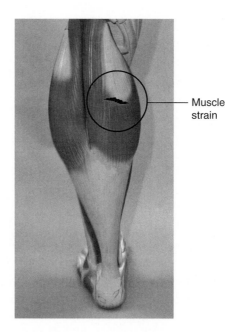

Muscle
strain

**Figure 13-8**

A muscle strain results in
separation or tearing of
fibers.

- *Grade 2 strain*. A number of muscle fibers have been torn, and
active contraction of the muscle is extremely painful. Usually a
depression or divot can be felt somewhere in the muscle belly at
the place at which the muscle fibers have been torn. Some swelling
may occur because of capillary bleeding; therefore, some
discoloration is possible.
- *Grade 3 strain*. A complete rupture of a muscle has occurred in the
area of the muscle belly at the point at which muscle becomes
tendon or at the tendinous attachment to the bone. There is
significant impairment to or perhaps total loss of movement.
Initially, pain is intense but quickly diminishes because of complete
nerve fiber separation.

Muscle strains can occur in any muscle and usually result from some
uncoordinated activity between muscle groups.[3] Grade 3 strains are most
common in the biceps tendon of the upper arm or in the Achilles heel
cord in the back of the calf. When either of these tendons tears, the muscle tends to bunch toward its attachment at the bone site. Grade 3 strains
involving large tendons that produce great amounts of force must be surgically repaired. Smaller musculotendinous ruptures such as those that
occur in the fingers may heal by immobilization with a splint.

Regardless of the severity of the strain, the time required for rehabilitation is lengthy.[14] In many instances muscle strains are incapacitating, making rehabilitation time for a muscle strain even longer than
for a ligament sprain. Incapacitating muscle strains occur most frequently
in the large, force-producing hamstring and quadriceps muscles of the

**13-3 Critical Thinking**
Exercise

A football player sustains
repeated contusions to the left
quadriceps muscle.

**?** What should he be most
concerned about?

lower extremity. The treatment of hamstring strains requires a healing period of 6 to 8 weeks and a considerable amount of patience. Trying to return to activity too soon often causes reinjury to the area of the muscle that has been strained, and the healing process must begin again.

### Muscle Guarding

Following injury, the muscles that surround the injured area contract to, in effect, splint that area, thus minimizing pain by limiting movement. Quite often this "splinting" is incorrectly referred to as a muscle spasm. The terms *spasm* and *spasticity* are more correctly associated with increased tone or contractions of muscle that occur because of some upper motor neuron lesion in the brain. Thus **muscle guarding** is a more appropriate term for the involuntary muscle contractions that occur in response to pain following musculoskeletal injury.[14]

> **muscle guarding**
> Muscle contraction in response to pain.

### Muscle Cramps

**Muscle cramps** are extremely painful involuntary muscle contractions that occur most commonly in the calf, abdomen, or hamstrings, although any muscle can be involved.[13] The occurrence of heat cramps is related to excessive loss of water and, to some extent, several electrolytes or ions (sodium, chloride, potassium, magnesium, and calcium) that are essential elements in muscle contraction (see Chapter 9).

> **muscle cramps**
> Involuntary muscle contraction.

### Muscle Soreness

Overexertion in strenuous muscular exercise often results in muscular pain. All active people at one time or another have experienced **muscle soreness** usually resulting from some physical activity to which they are unaccustomed. The older a person gets, the more easily muscle soreness seems to develop.

> **muscle soreness**
> Pain caused by overexertion in exercise.

There are two types of muscle soreness. The first type of muscle pain is *acute-onset muscle soreness,* which accompanies fatigue. It is transient and occurs during and immediately after exercise. The second type of soreness involves delayed muscle pain that appears approximately 12 hours after injury. This *delayed-onset muscle soreness (DOMS)* becomes most intense after 24 to 48 hours and then gradually subsides so that the muscle becomes symptom-free after 3 or 4 days. DOMS is described as a syndrome of delayed muscle pain leading to increased muscle tension, swelling, and stiffness and to resistance to stretching.[13]

DOMS is thought to result from several possible causes. It may occur from very small tears in the muscle tissue, which seems to be more likely with eccentric or isometric contractions. It may also occur because of disruption of the connective tissue that holds muscle tendon fibers together.

Muscle soreness may be prevented by beginning exercise at a moderate level and gradually progressing the intensity of the exercise over time. Treatment of muscle soreness usually also involves static or PNF stretching activity. Another important treatment for muscle soreness, as for other conditions discussed in this chapter, is ice applied within the first 48 to 72 hours.[14]

## Nerve Injuries

In athletics, nerve injuries usually involve either compression or tension. Nerve injuries, as with injuries to other tissues in the body, can be acute or chronic. Trauma directly affecting nerves can produce a variety of sensory responses, including hypoesthesia (diminished sense of feeling), hyperesthesia (increased sense of feelings such as pain or touch), or paresthesia (numbness, prickling, or tingling, which may occur from a direct blow or stretch to an area). For example, a sudden nerve stretch or pinch can produce both a sharp burning pain that radiates down a limb and muscle weakness as happens in a "burner" or "stinger" in the shoulder from injury to the brachial plexus. **Neuritis**, a chronic nerve problem, can be caused by a variety of forces that usually have been repeated or continued for a long time. Symptoms of neuritis can range from minor nerve problems to paralysis. More serious injuries involve the crushing of a nerve or complete division (severing). This type of injury may produce a lifelong physical disability, such as paraplegia or quadriplegia, and should therefore not be overlooked in any circumstance.

> **neuritis**
> Chronic nerve irritation.

Specialized tissue, such as nerve cells, cannot regenerate once the nerve cell dies. In an injured peripheral nerve, however, the nerve fiber can regenerate significantly if the injury does not affect the cell body. For regeneration to occur, an optimal environment for healing must exist.

Regeneration is slow, at a rate of only 3 to 4 mm per day. Damaged nerves within the central nervous system regenerate very poorly compared to nerves in the peripheral nervous system.[14]

## CHRONIC OVERUSE INJURIES

### The Importance of Inflammation in Healing

For most people, the word *inflammation* has negative connotations. However, inflammation is an essential part of the healing process.[15] Once a structure is damaged or irritated, inflammation must occur to initiate the healing process. *Signs and symptoms of inflammation include pain, swelling, warmth, loss of function, and perhaps redness.*[8] Inflammation is supposed to be an acute process that ends when its role in the healing process has been accomplished. However, if the source of irritation (e.g., the repetitive movements that cause stress to the tendon) is not removed, then the inflammatory process becomes chronic rather than acute.[15] When this situation occurs, an acute condition may become a chronic disabling problem.

Signs of inflammation:
- pain
- warmth
- swelling
- loss of function
- redness

### Tendinitis

Of all the overuse problems associated with sport activity, **tendinitis** is probably the most common.[6] Any term ending in the suffix *-itis* means inflammation is present. Tendinitis means inflammation of a **tendon**. During muscle activity, a tendon must move or slide on other structures around it whenever the muscle contracts. If a particular movement is performed repeatedly, the tendon becomes irritated and inflamed.[4] This

> **tendinitis**
> Inflammation of a tendon.

The suffix *-itis* means "inflammation of."

> **tendon**
> Tough band of connective tissue that attaches muscle to bone.

**crepitus**
A crackling feel or sound.

inflammation is manifested by pain on movement, swelling, possibly some warmth, and usually crepitus. **Crepitus** is a crackling sound. It is usually caused by the tendon's tendency to stick to the surrounding structure while it slides back and forth. This sticking is caused primarily by the chemical products of inflammation that accumulate on the irritated tendon.

The key to the treatment of tendinitis is rest.[14] If the repetitive motion causing irritation to the tendon is eliminated, the inflammatory process will allow the tendon to heal. Unfortunately, athletes find it difficult to totally stop activity and rest for 2 or more weeks while the tendinitis subsides. The athlete should substitute some form of activity, such as bicycling or swimming, to maintain present fitness levels while avoiding continued irritation of the inflamed tendon. In runners, tendinitis most commonly occurs in the Achilles tendon in the back of the lower leg; in swimmers, it often occurs in the muscle tendons of the shoulder joint. However, tendinitis can flare up in any activity in which overuse and repetitive movements occur.

### Tenosynovitis

**tenosynovitis** (ten oh sin oh **vie** tis)
Inflammation of a tendon and its synovial sheath.

**Tenosynovitis** is very similar to tendinitis in that the muscle tendons are involved in inflammation. However, many tendons are subject to an increased amount of friction because of the tightness of the space through which they must move. In these areas of high friction, tendons are usually surrounded by synovial sheaths that reduce friction on movement. If the tendon sliding through a synovial sheath is subjected to overuse, inflammation is likely to occur (Figure 13-9).[2] As with tendinitis, the inflammatory process produces by-products that are "sticky" and tend to cause the sliding tendon to adhere to the synovial sheath surrounding it.

Tenosynovitis occurs most commonly in the long flexor tendons of the fingers as they cross over the wrist joint and in the biceps tendon around the shoulder joint. Treatment for tenosynovitis is the same as for tendinitis. Because both conditions involve inflammation, anti-inflammatory drugs may be helpful in chronic cases.

**Figure 13-9**

Tenosynovitis is an inflammation of the sheath covering a tendon. The left Achilles tendon is swollen and inflamed.

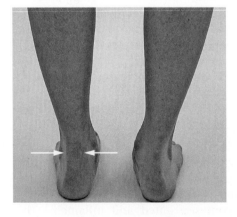

## Bursitis

Bursitis occurs around joints, where there is friction between tendon and bone, skin and bone, or muscle and other muscles. Without some mechanism of protection in these high-friction areas, chronic irritation would exist.

**Bursae** are pieces of synovial membrane that contain a small amount of fluid (synovial fluid). Just as oil lubricates a hinge, these small pieces of synovium permit motion of these structures without friction.

If excessive movement or perhaps some acute trauma occurs around the bursae, they become irritated and inflamed and begin producing large amounts of synovial fluid.[9] The longer the irritation continues or the more severe the acute trauma, the more fluid is produced. As fluid continues to accumulate in the limited space available, pressure increases, causing pain in the area. Bursitis can be an extremely painful condition that may severely restrict movement, especially if it occurs around a joint. Synovial fluid continues to be produced until the movement or trauma producing the irritation is eliminated.

Occasionally, a bursa or synovial sheath completely surrounds a tendon, allowing more freedom of movement in a tight area. Irritation of this synovial sheath may restrict tendon motion. All joints have many bursae surrounding them. The three bursae that are most commonly irritated as a result of various types of physical activity are the subacromial bursa in the shoulder joint under the distal clavicle and acromion process; the olecranon bursa on the tip of the elbow; and the prepatellar bursa on the front surface of the patella. All three of these bursae produce large amounts of synovial fluid, affecting motion at their respective joints.

> **bursae**
> Pieces of synovial membrane that contain a small amount of fluid.

## Osteoarthritis

Any mechanical system wears out with time. The joints in the body are mechanical systems, and wear and tear, even from normal activity, is inevitable. The most common result of this wear and tear, a degeneration of the articular or hyaline cartilage, is referred to as **osteoarthritis**.[9] The cartilage may be worn away to the point of exposing, eroding, and polishing the underlying bone (Figure 13-10).

Any process that changes the mechanics of the joint eventually leads to degeneration of that joint. Degeneration is a result of repeated trauma to the joint and to tendons, ligaments, and fasciae surrounding the joint. Such injuries may be caused by a direct blow or fall, by pressure of carrying or lifting heavy loads, or by repeated trauma to the joint as in running or cycling.

Osteoarthritis most often affects the weight-bearing joints: the knees, hips, and lumbar spine. Also affected are the shoulders and cervical spine. Although many other joints may show pathological degenerative change, clinically the disease only occasionally produces symptoms in them. Any joint that is subjected to acute or chronic trauma may develop osteoarthritis.[14]

> **osteoarthritis**
> A wearing down of hyaline cartilage.

**Osteoarthritis**

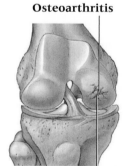

**Eroding Underlying bone**

**Figure 13-10**

Osteoarthritis is a degeneration and erosion of the hyaline cartilage.

The symptoms of osteoarthritis are relatively local. Osteoarthritis may be localized to one side of the joint or may be generalized about the joint. One of the most distinctive symptoms is pain, which is brought about by friction that occurs with use and which is relieved by rest. Stiffness is a common complaint that occurs with rest and is quickly loosened with activity. This symptom is prominent upon rising in the morning. Joints may also show localized tenderness, or grating that may be heard and felt.[8]

### Myofascial Trigger Points

> **trigger point**
> Area of tenderness in a tight band of muscle.

A **trigger point** is an area of tenderness in a tight band of muscle. In the athlete, painful or active trigger points most often develop because of some mechanical stress to the muscle.[14] This stress could involve either an acute muscle strain or static postural positions that produce constant tension in the muscle. Trigger points occur most typically in the neck, upper back, and lower back. Palpation of the trigger point produces pain in a predictable distribution of referred pain. The pain may also cause some restricted range of motion. Pressure on the trigger point produces a twitch or a jump response from the pain. Pain can be increased by passive or active stretching of the involved muscle.

## THE IMPORTANCE OF THE HEALING PROCESS FOLLOWING INJURY

It is essential to have some understanding of both the sequence and time frames for the various phases of healing, realizing that certain physiological events occur during each of the phases. Any interference with the healing process during a rehabilitation program will likely slow return to full activity. The healing process must have an opportunity to accomplish what it is supposed to. At best, you can only try to create an environment that is conducive to the healing process. Little can be done to speed up the process physiologically, but many things may be done during rehabilitation to impede healing.

Phases of the healing process:
• inflammatory response phase
• fibroblastic repair phase
• maturation-remodeling phase

The healing process consists of three phases: the inflammatory response phase, the fibroblastic repair phase, and the maturation-remodeling phase.[1] Although the phases of healing are often discussed as three separate entities, the healing process is a continuum. Phases of the healing process overlap one another and have no definitive beginning or end (Figure 13-11).[14]

### Inflammatory Response Phase

The inflammatory response phase begins immediately following injury (Figure 13-12A). The inflammatory response phase is perhaps the most critical phase of the healing process. Without the physiological changes that take place during the inflammatory process, the later stages of healing cannot occur. The destruction of tissue produces direct injury to the cells of the various soft tissues. During this phase, phagocytic cells clean up the mess created by the injury. Injured cells release chemicals that

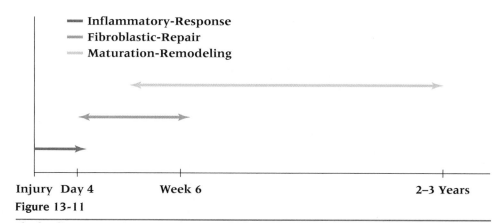

**Figure 13-11**

The healing process is a continuum in which the three phases of healing overlap one another.

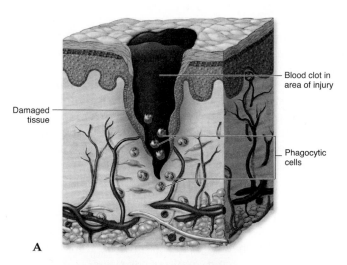

A

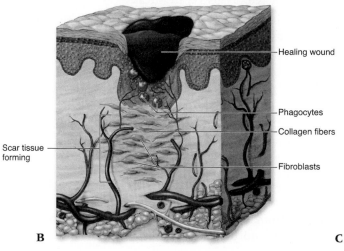

B

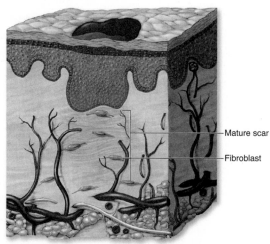

C

**Figure 13-12**

Tissue Healing:
(A) Inflammatory-response phase—blood clot forms in the area of injury and phagocytic cells clean up damaged tissue cells.
(B) Fibroblastic repair phase—Fibroblasts lay down collagen fibers forming scar.
(C) Maturation-remodeling phase—scar tissue remodels and realigns along lines of stress and strain.

facilitate the healing process. As indicated previously this phase is characterized symptomatically by redness, swelling, tenderness, increased temperature, and loss of function. This initial inflammatory response lasts for approximately 2 to 4 days following initial injury.

### Fibroblastic Repair Phase

During the fibroblastic phase of healing, proliferative and regenerative activity leading to scar formation and repair of the injured tissue occurs (Figure 13-12B). The period of scar formation, referred to as *fibroplasia*, begins within the first few hours following injury and may last for as long as 4 to 6 weeks. During this period many of the signs and symptoms associated with the inflammatory response subside. The athlete may still indicate some tenderness to touch and usually complains of pain when particular movements stress the injured structure. As scar formation progresses, complaints of tenderness or pain gradually disappear.

### Maturation-Remodeling Phase

The maturation-remodeling phase of healing is a long-term process (Figure 13-12C). This phase features a realignment or remodeling of the scar tissue according to the tensile forces to which that scar is subjected. With increased stress and strain, the collagen fibers that make up the scar realign in a position of maximum efficiency parallel to the lines of tension. The tissue gradually assumes normal appearance and function, although a scar is rarely as strong as the normal uninjured tissue. Usually after about 3 weeks, a firm, strong, contracted, nonvascular scar exists. The maturation phase of healing may require several years to be totally complete.

## SUMMARY

- Fractures may be classified as either greenstick, transverse, oblique, spiral, comminuted, impacted, avulsive, or stress.
- Dislocations and subluxations are disruptions of the joint capsule and ligamentous structures surrounding the joint.
- Ligament sprains involve stretching or tearing the fibers that provide stability at the joint.
- Repeated contusions may lead to the development of myositis ossificans.
- Muscle strains involve a stretching or tearing of muscle fibers and their tendons and cause impairment to active movement.
- Muscle soreness may be caused by spasm, connective tissue damage, muscle tissue damage, or some combination of these factors.
- Tendinitis, an inflammation of a muscle tendon that causes pain on movement, usually occurs because of overuse.
- Tenosynovitis is an inflammation of the synovial sheath through which a tendon must slide during motion.

- Bursitis is an inflammation of the synovial membranes located in areas in which friction occurs between various anatomical structures.

- Osteoarthritis involves degeneration of the articular cartilage or subchondral bone.

- A trigger point is an area of tenderness in a tight band of muscle that develops from some mechanical stress to the muscle.

- The three phases of the healing process, the inflammatory response phase, the fibroblastic repair phase, and the maturation-remodeling phase, occur in sequence but overlap one another in a continuum.

---

*Solutions to Critical Thinking* Exercises

**13-1** A stress fracture is not an actual break of the bone; it is simply an irritation of the bone. Treatment of a stress fracture requires about 14 days of rest. However, the coach should point out that a stress fracture can become a true fracture if it is not rested; if that happens, 4 to 6 weeks of immobilization in a cast is necessary. Thus, it is critical that this athlete rest for the required amount of time.

**13-2** Little can be done to speed up the healing process physiologically. This athlete must realize that certain physiological events must occur during each phase of the healing process. Any interference with this healing process during a rehabilitation program will likely slow return to full activity. The healing process must have an opportunity to accomplish what it is supposed to.

**13-3** Repeated contusion of any muscle may lead to the development of myositis ossificans. The key to treating myositis ossificans is prevention. An initial contusion to any muscle should be immediately protected with padding to prevent reinjury.

## REVIEW QUESTIONS AND CLASS ACTIVITIES

1. What is the difference between an acute injury and a chronic injury? Give examples of each.
2. Describe various types of fractures and the mechanisms that cause fractures to occur.
3. How does a stress fracture differ from a regular fracture?
4. Differentiate between a subluxation and a dislocation.
5. What structures are found at a joint? What are their functions?
6. How do the three grades of ligament sprains differ?
7. What is myositis ossificans and how can it be prevented?
8. Differentiate between muscle strains, muscle cramps, muscle guarding, and muscle soreness.
9. How does a damaged nerve heal?
10. How are tendinitis, tenosynovitis, and bursitis related to one another?
11. Explain how osteoarthritis develops.
12. What are myofascial trigger points, where are they most likely to occur, and what are the signs and symptoms?
13. Discuss the physiological events that occur during each of the different phases of the healing process.
14. Invite an orthopedist to class to discuss common injuries to the musculoskeletal system.

## REFERENCES

1. American Orthopaedic Society for Sports Medicine: 1990. *Sports-induced inflammation,* Park Ridge, IL, American Academy of Orthopaedic Surgeons.
2. Blauvelt, CT, Nelson, FRT: 1998. *A manual of orthopaedic terminology,* 4th ed. St Louis, Mosby–Year Book.
3. Brukner, P, Khan, K: 2002. Sports injuries. In Brukner, P (ed), *Clinical sports medicine,* 2nd ed, Sydney, McGraw-Hill.
4. Cailliet, R: 2004. *Medical orthopedics: conservative management of musculoskeletal impairments,* Chicago, AMA Press.
5. Delforge, G (ed): 2003. *Musculoskeletal trauma: implications for sports injury management,* Champaign, IL, Human Kinetics.
6. DiFiori, JP: 2002. Overuse injuries in young athletes: an overview, *Athletic therapy today* 7(6):25–29.
7. Drake, DF: 2004. Sports and performing arts medicine. 4. traumatic injuries in sports, *Archives of physical medicine and rehabilitation* 85 (3 Suppl):S67–S71.
8. Gallaspie, J, May, D: 2001. *Signs and symptoms of athletic injuries,* St Louis, Mosby.
9. Green, WB: 2005. *Essentials of musculoskeletal care.* 3rd ed, Rosemont, IL, American Academy of Orthopaedic Surgeons.
10. Hutson, M: 2002. *Sports injuries—recognition and management,* 3rd ed, Oxford, England, Oxford University Press.
11. Kjaer, M: 2003. *Textbook of sports medicine: basic science and clinical aspects of sports injury and physical activity,* Oxford, Blackwell Science.
12. Maehlum, S, Mhlum, S: 2004. *Clinical guide to sports injuries,* Champaign, IL, Human Kinetics.
13. Prentice, WE: 2009. *Arnheim's Principles of athletic training,* New York, McGraw-Hill.
14. Prentice, W: 2010. *Rehabilitation techniques in sports medicine and athletic training,* New York, McGraw-Hill.
15. Scott, A; Khan, KM; Roberts, CR: 2004. What do we mean by the term "inflammation": a contemporary basic science update for sports medicine, *British journal of sports medicine* 38(3):372–380.
16. Shamus, E, Shamus, J: 2001. *Sports injury: prevention and rehabilitation,* New York, McGraw-Hill.
17. Strauss, R: 1996. *Sports medicine,* Philadelphia, WB Saunders.
18. Wilder, RP, Sethi, S: 2004. Overuse injuries: tendinopathies, stress fractures, compartment syndrome, and shin splints, *Clinics in sports medicine* 23(1):55–81.

## ANNOTATED BIBLIOGRAPHY

Booher, JM, Thibodeau, GA: 2000. *Athletic injury assessment,* Boston, McGraw-Hill.

    *An excellent guide to the recognition, assessment, classification, and evaluation of athletic injuries.*

Griffith, HW, Pederson, M: 2004. *Complete guide to sports injuries: how to treat fractures, bruises, sprains, dislocations, and head injuries,* New York, Perigee.

    *Tells readers how to treat, avoid, and rehabilitate nearly 200 of the most common sports injuries, including fractures, bruises, sprains, strains, dislocations, and head injuries.*

Kjaer, M: 2003. *Textbook of sports medicine: basic science and clinical aspects* of sports injury and physical activity, Oxford, Blackwelll Science.

*Provides capsule summaries of the history, diagnosis, and treatment of orthopedic problems that respond to nonsurgical intervention in this primer for clinicians. Brief yet detailed entries explain the causes and treatment of impairments of the musculoskeletal system.*

Maehlum, S, Mhlum, S: 2004. *Clinical guide to sports injuries,* Champaign, Ill., Human Kinetics.

*This text and reference for sports medicine practitioners covers each step of the injury management process, beginning with the patient's presentation.*

Peacinn, M, Bojanic, I: 2003. *Overuse injuries of musculoskeletal system,* Boca Raton, FL, CRC Press.

*A comprehensive text describing overuse injuries of the tendon, tendon sheath, bursae, muscle, muscle-tendon function, cartilage, and nerve.*

Williams, JGP: 1990. *Color atlas of injury in sport,* Chicago, Mosby–Year Book.

*An excellent visual guide to the area of sports injuries, covering the nature and incidence of sport injury, types of tissue damage, and regional injuries caused by a variety of sports activities.*

**WEB SITES**

American Red Cross:
www.redcross.org
National Institute of Health:
www.nih.gov

Wheeless' Textbook of Orthopedics:
www.wheelessonline.com/

# The Foot

## CHAPTER 14

*When you finish this chapter you will be able to:*

- Briefly describe the anatomy of the foot.
- Explain the process of injury assessment for the foot.
- Formulate steps that can be taken to minimize foot injuries.
- Identify the causes of various foot injuries commonly seen in athletes.
- Describe the appropriate care for injuries incurred in the foot.

## FOOT ANATOMY

### Bones

The human foot must function both to absorb forces and to provide a stable base of support during walking, running, and jumping. It contains twenty-six bones (seven tarsal, five metatarsal, and fourteen phalangeal) that are held together by an intricate network of ligaments and fascia and moved by a complicated group of muscles (Figure 14-1). The tarsal bones that form the ankle include the talus and calcaneous. The navicular, cuboid, and three cuneiform bones form the instep of the foot.

### Ligaments

#### Arches of the Foot

The foot is structured, by means of ligamentous and bony arrangements, to form several arches. The arches assist the foot in supporting the body weight and in absorbing the shock of weight bearing. There are four arches: the medial longitudinal, the lateral longitudinal, the metatarsal, and the transverse (Figure 14-2).

The *metatarsal arch* is shaped by the distal heads of the metatarsals. The arch stretches from the first to the fifth metatarsal. The *transverse arch* extends across the transverse tarsal bones and forms a half dome. The *medial longitudinal arch* originates along the medial border of the calcaneus and extends forward to the distal head of the first metatarsal. The main supporting ligament of the medial longitudinal arch is the plantar calcaneonavicular ligament, which acts as a spring by returning the arch to its normal position after it has been stretched. The *lateral longitudinal arch* is on the lateral aspect of the foot and follows the same

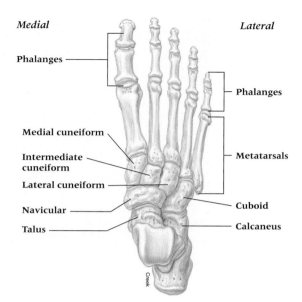

Medial

Lateral

Phalanges

Phalanges

Medial cuneiform

Metatarsals

Intermediate
cuneiform

Lateral cuneiform

Cuboid

Navicular

Talus

Calcaneus

Creek

**Figure 14-1**

Bony structure of the foot,
dorsal aspect.

pattern as the medial longitudinal arch. It is formed by the calcaneus, cuboid, and fifth metatarsal.

### Plantar Fascia (Plantar Aponeurosis)

The plantar fascia is a thick white band of fibrous tissue originating from the medial aspect of the calcaneus and ending at the distal heads of the metatarsals. Along with ligaments, the plantar fascia supports the foot against downward forces (Figure 14-3).

## Muscles

The medial movements include adduction (medial movement of the forefoot—metatarsals) and supination (a combination of inversion and adduction). Muscles that produce these movements pass both behind and in front of the medial malleolus. Muscles passing behind are the tibialis posterior, flexor digitorum longus, and flexor hallucis longus. Muscles passing in front of the medial malleolus are the tibialis anterior and the extensor hallucis longus (Figure 14-4A).

The lateral movements of the foot include abduction (lateral movement of the forefoot—metatarsals) and pronation (a combination of eversion and abduction). Muscles passing behind the lateral malleolus are the peroneus longus and the peroneus brevis. Muscles passing in front of the lateral malleolus are the peroneus tertius and extensor digitorum longus (Figure 14-4 A&B).

In general the small intrinsic muscles on the plantar surface of the foot cause toe flexion whereas those muscles on the dorsum of the foot cause toe extension and abduction (Figure 14-5) (Table 14-1).

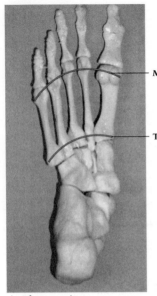

Metatarsal arch

Transverse arch

**A** Plantar view

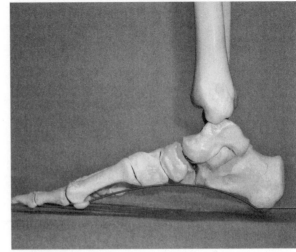

Medial longitudinal arch

**B** Medial view

**Figure 14-2**

Arches of the foot:
(A) Metatarsal and transverse arches. (B) Medial longitudinal arch. (C) Lateral longitudinal arch.

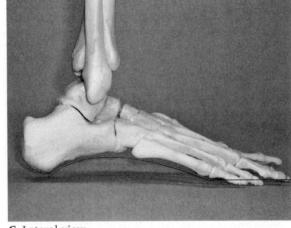

Lateral longitudinal arch

**C** Lateral view

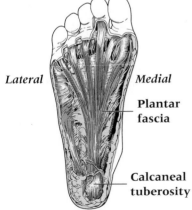

*Lateral*  *Medial*

**Plantar fascia**

**Calcaneal tuberosity**

**Figure 14-3**

Plantar fascia

## PREVENTION OF FOOT INJURIES

Understanding the foot's structure and mechanics, types of footwear (see Chapter 6), and surface concerns is important in preventing foot injuries.[16] Particular attention should be given to athletes who may be predisposed to injuries caused by muscular or tendinous tightness or, conversely, weakness or hypermobility. Such situations, when recognized early, can usually be remedied by exercise, by the use of appropriate shoe inserts or **orthotics,** or by selecting appropriate shoes.[11,12] Many injuries to the foot can be prevented by using an orthotic device

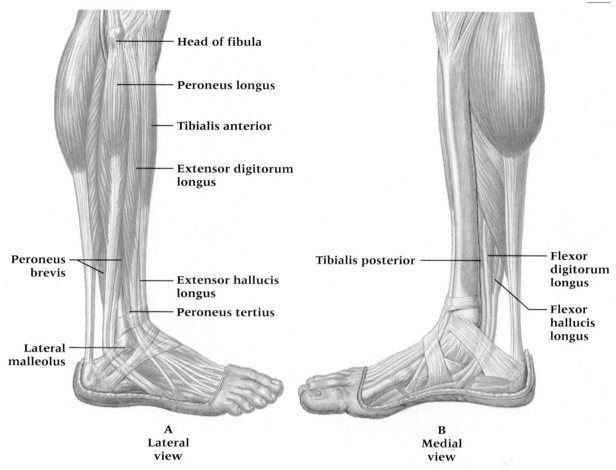

**A**
**Lateral**
**view**

**B**
**Medial**
**view**

Head of fibula

Peroneus longus

Tibialis anterior

Extensor digitorum longus

Peroneus brevis

Extensor hallucis longus

Peroneus tertius

Lateral malleolus

Tibialis posterior

Flexor digitorum longus

Flexor hallucis longus

**Figure 14-4**

Muscles originating in the lower leg that produce movements in the foot: (A) Lateral view. (B) Medial view.

---

**Orthotic**
A custom designed insert that can be placed in the shoe and worn to correct a variety of biomechanical abnormalities that can potentially lead to injury.

---

to correct biomechanical problems that may exist in the foot and that can potentially cause an injury. The orthotic is a plastic, rubber, or leather support that is placed in the shoe as a replacement for the existing insert. Ready-made orthotics can be purchased in sporting goods or shoe stores. Some patients will need to have orthotics that are custom fitted or made by the athletic trainer or podiatrist.

Not everyone has the same kind of foot and can wear the same type of shoe. Each individual should select a shoe that is most appropriate for him or her. Strengthening, stretching, and mobility exercises should be performed routinely by athletes in sports that place a great deal of stress and strain on the feet.[26]

The foot must continually adapt to the contact surface. Training on surfaces that are irregular and variable in resilience can ultimately serve to strengthen the foot over time. However, a nonyielding surface may in some cases overstress joints and soft tissue, eventually leading to an acute or chronic pathological condition in the foot or somewhere in the kinetic chain. In contrast, a surface that is too resilient and absorbs too

**Figure 14-5**

Intrinsic muscles of the foot.
(A) Muscles on the plantar
(bottom) surface of the foot
that produce flexion of the
toes. (B) Muscles on the
dorsal (top) surface of the
foot that produce extension
of the toes.

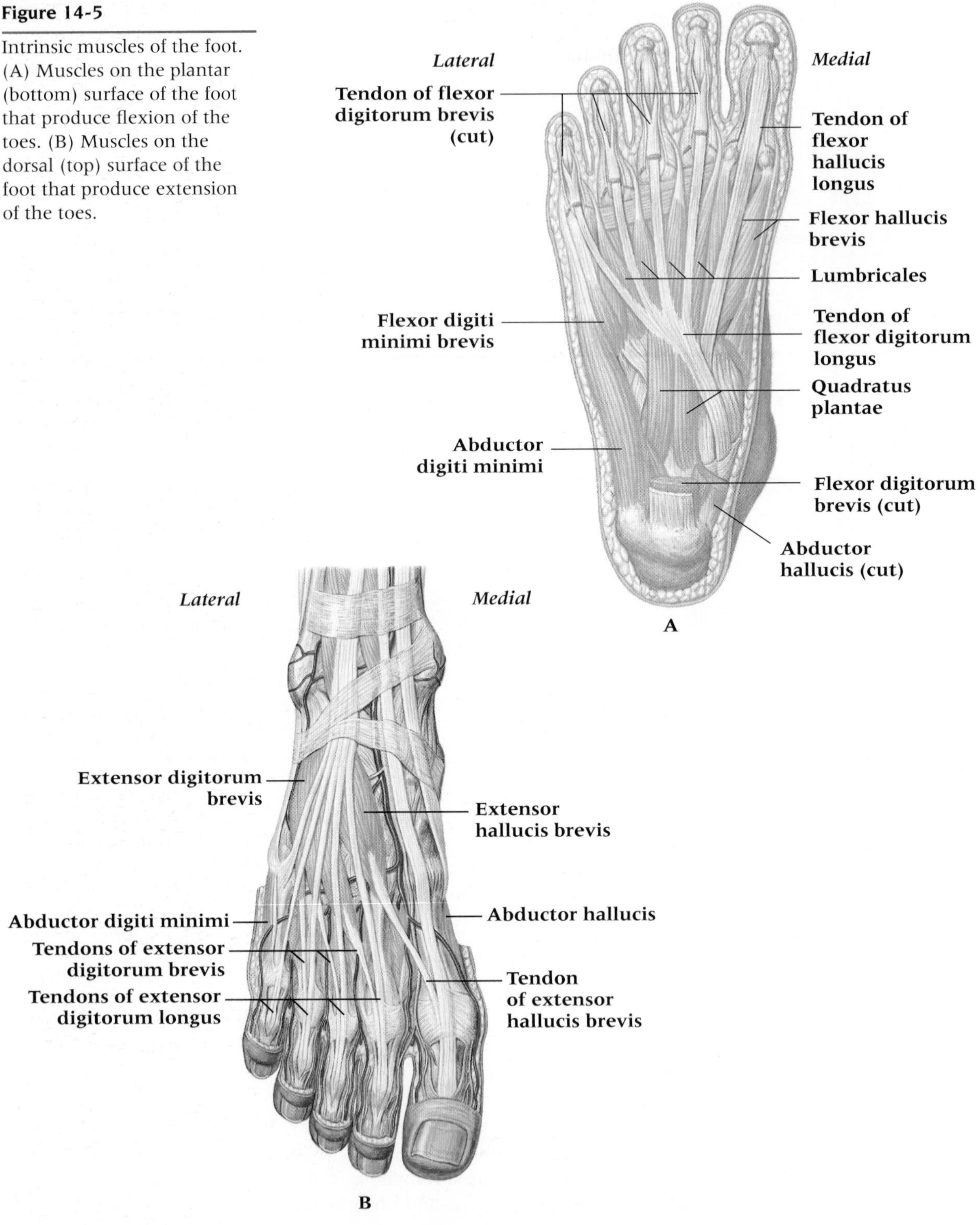

*Lateral*

Tendon of flexor
digitorum brevis
(cut)

*Medial*

Tendon of
flexor
hallucis
longus

Flexor hallucis
brevis

Lumbricales

Flexor digiti
minimi brevis

Tendon of
flexor digitorum
longus

Quadratus
plantae

Abductor
digiti minimi

Flexor digitorum
brevis (cut)

Abductor
hallucis (cut)

**A**

*Lateral*

*Medial*

Extensor digitorum
brevis

Extensor
hallucis brevis

Abductor digiti minimi

Abductor hallucis

Tendons of extensor
digitorum brevis

Tendon
of extensor
hallucis brevis

Tendons of extensor
digitorum longus

**B**

**TABLE 14-1** Muscles of the Foot

| | |
|---|---|
| Adduction and supination | Tibialis posterior |
| | Flexor digitorum longus |
| | Flexor hallucis longus |
| | Tibialis anterior |
| | Extensor hallucis longus |
| Abduction and pronation | Peroneus longus |
| | Peroneus brevis |
| | Peroneus tertius |
| | Extensor digitorum longus |
| Toe flexion | Flexor digitorum brevis |
| | Flexor digitorum longus |
| | Flexor hallucis brevis |
| | Flexor hallucis longus |
| | Flexor digiti minimi brevis |
| | Quadratus plantae |
| | Lumbricales |
| Toe extension | Extensor digitorum brevis |
| | Extensor digitorum longus |
| | Extensor hallucis longus |
| Toe abduction | Abductor hallucis |
| | Dorsal interrosi |
| | Abductor digiti minimi |
| Toe adduction | Adduction hallucis |
| | Plantar interossi |

much of the impact energy may lead to early fatigue in sports such as basketball and indoor tennis.

The majority of foot skin conditions are preventable.[2] The athlete should be instructed on proper foot hygiene, which includes proper washing and drying of the feet following activity and changing to clean socks daily. Wearing properly fitting shoes and socks (see Chapter 6) should be emphasized. Athletes who have abnormal foot stresses caused by faulty mechanics may find the use of custom orthotics to be helpful.[12]

Nearly all blisters, calluses, corns, and ingrown toenails are preventable.

## FOOT ASSESSMENT

**Generally fitness professionals, coaches, and others working in areas related to exercise and sport science are not adequately trained to evaluate injuries. It is strongly recommended that injured athletes be referred to qualified medical personnel (i.e., physicians, athletic trainers, physical therapists) for injury evaluation.** Information on the following special tests has been included simply to give some idea about the different basic tests that nonmedical personnel may do to determine the nature and severity of the athlete's injury. The primary responsibility of those who are not health care personnel is to be able to recognize any potential "red flags" associated with the injury, provide appropriate first aid for the injury, and make correct decisions about how the injury should be managed initially, including immediate return to play or activity decisions. (Refer to Chapter 7.)

## History

When deciding how to manage a foot injury an assessment must be made to determine the type of injury and its history.[25] The following questions should be asked:

- How did the injury occur?
- Did it occur suddenly or come on slowly?
- Was the mechanism a sudden strain, twist, or blow to the foot?
- What type of pain is there? Is there muscle weakness? Are there noises such as crepitation during movement? Is there any alteration in sensation?
- Can the athlete point to the exact site of pain? When is the pain or other symptoms more or less severe?
- On what type of surface has the athlete been training? What type of footwear was being used during training? Is it appropriate for the type of training? Is discomfort increased when footwear is worn?
- Is this the first time this condition has occurred, or has it happened before? If so, when, how often, and under what circumstances?

## Observation

The athlete should be observed to determine the following:

- Whether he or she is favoring the foot, is walking with a limp, or is unable to bear weight.
- Whether the injured part is deformed, swollen, or discolored.
- Whether the foot changes color when bearing weight and not bearing weight (changing rapidly from a darker to a lighter pink when not bearing weight).
- Whether the foot is well aligned and whether it maintains its shape when bearing weight.
- What the wear patterns look like on the sole of the shoe. Is there symmetry between the two shoes?
- Whether the athlete has a high arch (pes caus) or a flat foot (pes planus).

## Palpation

**point tenderness**
Pain is produced when the site of injury is palpated.

Palpation of the bony structures should be done first to check for deformities or areas of point tenderness. Palpation of the muscles and their tendons in the foot is essential to detect **point tenderness,** abnormal swelling or lumps, muscle spasm, or muscle guarding.[4] The dorsal pedal pulse, located on the anterior surface of the ankle and foot, should be palpated to check for normal circulation.

# RECOGNITION AND MANAGEMENT OF FOOT INJURIES

## Retrocalcaneal Bursitis (Pump Bump)

**Cause of injury**   The retrocalcaneal bursa lies between the calcaneous and the Achilles tendon on the back of the heel. This bursa can become chronically irritated and inflamed by constant rubbing or pressure from the heel counter of a shoe.[27] If inflammation continues for many months, a bone callus, or **exostosis,** is likely to form on the back of the heel (Figure 14-6A). This exostosis has been referred to as a ***pump bump.*** (A pump is a type of woman's shoe with a heel counter that tends to cross right over the retrocalcaneal bursa.) This condition should be differentiated from **Sever's disease,** which involves a chronic inflammation at the attachment of the Achilles tendon on the posterior calcaneous in young athletes.

**Signs of injury**   All the signs of bursitis—tenderness, swelling, warmth, and redness—will be present and will progress eventually to a palpable and tender bony bump on the back of the calcaneous.

| |
|---|
| **exostosis (ek sosto sis)** |
| A bony outgrowth. |

| |
|---|
| **Sever's disease** |
| Chronic inflammation of Achilles tendon attachment. |

**Figure 14-6**

(A) A pump bump that develops from retrocalcaneal bursitis (B) can be protected using a doughnut-type pad.

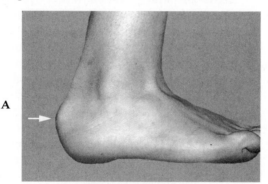

**A**

**Lateral view**

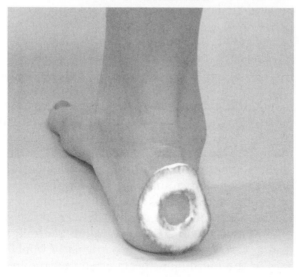

**B**

Recognition and
Management of Specific
Injuries and Conditions

**Care**  A doughnut-type pad should be constructed and placed around the area of tenderness to disperse pressure created by the heel counter (Figure 14-6B). Also, a heel lift can help to change the site of pressure. The athlete may also want to choose a shoe with a heel counter that is either a little higher or lower than the one presently being worn.

### Heel Bruise

The athlete who is prone to heel bruises should routinely wear a padded heel cup.

**Cause of injury**  Of the many contusions and bruises that an athlete may receive, none is more disabling than the heel bruise on the bottom of the calcaneous.[27] Sport activities that demand a sudden stop-and-go response or a sudden change from a horizontal to a vertical movement, such as basketball jumping, high jumping, and vaulting in gymnastics, are particularly likely to cause heel bruises.[9] The heel has a thick, cornified skin layer and a heavy fat pad covering, but even this thick padding cannot protect against a sudden abnormal force directed to this area.

**Signs of injury**  When injury occurs, the athlete complains of severe pain in the heel and is unable to tolerate the stress of weight bearing. An acute bruise of the heel may progress to chronic inflammation of the bone covering (periosteum).

**Care**  Initially, cold is applied to the heel bruise, and if possible, the athlete should not step on the heel for at least 24 hours. If pain when walking has subsided by the third day, the athlete may resume moderate activity—with the protection of a heel cup or protective doughnut (Figure 14-7). An athlete who is prone to or who needs protection from a heel bruise should routinely wear a heel cup with a foam rubber pad as a preventive aid. Surrounding the heel with a firm heel cup diffuses traumatic forces and compresses the fat pad under the calcaneous providing additional cushioning. This can also be accomplished by applying athletic tape as if it were a heel cup.

**14-1 Critical Thinking**
Exercise

A distance runner is complaining of pain that started on the bottom of her heel and now seems to also be bothering the long arch. She states that pain seems to be the worst in the morning when she first gets out of bed.

? What condition usually results in these complaints and how should this problem be managed?

### Plantar Fasciitis

**Cause of condition**  Heel pain is a very common problem in both the athletic and nonathletic populations. The plantar fascia runs the length of the sole of the foot (refer to Figure 14-3). It assists in maintaining the stability of the foot and in supporting the medial longitudinal arch.[8] A number of conditions have been studied as possible causes of plantar fasciitis. They include leg length discrepancy, inflexibility of the medial longitudinal arch, tightness of the gastrocnemius-soleus unit, wearing shoes without sufficient arch support, a lengthened stride during running, and running on soft surfaces.[8]

**Signs of condition**  The athlete complains of pain in the anterior medial heel, usually at the attachment of the plantar fascia to the calcaneus that eventually moves more centrally into the middle of the plantar fascia.[23] This pain is particularly troublesome when the athlete rises in the morning or bears weight on the foot after sitting for a long

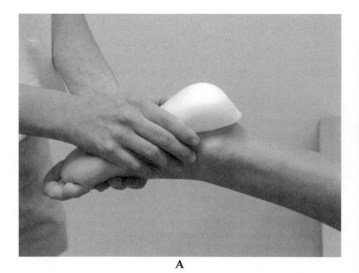

A

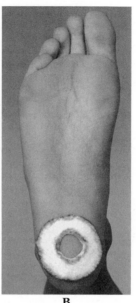

B

**Figure 14-7**

Protection of a heel
bruise using (A) A
heel cup. (B) A felt
doughnut pad.

period. However, the pain lessens after a few steps. Pain also is intensified when the toes and forefoot are forcibly dorsiflexed.

**Care** Management of plantar fasciitis generally requires an extended period of treatment.[22] It is not uncommon for symptoms to persist for as long as 8 to 12 weeks. Vigorous heel cord stretching should be done, along with exercises to stretch the plantar fascia in the arch.[23] Wearing a night splint that gently dorsiflexes the foot and stretches the plantar fascia during sleep is recommended and widely used[22] (Figure 14-8). Use of a heel cup compresses the fat pad under the calcaneous and provides a cushion under the area of irritation (refer to Figure 14-7). A simple arch taping often allows pain-free ambulation. Orthotic therapy is very useful in the treatment of this problem. In some cases, particularly during a competitive season, the athlete may continue to train and compete if symptoms and associated pain are not prohibitive.

### Fractures of the Metatarsals

**Cause of injury** Fractures of the metatarsals can be caused by direct force, such as having the foot stepped on by another player, by being kicked or kicking another object, or by twisting or torsional stresses.[27] The most common acute fracture is to the neck of the fifth metatarsal (Jones fracture).[3]

**Signs of injury** It is very difficult to differentiate a fracture from a sprain of the metatarsal ligaments. Fractures of the metatarsals are characterized by swelling and pain. A fracture may be more point tender and occasionally it may be possible to palpate a deformity. The most definitive way to distinguish a fracture from a sprain is to get an x-ray.[5]

Throughout the remainder of this text, when the Dr. Icon appears, the athlete should be referred to a physician for injury management.

**Figure 14-8**

A night splint for plantar fasciitis is worn while sleeping.

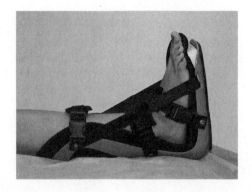

**Care**  Treatment is usually symptomatic, with PRICE used to control swelling. Once swelling has subsided, a short leg walking cast is applied for 3 to 6 weeks. Ambulation is usually possible by the second week. A shoe with a large toe box should be worn.[20]

### Jones Fracture

**Cause of injury**  A Jones fracture involves a fracture at the neck of the fifth metatarsal that can occur from overuse, acute inversion, or high-velocity rotational forces (Figure 14-9). A Jones fracture occurs most often as a sequela of a stress fracture.[3]

**Signs of injury**  The athlete complains of a sharp pain on the lateral border of the foot and usually reports hearing a "pop." Because of a history of poor blood supply and delayed healing, a Jones fracture may result in nonunion, requiring an extended period of rehabilitation.[9]

**Care**  A Jones fracture of the fifth metatarsal usually requires a non-weight-bearing short leg cast for 6 to 8 weeks for nondisplaced fractures. With cases of delayed union, nonunion, or especially displaced fractures, the Jones fracture requires internal fixation, with or without bone grafting. In the highly competitive athlete, immediate surgical internal fixation should be recommended.[15]

### Second Metatarsal Stress Fractures

**Cause of injury**  Second metatarsal stress fractures, also referred to as *march fractures,* occur most often in running and jumping sports. As with other overuse injuries in the foot, the most common causes include structural deformities in the foot, training errors, changes in training surfaces, and wearing inappropriate shoes.[9]

*Morton's toe* is a condition in which the first metatarsal is abnormally short, making the second toe appear longer than the great toe (Figure 14-10). In a normal walking gait, the first metatarsal bears most of the weight. However, because the first metatarsal in a Morton's toe is short, the second metatarsal must bear a greater percentage of the forces during walking and even greater forces in a running gait. Thus a Morton's toe increases the chance of a stress fracture of the second metatarsal.[27]

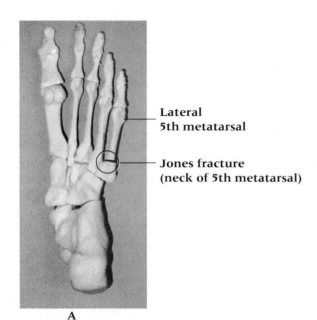

Lateral
5th metatarsal

Jones fracture
(neck of 5th metatarsal)

**A**

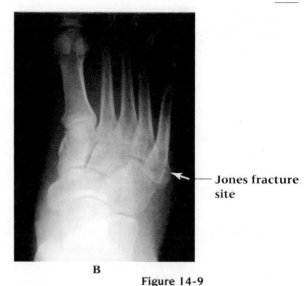

**B**

Jones fracture
site

**Figure 14-9**

(A) A Jones fracture occurs
at the neck of the fifth
metatarsal. (B) X-ray.

**Signs of injury**   The athlete usually complains of pain and point tenderness along the second metatarsal. Commonly the athlete indicates the presence of pain during running and perhaps also during walking. The athlete may also feel ongoing pain and aching during non-weight-bearing movements.[20]

**Care**   Treatment for stress fractures should focus on determining the precipitating cause or causes and alleviating those that created the problem. Athletes with second metatarsal stress fractures tend to do well with modified rest and non-weight-bearing exercises such as pool running or using an upper body ergometer or stationary bike to maintain cardiorespiratory fitness for 2 to 4 weeks. These exercises are followed by the athlete's progressive return to running and jumping sports over a 2- to 3-week period using appropriate shoes.

**Figure 14-10**

In a Morton's toe, the first
metatarsal is abnormally
short.

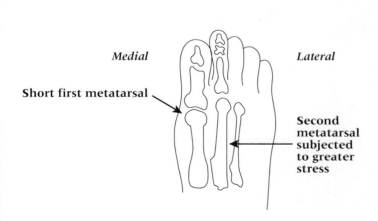

*Medial*

*Lateral*

**Short first metatarsal**

**Second
metatarsal
subjected
to greater
stress**

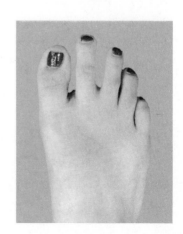

Fatigue, poor posture,
overuse, excessive weight, or
improperly fitting shoes may
damage the supporting tissue
of the arch.

---

**metatarsalgia** (metah
tar **sal** gee ah)
Pain on the bottom of
the foot.

---

As long as an existing
condition in the foot is *not*
causing pain, don't try to
fix it.

---

**pes planus (pees** plan is)
Flat feet.

---

## Metatarsal Arch Strain

**Cause of injury**    Athletes with hypermobility of the metatarsals caused by laxity in the ligaments are prone to sprain of the metatarsal arch.[9] Hypermobility allows the metatarsals in the foot to spread apart (splayed foot), giving the appearance of a fallen metatarsal arch.[14]

**Signs of injury**    The athlete has pain or cramping in the metatarsal region. There is point tenderness, with signs of inflammation and weakness in the area. Pain in this region is called **metatarsalgia.**[13] Although metatarsalgia is a general term to describe pain or cramping in the ball of the foot, it is more commonly associated with pain under the second and sometimes the third metatarsal head. A heavy callus often forms in the area of pain.

**Care**    Treatment of acute metatarsalgia usually consists of applying a pad to elevate the depressed metatarsal heads. The pad is placed in the center and just behind the ball of the foot (metatarsal heads) (Figure 14-11). A daily regimen of exercise should concentrate on strengthening foot muscles and stretching the heel cord.

## Longitudinal Arch Strain

**Cause of injury**    Longitudinal arch strain is usually caused by subjecting the musculature on the plantar surface of the foot to unaccustomed stresses and forces when coming in contact with hard playing surfaces. In this condition, there is a flattening or depression of the longitudinal arch **(pes planus)** while the foot is in the midsupport phase, resulting in a strain to the arch.[24] Such a strain may appear

### Figure 14-11

A metatarsal bar (felt pad)
placed just proximal to
(behind) the metatarsal heads
is used to reduce
metatarsalgia (plantar view).

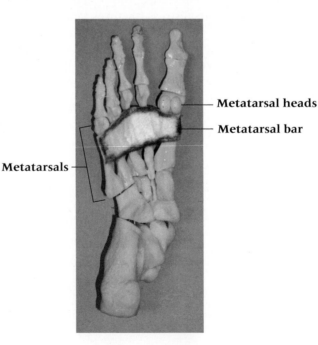

Metatarsal heads

Metatarsal bar

Metatarsals

**Figure 14-12**

Fallen medial longitudinal arch

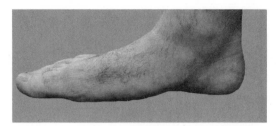

suddenly, or it may develop slowly over a considerable length of time. It should be added that some people have a congenital pes planus or pes carus (high arch) which do not cause pain.

**Signs of injury** As a rule, pain is experienced only when running is attempted and usually appears just below the medial malleolus and the posterior tibial tendon, accompanied by swelling and tenderness along the medial aspects of the foot. Prolonged strain will also involve the calcaneonavicular ligament and first cuneiform with the navicular. The flexor muscle of the great toe (flexor hallucis longus) often develops tenderness as a result of overuse in compensating for the stress on the ligaments.

Many people have what appears to be a flat foot or a fallen longitudinal arch with no associated symptoms or pain whatsoever. In these cases the rule that should always be followed is "If it's not broken, don't try to fix it" (Figure 14-12).

**Care** The management of a longitudinal arch strain involves immediate care consisting of PRICE followed by appropriate therapy and reduction of weight bearing. Weight bearing must be performed pain-free. Arch taping might be used to allow earlier pain-free weight bearing.

### Fractures and Dislocations of the Toes (Phalanges)

**Cause of injury** Fractures of the phalanges may be incurred by kicking an object or stubbing a toe or dropping a heavy object on the toes.

**Signs of injury** Generally fractures and dislocations of the phalanges are accompanied by swelling and discoloration. If the fracture is to the proximal phalanx of the great toe or to the distal phalanx and also involves the interphalangeal joint, the injury should be referred to a physician.

**Care** If the break is in the bone shaft, adhesive tape is applied. However, if more than one toe is involved, a cast may be applied for a few days. As a rule, 3 or 4 weeks of inactivity permit healing, although tenderness may persist for some time. A shoe with a wide toe box should be worn; in cases of great toe fracture, a stiff sole should be worn.

Dislocations of the phalanges are less common than fractures. If one occurs, it is usually a dislocation of the proximal joint of the middle phalanx. The mechanism of injury is the same as for fractures. Reduction is usually performed easily without anesthesia by a physician.

Fractures and dislocations of the toes can be caused by kicking an object or stubbing a toe.

**14-2 Critical Thinking**
Exercise

A field hockey player complains of swelling, tenderness, and aching in the head of the first metatarsophalangeal joint of her left foot. On inspection, the great toe is deviated laterally.

? What is this condition commonly called, and why does it occur?

**Figure 14-13**

A hallux valgus deformity
with a bunion

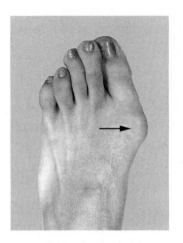

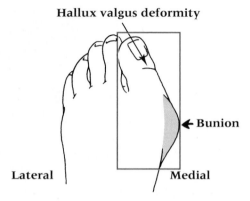

Hallux valgus deformity

← Bunion

Lateral          Medial

## Bunions (Hallux Valgus Deformity)

**Cause of injury**  A bunion, also referred to as an exostosis, is a painful deformity of the head of the first metatarsal.[10] A bunion involves bony enlargement of the head of the first metatarsal that progresses to the point at which the great toe becomes malaligned and moves laterally toward the second toe, sometimes to such an extent that it eventually overlaps the second toe, creating what is called a hallux valgus deformity (Figure 14-13).[14] This type of bunion may also be associated with a depressed or flattened transverse arch. Often the bunion occurs from wearing shoes that are pointed, too narrow, too short, or have high heels.

**Signs of injury**  A bunion is one of the most frequent painful deformities of the great toe. As the bunion is developing, there is tenderness, swelling, and enlargement with calcification of the head of the first metatarsal. Poorly fitting shoes increase the irritation and pain.

**Care**  Shoe selection plays an important role in the treatment of bunions. Shoes of the proper width cause less irritation to the bunion. Protective devices such as some type of doughnut pad over the bunion help disperse pressure, and tape can also be used. If the condition progresses, a special orthotic device may help normalize foot mechanics and significantly reduce the symptoms and progression of a bunion. Surgery to correct the hallux valgus deformity is very common during the later stages of this condition.[10]

## Morton's Neuroma

**Cause of condition**  A **neuroma** is a mass occurring in the common plantar nerve. It occurs most commonly between the third and fourth metatarsal heads, where the nerve is the thickest because it is receiving both branches from the medial and lateral plantar nerves (Figure 14-14).[14]

---

**14-3 Critical Thinking**
Exercise

A soccer player complains of intermittent pain in the region between the third and fourth toes of the left foot. Pain along with tingling and numbness seems to radiate from the base to the tip of the toes during weight bearing.

? What condition usually causes these symptoms and how can it be managed?

---

**neuroma**
Enlargement of a nerve.

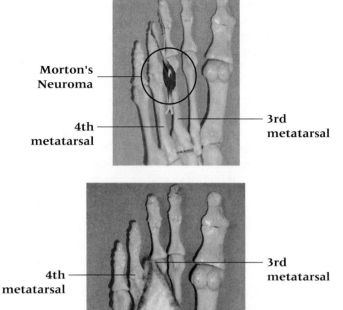

**Figure 14-14**

A Morton's neuroma usually occurs between the third and fourth metatarsal heads.

Morton's Neuroma

4th metatarsal

3rd metatarsal

**Figure 14-15**

A teardrop-shaped pad placed between the 3rd and 4th matatarsal heads will spread them apart during weight bearing, taking pressure off the neuroma.

4th metatarsal

3rd metatarsal

**Signs of condition**   The athlete complains of severe intermittent pain radiating from the distal metatarsal heads to the tips of the toes; the pain is often relieved when the foot is not bearing weight.[18] The athlete complains of a burning numbness in the forefoot that is often localized to the third web space and radiating to the toes.[13] Hyperextension of the toes on weight bearing, as in squatting, stair climbing, or running, can increase the symptoms. Wearing shoes with a narrow toe box or high heel can increase the symptoms.

**Care**   Either a metatarsal bar (see Figure 14-11) is placed just proximal to the metatarsal heads or a teardrop-shaped pad is placed between the heads of the third and fourth metatarsals in an attempt to have these toes splay apart with weight bearing (Figure 14-15). Shoe selection also plays an important role in treatment of neuromas. A shoe that is wide in the toe box area should be selected.

## Turf Toe

**Cause of injury**   Turf toe is a hyperextension injury resulting in a sprain of the great toe, either from repetitive overuse or trauma.[16] Typically, these injuries occur on unyielding synthetic turf, although they can occur on grass also.[17] Many of these injuries occur because artificial turf shoes often are more flexible and allow more dorsiflexion of the great toe.

Some shoe companies have addressed this problem by adding steel or other materials to the forefoot of their turf shoes to stiffen them. A sprain of the great toe can also occur from kicking some nonyielding object.[4]

**Care**   Flat insoles that have thin sheets of steel under the forefoot are available. When commercially made products are not available, a thin, flat piece of thermoplastic material may be placed under the shoe insole or may be molded to the foot. Taping the toe to prevent dorsiflexion may be done separately or in addition to one of the shoe-stiffening suggestions (refer to Figure 11-14). In less severe cases, the athlete can continue to play with the addition of a rigid insole. With more severe sprains, 3 to 4 weeks may be required for pain to subside to the point at which the athlete can push off on the great toe.[17]

## Calluses

**Cause of condition**   Foot calluses may be caused by shoes that are too narrow or too short. Calluses that develop from friction can be painful because the fatty layer loses its elasticity and cushioning effect. The excess callus moves as a gross mass, becoming highly vulnerable to tears, cracks, and, ultimately, infections.[6] It is not uncommon for blisters to develop underneath a callus.

**Care**   Athletes who are prone to excess calluses should be encouraged to use an emery callus file after each shower. Massaging small amounts of lanolin into devitalized calluses once or twice a week after practice may help maintain some tissue elasticity. The coach may have the athlete decrease the calluses' thickness and increase their smoothness by sanding or pumicing. NOTE: *Great care should be taken not to remove the callus totally and the protection it affords at a given pressure point.*

Athletes whose shoes are properly fitted but who still develop heavy calluses commonly have faulty foot mechanics that may require special orthotics. Special cushioning devices such as wedges, doughnuts, and arch supports may help to distribute the weight on the feet more evenly and thus reduce skin stress. Excessive callus accumulation can be prevented by (1) wearing at least one layer of socks, (2) wearing shoes that are the correct size and in good condition, and (3) routinely applying materials such as petroleum jelly to reduce friction.

## Blisters

**Cause of injury**   As a result of shearing forces acting on the skin, blisters develop in which fluid accumulates below the outer skin layer. This fluid may be clear, or bloody. Soft feet coupled with this shearing skin stress can produce severe blisters. The application of a skin lubricant can protect the skin against abnormal friction. Wearing socks with no folds or wrinkles can protect the athlete with sensitive skin or the one who perspires excessively.[2] Wearing the correct-size shoe is essential. Shoes should be broken in before being used for long periods.

**Care**   If a blister or hot spot arises, the athlete has several options: (1) cover the irritated skin with a friction-proofing material, such as skin

◁◯ **14-4 Critical Thinking**
Exercise

A football player who both practices and plays on artificial turf complains of pain in his right great toe.

? What type of injury frequently occurs to the great toe when competing on artificial turf?

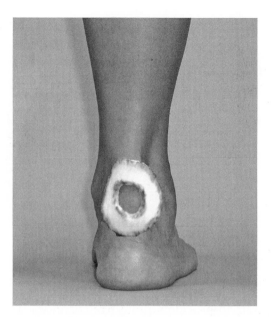

**Figure 14-16**

A blister should be padded using a felt doughnut pad to take pressure off the blister and provide relief.

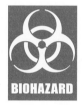

lubricant, (2) cover the blister with an adhesive bandage, or (3) apply a doughnut pad that surrounds the blister.

When caring for a blister, there is always a possibility of infection from contamination. Any blister that appears to be infected requires medical attention. In sports, two approaches are generally used to care for blisters. The conservative approach is that a blister should not be contaminated by cutting or puncturing but should be protected from further insult by a small doughnut until the initial irritation has subsided (Figure 14-16). However, the pressure of the fluid inside the blister can often be extremely painful and in some cases debilitating. Puncturing may be necessary to allow the athlete to continue to play or practice but should only be done by athletic trainers or physicians. Focus Box 14-1 details the technique for opening a blister. Conservative care of blisters is

---

14-1    *Focus Box*

**Caring for a Torn Blister**

1. Cleanse the blister and surrounding tissue with soap and water; rinse with an antiseptic.
2. If the blister is open, drain the fluid using a sterile gauze pad.
3. Apply antibiotic ointment under and around the loose skin; cover the area with a sterile dressing.
4. Apply a doughnut pad around blister.
5. Change dressing daily and check for signs of infection.
6. Within 2 or 3 days, or when the underlying tissue has hardened sufficiently, remove the dead skin by trimming as close as possible to the perimeter of the blister.

**Figure 14-17**

(A) Hard corns appear on the top of a toe and are usually associated with hammer toes. (B) Soft corns usually appear between the fourth and fifth toes.

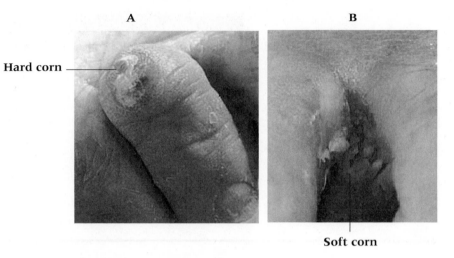

**A**   **B**

Hard corn ——————

Soft corn

preferred when there is little danger of tearing or aggravation through activity. A product called Second Skin by Spenco is widely used on blisters to provide a protective coating.

## Corns

**Cause of condition**   The hard corn is the most serious type of corn. It is caused by the pressure of improperly fitting shoes, the same mechanism that causes calluses. Hammer toes and hard corns are usually associated; the hard corns form on the tops of the deformed toes. The soft corn is the result of a combination of wearing narrow shoes and excessive foot perspiration (Figure 14-17).[6]

**Signs of condition**   The corn usually forms between the fourth and fifth toes. A circular area of thickened, white, macerated skin appears between and at the base of the toes. There also appears to be a black dot in the center of the corn. Both pain and inflammation are likely to be present. Symptoms are local pain and disability, with inflammation and thickening of soft tissue.

**Care**   When caring for a soft corn, the best procedure is to have the athlete wear properly fitting shoes, keep the skin between the toes clean and dry, and decrease pressure by keeping the toes separated with cotton or lamb's wool. The athlete, to treat a hard corn, should soak feet daily in warm, soapy water to soften the corn. To alleviate further irritation, the corn should be protected by a small felt or sponge rubber doughnut.

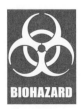

BIOHAZARD

## Ingrown Toenails

**Cause of condition**   An ingrown toenail is a condition in which the leading side edge of the toenail has grown into the soft tissue nearby, usually resulting in severe inflammation and infection[1] (Figure 14-18).

**Signs of condition**   The classic signs of infection are swelling, heat, aching, redness, and accumulation of pus.

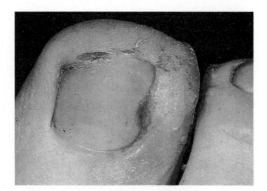

**Figure 14-18**

Ingrown toenail

**Care**   It is important that the athlete's shoes be of the proper length and width, because continued pressure on a toenail can lead to serious irritation or cause it to become ingrown. In most cases, ingrown toenails can be prevented by trimming the nails correctly. The nail must be trimmed so that its margins do not penetrate the tissue on the sides. Also, the nail should be left sufficiently long that it is clear of the underlying tissue but should be cut short enough that it is not irritated by either shoes or socks. Cutting a "V" notch in the toenail toward the infected side will allow the nail to grow more toward the middle. Focus Box 14-2 details the care for an ingrown toenail.

## Blood under the Toenail (Subungual hematoma)

**Cause of injury**   Blood can accumulate under a toenail as a result of the toe being stepped on, of dropping an object on the toe, or of kicking another object. Repetitive shearing forces on toenails, as may occur in the shoe of a long-distance runner, may also cause bleeding into the nail bed. In any case, blood that accumulates in a confined space underneath the nail is likely to produce extreme pain and can ultimately cause loss of the nail[1] (Figure 14-19).

**Signs of injury**   Bleeding into the nail bed may be either immediate or slow, producing considerable pain. The area under the toenail

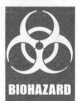

**BIOHAZARD**

---

**14-2**   *Focus Box*

**Managing the Ingrown Toenail**

1. Soak the toe in hot water (110° to 120° F) (43.3° to 48.8°C) for approximately 20 minutes, two or three times daily.
2. When the nail is soft and pliable, use forceps to insert a wisp of cotton under the edge of the nail and lift it from the soft tissue.
3. Continue this procedure until the nail has grown out sufficiently to be trimmed straight across.

An ingrown toenail can easily become infected. If this occurs, the athlete should be immediately referred to a physician for treatment.

**Figure 14-19**

A subungual hematoma is blood accumulating under the nail.

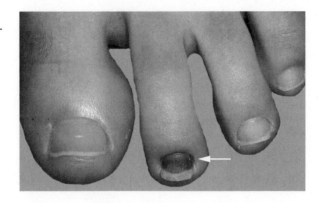

assumes a bluish-purple color and gentle pressure on the nail greatly exacerbates pain.

**Care** An ice pack should be applied immediately, and the foot should be elevated to decrease bleeding. Within the next 12 to 24 hours, the pressure of the blood under the nail should be released by drilling a small hole though the nail into the nail bed. This drilling must be done under sterile conditions and is best done by either a physician or an athletic trainer. It is not uncommon to have to drill the nail a second time because more blood is likely to accumulate.

## SUMMARY

- The human foot must function both to absorb forces and to provide a stable base of support during walking, running, and jumping.
- The twenty-six bones in the foot are held together by an intricate network of ligaments and fascia and are moved by a complicated group of muscles.
- Foot injuries may be prevented by selecting appropriate footwear and using various orthotic devices inserted into the shoe to protect the foot from abnormal forces, stresses, and strains.
- A pump bump develops from chronic retrocalcaneal bursitis on the back of the heel.
- Plantar fasciitis is pain in the anterior medial heel, usually at the attachment of the plantar fascia to the calcaneus. Orthotics in combination with stretching exercises can significantly reduce pain.
- A Jones fracture is a fracture of the neck of the fifth metatarsal that often results in delayed healing.
- The most common stress fracture in the foot involves the second metatarsal (march fracture).
- Metatarsal and longitudinal arch sprains are best treated by inserting appropriate support pads into the shoes.

- A bunion is a deformity of the head of the first metatarsal in which the large toe assumes a hallux valgus position.
- To treat a Morton's neuroma, a metatarsal bar is placed just proximal to the metatarsal heads or a teardrop-shaped pad is placed between the heads of the third and fourth metatarsals in an attempt to have these toes splay apart with weight bearing.
- Turf toe is a hyperextension injury resulting in a sprain of the great toe.
- The foot within the shoe can sustain forces that produce calluses, blisters, corns, or ingrown toenails.

---

*Solutions to Critical Thinking* Exercises

---

**14-1** These complaints are most typically associated with plantar fasciitis, which can be treated with a combination of vigorous heel cord stretching, stretching the plantar fascia in the arch, using a heel cup, arch taping, and using an orthotic with increased arch support.

**14-2** This condition is a bunion or hallux valgus deformity. It is associated with wearing shoes that are too pointed, narrow, or short. It may begin with an inflamed bursa over the metatarsophalangeal joint. It can be associated with a depressed transverse arch or a pronated foot.

**14-3** Most likely the athlete has a Morton's neuroma. A metatarsal bar or a teardrop-shaped pad applied in the correct position on the sole of the foot can help to spread the metatarsal heads apart and take pressure off the neuroma, reducing the symptoms.

**14-4** A sprain of the great toe is often referred to as turf toe. It results from a hyperextension of the great toe and usually occurs in athletes playing on artificial turf.

## REVIEW QUESTIONS AND CLASS ACTIVITIES

1. Briefly describe the anatomy of the foot.
2. In evaluating an acute condition in the foot region, what general observations can be made?
3. What measures can be taken to prevent foot injuries?
4. What is the relationship between a pump bump and retrocalcaneal bursitis?
5. What is a Jones fracture, and why does it take so long to heal?
6. How is it possible for a heel bruise to lead to plantar fasciitis?
7. How are stress fractures of the second metatarsal managed?
8. Discuss how various arch sprains can be treated.
9. What injuries may potentially result from wearing shoes that are too tight?
10. How does a Morton's toe differ from a Morton's neuroma?
11. How would you care for a chronic case of turf toe?
12. What is the recommended procedure in caring for a blister on the foot?

### REFERENCES

1. Adams BB: 1999. Running-related toenail abnormality, *Physician and sportsmedicine* 27(13):85.
2. Are you taking good care of your feet? Over-the-counter remedies can relieve minor aches and pains,

2002. *Tufts University health & nutrition letter* 20(7):6.

3. Bender, JA: 2000. Fifth metatarsal fractures: diagnosis and management, *Sports medicine alert* 6(3):18–20.

4. Bender, JA: 2000. Turf toe injuries: correctly diagnosing an uncommon injury, *Sports medicine alert* 6(4):28–29.

5. Brukner, P: 2002. Foot pain. In Brukner, P (ed), *Clinical sports medicine*, 2nd ed, pp. 584–601, Sydney, McGraw-Hill.

6. Burkhart, CG: 1999. Skin disorders of the foot in active patients, *Physician and sportsmedicine* 27(2): 88.

7. Cornwall, MW: 2000. Common pathomechanics of the foot, *Athletic therapy today* 5(1):10.

8. Cornwall, MW, McPoil, TG: 1999. Plantar fasciitis: etiology and treatment, *The journal of orthopaedic & sports physical therapy* 29(12):756.

9. Coughlin, MI: 1995. Forefoot disorders. In Baxter DE, editor: *The foot and ankle in sports*, St Louis, Mosby.

10. Coughlin, M, Jones, C: 2007. Hallux valgus: demographics, etiology, and radiographic assessment. *Foot & ankle international* 28(7):759–777.

11. Dolan, MG: 2000. The use of foot orthotic devices in clinical practice, *Athletic therapy today* 5(1):17.

12. Finestone, A, Novack, V, Farfel, A: 2004. A prospective study of the effect of foot orthoses composition and fabrication on comfort and the incidence of overuse injuries, *Foot & ankle international* 25(7):462–466.

13. Gulick, DT: 2002. Differential diagnosis of Morton's neuroma, *Athletic therapy today* 7(1):39–42.

14. Hunter, S, Prentice, W, Zinder, S: 2010. Rehabilitation of ankle and foot injuries. In Prentice, WE, editor: *Rehabilitation techniques in sports medicine and athletic training*, ed 4, New York, McGraw-Hill.

15. Jaivin, JS: 2000. Foot injuries and arthroscopy in sport, *Sports Medicine* 29(1):65.

16. Mann, RA: 1995. Great toe disorders. In Baxter, DE, editor: *The foot and ankle in sports*, St Louis, Mosby.

17. McGraw, E: 2008. Turf toe, *Coach & athletic director* 77(7):34.

18. Metzl, J: 2008. Morton's neuroma: A common cause of foot pain. *Triathlete* 293:30.

19. Peterson, JA: 2002. 10 steps for preventing and treating foot problems, *ACSM's health & fitness journal* 6(2):44.

20. Petrisor, B, Ekrol, I: 2006. The epidemiology of metatarsal fractures. *Foot & ankle international* 27(3):172–174.

21. Pfeffer, GB: 1995. Plantar heel pain. In Baxter, DE, editor: *The foot and ankle in sport*, St Louis, Mosby.

22. Ryan, G: 2007. How to manage plantar fasciitis. In MacAuley, D. (ed.). Evidence-based sports medicine, Malden, MA, Blackwell.

23. Shea, M: 2002. Plantar fasciitis: prescribing effective treatments, *Physician and sports medicine* 30(7):21–25.

24. Sherman, KP: 1999. The foot in sport, *British journal of sports medicine* 33(1):6.

25. Springer, BL: 2004. Time wounds all heels: learn to recognize symptoms of common foot injuries before they turn into problems for you or your clients, *IDEA fitness journal* 1(4):58–65.

26. Tiller, R: 2002. Prevention of common pes problems, *Athletic therapy today* 7(6):52–53.

27. Weatherford, ML: 2001. *Podiatry sourcebook*, Detroit, Omnigraphics.

## ANNOTATED BIBLIOGRAPHY

Alexander, I: 1997. *The foot: examination and diagnosis,* New York, Churchill-Livingston.

*Practical guide to clinical care of the foot and ankle. Presents anatomy, biomechanics, and a systematic approach to evaluation. Discusses common complaints.*

Baxter, DE: 1995. *The foot and ankle in sport,* St Louis, 1995, Mosby.

*A complete medical text on all aspects of the foot and ankle. It covers common sports syndromes, anatomical disorders in sports, unique problems, shoes, orthoses, and rehabilitation.*

Tremaine, MD, Elias, M: 1998. *The foot and ankle source book: everything you need to know,* Lowell House.

*Discusses common problems affecting feet and ankles; from bunions and corns to flat feet and sports injuries. Surveys the range of problems, preventive treatments, orthopedic inserts, and other health solutions to foot ailments, providing an uncommon range of disorders and treatments ranging from self-help to surgery.*

Weatherford, ML: 2001. *Podiatry sourcebook,* Detroit, Omnigraphics.

# The Ankle and Lower Leg

*When you finish this chapter you will be able to:*

- Describe the bony, ligamentous, and muscular anatomy of the ankle and lower leg.
- List considerations for preventing injuries to the ankle and lower leg.
- Explain how to assess common ankle and lower leg injuries.
- Identify the possible causes and signs of various injuries that can occur in the ankle and lower leg.
- Examine the procedures that can be used in caring for ankle and lower leg injuries.

The ankle joint is composed of the
- tibia
- fibula
- talus

## ANKLE AND LOWER LEG ANATOMY

### Bones

The portion of the anatomy below the knee and above the ankle is the lower leg. It is composed of the thicker tibia, which is more medial, and the thinner fibula, which is more lateral. The ankle joint or *talocrural joint* is formed by the thickened distal portion of the fibula, called the lateral malleolus; the thickened distal portion of the tibia, called the medial malleolus; and the more-or-less cube-shaped tarsal bone, called the talus, that fits between the two malleoli. The ankle joint allows two motions: plantarflexion and dorsiflexion. The joint between the talus and the calcaneous is called the *subtalar joint*. Inversion and eversion take place at the *subtalar joint* (Figure 15-1).

The talocrural joint allows two motions:
- plantarflexion
- dorsiflexion

### Ligaments

The tibia and fibula are held together by the interosseous membrane, which extends the entire length of the two bones. The anterior and posterior tibiofibular ligaments bridge the tibia and fibula and form the distal portion of the interosseous membrane. The medial aspect of the ankle is relatively stable because of the thick deltoid ligament. The presence of this strong deltoid ligament combined with the fact that the lateral malleolus of the fibula extends further distally than the medial malleolus limits the ability of the ankle to evert. Thus eversion ankle sprains are considerably less common than inversion sprains. The three lateral ligaments include the anterior talofibular, the posterior talofibular, and the calcaneofibular. The lateral ligaments collectively limit inversion and are much more susceptible to injury (Figure 15-2).

The subtalar joint allows two motions:
- inversion
- eversion

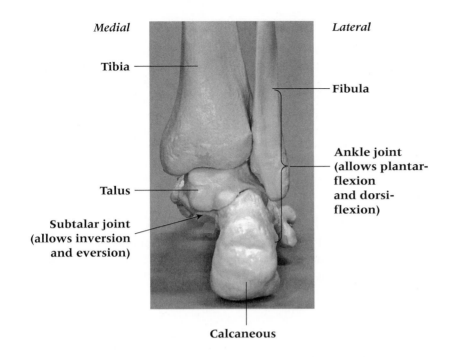

*Medial*        *Lateral*

Tibia

Fibula

Ankle joint
(allows plantar-
flexion
and dorsi-
flexion)

Talus

Subtalar joint
(allows inversion
and eversion)

Calcaneous

**Figure 15-1**

The ankle joint is formed by
the tibia, fibula, and talus.
The subtalar joint is formed
by the talus and calcaneus.

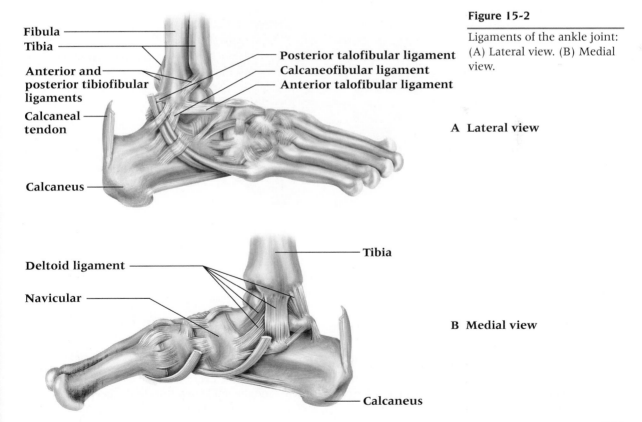

Fibula
Tibia

Anterior and
posterior tibiofibular
ligaments

Calcaneal
tendon

Posterior talofibular ligament
Calcaneofibular ligament
Anterior talofibular ligament

Calcaneus

**A  Lateral view**

Deltoid ligament

Navicular

Tibia

**B  Medial view**

Calcaneus

**Figure 15-2**

Ligaments of the ankle joint:
(A) Lateral view. (B) Medial
view.

Recognition and
Management of Specific
Injuries and Conditions

Medial ligament includes the
deltoid.

Lateral ligaments include the
• anterior talofibular
• posterior talofibular
• calcaneofibular

Preventing lower leg and
ankle injuries:
• heel cord stretching
• strength training
• neuromuscular control
• appropriate footwear
• ankle taping and bracing

## Muscles

Contraction of the muscles in the lower leg produces movement at the ankle joint. The muscles of the lower leg are divided into four distinct groups (Figure 15-3). Each of the four muscle groups is contained separately within a compartment by thick sheets of fascia (connective tissue) which surround them. Essentially the muscles that dorsiflex the ankle are contained within the anterior compartment, the muscles that plantarflex the ankle are in the superficial posterior compartment, the muscles that evert the ankles are in the lateral compartment, and the muscles that invert the ankle are found in the deep posterior compartment (Table 15-1).

## PREVENTION OF LOWER LEG AND ANKLE INJURIES

Many lower leg and ankle injuries, especially sprains, can be reduced by Achilles tendon stretching, strengthening of key muscles, improving neuromuscular control, choosing appropriate footwear, and, when necessary, proper taping or bracing.[3,12,13]

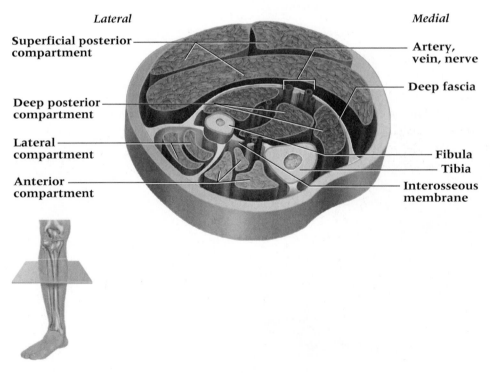

**Figure 15-3**

The muscles of the lower leg are divided into four distinct groups contained separately within individual compartments: the ankle dorsiflexors in the anterior compartment, the ankle evertors in the lateral compartment, the ankle plantar flexors in the superficial posterior compartment, and the ankle invertors in the deep posterior compartment.

| TABLE 15-1 Muscles of the Ankle Joint | |
|---|---|
| Ankle dorsiflexion (Anterior compartment) | Extensor digitorum longus<br>Extensor hallucis longus<br>Tibialis anterior (primary dorsiflexor) |
| Ankle plantarflexion (Superficial posterior compartment) | Soleus<br>Gastrocnemius |
| Ankle inversion (Deep posterior compartment) | Tibialis posterior<br>Flexor digitorum longus<br>Flexor hallucis longus |
| Ankle eversion (Lateral compartment) | Peroneus longus<br>Peroneus brevis |

### Achilles Tendon Complex Stretching

The athlete with a tight Achilles tendon complex should routinely stretch before and after practice.[20] To properly stretch the Achilles tendon complex, the ankle should be dorsiflexed and the knee fully extended to stretch the gastrocnemius muscle, and then the knee should be flexed to about 30 degrees to stretch the soleus muscle (Figure 15-4). There should be at least 10 degrees of dorsiflexion for normal ankle motion to occur.

### Strength Training

Achieving both static and dynamic joint stability through strength training is critical in preventing ankle injury (Figure 15-5). A balance in

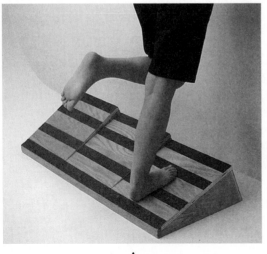
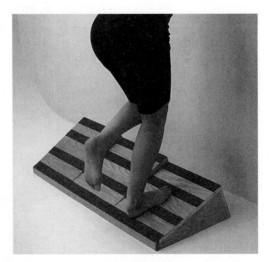

A                                                    B

**Figure 15-4**

Stretching techniques for the left Achilles tendon complex: (A) Stretching position for the gastrocnemius muscle. (B) Stretching position for the soleus muscle.

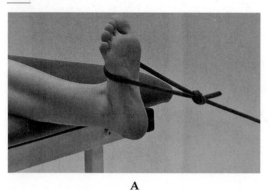 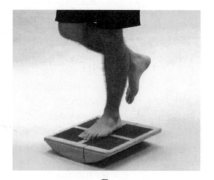

| A | B |

**Figure 15-5**

Strengthening exercises are important in prevention of ankle sprains and may be done using (A) surgical tubing resistance or (B) a wobble board.

strength throughout the full range of motion must be developed and maintained in each of the four muscle groups that surround the ankle joint.[28] Strengthening exercises should be done in eversion and inversion, which can be done by rocking the ankle back and forth on a wobble board, and also in using surgical tubing.

## Neuromuscular Control

As is the case with strength training, maintaining neuromuscular control is critical to prevention of injury to the ankle joint. Neuromuscular control relies on the central nervous system to interpret and integrate proprioceptive and kinesthetic information and then to control individual muscles and joints to produce coordinated movements that collectively protect the joint from injury. Thus, the foot and ankle must respond quickly to any uneven surface condition. Ankle joint position sense can be enhanced by training on uneven surfaces or by spending time each day on a balance board (Figure 15-6).

## Footwear

As discussed in Chapters 6 and 14, proper footwear can be an important factor in reducing injuries to both the foot and the ankle. Shoes should not be used in activities for which they were not intended—for example, running shoes, which are designed for straight-ahead activity,

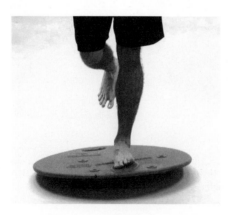

**Figure 15-6**

Unilateral stance on BAPS board.

should not be worn to play basketball, a sport demanding a great deal of lateral movement.

## Preventive Ankle Taping and Bracing

There is some doubt about whether it is beneficial to routinely tape ankles that have no history of sprain. Tape, properly applied, can provide some prophylactic protection. Poorly applied tape does more harm than good. Tape that constricts soft tissue and blood circulation or disrupts normal biomechanical function can, in time, create unnecessary problems.[8]

Ankle bracing can also offer protection to the ankle joint (Figure 15-7).[7] Braces may prevent lateral and inversion movement of the foot without inhibiting plantarflexion (see Chapter 6).[10] Lace-up supports and semirigid ankle braces are increasingly being used instead of tape to prevent recurrent ankle sprains.

## ASSESSING THE ANKLE JOINT

**Generally fitness professionals, coaches, and others working in areas related to exercise and sport science are not adequately trained to evaluate injuries. It is strongly recommended that injured athletes be referred to qualified medical personnel (i.e., physicians, athletic trainers, physical therapists) for injury evaluation.** Information on the following special tests has been included simply to give some idea about the different basic tests that nonmedical personnel may do to determine the nature and severity of the athlete's injury. The primary responsibility of those who are not health care personnel is to be able to recognize any potential "red flags" associated with

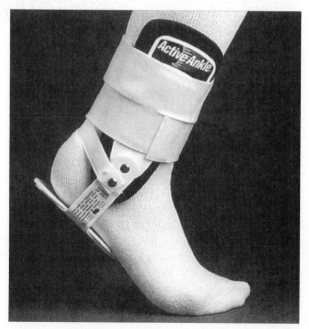

**Figure 15-7**

Ankle braces may be used to support weak ankles.

the injury, provide appropriate first aid for the injury, and make correct decisions about how the injury should be managed initially, including immediate return to play or activity decisions (refer to Chapter 7).

## History

The athlete's history may vary, depending on whether the problem is the result of sudden trauma or is chronic. The athlete with an acute sudden trauma to the ankle should be asked the following questions:

- What trauma or mechanism occurred?
- What was heard when the injury occurred—a crack, snap, or pop?
- What were the duration and intensity of pain?
- How disabling was the occurrence? Could the athlete walk right away, or was he or she unable to bear weight for a time?
- Has a similar injury occurred before?
- Was there immediate swelling, or did the swelling occur later (or at all)? Where did the swelling occur?
- What past ankle injuries have occurred?

## Observation

In an initial look at the ankle, the athletic trainer determines the following:

- Is there an obvious deformity?
- Are the bony contours of the ankle normal and symmetrical, or is there a deviation such as a bony deformity?
- Is there any discoloration?
- Is there crepitus or abnormal sound in the ankle joint?
- Is heat, swelling, or redness present?
- Is the athlete in obvious pain?
- Does the athlete have a normal ankle range of motion?
- If the athlete is able to walk, is there a normal walking pattern, or does the athlete walk with a limp?

## Palpation

Palpation in the ankle region should start with key bony landmarks and ligaments and progress to the musculature, especially the major ligaments that surround the ankle. The purpose of palpation in this region is to detect obvious structural deformities, swelling, and localized tenderness.

## Special Tests for Ankle Injuries

**Bump test**   When fracture is suspected, a gentle percussive blow can be applied upward on the bottom of the heel. Such blows set up a vibratory force that resonates at the fracture, causing pain (Figure 15-8A).

**Anterior drawer test**   The anterior drawer test is used to determine the extent of injury to the anterior talofibular ligament primarily and to the other lateral ligaments secondarily (Figure 15-8B). The coach grasps

**◁◁ 15-1 Critical Thinking**
Exercise

A basketball player sustains a grade 1 inversion sprain of her left ankle during a game. There is immediate pain and swelling, and she is unable to bear weight.

? What is the most important first-aid goal immediately following injury, and how may that first-aid goal best be accomplished?

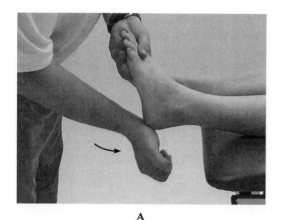

**A**

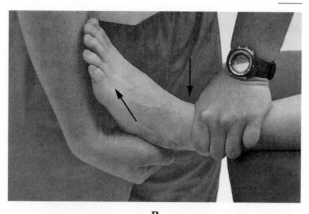

**B**

**C**

**Figure 15-8**

Special tests for ankle
injuries: (A) Bump test.
(B) Anterior drawer test.
(C) Talar tilt test.

the lower tibia in one hand and the calcaneus in the palm of the other hand. The tibia is then pushed backward as the calcaneus is pulled forward. A positive anterior drawer sign occurs when the foot slides forward.

**Talar tilt test** Talar tilt tests are used to determine the extent of inversion or eversion injuries. With the foot positioned at 90 degrees to the lower leg and stabilized, the calcaneus is inverted. Excessive motion of the talus at 90° indicates injury to the calcaneofibular and possibly the anterior and posterior talofibular ligaments as well (Figure 15-8C). Excessive motion in inversion with the ankle plantarflexed indicates a sprain of the anterior talofibular ligament.

## Functional Examination

Muscle function is important in evaluating the ankle injury. If the athlete cannot execute or has difficulty performing the following functional activities, the athlete is not ready to return to activity:

- Walk on toes.
- Walk on heels.

- Hop on affected foot without heel touching surface.
- Start or stop the running motion.
- Change direction rapidly.
- Run figure eights.

## RECOGNITION AND MANAGEMENT OF INJURIES TO THE ANKLE

### Ankle Sprains

**Cause of injury**  Ankle sprains are among the more common injuries seen in athletics (Figure 15-9).[21] Injuries to the ligaments of the ankle may be classified by the mechanism of injury.[18]

**Inversion sprains**  An inversion ankle sprain is most common and often results in injury to the lateral ligaments. The anterior talofibular ligament is the weakest of the three lateral ligaments. It is injured in an inverted and plantarflexed position (Figure 15-10). The calcaneofibular and posterior talofibular ligaments are also likely to be injured in inversion sprains as the force of inversion is increased. Increased inversion force is needed to tear the calcaneofibular ligament (Figure 15-11).[13]

**Eversion sprains**  Eversion ankle sprains are less common than inversion ankle sprains largely because of the bony and ligamentous anatomy. Eversion injuries may involve an avulsion fracture of the tibia before the deltoid ligament tears. The deltoid ligament may also be contused in inversion sprains because of impingement between the medial malleolus and the calcaneus. Although eversion sprains are less common, these sprains may take longer to heal than do inversion sprains (Figure 15-12).[13]

**High ankle sprains**  The anterior and posterior tibiofibular ligaments and the distal portion of the interosseous membrane holding the tibia and fibula together are torn with forced hyperdorsiflexion and external rotation of the foot as when twisting on a planted foot. These structures are often injured in conjunction with a severe sprain of the medial and lateral ligament complexes. Sprains of these ligaments are

Ankle sprain classifications:
- inversion sprain
- eversion sprain
- high ankle sprain

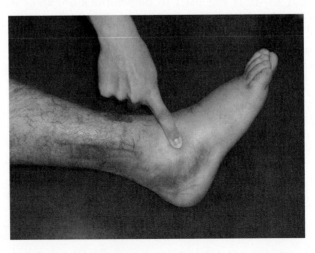

**Figure 15-9**

The ankle and usually the foot are swollen and discolored following an ankle sprain.

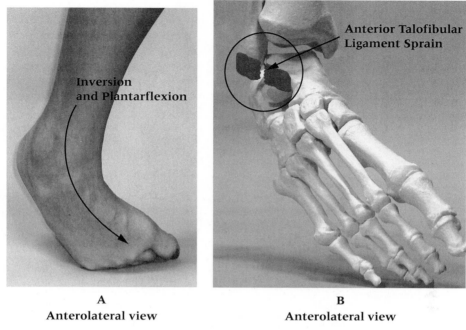

**A**
**Anterolateral view**

**B**
**Anterolateral view**

**Figure 15-10**

A mechanism of injury that involves (A) plantarflexion and inversion can (B) cause a sprain of the anterior talofibular ligament.

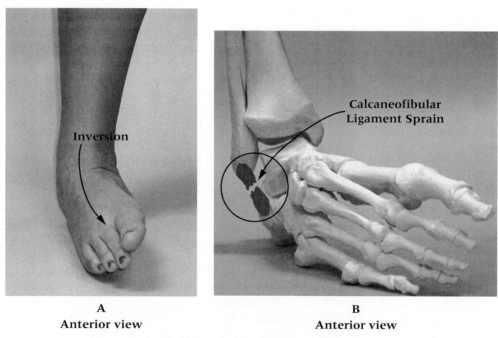

**A**
**Anterior view**

**B**
**Anterior view**

**Figure 15-11**

A mechanism of injury that involves (A) inversion can (B) cause a sprain of the calcaneofibular ligament.

**Figure 15-12**

A mechanism of injury that involves (A) eversion can (B) cause a sprain of the deltoid ligament.

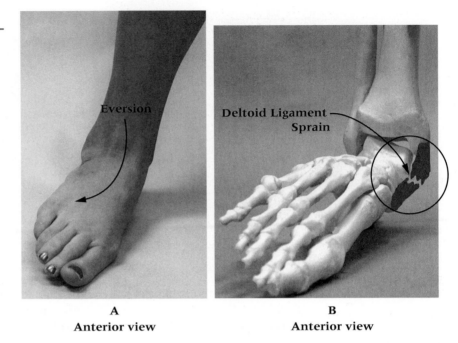

| A | B |
|---|---|
| **Anterior view** | **Anterior view** |

extremely hard to treat and often take months to heal. Return to sport may be delayed for a longer time than for inversion or eversion sprains (Figure 15-13).[13,27]

**Signs of injury**   In a grade 1 sprain, there is some stretching or perhaps tearing of the ligamentous fibers with little or no joint instability. Mild pain, little swelling, and joint stiffness may be apparent.

With a grade 2 sprain, there is some tearing and separation of the ligamentous fibers and moderate instability of the joint. Moderate-to-severe pain, swelling, and joint stiffness should be expected.

Grade 3 sprains involve total rupture of the ligament, manifested primarily by gross instability of the joint. Severe pain may be present initially, followed by little or no pain because of total disruption of nerve fibers. Swelling may be profuse, and thus the joint tends to become very stiff some hours after the injury. A grade 3 sprain with marked instability usually requires some form of immobilization lasting several weeks.[28] Surgical repair or reconstruction may be necessary to correct an instability.

**Care**   For ankle sprains, as for all acute musculoskeletal injuries, initial treatment efforts should be directed toward limiting the amount of swelling. This treatment is more essential for ankle sprains than for any other injury. Controlling initial swelling is the single most important treatment measure that can be taken during the entire rehabilitation process. Limiting the amount of acute swelling can significantly reduce the time required for rehabilitation. Initial management includes PRICE: protection, rest, ice, compression, and elevation.[13]

The technique described in Focus Box 15-1 should be followed exactly to be maximally effective in limiting swelling following ankle sprain.

The most important factor in rehabilitation of an ankle sprain is controlling initial swelling with PRICE.

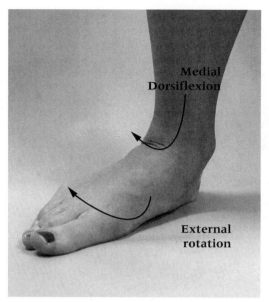

**A**
**Anteromedial view**

Medial
Dorsiflexion

External
rotation

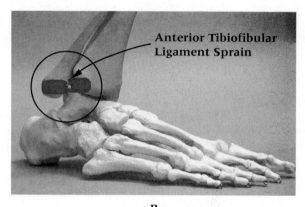

**Anterior Tibiofibular
Ligament Sprain**

**B**
**Anterolateral view**

**Figure 15-13**

A mechanism of injury that
involves (A) hyperdorsiflexion
and external rotation of the
foot can (B) cause a sprain of
the anterior tibiofibular
ligament.

---

**15-1 ▷ Focus Box**

---

**Technique for Controlling Swelling Immediately Following Injury**

- As soon as possible following the injury, cut out a horseshoe-shaped pad made of felt or foam and fit it around the malleolus on the side of injury. The horseshoe will provide focal compression in the injured area[24] (Figure 15-14A).

- Apply a wet compression wrap over this pad. Wetting the elastic wrap helps facilitate the passage of cold from ice packs. Wrapping should begin covering the toes and progress proximally, completely compressing the ankle joint and ending just below the level of the gastrocnemius muscle (Figure 15-14A).

- Surround the ankle joint entirely with ice bags and secure them in place with a second, dry, elastic wrap. Ice bags should be left on for 20 minutes initially and then 1 hour off and 20 minutes on as much as possible over the next 24 hours. During the following 72-hour period, ice should be applied as often as possible (Figure 15-14B).

- The foot and ankle should be elevated to a minimum of 45 degrees while icing. The ankle should be elevated as much as possible during the 72-hour period after injury. Keeping the injured part elevated while sleeping is particularly important (Figure 15-14C).

- The athlete should be placed on crutches to avoid weight bearing for a minimum of 24 hours following injury to allow the healing process to accomplish what it needs to (see Chapter 7). After 24 hours the athlete should be encouraged to begin weight bearing as soon as tolerated.

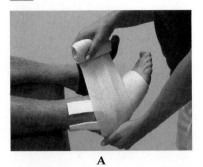
A

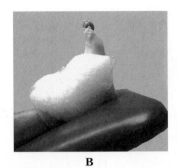
B

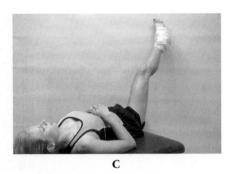
C

**Figure 15-14**

PRICE technique: (A) A wet compression wrap should be applied over the horseshoe pad; (B) Ice bags should be secured in place by a dry compression wrap; and (C) The leg should be elevated during the initial treatment period.

In the past, athletes were simply returned to sports once the pain was low enough to tolerate the activity. Returning to full activity should include a gradual progression of functional activities (i.e., walking, jogging, running, cutting, etc.) that slowly increase the stress on the ligament. The specific demands of each individual sport dictate the individual drills of this progression.[14,21]

Ideally, the athlete should return to sport without the aid of ankle support. However, it is common practice to wear some type of ankle support initially.[10] Ankle taping has a stabilizing effect on unstable ankles without interfering with motor performance. High-topped footwear may further stabilize the ankle. If cleated shoes are worn, cleats should be outset along the periphery of the shoe to provide stability. A protective ankle brace can also be worn for support as a substitute for taping.[10,13]

### Ankle Fractures

**Cause of injury** When assessing an ankle injury always be cautious about suspecting an ankle sprain when a fracture actually exists. Ankle fractures can occur from several mechanisms that are similar to those that cause ankle sprains.[17] In an inversion injury, medial malleolus fractures often occur along with a sprain of the lateral ligaments of the ankle. A fracture of the lateral malleolus is often more likely to occur than a sprain if an eversion force is applied to the ankle. With a fracture of the lateral malleolus, however, there may also be a sprain of the deltoid ligament. With avulsion injuries it is often the injured ligaments rather than the fracture that prolong the rehabilitation period (Figure 15-15).

**Signs of injury** A fracture of the malleoli generally results in immediate swelling. There is point tenderness over the bone and the athlete is apprehensive when asked to bear weight.

**Care** If the possibility of a fracture exists, splint the ankle and refer the athlete to the physician for x-ray examination and immobilization. Usually a physician treats fractures by casting the leg in a short walking cast for 6 weeks with early weight bearing. The course of rehabilitation following this period of immobilization is generally the same as for ankle sprains. Once near-normal levels of strength, flexibility, and

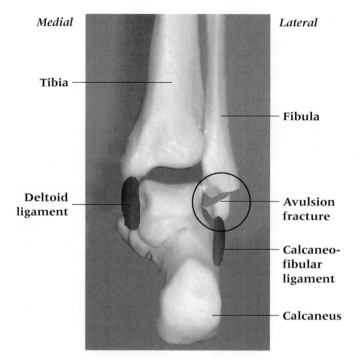

*Medial*

*Lateral*

Tibia

Fibula

Deltoid
ligament

Avulsion
fracture

Calcaneo-
fibular
ligament

Calcaneus

**Figure 15-15**

The mechanism that
produces an inverson ankle
sprain can also cause an
avulsion fracture of the fibula

neuromuscular control have been regained and the injured athlete can
perform functional activities, full activity may be resumed.[13]

## Tendinitis

**Cause of injury**  Inflammation of the tendons surrounding the
ankle joint is a common problem in athletes. The tendons most often
involved are the posterior tibialis tendon behind the medial malleolus, the anterior tibialis on the dorsal surface of the ankle, and the
peroneal tendons behind the lateral malleolus (Figure 15-16). Tendinitis in these tendons may result from one specific cause or from a
collection of mechanisms including faulty foot mechanics, inappropriate or poor footwear that can create faulty foot mechanics, acute
trauma to the tendon, tightness in the heel cord complex, or training
errors.[31]

**Signs of injury**  Athletes who develop tendinitis are likely to complain of pain with both active movement and passive stretching;
swelling around the area of the tendon caused by inflammation of the
tendon; crepitus on movement; and stiffness and pain following periods
of inactivity but particularly in the morning.[29]

**Care**  Techniques that reduce or eliminate inflammation, including rest, therapeutic modalities (ice), and anti-inflammatory medications, should be used. The use of an orthotic device to correct the
biomechanics or taping the foot may also be helpful in reducing stress
on the tendons.

common sites for tendinitis:
• Anterior tibialis
• Posterior tibialis
• Peroneals

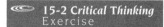

**15-2 Critical Thinking**
Exercise

A jogger, after running downhill
for an extended period, experiences pain in the anterior
medial aspect of the left foot.
The condition is diagnosed as
anterior tibialis tendinitis.

? How should this condition be
managed?

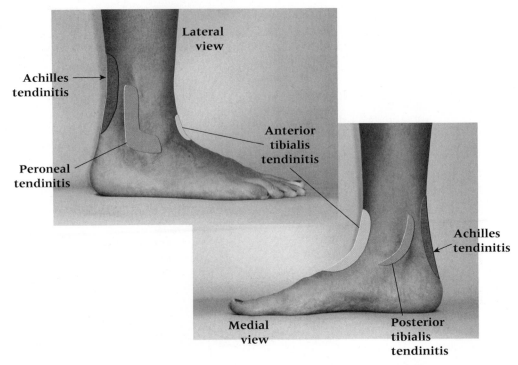

Lateral view

Achilles tendinitis

Peroneal tendinitis

Anterior tibialis tendinitis

Achilles tendinitis

Medial view

Posterior tibialis tendinitis

**Figure 15-16**

Common sites of tendinitis around the ankle

In many instances, if the mechanism that is causing the irritation and inflammation of the tendon is removed and the inflammatory process is allowed to run its normal course, the tendinitis will resolve within 10 days to 2 weeks. It is best to allow the athlete to rest for a sufficient time for tendon healing to take place.

## ASSESSING THE LOWER LEG

### History

An athlete who complains of discomfort in the lower leg region should be asked the following questions:

- How long has it been hurting?
- Where is the pain or discomfort?
- Has the feeling changed or is there numbness?
- Is there a feeling of warmth?
- Is there any sense of muscle weakness or difficulty in walking?
- How did the problem occur?

### Observation

The athlete is generally observed for the following:

- Any postural deviations, such as toeing in, should be noted.
- Any walking difficulty should be noted, along with leg deformities or swelling.

Palpation

Palpation should be done over the musculature in each of the four compartments. When fracture is suspected, a gentle percussive blow can be given to the tibia or fibula below or above the suspected site. Percussion can also be applied upward on the bottom of the heel. Such blows set up a vibratory force that resonates at the fracture, causing pain.

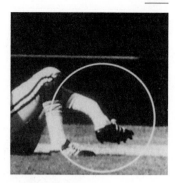

**Figure 15-17**

Fractures of the lower leg can be serious injuries.

## RECOGNITION AND MANAGEMENT OF INJURIES TO THE LOWER LEG

### Tibial and Fibular Fractures

**Cause of injury** The tibia and fibula constitute the bony components of the lower leg and are primarily responsible for weight bearing and muscle attachment. The tibia is the most commonly fractured long bone in the body; this injury is usually the result either of direct trauma to the area or of indirect trauma, such as a combination rotatory/compressive force. Fractures of the fibula are usually seen in combination with a tibial fracture or as a result of direct trauma to the area (Figure 15-17).

The tibia is more commonly fractured than the fibula.

**Signs of injury** Tibial fractures present with immediate pain, swelling, and possible deformity and may be open or closed. Fibular fractures alone are usually closed and present with pain and point tenderness on palpation and with ambulation.

**Care** Immediate treatment should include applying a splint to immobilize the fracture along with ice followed by immediate medical referral. Most likely a period of immobilization and restricted weight bearing is necessary for weeks to possibly months, depending on the severity and involvement of the injury.

### Tibial and Fibular Stress Fractures

**Cause of injury** Stress fractures of the tibia and fibula are common in sports. Studies indicate that tibial stress fractures occur at a higher rate than those of the fibula. Stress fractures in the lower leg are usually the result of repetitive loading during training and conditioning (Figure 15-18). Tibial stress fractures are prevalent in athletes involved with jumping.[2] (The progression of a stress fracture was discussed in Chapter 13.)

**Signs of injury** The athlete complains of pain with activity that sometimes becomes worse when activity is stopped. Focal point tenderness on the bone helps differentiate a stress fracture from medial tibial stress syndrome, which is located in the same area but is more diffuse. Tibial stress fractures usually occur in the middle of the shaft whereas fibular stress fractures are more likely to occur in the distal part of the bone.[11]

**Care** An athlete with a suspected stress fracture should be referred to a physician for diagnosis. The physician will most likely do a bone scan, looking for signs of inflammation. Immediate elimination of the

**Figure 15-18**

X-ray film of a stress fracture in the tibia

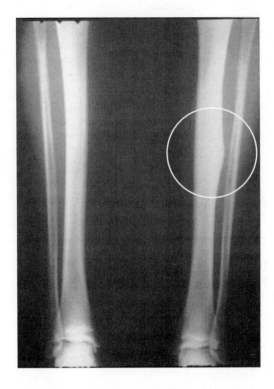

offending activity is most important. Generally recuperation requires about a 2-week period during which the athlete can continue to be weight bearing but must not engage in the activity that caused the problem in the first place. The athlete must be educated on the importance of adhering to this advice to prevent further damage to the bone. Progressively increasing stresses and strains can be placed on the bone so the athlete can gradually return to normal training.[4,9,29,32]

### Shin Splints (Medial Tibial Stress Syndrome)

| shin splints |
| --- |
| Medial tibial stress syndrome; anterior lower leg pain. |

**Cause of injury**  The term **shin splints** is a catchall that has traditionally referred to any type of pain in the anterior aspect of the lower leg. *Medial tibial stress syndrome,* as it is more correctly called, is a condition that involves increasing pain specifically at the distal two-thirds of the posterior medial aspect of the tibia[13,24] (Figure 15-19). A strain of the posterior tibialis muscle and its fascial sheath at its attachment to the periosteum of the distal tibia during running activities is the most likely mechanism for this injury.[9] Pain in the anterior shin could also be caused by other injuries or conditions, including stress fractures, compartment syndromes, or tendinitis.[9] Pain can arise secondary to a combination of faulty foot mechanics, tightness of the heel cord, muscle weakness, improper footwear, and training errors usually involving a change in running surfaces.[21,26]

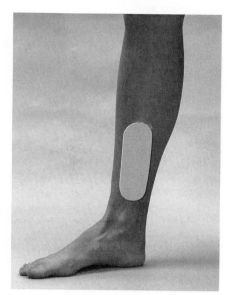

**Figure 15-19**

In medial tibial stress syndrome, the pain is usually located on the medial aspect of the lower leg just posterior to the tibia (shaded area). Pain is most often associated with the posterior tibialis muscle.

**Signs of injury** Pain is usually diffuse about the distal medial tibia and the surrounding soft tissues. Initially, the area may only hurt after an intense workout. As the condition worsens, daily ambulation may be painful and morning pain and stiffness may be present. Medial tibial stress syndrome can progress to a stress fracture if not treated appropriately.[19]

**Care** Management of this condition should include physician referral to rule out the possibility of stress fracture via the use of bone scan and plain films. Activity modification along with measures to maintain cardiovascular fitness are set in place immediately. Correction of abnormal foot mechanics during walking and running must also be addressed with shoes and, if needed, custom foot orthotics. Ice massage to the area may be helpful in the reduction of localized pain and inflammation. A stretching program for the heel cord should be initiated (refer to Figure 15-4). Occasionally, supportive taping to the longitudinal arch might be helpful[12] (refer to Figure 11-12).

### Shin Contusions

**Cause of injury** The shin (tibia), lying just under the skin, is exceedingly vulnerable and sensitive to blows or bumps. Because of the absence of muscular or adipose padding, force is not dissipated and the periosteum receives the impact delivered to the shin. Shin contusions occur frequently in soccer, and the incidence can be minimized by wearing appropriate shin guards (refer to Figure 6-23).

**Signs of injury** The athlete complains of intense pain, swelling, and increased warmth. A bulging hematoma with a jellylike consistency develops rapidly. In some instances the hematoma may increase to the size of a golf ball (Figure 15-20).

Severe blows to an unprotected shin can lead to a chronic inflammation.

**Figure 15-20**

A serious shin contusion can cause a compartment syndrome.

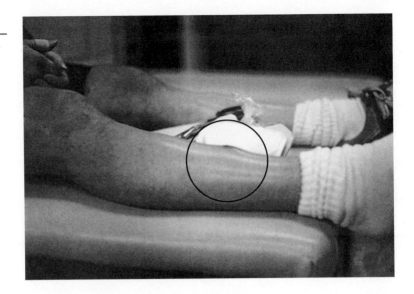

**Care** A compressive wrap along with ice and elevation should be applied immediately to minimize swelling. Occasionally a physician may decide to aspirate the hematoma. A protective doughnut pad constructed to disperse pressure away from the contusion should be worn to protect the area from additional injury.

## Compartment Syndromes

Compartment syndrome classifications:
- acute compartment syndrome
- acute exertional compartment syndrome
- chronic compartment syndrome

**Cause of injury** Compartment syndromes are conditions in which increased pressure within one of the four compartments of the lower leg causes compression of muscular and neurovascular structures within that compartment (refer to Figure 15-3).[22] The anterior and deep posterior compartments are usually involved.[6]

Compartment syndromes can be divided into three categories: acute compartment syndrome, acute exertional compartment syndrome, and chronic compartment syndrome.[5] *Acute compartment syndrome* occurs secondary to direct trauma to the area, such as being kicked in the anterior aspect of the lower leg. Acute compartment syndrome is considered to be a medical emergency because of the possibility of compression of arterial and nerve supply, which could result in additional injury to structures distal to the compartment. *Acute exertional compartment syndrome* occurs without any precipitating trauma and can evolve with minimal to moderate activity. *Chronic compartment syndrome* is activity related in that the symptoms arise rather consistently at a certain point in the activity. Chronic compartment syndrome usually occurs during running and jumping activities, and symptoms cease when activity stops.[6,31]

**Signs of injury** Because of increased intracompartmental pressure associated with compartment syndromes, the athlete complains of a deep aching pain, tightness and swelling of the involved compartment, and

**15-3 Critical Thinking**
Exercise

A soccer player who is not wearing shin guards is kicked on the outside shin of his right leg. After several minutes the pain begins to increase and he feels some tingling and numbness in his foot.

? What is the primary concern with this injury, and what steps should be taken to manage this situation?

pain with passive stretching of the involved muscles.[22] Reduced circulation and sensory changes can be detected in the foot. Intracompartmental pressure measurements further define the severity of the condition. A compartment syndrome that is not recognized, diagnosed, and treated properly can lead to a poor functional outcome for the athlete.[12]

**Care**  Immediate first aid for acute compartment syndrome should include the application of ice and elevation. However, in this situation a compression wrap should not be used to control swelling because there is already a problem with increased pressure in the compartment. Using a compression wrap only acts to increase the pressure.

In the case of both acute compartment syndrome and acute exertional compartment syndrome, measurement of intracompartmental pressures by a physician confirms the diagnosis with emergency fasciotomy to release the pressure within that compartment being the definitive treatment. Athletes undergoing anterior or deep posterior compartment fasciotomy may not return to full activity for 2 to 4 months post surgery.[15]

Management of chronic compartment syndrome is initially conservative, with activity modification, icing, and stretching of the anterior compartment musculature and heel cord complex. If conservative measures fail, fasciotomy of the affected compartments has shown favorable results in an athlete's return to higher levels of activity.

## Achilles Tendinitis

**Cause of injury**  The Achilles tendon is the largest tendon in the human body. It serves as a common tendon for the gastrocnemius and soleus muscles and inserts on the calcaneus. This Achilles tendon complex produces plantarflexion of the ankle. Achilles tendinitis is an inflammatory condition that occurs because of repetitive stresses and strains placed on the tendon such as with running or jumping activities.[15] Repetitive weight-bearing activities such as running or early season conditioning in which the duration and intensity are increased too quickly with insufficient recovery time worsen the condition. Uphill running or hill workouts usually aggravate the condition. The athlete may experience reduced gastrocnemius and soleus muscle flexibility in general that may worsen as the condition progresses and adaptive shortening occurs. Chronic Achilles tendinitis may eventually lead to rupture of the Achilles tendon.[16]

**Signs of injury**  The athlete often complains of generalized pain and stiffness about the Achilles tendon just proximal to the calcaneal insertion. Achilles tendinitis often begins with a gradual onset over time. Symptoms may progress to morning stiffness and discomfort with walking after periods of prolonged sitting. The tendon may be warm and painful to palpation, and if the inflammation persists, the tendon may thicken[1] (see Figure 13-9).

**Care**  Achilles tendinitis generally takes a long time to resolve. It is important to create a proper healing environment by limiting or

**15-4 Critical Thinking**
Exercise

A 35-year old racquetball player feels a pop and severe immediate pain in the back of his left lower leg. He actually felt like someone kicked him, but when he turned around no one was there. Then he realized he could not push off on his foot.

**?** What injury does he most likely have, and how should it be managed?

---

**tennis leg**
Strain of gastrocnemius muscle.

restricting the activity that caused the inflammation. Aggressive stretching of the Achilles tendon complex (refer to Figure 15-4), inserting a heel lift under the calcaneus, using taping techniques to provide support to the Achilles tendon (refer to Figure 11-16), and using anti-inflammatory medication have all been recommended as treatments.[12] Chronic Achilles tendinitis may eventually predispose the athlete to rupture of the Achilles tendon.

### Achilles Tendon Rupture

**Cause of injury**   Injury may range from a grade 1 strain of the muscle to complete rupture of the tendon. A tight Achilles tendon is prone to strain, particularly of the gastrocnemius muscle. Achilles tendon rupture is usually caused by a sudden, forceful plantarflexion of the ankle.[20] A rupture of the Achilles tendon is more common in athletes above the age of 30 years and occurs in activities requiring ballistic movement, such as tennis and basketball[16] (Figure 15-21).

**Signs of injury**   Athletes may feel or hear a pop and feel as if they have been kicked in the back of the leg. Plantarflexing the ankle will be painful and limited but still possible with the assistance of the tibialis posterior and the peroneals. A palpable defect will be noted along the length of the tendon. The athlete will require the use of crutches to continue ambulation without an obvious limp.[16]

**Care**   After an Achilles tendon rupture, the question of surgical repair versus cast immobilization arises.[11] Surgical repair of the tendon is recommended to allow the athlete to return to previous levels of activity. Surgical repair of the Achilles tendon may require a period of immobilization for 6 to 8 weeks to allow for proper tendon healing. It is

*Achilles tendinitis generally takes a long time to resolve.*

*A ruptured Achilles tendon can occur following chronic inflammation.*

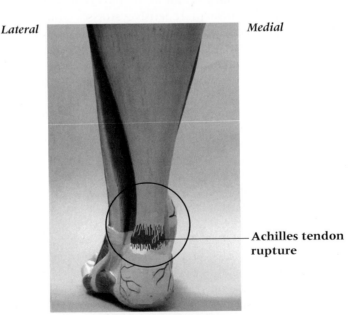

*Lateral*                    *Medial*

**Achilles tendon rupture**

**Figure 15-21**

Achilles tendon rupture
involves tearing and
separation of fibers.

important that the athlete not only regain full range of motion without harming the repair, but also regain normal muscle function through controlled progressive strengthening exercises.[12]

## SUMMARY

- The movements that take place at the talocrural joint are ankle plantarflexion and dorsiflexion. Inversion and eversion occur at the subtalar joint.

- Many lower leg and ankle injuries, especially sprains, can be reduced by Achilles tendon stretching, strengthening of key muscles, improving neuromuscular control, choosing appropriate footwear, and, when necessary, proper taping or bracing.

- Ankle sprains are very common. Inversion sprains usually involve the lateral ligaments of the ankle, and eversion sprains frequently involve the medial ligaments of the ankle. Dorsiflexion injuries often involve the tibiofibular ligaments and may be very severe.

- The early phase of treatment following an ankle sprain uses protection, rest, ice, compression, and elevation, all of which are critical components in preventing swelling.

- Tendinitis in the posterior tibialis, anterior tibialis, and the peroneal tendons may result from one specific cause or from a collection of mechanisms. Techniques that act to reduce or eliminate inflammation, including rest, ice, and anti-inflammatory medications, should be incorporated into rehabilitation.

- Although some injuries that occur in the region of the lower leg are acute, the majority of injuries seen in an athletic population result from overuse, most often from running.

- Tibial fractures can create long-term problems for the athlete if inappropriately managed, whereas fibular fractures generally require much shorter periods for immobilization. Treatment of these fractures is immediate medical referral and most likely a period of immobilization and restricted weight bearing.

- Stress fractures in the lower leg are usually the result of the bone's inability to adapt to the repetitive loading response during training and conditioning of the athlete and are more likely to occur in the tibia.

- Care for medial tibial stress syndrome must be comprehensive and must address several factors, including musculoskeletal training and conditioning as well as proper footwear and orthotics intervention.

- Compartment syndromes can occur from acute trauma or from repetitive trauma or overuse. They can occur in any of the four compartments but are most likely to occur in the anterior compartment or deep posterior compartment.

- Achilles tendinitis often presents with a gradual onset over time and may be resistant to a quick resolution.

- Perhaps the greatest question after an Achilles tendon rupture is whether surgical repair or cast immobilization is the best method of treatment. Regardless, the time required for rehabilitation is significant.

---

### Solutions to Critical Thinking Exercises

**15-1** The most important care that can be given immediately following ankle sprain is to control or minimize the swelling. This goal is accomplished by using a combination of ice, compression, elevation, and rest beginning immediately and continuing for at least the next 72 hours.

**15-2** The athlete is instructed to rest or reduce the stress of running. Application of ice packs followed by stretching is carried out before and after activity. A strengthening program is implemented along with treatment by oral anti-inflammatory medications as needed.

**15-3** This athlete may be developing an acute compartment syndrome in the anterior compartment. If so, this condition should be handled as an emergency. The coach should immediately elevate the leg and apply ice but no compression wrap, and the athlete should be given medical attention as soon as possible.

**15-4** This scenario is a classic description of a ruptured Achilles tendon. In cases of a complete rupture, surgery is necessary to repair the tendon, followed by a reasonably long period of rehabilitation.

## REVIEW QUESTIONS AND CLASS ACTIVITIES

1. Describe the anatomy of the ankle and lower leg.
2. How can ankle and lower leg injuries be prevented?
3. What questions should be asked when assessing injuries to the lower leg or ankle?
4. Describe the common mechanisms of injury for acute ankle sprains. What structures are damaged?
5. How can fractures in the lower leg and ankle be ruled out?
6. What is the appropriate care for stress fractures of the tibia and fibula?
7. Which of the tendons surrounding the ankle joint can potentially develop tendinitis?
8. What are some indications of a heel cord rupture? How is a heel cord rupture cared for?
9. How does Achilles tendinitis develop? How should it be cared for?
10. Contrast acute compartment syndrome with chronic compartment syndrome.
11. What exactly are shin splints and what measures can be taken to eliminate this problem?
12. What is the most important thing that can be done in caring for a shin contusion?

## REFERENCES

1. Allredson, H, Lorentzon, R: 2000. Chronic Achilles tendinosis: recommendations for treatment and prevention, *Sports medicine* 29(2): 135.

2. Anderson, SJ: 2002. Acute ankle sprains: keys to diagnosis and return to play, *Physician and sportsmedicine* 30(12):29–35.

3. Bahr, R: 2002. Can we prevent ankle sprains? In MacAuley, D (ed), *Evidence-based sports medicine*, pp. 470–490, London, BMJ Books.

4. Blackman, PG: 2000. A review of chronic exertional compartment syndrome in the lower leg, *Medicine and science in sports & exercise* 32 (3 suppl):S4.

5. Bong, M, Polatsch, D, Jazrawi, L: 2005. Chronic exertional compartment syndrome diagnosis and management, *Bulletin—hospital for joint diseases* 62(3/4):77.

6. Bot, SDM, van Mechelen, W: 1999. The effect of ankle bracing on athletic performance, *Sports medicine* 27(3):171.

7. Cordova, ML: 2002. Efficacy of prophylactic ankle support: an experimental perspective, *Journal of athletic training,* 37(4):446–457.

8. Couture, CJ: 2002. Tibial stress injuries: decisive diagnosis and treatment of "shin splints," *Physician and sportsmedicine* 30(6): 29–36.

9. Gross, MT, Liu, HY: 2003. The role of ankle bracing for prevention of ankle sprain injuries, *The journal of orthopaedic & sports physical therapy* 33(10):572–577.

10. High alert for Achilles tendon rupture? 2001. *Physician and sportsmedicine* 29(12):11–12.

11. Hirth, C: 2010. Rehabilitation of lower leg injuries. In Prentice WE, editor: *Rehabilitation techniques in sports medicine and athletic training,* 4th ed. New York, McGraw-Hill.

12. Hunter, S, Prentice, W, Zinder, S: 2010. Rehabilitation of foot and ankle injuries. In Prentice WE, editor: *Rehabilitation techniques in sports medicine and athletic training,* 5th ed. New York, McGraw-Hill.

13. Kohn, H: 1997. Shin pain and compartment syndromes in running. In Guten G, editor: *Running injuries,* Philadelphia, WB Saunders.

14. Kovaleski, J: 2006. Functional rehabilitation after lateral ankle injury. *Athletic therapy today* 11(3): 52.

15. Johnston, R: 2003. Achilles tendon: tendinitis and tears, *Hughston health alert* 15(1):7.

16. Kortebein, PM et al.: 2000. Medial tibial stress syndrome, *Medicine and science in sports & exercise* 32(3 suppl): S27.

17. McAlindon, R: 2007: Ankle fractures, *Hughston Health Alert* 19(2):1.

18. McKeon, P, Mattacola, C: 2008. Interventions for the prevention of first time and recurrent ankle sprains. *Clinics in sports medicine* 27(3):371.

19. Madras, D: 2003. Rehabilitation for functional ankle instability, *Journal of sport rehabilitation* 12(2): 133–142.

20. Metz, R, Verleisdonk, E: 2008. Acute Achilles tendon rupture. *American journal of sports medicine* 36(9):1688.

21. Nyska, M (ed): 2002. *The unstable ankle,* Champaign, IL, Human Kinetics.

22. Ray, T, Robertson, J: 2005. Exercise-induced shin pain. *Athletic therapy today* 10(5):72.

23. Renstrom, P, Lynch, SA: 2002. Management of acute ankle sprains, In Nyska, M. *The unstable ankle,* Champaign, Ill., Human Kinetics, pp. 168–178.

24. Robertson, K, Molloy, L: 2007. Medial tibial stress syndrome or 'shin splints.' *Modern athlete & Coach* 45(3):31.

25. Shin splint prevention warmup routine, *Physical education digest* 20(4):56–57, 2004.
26. Silvestri, PG: 2002. Management of syndemotic ankle sprains, *Athletic therapy today* 7(5):48–49.
27. Thacker, SB et al.: 1999. The prevention of ankle sprains in sports: a systematic review of the literature, *American journal of sports medicine* 27(6):753.
28. Wilder, RP, Sethi, S: 2004. Overuse injuries: tendinopathies, stress fractures, compartment syndrome, and shin splints, *Clinics in sports medicine* 23(1):55–81.
29. Wilkerson, GB: 1991. Treatment of the inversion ankle sprain through synchronous application of focal compression and cold, *Athletic training* 26(3):220.
30. Willy C, Becker B, Evers, H: 1996. Unusual development of acute exertional compartment syndrome due to delayed diagnosis: a case report, *International journal of sports medicine* 17(6):458.
31. Wright, IC et al.: 2000. The effects of ankle compliance and flexibility on ankle sprains, *Medicine and science in sports & exercise* 32(2): 260.
32. Young, A, McAllister, D: 2006. Evaluation and treatment of tibial stress fractures, *Clinics in sports medicine* 25(1):117.

**ANNOTATED BIBLIOGRAPHY**

Baxter, D: 1995. *The Foot and Ankle in Sport,* St Louis, Mosby.
> *Discusses all aspects of dealing with foot and ankle injuries as they occur in an athletic population.*

Nyska, M, Mann, G (eds): 2002. *The unstable ankle,* Champaign, IL, Human Kinetics.
> *This book does a nice job of covering a variety of topics without going into a lot of detail.*

Pfeffer, R: 2000. *Athletic injuries to the foot and ankle,* Park Ridge, IL, American Academy of Orthopedic Surgeons.
> *This book goes into great detail on a wide variety of injuries that occur in the ankle joint.*

**WEB SITES**

Gray's Anatomy of The Human Body: www.bartleby.com/107

American Orthopaedic Foot and Ankle Society: http://aofas.org

World Ortho: www.worldortho.com
> *Use the search engine in this site to locate relevant information.*

American Podiatric Medical Association: www.apma.org
> *Provides a variety of information on foot and ankle injuries from the APMA.*

AAOS Online Service: Foot and Ankle http://orthoinfo.aaos.org/category.cfm?topcategory=Foot
> *Provides answers to a wide range of questions on foot and ankle injuries from the American Academy of Orthopedic Surgeons.*

# The Knee and Related Structures

*When you finish this chapter you will be able to:*

- Describe the anatomical relationships of the bones, ligaments, and muscles that surround the knee joint.
- Explain how to prevent knee injuries.
- Briefly describe how to assess an injury of the knee joint.
- Recognize injuries to the stabilizing structures of the knee.
- Differentiate between acute and overuse injuries that occur at the knee joint.
- Identify injuries that can occur to the patella.
- Describe injuries that can occur to the extensor mechanism.

The knee is considered one of the most complex joints in the human body. Because so many sports place extreme stress on the knee, it is also one of the most frequently injured joints. The knee is commonly considered a hinge joint because its two principal movements are flexion and extension. However, because rotation of the tibia is an essential component of knee movement, the knee is not a true hinge joint. The stability of the knee joint depends primarily on the ligaments, the joint capsule, and the muscles that surround the joint. The knee functions to provide stability in weight bearing and mobility in locomotion.

## KNEE ANATOMY

### Bones

The knee joint consists of four bones: the femur, the tibia, the fibula, and the patella (Figure 16-1). These four bones form several articulations between the femur and the tibia, the femur and the patella, the femur and the fibula, and the tibia and fibula. The articular surfaces of the knee joint are completely enveloped by the largest joint capsule in the body. Synovial membrane lines the inner surface of the joint capsule.

*Muscles and ligaments provide the main source of stability in the knee.*

The distal end of the femur expands into the lateral and medial femoral condyles, which are designed to articulate with the tibia and the patella. The patella, or kneecap, is located in the tendon of the quadriceps muscle group on the front of the knee and moves up and down in a groove between the two femoral condyles as the quadriceps muscle group contracts and relaxes. The proximal end of the tibia, or the tibial plateau, is very flat and must articulate with the round condyles of the femur.

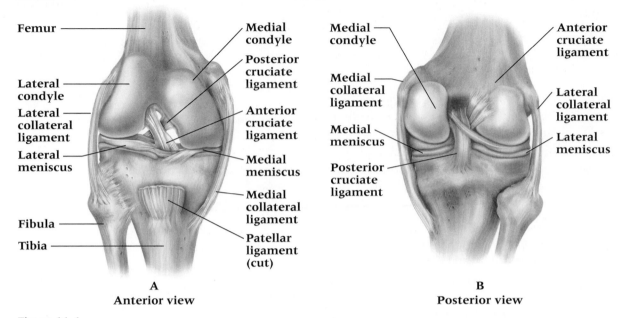

**A**
**Anterior view**

**B**
**Posterior view**

**Figure 16-1**

Bone, ligaments, and menisci in the knee.
(A) Anterior view.
(B) Posterior view.

Generally the meniscus has a poor blood supply that can impair healing in a torn meniscus.

The medial meniscus and lateral meniscus are fibrocartilage disks that are shaped like bowls, thicker on the outside border and thinner on the inside (Figure 16-2). They lie on top of the flat tibial plateau and function to make the rounded femoral condyles fit better on the flat tibial plateau, thus increasing the stability of the joint. They also help cushion any stresses placed on the knee joint by keeping the bony surface of the femur separated from the tibial plateau.

### Ligaments

The major stabilizing ligaments of the knee include the cruciate ligaments and the collateral ligaments (refer to Figure 16-1).

**Figure 16-2**

Menisci of the knee

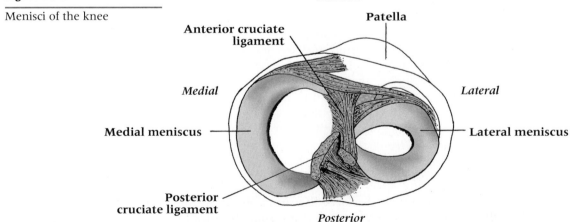

The anterior and posterior cruciate ligaments account for a considerable amount of stability in the knee. In general, the anterior cruciate ligament (ACL) prevents the femur from moving posteriorly during weight bearing. It also stabilizes the tibia against excessive internal rotation and serves as a secondary stabilizer when there is injury to the collateral ligaments. The posterior cruciate ligament (PCL) prevents the femur from sliding forward during weight bearing.

The medial and lateral collateral ligaments function to stabilize the knee against the side to side (valgus/varus) forces at the knee joint. The medial collateral ligament (MCL) attaches above the joint line on the medial condyle of the femur and inserts well below the joint line on the tibia. Its major purpose is to protect the knee from valgus forces that are applied to the lateral surface of the joint and to resist external tibial rotation. There are two parts of the MCL: the superficial portion and the deep portion, which is actually a thickened part of the medial joint capsule. The medial meniscus is attached to the deep portion of the medial collateral ligament.

The lateral collateral ligament (LCL) is attached to the lateral condyle of the femur and to the head of the fibula. The lateral collateral ligament resists varus forces that are applied to the medial surface of the knee. Both the medial and lateral collateral ligaments are tightest during knee extension but relaxed during flexion.

Major movements of the knee:
- flexion
- extension
- rotation

## Muscles

For the knee to function properly, a number of muscles must work together in a highly complex fashion (Figure 16-3). In general, contraction of the quadriceps muscle group (the rectus femoris, and the vastus medialis, intermedialis, and lateralis) on the front of the thigh causes knee extension. Contraction of the hamstring muscle group (the biceps femoris, semitendinosus, and semimembranosus) on the back of the thigh, along with the gracilis, sartorius, popliteus, gastrocnemius, and plantaris, causes knee flexion. The hamstrings, popliteus, sartorius, and gracilis contribute to tibial rotation. Table 16-1 summarizes all of the muscles that produce various movements at the knee joint.

# PREVENTION OF KNEE INJURIES

Preventing knee injuries in sports is a complex problem. Of major importance are effective physical conditioning, rehabilitation, and skill development, as well as shoe type. The routine use of protective bracing may be a questionable practice.

## Physical Conditioning and Rehabilitation

To avoid knee injuries, the athlete must be as highly conditioned as possible, meaning total body conditioning that includes strength, flexibility, cardiovascular and muscle endurance, agility, speed, and balance.[31] Specifically, the muscles surrounding the knee joint must be as strong as possible. Depending on the requirements of a sport, some balance in

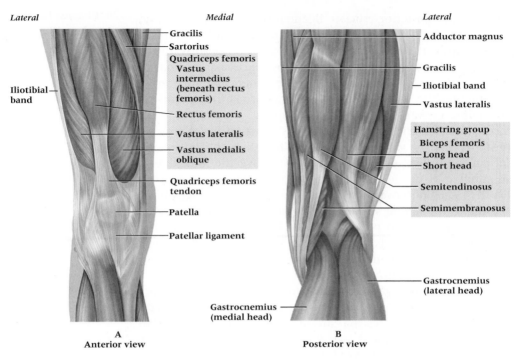

**Figure 16-3**

Muscles of the knee.
(A) Anterior view.
(B) Posterior view.

**TABLE 16-1** Muscles of the Knee Joint

| | |
|---|---|
| Knee flexion | Hamstring group |
| | Biceps femoris |
| | Semitendinosus |
| | Semimembranosus |
| | Gracilis |
| | Sartorius |
| | Gastrocnemius |
| | Popliteus |
| | Plantaris |
| Knee extension | Quadriceps muscle group |
| | Vastus medialis |
| | Vastus lateralis |
| | Vastus intermedius |
| | Rectus femoris |
| External tibial rotation | Biceps femoris |
| Internal tibial rotation | Popliteus |
| | Semitendinosus |
| | Semimembranosus |
| | Sartorius |
| | Gracilis |

strength should exist between the quadriceps and hamstring muscle groups. For example, in football players the hamstring muscles should have about 60–75 percent of the strength of the quadriceps muscles.[21] The gastrocnemius muscle should also be strengthened to help stabilize the knee. Although maximizing muscle strength may prevent some injuries, it fails to prevent rotational injuries.

Knees that have been injured must be properly rehabilitated. Once the ligaments that stabilize the knee have been injured, the knee relies to a great extent on the strength of all the muscles that surround the joint to provide the inherent stability that was lost with the injury. Thus strengthening exercises are essential in preventing reinjury. Repeated minor injuries to a knee make it susceptible to a major injury.

## Shoe Type

During recent years, collision sports such as football have been using soccer-style shoes. The change from a few long conical cleats to a large number of cleats that are short and broad has significantly reduced knee injuries in football.[23] The more numerous and shorter cleats are better because the foot does not become fixed to the surface and the shoe still allows controlled running and cutting.[23]

## Functional and Prophylactic Knee Braces

Functional and prophylactic knee braces were discussed in Chapter 6. These braces have been designed to prevent or reduce the severity of knee injuries.[18] Prophylactic knee braces are worn on the lateral surface of the knee to protect the medial collateral ligament (Figure 16-4A).[31] Their usefulness, however, is questionable and some studies have even shown that they increase the chance of injury.

Functional knee braces are worn to provide some degree of support to the unstable knee once an athlete returns to activity following injury.[27] All functional braces are custom fitted to some degree and use hinges and posts for support. Some braces use custom-molded thigh and calf enclosures to hold the brace in place, whereas others rely on straps for suspension (Figure 16-4B). These braces are designed to control excessive rotational stress or tibial translation.[5] The effectiveness of protective knee braces is at best controversial.[34] However, if combined with an appropriate rehabilitation program, these braces have been shown to restrict anterior/posterior translation of the tibia at low loads.[32]

## ASSESSING THE KNEE JOINT

**Generally fitness professionals, coaches, and others working in areas related to exercise and sport science are not adequately trained to evaluate injuries. It is strongly recommended that injured athletes be referred to qualified medical personnel (i.e., physicians, athletic trainers, physical therapists) for injury evaluation.** Information on the following special tests has been included simply to give some idea about the different basic tests that

**Figure 16-4**

(A) Prophylactic knee brace.

(B) Functional knee brace.

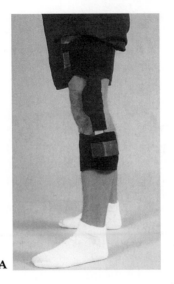

**A**

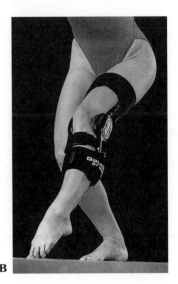

**B**

nonmedical personnel may do to determine the nature and severity of the athlete's injury. The primary responsibility of those who are not health care personnel is to be able to recognize any potential "red flags" associated with the injury, provide appropriate first aid for the injury, and make correct decisions about how the injury should be managed initially, including immediate return to play or activity decisions. (Refer to Chapter 7.) Unquestionably, the most important aspect of understanding what pathological process has taken place is to become familiar with the traumatic sequence and mechanisms of injury, either through having seen the injury occur or through learning its history.

## History

To determine the history and major complaints involved in a knee injury, the following questions should be asked.

### Current Injury

- What were you doing when the knee was hurt?
- What position was your body in?
- Did the knee collapse?
- Did you hear a noise or feel any sensation at the time of injury, such as a pop or crunch? (A pop could indicate an anterior cruciate tear, a crunch could be a sign of a torn meniscus, and a tearing sensation might indicate a capsule tear.)
- Could you move the knee immediately after the injury? If not, was it locked in a bent or extended position? (Locking could mean a meniscal tear.) After being locked, how did it become unlocked?
- Did swelling occur? If yes, was it immediate, or did it occur later? (Immediate swelling could indicate a cruciate or tibial fracture,

whereas later swelling could indicate a capsular, synovial, or meniscal tear.)

■ Where was the pain? Was it local, all over, or did it move from one side of the knee to the other?

■ Have you hurt the knee before?

When first assessing the injury, observe whether the athlete is able to support body weight flat-footed on the injured leg or whether the athlete finds it necessary to stand and walk on the toes. Toe walking is an indication that the athlete is holding the knee in a splinted position to avoid pain or that the knee is being held in a flexed position by a wedge of dislocated meniscus.

In first-time acute knee sprains, fluid and blood effusion is not usually apparent until after a 24-hour period. However, in an anterior cruciate ligament sprain, blood may accumulate in the joint (hemarthrosis) during the first hour after injury. Swelling and discoloration (ecchymosis) will occur unless the swelling is controlled through the use of compression, elevation, and ice.

### Recurrent or Chronic Injury

■ What is your major complaint?

■ When did you first notice the condition?

■ Is there recurrent swelling?

■ Does the knee ever lock or catch? (If yes, it may be a torn meniscus or a loose body in the knee joint.)

■ Is there severe pain? Is it constant, or does it come and go?

■ Do you feel any grinding or grating sensations? (If yes, it could indicate chondromalacia or traumatic arthritis.)

■ Does your knee ever feel like it is going to give way or has it actually done so? (If yes and often, it may be a capsular, cruciate, or meniscal tear, a loose body, or a subluxating patella.)

■ What does it feel like to go up and down stairs? (Pain may indicate a patellar irritation or meniscal tear.)

■ What past treatment, if any, have you received for this condition?

## Observation

A visual examination should be performed after the major complaints have been determined. The athlete should be observed in a number of situations: walking, half-squatting, and going up and down stairs. The leg also should be observed for asymmetry. Establish whether both the athlete's knees look the same:

■ Do the knees appear symmetrical?

■ Is one knee obviously swollen?

■ Is muscle atrophy apparent?

If possible, the athlete with an injured knee should be observed in the following actions:
• walking
• half-squatting
• going up and down stairs

## Walking

- Does the athlete walk with a limp, or is the walk free and easy? Is the athlete able to fully extend the knee during heel strike?
- Can the athlete fully bear weight on the affected leg?
- Is the athlete able to perform a half-squat to extension?
- Can the athlete go up and down stairs with ease? (If stairs are unavailable, stepping up on a box or stool will suffice.)

## Palpation

For palpation to yield any valuable information about the nature of the injury, at least a basic knowledge of the anatomy of the bones, ligaments, and the muscles must exist. The athlete should either be lying on the back (supine) or sitting on the edge of the training table or a bench with the knee flexed to 90 degrees.

The bony structures of the knee are palpated for areas of tenderness or pain or for deformities, which might indicate a fracture or dislocation.

After palpation of the bony structures, the lateral collateral ligament and medial collateral ligament should be palpated for areas of tenderness. Because the anterior and posterior cruciate ligaments are inside the joint capsule they cannot be palpated. However the joint line, which is the articulation between the femoral condyles and the flat tibial plateau, should be palpated all around the knee joint. Tenderness at the joint line may indicate injury to either the medial or lateral menisci or the joint capsule.

## Special Tests

Both acute and chronic injury to the knee can produce ligamentous instability.[31] It is critical that the injured knee's stability be evaluated as soon after injury as possible. To be able to correctly conduct a series of stability tests and then determine the exact nature of the injury takes a considerable amount of training.[9]

Perhaps the simplest test is to compare the injured knee with the uninjured knee to determine any differences in stability. Determination of the degree of instability is made by the endpoint feel during stability testing. As stress is applied to a joint, some motion is limited by an intact ligament. In a normal joint, the endpoint is abrupt with little or no give and no reported pain. With a grade 1 sprain, the endpoint is still firm with little or no instability and some pain is present. With a grade 2 sprain, the endpoint is soft with some instability present and a moderate amount of pain. In a grade 3 complete rupture, the endpoint is very soft with marked instability, and pain is severe initially, then mild.

There are many different tests that should be performed by a trained individual to accurately assess ligament stability. However, the valgus/varus stress test, Lachman's test, and Apley's compression test may be easily done to determine the degree of instability in the knee caused by

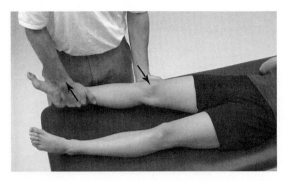

**Figure 16-5**

Valgus knee stress test for injury to the MCL

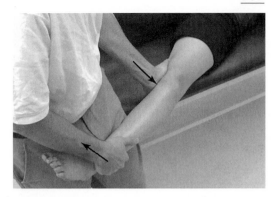

**Figure 16-6**

Varus knee stress test for injury to the LCL

ligament or meniscal injury. These tests are not definitive but rather are possible indicators of injury.[9] If they appear to be positive the athlete should be referred to a physician.

### Valgus/Varus Stress Tests

Valgus and varus stress tests are intended to reveal laxity of the medial and lateral collateral ligaments. The athlete lies supine with the leg extended. To test the medial collateral ligament, valgus stress is applied with the knee fully extended and at 30 degrees of flexion (Figure 16-5).

To test the lateral collateral ligament, the examiner holds the ankle firmly with one hand while placing the other over the medial joint line. The examiner then places a varus force laterally in an attempt to open the lateral side of the knee (Figure 16-6).

### Lachman's Test

The Lachman's test is the most commonly used test for checking the integrity of the anterior cruciate ligament (Figure 16-7). The test is administered by positioning the knee in approximately 30 degrees of flexion with the athlete lying on their back. One hand of the examiner stabilizes the leg by grasping the distal end of the thigh, and the other hand grasps the proximal aspect of the tibia, attempting to move it anteriorly. If there is unchecked anterior movement of the tibia, this is a positive Lachman's test which indicates damage to the anterior cruciate.

### Apley's Compression Test

The Apley's compression test (Figure 16-8) is used to detect a meniscus tear. It is performed with the athlete lying face down and the affected leg flexed to 90 degrees. While stabilizing the thigh, a hard downward pressure is applied to the leg. The leg is then rotated back and forth. If pain results, a meniscal injury may have occurred. A medial meniscal tear is noted by external rotation, and a lateral meniscal tear is noted by internal rotation of the lower leg.

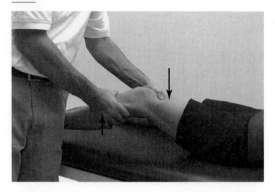

**Figure 16-7**

Lachman's test for anterior cruciate ligament injury

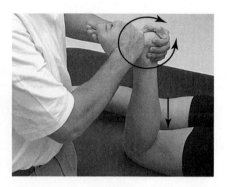

**Figure 16-8**

Apley's compression test for meniscal injury

### Functional Tests

It is important that the athlete's knee also be tested for function. The athlete should begin with walking (forward, backward, straight line, curve) and progress to jogging (straight, curve, uphill, downhill), running (forward, backward), and then sprinting (straight, curve, large figure eight, small figure eight, zig-zag, carioca).

## RECOGNITION AND MANAGEMENT OF INJURIES TO THE KNEE

### Ligament Injuries

The major ligaments of the knee can be torn in isolation or in combination.[3] Depending on the application of forces, injury can occur from a direct straight-line or single-plane force, from a rotary force, or from a combination of the two.

### Medial Collateral Ligament Sprain

**Cause of injury**   Injury to the MCL most often occurs either as a result of a medially directed valgus force from the lateral side or from external rotation of the tibia (Figure 16-9).[19] MCL tears resulting from rotation combined with valgus stress with the foot fixed frequently result in ACL and occasionally PCL tears.[21]

More significant injuries usually occur with medial sprains than from lateral sprains because of the increased potential of injury to the joint capsule and the medial meniscus. Many mild-to-moderate sprains leave the knee unstable and thus vulnerable to additional internal derangements.

**Signs of injury**   The force and angle of the trauma usually determine the extent of injury. Even after witnessing the occurrence of a knee injury, it is difficult to predict the extent of tissue damage. The most revealing time for testing joint stability is immediately after injury before effusion masks the extent of derangement.[19]

*Lateral*                          *Medial*

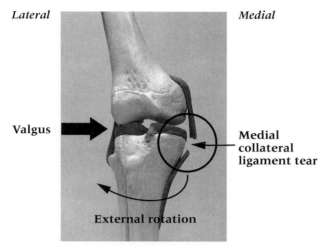

**Valgus**

**Medial collateral ligament tear**

**External rotation**

**Figure 16-9**

A valgus force with the tibia in external rotation injures the medial collateral and capsular ligaments, the medial meniscus, and sometimes the anterior cruciate ligaments.

In a grade 1 MCL sprain, a few ligament fibers are torn or stretched; the joint is stable during valgus stress tests; there is little or no joint effusion; there may be some joint stiffness and point tenderness just below the medial joint line; even with minor stiffness, there is almost full passive and active range of motion (Figure 16-10A).

*Anterior*                  *Posterior*

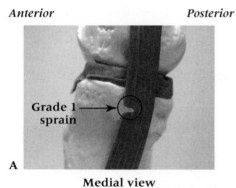

**Grade 1 sprain**

**A**

**Medial view**

*Anterior*                  *Posterior*

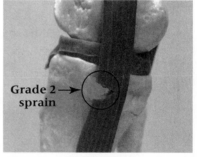

**Grade 2 sprain**

**B**

**Medial view**

*Anterior*                  *Posterior*

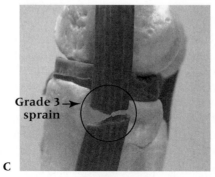

**Grade 3 sprain**

**C**

**Medial view**

**Figure 16-10**

Medial collateral ligament sprain: (A) Grade 1. (B) Grade 2. (C) Grade 3.

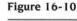

A grade 2 MCL sprain involves moderate tearing or partial separation of ligament fibers; no gross instability, but minimum or slight laxity during full extension; slight or absent swelling unless the meniscus or ACL has been torn; moderate-to-severe joint tightness with an inability to actively extend the knee completely (the athlete is unable to place the heel flat on the ground); definite loss of passive range of motion; and pain in the medial aspect with general weakness and instability (Figure 16-10B).

A grade 3 MCL sprain means a complete tear of the ligament; complete loss of medial stability; minimum-to-moderate swelling; immediate severe pain followed by a dull ache; loss of motion because of effusion and hamstring guarding; a valgus stress test that reveals some joint opening in full extension and significant opening at 30 degrees of flexion (Figure 16-10C). A medial meniscus tear may also exist since the meniscus is attached to the medial joint capsule portion of the deep medial collateral ligament.

**Care** Immediate care consists of PRICE for at least 24 hours. Crutches may be used if the athlete is unable to walk without a limp. Depending on the severity and possible complications, a postoperative knee immobilizer may be applied by the physician (Figure 16-11) for 2 to 5 days, after which range-of-motion exercises are begun. Isometric exercise emphasizing quadriceps strengthening (quad sets, straight leg lifts) should progress to active, resisted, full-range exercise as soon as possible. The athlete then graduates to stationary biking, stair climbing, and resisted flexion/extension exercises as soon as possible. Use of tape or perhaps a hinged brace when attempting to return to running activities is encouraged.

Conservative nonoperative treatment is recommended for isolated grade 2 and even grade 3 MCL sprains. Conservative treatment usually involves limited immobilization with range-of-motion and progressive weight bearing for 2 weeks followed by protection with a functional hinged brace for another 2 to 3 weeks.

The athlete is allowed to return to full participation when the knee has regained normal strength, power, flexibility, endurance, and coordination. Usually 1 to 3 weeks is necessary for recovery. When returning to activity, the athlete may require tape support for a short period.

### Lateral Collateral Ligament Sprain

**Cause of injury** Injury to the LCL most often occurs either as a result of a laterally directed varus force from the medial side or from internal rotation of the tibia (Figure 16-12). If the force is great enough, bony fragments can be avulsed from the femur or tibia. Sprain of the LCL is much less prevalent than sprain of the MCL.

**Signs of injury** An LCL sprain causes pain and tenderness over the ligament; swelling and effusion; some joint laxity with a varus stress test at 30 degrees (if laxity exists in full extension, ACL and possibly PCL injury should be evaluated); and pain is greatest with grade 1 and grade 2 sprains. In grade 3 sprains, pain is intense initially, then subsides to a dull ache.

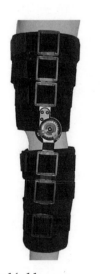

**Figure 16-11**

An adjustable knee immobilizer may be used, depending on whether full extension or some other angle is desired.

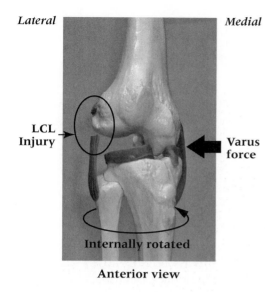

*Lateral*    *Medial*

**LCL
Injury**

**Varus
force**

**Internally rotated**

**Anterior view**

**Figure 16-12**

A varus force with the tibia
internally rotated injures the
lateral collateral ligament; in
some cases both the cruciate
ligaments and the attachments
of the iliotibial band and biceps
muscle of the thigh may be
torn.

A lateral knee sprain can be
caused by a varus force when
the tibia is internally rotated.

**Care**    Management of the LCL injury should follow the same
procedures as for MCL injuries.

## Anterior Cruciate Ligament Sprain

**Cause of injury**    Unfortunately, ACL injuries are fairly common in
sports. In recent years it has become clear that ACL tears are more likely
to occur in females than in males.[29] A great deal of research has focused on trying to explain why this is the case. Contributing factors that
have been investigated include hormonal influences, a variety of
anatomical factors, and level of conditioning—to name only a few. To
date, none of these explanations has proven to be definitive.[31]

It appears that certain biomechanical differences between males and
females offer the most plausible explanation. ACL injuries are most likely
to occur with deceleration, rotation, and valgus stress to the knee.[13] This
mechanism is very common when the athlete lands from a jump with
the knee extended as opposed to flexed. The most common noncontact
mechanism for tearing the ACL is when the athlete decelerates, with the
foot planted on the ground, and turns in the direction of the planted
foot forcing the tibia into internal rotation[33] (Figure 16-13). Generally,
females tend to land with their knees more extended and this factor
combined with the fact that females tend to have greater differences in
hamstring/quadriceps strength ratios seems to offer the most likely explanation for this trend.[27] There is still a great deal of research being conducted in this area.[31] Tears of the anterior cruciate are often associated
with injury to other supporting structures in the knee. For example, a
tear of the ACL, MCL, and medial meniscus has been referred to as the
"unhappy triad."

**Signs of injury**    The athlete with a torn ACL experiences an audible pop followed by immediate disability and will complain that the

**16-2 Critical Thinking**
Exercise

A lacrosse player carrying the
ball attempts to avoid a de-
fender by planting his right foot
firmly on the ground and cutting
hard to his left. His knee immediately gives way, and he hears a
loud pop. He has intense pain
immediately but after a few minutes he feels as if he can get up
and walk.

**?**  What ligament has most
likely been injured? What stability tests should be done to
determine the extent of the
injury to this ligament?

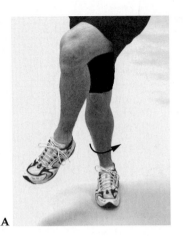

*Lateral*            *Medial*

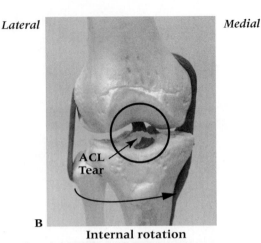

ACL
Tear

**A**          **B**      **Internal rotation**

**Figure 16-13**

The primary mechanism of a noncontact ACL sprain is cutting in the same direction as the planted foot (internal rotation of the tibia).

knee feels like it is coming apart. ACL tears produce rapid swelling at the joint line. Usually the athlete experiences intense pain initially. However, within minutes the athlete begins to feel that the knee is not badly hurt and will profess an ability to get up and walk. The athlete with an ACL tear will exhibit a positive Lachman's Test.

**Care** Even with application of proper first aid and immediate PRICE, swelling begins within 1 to 2 hours and peaks within 4 to 6 hours.[3] The athlete typically cannot walk without help.

Anterior cruciate ligamentous injury can lead to serious knee instability; an intact ACL is necessary for a knee to function in high-performance situations.[22] Controversy exists among physicians about how best to treat an acute ACL rupture and when surgery is warranted. Surgery may involve joint reconstruction to replace the lost anterior cruciate support. This type of surgery involves 3 to 5 weeks in some type of brace, and 4 to 6 months of rehabilitation.[13] Little scientific evidence exists to support the use of functional knee braces following ACL injury, yet many physicians feel that the braces can provide some protection during activity.[34]

### Posterior Cruciate Ligament Sprain

**Cause of injury** The PCL is most likely to be injured when the knee is hyperflexed from falling with full weight on the anterior aspect of the bent knee with the foot in plantar flexion[24] (Figure 16-14). In addition, it can be injured by a rotational force, which also affects the medial or lateral side of the knee.[20]

**Signs of injury** The athlete will report feeling a pop in the back of the knee; tenderness and relatively little swelling will be evident in the popliteal fossa; laxity will be demonstrated in a posterior drawer test.[24]

**Care** PRICE should be initiated immediately. Nonoperative rehabilitation of grade 1 and 2 injuries should focus on quadriceps strengthening. Controversy exists as to whether a grade 3 PCL tear should be treated nonoperatively or with surgical intervention.[16] Unlike the

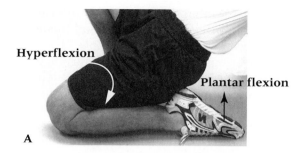

A

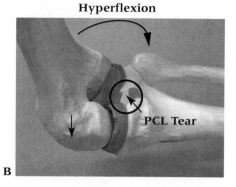

B

situation faced by athletes with ACL tears, many high-level athletes can do very well without the PCL. Rehabilitation following surgery generally involves 6 weeks of immobilization in extension with full weight bearing on crutches. Range of motion exercises begin at 6 weeks, progressing to the use of progressive resistance exercise at 4 months.[11]

## Meniscus Injuries

**Cause of injury**   A tear of the meniscus most often results from weight bearing combined with a rotational force while extending or flexing the knee (Figure 16-15).[25] The medial meniscus has a much higher incidence of injury than does the lateral meniscus. Because of its attachment to the deep portion of the MCL, the medial meniscus is prone to disruption from valgus and rotational forces. The lateral meniscus does not attach to the capsule and is more mobile during knee movement.

A large number of medial meniscus lesions are the outcome of a sudden, strong, internal rotation of the femur with a partially flexed knee while the foot is firmly planted.[3] As a result of the force of this action, the meniscus is pulled out of its normal bed and pinched

**Figure 16-14**

The primary mechanism of a PCL tear is falling on the knee and forcing it into hyperflexion with the ankle plantar flexed.

**Figure 16-15**

(A) The primary mechanism for a meniscus tear is rotation from a cutting maneuver creating a valgus force. (B) This often results in a "bucket handle" tear.

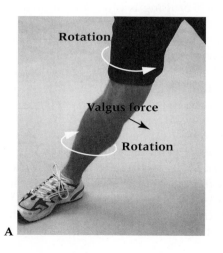

A

Rotation

Valgus force

Rotation

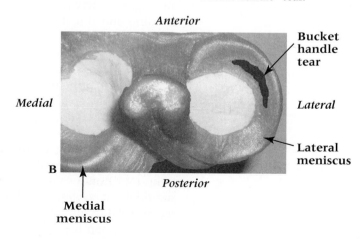

B

Anterior

Bucket handle tear

Medial

Lateral

Lateral meniscus

Medial meniscus

Posterior

between the femoral condyles. Tears within the cartilage fail to heal because of inadequate blood supply. However, some peripheral meniscus tears do heal when an adequate supply of blood is available.

**Signs of injury**   An absolute diagnosis of meniscal injury is difficult. A meniscal tear may result in the following symptoms: effusion developing gradually over 48 to 72 hours; joint-line pain and loss of motion; intermittent locking and giving way; and pain when squatting. Chronic meniscal lesions may also display recurrent swelling and obvious muscle atrophy around the knee. Often the athlete complains of an inability to perform a full squat or to change direction quickly when running without experiencing pain, a sense of the knee collapsing, or a popping sensation.

**Care**   Immediate care involves PRICE. Even if the knee is not locked but shows indications of a tear, the athlete should be sent to a physician for diagnosis. The knee that is locked by a displaced meniscus may require unlocking with the athlete under anesthesia so that a detailed examination can be conducted. Management of the nonlocking acute meniscus tear should follow a course similar to that for MCL injuries and does not necessarily require surgery.[25]

If discomfort, disability, and locking of the knee continue, arthroscopic surgery may be required to remove a portion of the meniscus. In certain cases a torn meniscus can be repaired using sutures. Surgical management of meniscal tears should make every effort to minimize loss of any portion of the meniscus.

## Joint Contusions (Bruises)

**Cause of injury**   A blow struck against the muscles crossing the knee joint can result in a handicapping condition. One of the muscles frequently involved is the vastus medialis of the quadriceps group, which is primarily involved in locking the knee in a position of full extension.

**Signs of injury**   Bruises of the vastus medialis produce all the appearances of a knee sprain, including severe pain, loss of movement, and signs of acute inflammation. Such bruising is often manifested by swelling and discoloration caused by the tearing of muscle tissue and blood vessels. If adequate first aid is given immediately, the knee usually returns to functional use 24 to 48 hours after the trauma.

**Care**   Care of a bruised knee depends on many factors. However, management principally depends on the location and severity of the contusion. The following procedures are suggested. Apply compression bandages and cold until resolution has occurred. Recommend inactivity and rest for 24 hours. If swelling occurs, continue cold application for 72 hours. If swelling and pain are intense, refer the athlete to the physician. Once the acute stage has ended and the swelling has diminished to little or none, cold application with active range-of-motion exercises should be conducted within a pain-free range. Allow the athlete to return to normal activity with protective padding when pain and the initial irritation have subsided. If swelling is not resolved within a week,

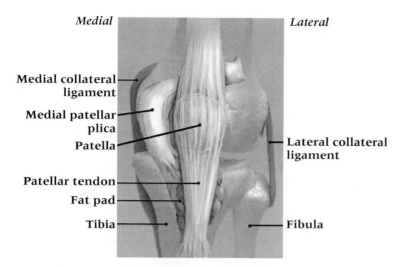

*Medial*        *Lateral*

Medial collateral ligament
Medial patellar plica
Patella
Patellar tendon
Fat pad
Tibia
Lateral collateral ligament
Fibula

**Figure 16-16**

Knee Plica

a chronic condition of either synovitis or bursitis may exist, indicating the need for rest and medical attention.

## Knee Plica

**Cause of injury**   A plica is a thickened fold of synovial membrane. There are three of them around the knee joint: the infrapatellar plica, the suprapatellar plica, and the mediopatellar plica, which is the least common but most subject to injury. It is located medial to the patella just above the joint line (Figure 16-16). Although most plicae are asymptomatic, the mediopatellar plica may be thick, nonyielding, and fibrotic, causing a number of symptoms.[31]

**Signs of injury**   The patient may or may not have a history of knee injury. If symptoms are preceded by trauma, it is usually from blunt force, such as a fall on the knee, or from a twist with the foot planted. A major complaint is recurrent episodes of painful pseudolocking of the knee when the patient has been sitting for a period of time. As the knee flexes, a snap may be felt or heard. The patient complains of pain while ascending or descending stairs or when squatting.[31]

**Care**   A knee plica that becomes inflamed as a result of trauma is usually treated conservatively with rest, anti-inflammatory agents, and local heat. If the condition recurs, causing a chondromalacia of the femoral condyle or patella, the plica will require surgical excision.

## Bursitis

**Cause of injury**   Bursitis in the knee can be acute, chronic, or recurrent. Although any one of the numerous knee bursae can become inflamed, the prepatellar and the deep infrapatellar bursae on the front of the knee have the highest incidence of irritation in sports (Figure 16-17). The prepatellar bursa often becomes inflamed from continued kneeling or falling directly on the knee, whereas the deep infrapatellar becomes irritated from overuse of the patellar tendon.[21]

**Figure 16-17**

Common bursae of the knee in cross section

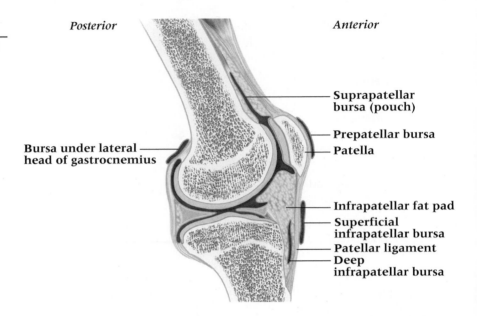

*Posterior*          *Anterior*

Suprapatellar bursa (pouch)

Prepatellar bursa
Patella

Bursa under lateral head of gastrocnemius

Infrapatellar fat pad
Superficial infrapatellar bursa
Patellar ligament
Deep infrapatellar bursa

The knee has many bursae; the prepatellar and deep infrapatellar bursae are most often irritated.

**Signs of injury**  Prepatellar bursitis results in localized swelling above the knee that is similar to a balloon. Swelling occurs outside the joint, and there may be some redness and increased temperature. Some inflamed bursae may be painful and disabling because of the swelling and should be treated accordingly. Swelling in the back of the knee does not necessarily indicate bursitis but could instead be a sign of Baker's cyst (Figure 16-18). A Baker's cyst develops swelling because of a problem in the joint and not because of bursitis. A Baker's cyst is commonly painless, causing no discomfort or disability.

**Figure 16-18**

Location of a Baker's cyst causes very little or no pain in the popliteal fossa on the back of the knee.

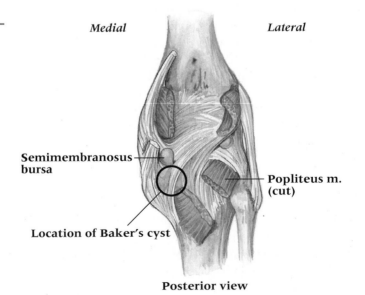

*Medial*          *Lateral*

Semimembranosus bursa

Popliteus m. (cut)

Location of Baker's cyst

**Posterior view**

**Care**   Management usually follows a pattern of eliminating the cause, prescribing rest, and reducing inflammation. Perhaps the two most important techniques for controlling bursitis are the use of elastic compression wraps and anti-inflammatory medication. When the bursitis is chronic or recurrent and the synovial lining of the joint capsule has thickened, a physician may cautiously use aspiration and a steroid injection.

## Loose Bodies within the Knee

**Cause of condition**   Because of repeated trauma to the knee during sports activities, loose bodies, sometimes called *joint mice,* can develop within the joint cavity. Loose bodies can result from osteochondritis dissecans (fragments of bone and cartilage), fragments from the menisci, pieces of torn synovial tissue, or a torn cruciate ligament.

**Signs of condition**   The loose bodies may move in the joint space and become lodged to cause locking and popping. The athlete complains of pain, instability, and a feeling that the knee is giving way.

**Care**   When the loose body becomes wedged between articulating surfaces, irritation can occur. If not surgically removed, the loose body can create conditions that lead to joint degeneration.

A knee that locks and unlocks during activity may indicate a torn meniscus.

## Iliotibial Band Friction Syndrome (Runner's Knee)

**Cause of injury   Iliotibial band friction syndrome** is an overuse condition commonly occurring in runners or cyclists that can be attributed to malalignment and structural asymmetries of the foot and lower leg. Irritation develops over the lateral femoral condyle or at the band's insertion on the lateral side of the knee where friction is created as the knee repeatedly flexes and extends.[32]

**Signs of injury**   There may be tenderness, some mild swelling, increased warmth, and possibly some redness over the lateral femoral condyle. Pain increases during running or cycling activities.[12]

**Care**   Treatment includes stretching the iliotibial band and performing techniques for reducing inflammation.[32] Management of runner's or cyclist's knee involves correction of foot and leg alignment problems. Therapy includes cold packs or ice massage before and after activity, proper warm-up and stretching, and avoiding activities that aggravate the problem, such as running on inclines.[12] Other procedures may include administering anti-inflammatory medications. A transverse friction massage done over the site of irritation can also help eliminate chronic inflammation.

> **iliotibial band friction syndrome**
> **(eel** e oh **tib** ee ul)
> Runner's knee.

## RECOGNITION AND MANAGEMENT OF INJURIES AND CONDITIONS OF THE EXTENSOR MECHANISM

The extensor mechanism of the knee consists of the quadriceps muscle group, the patellar tendon, the patella located within that tendon, and the tibial tubercle, which is the site of attachment for the patellar tendon.[11]

**◄ *16-3 Critical Thinking***
Exercise

A track athlete complains of pain in the anterior aspect of the knee while walking, running, ascending and descending stairs, or squatting. There is a grating sensation when flexing and extending the knee.

**?** What condition should be suspected and what should be the recommended treatment?

## Fracture of the Patella

**Cause of injury**   Fractures of the patella can be caused by either direct or indirect trauma. Most patellar fractures are the result of indirect trauma in which a severe pull of the patellar tendon occurs against the femur when the knee is semiflexed. This position subjects the patella to maximum stress from the quadriceps tendon and the patellar ligament. Forcible muscle contraction may then fracture the patella at its lower half. Direct injury most often produces fragmentation with little displacement. Falls, jumping, or running may result in a fracture of the patella.

**Signs of injury**   The fracture causes hemorrhage, resulting in generalized swelling. An indirect fracture causes tearing of the joint capsule, separation of bone fragments, and possible tearing of the quadriceps tendon. Direct fracture involves little bone separation.

**Care**   Diagnosis usually requires x-ray confirmation. As soon as the examiner suspects a patellar fracture, a cold wrap should be applied, followed by an elastic compression wrap and splinting. The athlete should then be referred to a physician. The athlete is normally immobilized for 2 to 3 months.

## Acute Patellar Subluxation or Dislocation

Knees that give way or catch
have a number of possible
pathological conditions:
- subluxating patella
- meniscal tear
- anterior cruciate
  ligamentous tear

**Cause of injury**   When an athlete plants the foot, decelerates, and simultaneously cuts in an opposite direction from the weight-bearing foot, the thigh rotates internally while the lower leg rotates externally, causing a medially directed valgus force at the knee.[2] The quadriceps muscle attempts to pull in a straight line and as a result pulls the patella laterally—a force that may dislocate the patella. As a rule, displacement takes place laterally, with the patella resting on the lateral condyle. This injury is more likely to occur in a female athlete than in a male because of a wider pelvis in a female.[1]

**Signs of injury**   The athlete experiences a complete loss of knee function along with pain and swelling; the patella rests in an abnormal position. A first-time patellar dislocation should always be suspected of being associated with a fracture.

**Care**   The knee should be immobilized in the position it is in (do not try to straighten the knee). Ice should be applied around the joint. The athlete should be taken to the physician, who will reduce the kneecap (put it back into place). After reduction, the knee is immobilized in extension for 4 weeks or longer, and the athlete is instructed to use crutches when walking. Muscle rehabilitation should involve strengthening all the muscles of the knee, thigh, and hip.[7]

The athlete may find it helpful to wear a neoprene brace that has a horseshoe-shaped felt pad designed to push the patella medially; the brace is worn while running or performing in sports (Figure 16-19).

## Chondromalacia Patella

**Cause of condition**   Chondromalacia patella is a softening and deterioration of the articular cartilage on the posterior surface of the

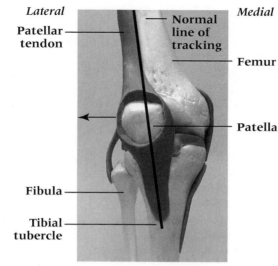

**Figure 16-19**

A special lateral pad in a
neoprene sleeve for the
dislocated patella

Lateral

Medial

Patellar
tendon

Normal
line of
tracking

Femur

Patella

Fibula

Tibial
tubercle

**Anterior view**

**Figure 16-20**

Lateral patellar tracking.
There is a tendency for the
patella to move laterally
when the knee goes into full
extension.

patella. The exact cause of chondromalacia is unknown but it is often
related to either abnormal movement of the patella within the femoral
groove or to overuse. Normally the patella moves up and down in the
femoral groove between the femoral condyles as the knee flexes and
extends. In some athletes the patella has a tendency to move or track
in a lateral direction as the quadriceps group contracts (Figure 16-20).[21]
This tracking most often occurs in athletes with weakness in the quadriceps muscle group or in female athletes who have a wider pelvis and
is generally referred to as patellofemoral syndrome.[18]

**Signs of condition**   The athlete may experience pain in the anterior aspect of the knee while walking, running, ascending and descending stairs, or squatting. There may be recurrent swelling around
the patella and a grating sensation when flexing and extending the
knee. The athlete may experience pain on the back of the patella or
when the patella is compressed within the femoral groove while the
knee is passively flexed and extended.

**Care**   Conservative treatment includes avoiding irritating activities
such as stair climbing and squatting; doing pain-free isometric exercises
that concentrate primarily on strengthening the quadriceps muscles; and
wearing a neoprene knee sleeve (Figure 16-21).[5] If conservative measures fail to help, surgery may be the only alternative.

## Jumper's Knee (Patellar Tendinitis)

**Cause of injury**   Jumping, kicking, or running may place extreme
tension on the knee extensor muscle complex. As a result of either a
single acute injury or, more commonly, repetitive injuries, **patellar
tendinitis** occurs in the patellar or quadriceps tendon.[17] On rare occasions, a patellar tendon may completely fail and rupture. Sudden or
repetitive forceful extension of the knee may begin an inflammatory
process that eventually leads to tendon degeneration.[27]

**16-4 Critical Thinking**
Exercise

A high jumper has been
diagnosed as having patellar
tendinitis or "jumper's knee." In
three weeks he has two important track meets and wants to
know what he can do to get rid
of the problems as soon as
possible.

? What options are there in
treating the athlete with patellar
tendinitis?

**patellar tendinitis
(pa teller)**
Jumper's knee.

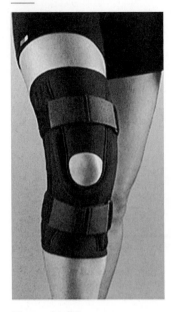

**Figure 16-21**

Neoprene sleeve

**Signs of injury** The athlete indicates vague pain and tenderness generally around the bottom of the patella on the posterior aspect that worsens when engaging in jumping or running activities. Quite often athletes say that if they could take their finger and reach under the kneecap at the bottom, the pain would be there.[14]

**Care** Any pain in the patellar tendon must preclude sudden explosive movement such as that characterized by heavy plyometric-type exercising. Several approaches to treating athletes with inflammation associated with jumper's knee have been reported, including rest, the use of ice, and anti-inflammatory medications.[10] A patellar tendon tenodesis brace or strap may also be used (Figure 16-22). An alternative to a commercial patellar strap is to use rolled-up prewrap or elastic tape around the knee just below the patella over the patellar tendon. Transverse friction massage has also been demonstrated to be an effective technique for care of jumper's knee.

## Osgood-Schlatter Disease

**Cause of condition** Osgood-Schlatter disease is a condition common to the rapidly growing immature adolescent's knee.[15] The most commonly accepted cause is the repeated pull of the patellar tendon at the tibial tubercle on the front of the tibia. The tibial tubercle is an important bony landmark because it is the site of attachment for the tendon of the entire quadriceps muscle group. Osgood-Schlatter disease is characterized by ongoing pain at the attachment of the patellar tendon at the tibial tubercle. Over time, a bony callus forms and the tubercle enlarges (Figure 16-23). This condition usually resolves when the athlete reaches the age of eighteen or nineteen. The only remnant is an enlarged tibial tubercle.[31]

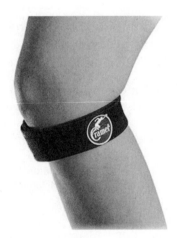

**Figure 16-22**

The tenodesis strap or brace for patellar tendinitis

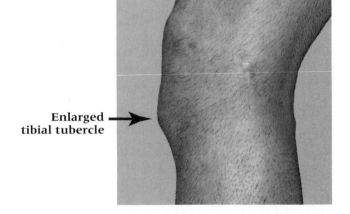

**Enlarged tibial tubercle** ➡

**Figure 16-23**

Osgood-Schlatter disease results in an enlarged tibial tubercle.

**Signs of condition**   Repeated irritation causes swelling, hemorrhage, and gradual degeneration at the tibial tubercle. The athlete complains of severe pain when kneeling, jumping, and running. There is point tenderness over the anterior proximal tibial tubercle.

**Care**   Treatment is usually conservative and includes the following: Stressful activities are decreased for approximately 6 months to 1 year; severe cases may require padding to protect the tibial tubercle from additional trauma; ice is applied to the knee before and after activities; and isometric strengthening of quadriceps and hamstring muscles is performed.[15]

## SUMMARY

- The knee is one of the most complex joints in the human body. Stability of the knee depends primarily on the bony articulations, ligaments, joint capsule, and muscles that surround the joint.

- Prevention of knee injuries involves maximizing muscle strength and wearing appropriate shoes. Use of protective knee bracing is questionable.

- Assessing an injury to the knee joint requires taking a history, observing both the appearance of the injured part and how the athlete moves, palpating the injured structures around the joint, and using special tests, including valgus/varus stress tests, Lachman's test, and Apley's compression test to determine the existing stability of the joint.

- The stabilizing structures most often injured are the medial and lateral collateral ligaments, the anterior and posterior cruciate ligaments, and the menisci.

- Other knee joint injuries that can occur either from acute trauma or from overuse are contusions, bursitis, joint mice, and iliotibial band friction syndrome.

- The patella and its surrounding area can develop a variety of injuries from sports activities, including fractures, subluxation and dislocation, and chondromalacia patella.

- The extensor mechanism of the knee consists of the quadriceps muscle group, the patellar tendon, the patella located within that tendon, and the tibial tubercle. Jumper's knee and Osgood-Schlatter disease are conditions associated with the extensor mechanism.

---

*Solutions to Critical Thinking* Exercises

---

**16-1**   A valgus stress test should be used to test the MCL. The examination in full extension tests the MCL, posteromedial capsule, and the cruciates. At 30 degrees of flexion the MCL is isolated. If there is some instability present with the knee in full extension, closely evaluate the integrity of the cruciate ligaments.

**16-2** This mechanism is typical for a sprain of the anterior cruciate ligament, although other ligamentous, capsular, and meniscal structures may be injured as well. An appropriate stability test for determining an injury to the ACL is the Lachman's test.

**16-3** It is likely that this athlete has chondromalacia patella. The athlete should avoid irritating activities such as stair climbing and squatting; do isometric exercises that are pain free to strengthen the quadriceps and hamstring muscles; and wear a neoprene knee sleeve. If conservative measures fail to help, surgery may be the only alternative.

**16-4** A conservative approach is to use normal techniques—reduce inflammation, rest, ice, ultrasound, anti-inflammatory medications, and so on. An alternative and more aggressive approach is to use a deep friction massage technique to increase the inflammatory response, which will ultimately facilitate healing. If successful, the more aggressive treatment may allow a quicker return to full activity.

## REVIEW QUESTIONS AND CLASS ACTIVITIES

1. What are the various structures that give the knee stability? What movements do these various structures prevent?
2. What motions can occur at the knee? Which muscles produce these movements?
3. Explain how a knee injury can best be prevented. What injuries are most difficult to prevent?
4. Demonstrate the steps that should be taken when assessing the knee.
5. Describe the mechanisms of injury for the collateral ligaments, the cruciate ligaments, and the menisci.
6. Contrast the signs and characteristics of grades 1, 2, and 3 medial collateral ligament sprains.
7. How might a contusion of the knee joint be related to bursitis of the knee?
8. How does a patellar subluxation or dislocation usually occur?
9. What factors can contribute to the development of chondromalacia?
10. What types of conditions can develop in the extensor mechanism? How are they cared for?
11. Invite an orthopedic physician to discuss the latest treatment and rehabilitation techniques for treating an injured knee.

### REFERENCES

1. Arendt, EA: 2002. Current concepts of lateral patella dislocation, *Clinics in sports medicine* 21(3): 499–519.
2. Baker, MM, Juhn, MS: 2000. Patello-femoral pain syndrome in the female athlete, *Clinical sports medicine* 19(2):315.
3. Bernstein, J: 2000. Meniscal tears of the knee: diagnosis and individualized treatment, *Physician and sportsmedicine* 28(3):83.
4. Boden, BP, Griffin, LY, Garrett, WE: 2000. Etiology and prevention of noncontact ACL injury, *Physician and sportsmedicine* 28(4):53.
5. Bolgla, L, Malone, T: 2005. Exercise prescription and patellofemoral pain: evidence for rehabilitation, *Journal of sport rehabilitation* 14(1): 72–88.
6. Carlson, L: 2002. Use of functional knee braces after ACL reconstruction, *Athletic therapy today* 7(3):48–49.

7. Cebesoy, O: 2007. Treatment of patellar instability. *Knee surgery, sports traumatology, arthroscopy* 15(6): 825.

8. Cosgarea, AJ: 2002. Evaluation and management of the unstable patella, *Physician and sportsmedicine* 30(10):33–40.

9. Curtis, N: 2006. Evidence-based knee evaluation and rehabilitation, *Athletic therapy today* 11(2):36.

10. Dale, B. Caswell, C: 2007. Functional rehabilitation for "jumper's knee." *Athletic therapy today* 12(5):7.

11. Edson, CJ, Feldmann, DD: 1999. Rehabilitation of posterior cruciate ligament injuries treated by operative methods, *Sports Med Arthroscop Rev* 7(4):303.

12. Ellis, R, Hing, W: 2007. Iliotibial band friction syndrome—A systematic review, *Manual Therapy* 12(3):200.

13. Fagenbaum, R: 2003. Jump landing strategies in male and female college athletes and the implications of such strategies for anterior cruciate ligament injury, *American journal of sports medicine* 31(2): 233–240.

14. Fredberg, U, Bolvig, L: 1999. Jumper's knee: review of the literature, *Scandinavian journal of medical science and sports* 9(2):66.

15. Gerbino, P: 2006. Adolescent anterior knee pain. *Operative techniques in sports medicine* 14(3): 203–211.

16. Grassmayr, M, Parker, D: 2008. Posterior cruciate ligament deficiency: biomechanical and biological consequences and the outcomes of conservative treatment: A systematic review. *Journal of science & medicine in sport* 11(5): 433.

17. Hale, S: 2005. Etiology of patellar tendinopathy in athletes. (Review), *Journal of sport rehabilitation* 14(3): 258–272.

18. Hamstra, L, Wright, K, Swanik, C: 2005. Joint stiffness and pain in individuals with patellofemoral syndrome, *Journal of orthopaedic & sports physical therapy* 35(8):495–501.

19. Jacobson, K, Chi, F: 2006. Evaluation and treatment of medial collateral ligament and medial-sided injuries of the knee. *Sports Med Arthroscop Rev* 14(2):58–66.

20. Janousek, AT et al.: 1999. Posterior cruciate ligament injuries of the knee joint, *Sports medicine* 28(6): 429.

21. Johnson, RM, Poppe, TR: 1999. Considering patellofemoral pain: exercise prescription, *Strength & conditioning journal* 21(1):73.

22. Kvist, J: 2004. Rehabilitation following anterior cruciate ligament injury: current recommendations for sports participation, *Sports medicine* 34(4):269–280.

23. Lambson, RB: 1996. Football cleat design and its effect on anterior cruciate ligament injuries: a three-year prospective study, *American journal of sports medicine* 24(2): 155–159.

24. Margheritini, F, Rihn, J, Musahl, V: 2002. Posterior cruciate ligament injuries in the athlete: an anatomical, biomechanical and clinical review, *Sports medicine* 32(6):393–408.

25. Mesiha, M, Zurakowski, D: 2007. Pathologic characteristics of the torn human meniscus. *American journal of sports medicine* 35(1):103–112.

26. Mullin, MJ: 2000. Functional rehabilitation of the knee, *Athletic therapy today* 5(2):28.

27. Myer, G, Ford, K, Hewett, T: 2004. Rationale and clinical techniques for anterior cruciate ligament injury prevention among female athletes, *Journal of athletic training* 39(4):352.

28. Oliver, C: 2002. Female athletes and ACL injuries, *Interscholastic athletic administration* 29(1):12–13.

29. Pellecchia, G, Hame, H, Behnke, P: 1994. Treatment of infrapatellar tendinitis: a combination of

modalities and transverse friction massage. *Journal of Sport Rehabilitation* 3(2):125.

30. Powers, CM et al.: 1999. Effect of bracing on patellar kinematics in patients with patellofemoral joint pain, *Medicine & Science in Sports & Exercise* 31(12):1714.

31. Prentice, W, Padua, D, Onate, J: 2010. Rehabilitation of the knee. In Prentice W, editor: *Rehabilitation techniques in sports medicine and athletic training*, New York, McGraw-Hill.

32. Racioppi, EA, Gulick, DT: 1999. Iliotibial band friction syndrome, *Athletic therapy today* 4(5):9.

33. Shimokochi, Y, Shultz, S: 2008. Mechanisms of noncontact anterior cruciate ligament injury. *Journal of athletic training* 43(4):396.

34. Styf, J: 1999. The effects of functional knee bracing on muscle function and performance, *Sports Medicine* 28(2):77.

## ANNOTATED BIBLIOGRAPHY

Darrow, M. Brazina, G: 2001. *The knee source book*, New York, McGraw-Hill.

*This straightforward guide discusses causes, symptoms, and treatments for common injuries and chronic conditions of the knee and explains what to do immediately after an injury to avoid more harm. Also discusses the benefits of rehab versus surgery.*

DeCarlo, M: 2004. Knee Rehabilitation, Philadelphia, Taylor & Francis, Inc.

*A complete guide to the most commonly encountered problems in sports medicine.*

Ellenbecker, T: 2000. *Knee ligament rehabilitation*, Philadelphia, Churchill-Livingston.

*Provides information to help diagnose and rehabilitate knee ligament injuries.*

Griffin, L: 1995. *Rehabilitation of the knee*, St Louis, Mosby.

*This text incorporates new advances in rehabilitation techniques and equipment and gives emphasis to sport-specific functional rehabilitation programs.*

# The Thigh, Hip, Groin, and Pelvis

*When you finish this chapter you will be able to:*

- Describe the major anatomical features of the thigh, hip, groin, and pelvis as they relate to sports injuries.
- Identify the major sports injuries to the thigh, hip, groin, and pelvis.
- Demonstrate appropriate emergency procedures for injuries to the thigh, groin, and pelvis.

Although the thigh, hip, groin, and pelvis have lower incidences of injury than do the knee and lower limb, they receive considerable trauma from a variety of sports activities.[2] Of major concern are thigh strains and contusions and chronic and overuse stresses affecting the thigh and hip.

## ANATOMY OF THE THIGH, HIP, GROIN, AND PELVIC REGION

### Bones

#### Thigh

The thigh is generally considered that part of the leg between the hip and the knee. The *femur* is the longest and strongest bone in the body (Figure 17-1). It is designed for maximum support and mobility during weight-bearing activity. The proximal head of the femur articulates with the acetabulum of the pelvis to form the hip joint and the distal femoral condyles articulate with the tibia at the knee joint.

#### Pelvis

The pelvis is a bony ring formed by two innominate bones, the sacrum, and the coccyx (Figure 17-2). The two innominate bones are each made up of an ilium, ischium, and pubis (Figure 17-3). The functions of the pelvis are to support the spine and trunk and to transfer their weight to the lower limbs. In addition to providing skeletal support, the pelvis serves as a place of attachment for the trunk and thigh muscles and protection for the pelvic organs.

Innominate bones:
- ilium
- ischium
- pubis

The hip and pelvis form the core for full body movement. The body's center of gravity is just in front of the upper part of the sacrum. Injuries to the hip or pelvis cause the athlete disability in the lower limb or trunk or both.[4]

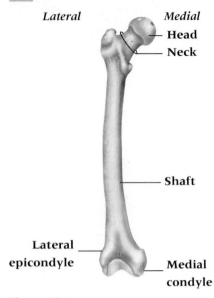

**Figure 17-1**

Femur (anterior view)

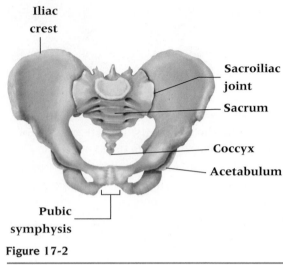

**Figure 17-2**

Pelvis (anterior view)

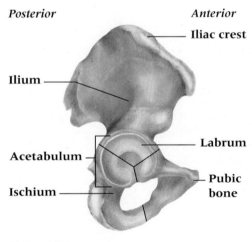

**Figure 17-3**

Innominate bone (lateral view)

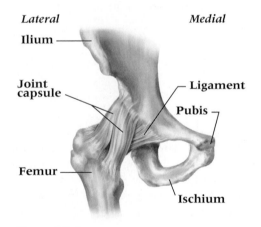

**Figure 17-4**

Hip joint ligaments and joint capsule (anterior view)

## Ligaments

The hip joint is formed by articulation of the femur with the innominate. The head of the femur fits into a deep socket, the acetabulum, and is stabilized by strong iliofemoral ligaments and a joint capsule (Figure 17-4). The sacrum is joined to other parts of the pelvis by strong sacrotuberous and sacrospinal ligaments, forming the sacroiliac joint. A small backward-forward movement is present at the sacroiliac junction. The sacroiliac joint is discussed in detail in Chapter 20.

## Muscles

### Thigh Muscles

The muscles located on the anterior thigh are the four quadriceps that function to extend the knee (Figure 17-5A). One of the quadriceps, the rectus femoris muscle, also acts to flex the hip. The sartorius muscle is also on the anterior thigh and acts to flex the hip and outwardly rotate the thigh (Figure 17-5A). The three hamstring muscles on the back of the thigh are flexors of the knee and act to extend the hip (Figure 17-5B). The five medial muscles are known as the adductor group and collectively act as adductors of the hip. They include the gracilis, pectineus, and the adductor magnus, longus, and brevis (Figure 17-5C).

### Hip Muscles

The muscles of the hip can be divided into anterior and posterior groups (Figure 17-5A). The anterior group includes the iliacus and psoas muscles,

**Figure 17-5**

Muscles of the thigh, hip, and groin: (A) Anterior view. (B) Posterior view.

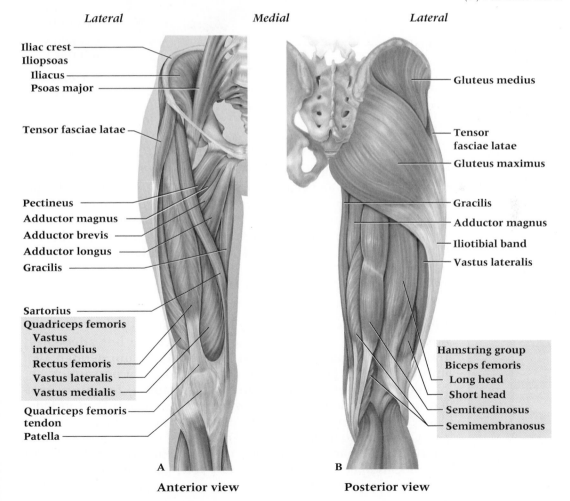

*Lateral*     *Medial*     *Lateral*

Iliac crest
Iliopsoas
Iliacus
Psoas major

Tensor fasciae latae

Pectineus
Adductor magnus
Adductor brevis
Adductor longus
Gracilis

Sartorius
Quadriceps femoris
  Vastus
  intermedius
  Rectus femoris
  Vastus lateralis
  Vastus medialis
Quadriceps femoris
tendon
Patella

Gluteus medius

Tensor
fasciae latae
Gluteus maximus

Gracilis
Adductor magnus
Iliotibial band
Vastus lateralis

Hamstring group
  Biceps femoris
   Long head
   Short head
  Semitendinosus
  Semimembranosus

**A**

**Anterior view**

**B**

**Posterior view**

**414**

**Figure 17-5 (continued)**

Muscles of the thigh, hip, and groin: (C) Deep muscles, posterior view.

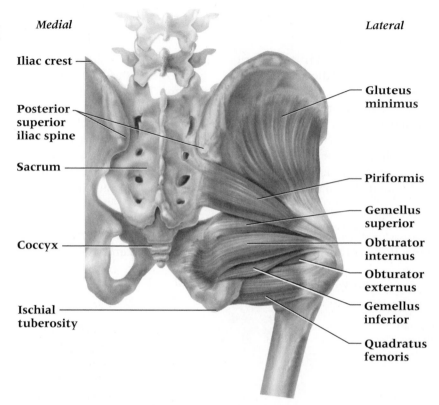

*Medial*  *Lateral*

Iliac crest

Posterior superior iliac spine

Sacrum

Coccyx

Ischial tuberosity

Gluteus minimus

Piriformis

Gemellus superior

Obturator internus

Obturator externus

Gemellus inferior

Quadratus femoris

**C Posterior view**

which flex the thigh on the trunk. The posterior group includes the tensor fasciae latae and gluteus medius, which abduct the thigh; the gluteus maximus, which extends the thigh; the gluteus minimus, which internally rotates the thigh; and the six deep outward rotators—the piriformis, superior gemellus, inferior gemellus, obturator internus, obturator externus, and quadratus femoris (Table 17-1).

## ASSESSING THIGH, HIP, GROIN, AND PELVIS INJURIES

**Generally fitness professionals, coaches, and others working in areas related to exercise and sport science are not adequately trained to evaluate injuries. It is strongly recommended that injured athletes be referred to qualified medical personnel (i.e., physicians, athletic trainers, physical therapists) for injury evaluation.** Information on the following special tests has been included simply to give some idea about the different basic tests that nonmedical personnel may do to determine the nature and severity of the athlete's injury. The primary responsibility of those who are not health care personnel is to be able to recognize any potential "red flags" associated with the injury, provide appropriate first aid for the injury, and make

| TABLE 17-1 Muscles of the Thigh, Hip, and Groin | |
|---|---|
| Hip flexion | Rectus femoris |
| | Sartorius |
| | Illiacus |
| | Psoas |
| Hip extension | Hamstrings |
| | Biceps femoris |
| | Semimembranosis |
| | Semitendinosis |
| | Gluteus maximus |
| Hip abduction | Gluteus medius |
| | Tensor fascia lata |
| Hip adduction | Gracilis |
| | Pectineus |
| | Adductor magnus |
| | Adductor longus |
| | Adductor brevis |
| Hip medial rotation | Gluteus minimus |
| Hip lateral rotation | Piriformis |
| | Superior gemellus |
| | Inferior gemellus |
| | Obturator internus |
| | Obturator externus |
| | Quadratus femoris |

correct decisions about how the injury should be managed initially, including immediate return to play or activity decisions. (Refer to Chapter 7.)

## History

- What mechanism do you think caused this injury to occur?
- When did you first notice this pain?
- Did the pain begin immediately, or did it occur gradually over a period of time?
- Have you ever had a problem in the area before?
- Has training intensity changed or increased recently?
- Where is the pain located?
- Describe the type of pain you have (e.g., sharp, dull, burning, aching).
- Does the pain radiate down the back or front of the legs or buttocks?
- When is the pain the worst (e.g., during activity, at rest, at night)?

## Observation

- The athlete should be observed for postural asymmetry while standing on one leg and during ambulation.

- From the front view, do the hips look even?
- From the side view, is the pelvis abnormally tilted anteriorly or posteriorly?
- The patella should also be noted for relative position and alignment.
- Does standing on one leg produce pain in the hip?
- The athlete should be observed during walking, bending, and sitting. Pain in the hip and pelvic region is normally reflected in movement distortions.

### Palpation

Bony palpation should include the iliac crest, hip joint, femur, sacrum, and coccyx, looking for point tenderness and discomfort. The soft tissues, including those on the anterior thigh, the posterior thigh, the groin, the buttocks, the lateral hip, and the anterior hip should be palpated to identify areas of tenderness or pain on active movement.[30]

### Special Tests

#### Thomas Test

The Thomas Test indicates whether there is tightness in the hip flexors (Figure 17-6). The athlete lies supine on a table, arms folded, legs together and fully extended, creating a normal curve in the low back. One thigh is brought to the chest, flattening the spine. In this position the extended thigh should be flat on the table. If not, there is tightness of the hip flexors. When the athlete fully extends the leg again, the curve in the low back returns.[30]

#### Straight Leg Raises

A straight leg raise can be used to test tightness in the hip extensors. The athlete lies supine and one leg is lifted flexing the hip (Figure 17-7). If the leg cannot be flexed to 90 degrees, there is tightness in the hip extensors. A positive straight leg test can also indicate a problem in the low back or sacroiliac joint.

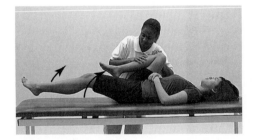

**Figure 17-6**

Thomas Test demonstrating
tight hip flexors

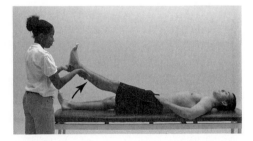

**Figure 17-7**

Straight leg raising test demonstrating
tightness of the hip extensors

## PREVENTION OF INJURIES TO THE THIGH, HIP, GROIN, AND PELVIC REGION

Despite the fact that the hip joint is one of the strongest and most stable joints in the body, primarily because of its strong ligaments and joint capsule and also its strong musculature, there are still many potential injuries that can occur in this region. While there are many muscles that produce a variety of movements throughout this region, they are extremely vulnerable to injury resulting from the dynamic power-producing contractions that occur. Success in dynamic running and jumping activities is largely dependent on the function of the muscles in this region. But at the same time, we rely on those same muscles working in conjunction with the pelvis, and the hip with its ligaments and capsule, to provide a base of stability on which the extremities function. Thus, to meet the demands of both dynamic force production and stabilization of the core of the body, the muscles, joints, and ligaments in this region are vulnerable to injury.

To prevent or at least minimize the chance of injury, it becomes essential to maintain strength and flexibility of those muscles of the hip, thigh, and pelvis. Athletes should concentrate on a dynamic stretching program that focuses on quadriceps, hamstrings, and groin muscles. Muscle strains in any of these muscle groups can have long-term consequences for healing and can prove to be disabling for the athlete. Likewise, muscles that are strong will be more resistant to injury, and thus a well-designed strengthening program can also help to minimize injuries. Strengthening exercises should routinely include squats, lunges, and leg presses as well as a variety of core strengthening exercises (see Chapter 4).[14]

*Flexibility and strengthening of the muscles in this region are the keys to preventing injury.*

## RECOGNITION AND MANAGEMENT OF INJURIES TO THE THIGH

Injuries to the thigh muscles are among the most common in sports. Contusions and strains occur often to the thigh, with the former having the highest incidence.

### Quadriceps Contusions

**Cause of injury** The quadriceps group is continually exposed to traumatic blows in a variety of sports. Contusions of the quadriceps display all the classic symptoms of most muscle bruises.

**Signs of injury** Quadriceps contusions usually develop as the result of a severe impact on the relaxed thigh, compressing the muscle against the hard surface of the femur.[6] At the instant of trauma, pain, a temporary loss of function, and the immediate bleeding of the affected muscles usually occur. The extent of the force and the degree of thigh relaxation determine the depth of the injury and the amount of structural and functional disruption that take place.[24]

Early detection and avoidance of profuse internal bleeding are vital, both in effecting a fast recovery by the athlete and in the prevention of widespread scarring of the muscle tissue. The athlete usually describes having been hit by a sharp blow to the thigh, which produced intense pain and weakness. The coach observes that the athlete is limping and holding the thigh. Palpation by the coach may reveal a swollen area that is painful to the touch. The seriousness or extent of injury is determined by the amount of weakness and decreased range of motion.

**Grade 1 (mild) contusions**   A Grade 1 quadriceps contusion can be either a very superficial intramuscular bruise or a slightly deeper one. The very superficial contusion creates a mild hemorrhage, minimal pain, no swelling, and mild point tenderness with no restriction of the range of motion. In contrast, a deeper first-degree contusion produces pain, mild swelling, point tenderness, and knee flexion of no more than 90 degrees.

**Grade 2 (moderate) contusions**   A Grade 2 quadriceps contusion is of moderate intensity, causing pain, swelling, and a range of knee flexion that is less than 90 degrees with an obvious limp present while walking.

**Grade 3 (severe) contusions**   A severe, or grade 3, quadriceps contusion represents a major disability. The blow may have been so intense as to split the fasciae, allowing the muscle to protrude (muscle herniation). Characteristically a deep intramuscular hematoma with an intermuscular spread is present. Pain is severe, and swelling may lead to the formation of a hematoma. Knee flexion is severely restricted and motion is limited to 45–90 degrees. The athlete has a decided limp.

**Care**   Immediate action includes compression by elastic bandage with the knee flexed to 120° to minimize the loss in range of motion for the first 12 hours.[3] This places the quadriceps in a stretched position and also helps to compress the injured area. The application of a cold medium can help control superficial hemorrhage (Figure 17-8). The thigh contusion should be handled conservatively with PRICE followed by a very gentle static stretch and crutch walking when a limp is present.

**Figure 17-8**

Immediate care of the thigh contusion: Applying a cold pack and pressure bandage along with a stretch may provide some relief.

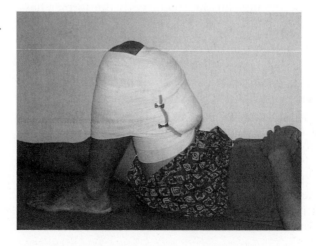

If an athlete has sustained a grade 2 or 3 thigh contusion, great care must be taken to avoid the occurrence of another one. The athlete should routinely wear a protective pad held in place by an elastic wrap while engaged in sports activity.

Isometric quadriceps contractions (quad sets) should begin as soon as they can be tolerated. Use of heat or massage should be avoided in the early stages of recovery.[14]

## Myositis Ossificans

**Cause of injury**   A severe blow or repeated blows to the thigh, usually the quadriceps muscle, can cause ectopic bone formation within the muscle, known as **myositis ossificans traumatica.**[23]

**Signs of injury**   Myositis ossificans commonly develops following bleeding into the quadriceps muscle and formation of a blood tumor. The contusion causes a disruption of muscle fibers, blood vessels, connective tissue, and the periosteum of the femur. Acute inflammation follows resolution of hemorrhage. The irritated tissue may produce tissue formations resembling cartilage or bone. In 2 to 4 weeks, formation of bone may be noted under x-ray examination. If the injury is to a muscle belly, complete absorption or a decrease in size of the formation may occur. This absorption is less likely if calcification is at a muscle origin or insertion. Some formations are completely free of the femur, whereas another may be stalklike and yet another broadly attached (Figure 17-9).

The following can cause the condition or, once present, aggravate it, causing it to become more pronounced:

- Attempting to run off a quadriceps contusion.
- Too vigorous treatment of a contusion—for example, massage directly over the contusion or superficial heat to the thigh.

> **myositis ossificans traumatica**
> Bone formation occurring in an abnormal place.

Myositis ossificans traumatica can occur following
- a single severe blow
- many blows to a muscle area
- improper care of a contusion

**17-1 Critical Thinking**
Exercise

A basketball player performing a layup shot receives a sharp blow to his right quadriceps muscle.

**?** How may the grade of this contusion be determined?

**Figure 17-9**

(A) Myositis ossificans is likely to develop in the anterior thigh following repeated contusion.
(B) X-ray view.

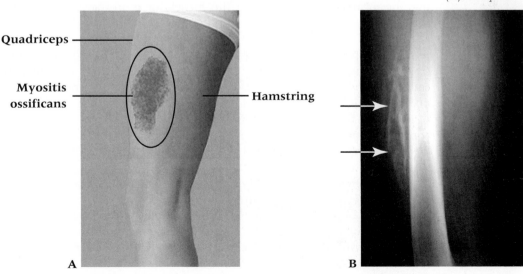

Quadriceps

Myositis ossificans

Hamstring

A    B

**Figure 17-10**

Rupture of the rectus femoris

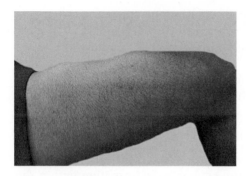

**Care** Improper care of a thigh confusion can lead to ossification in muscle. Once myositis ossificans traumatica is apparent, treatment should be extremely conservative. If the condition is painful and restricts motion, the formation may be surgically removed after 1 year with much less likelihood of its return. Too early removal of the formation may cause it to return. Recurrent myositis ossificans may indicate a problem with blood clotting.[16]

### Quadriceps Muscle Strain

**Cause of injury** The rectus femoris muscle of the quadriceps muscle group occasionally becomes strained by a sudden stretch (e.g., falling on a bent knee) or a sudden contraction (e.g., jumping in volleyball or kicking in soccer). Usually this muscle strain is associated with a muscle that is weakened or overly constricted.[21]

A tear in the region of the rectus femoris may cause partial or complete disruption of muscle fibers (Figure 17-10). The incomplete tear may be located centrally within the muscle or more peripheral to the muscle.

**Signs of injury** A peripheral quadriceps rectus femoris tear causes fewer symptoms than the deeper tear. In general, there is less point tenderness and little bleeding. A more centered partial muscle tear causes more pain and discomfort than does the peripheral tear. The deep tear causes a great deal of pain, point tenderness, spasm, and loss of function, but little discoloration from internal bleeding. In contrast, complete muscle tear of the rectus femoris may leave the athlete with little disability and discomfort but with some deformity of the anterior thigh.

**Care** On-site care of the quadriceps strain includes rest, cold application, and pressure to control internal bleeding. The extent of the tear should be ascertained as soon as possible before swelling masks the extent of injury (refer to Figure 17-10). To stabilize the muscle consider having the athlete wear a neoprene sleeve as healing occurs (Figure 17-11).

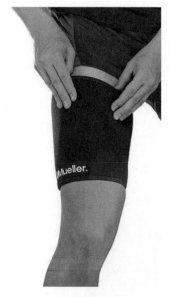

**Figure 17-11**

A neoprene sleeve may be worn for soft tissue support.

## Hamstring Muscle Strains

**Cause of injury**   Of all the thigh muscles subject to strain, the hamstring group has the highest incidence of strain. A quick change of the hamstring muscle function from knee stabilization to extension of the hip when running may be a primary cause of this strain (Figure 17-12).[27] What leads to this muscle failure and deficiency in the complementary action of opposing muscles is not clearly understood. Some possible reasons are muscle fatigue, sciatic nerve irritation, faulty posture, leg-length discrepancy, tight hamstrings, using improper form, and imbalance of strength between hamstring muscle groups.[14]

In most athletes, the hamstring muscle group should have at least 60 to 75 percent of the strength of the opposing quadriceps group. Stretching after exercise is imperative to avoid muscle tightness.[1]

Hamstring strain can involve the muscle belly or bony attachment. The extent of injury can vary from the pulling apart of a few muscle fibers to a complete rupture or an avulsion fracture.[27]

**Signs of injury**   Internal bleeding, pain, and immediate loss of function vary according to the degree of trauma. Discoloration may occur 1 or 2 days after injury.

**Grade 1 hamstring strain**   A grade 1 hamstring strain is usually evidenced by muscle soreness on movement and is accompanied by point tenderness. These strains are often difficult to detect when they occur. Irritation and stiffness do not become apparent until the athlete has cooled down after activity. The soreness of the mild hamstring strain in most instances can be attributed to muscle guarding rather than to the tearing of tissue.[12]

**Grade 2 hamstring strain**   A grade 2 muscle strain represents partial tearing of muscle fibers and can be identified by a sudden snap or tear of the muscle accompanied by severe pain and a loss of function

In order of incidence of sports injury to the thigh, quadriceps contusions rank first and hamstring strains rank second.

> ### 17-2 Critical Thinking
> Exercise
>
> A sprinter competing in a 100-yard dash experiences a sudden snap, severe pain, and weakness in the left hamstring muscle.
>
> **?** What kind of injury might the coach expect?

**Figure 17-12**

In many sports, stretching with excessive hip flexion of the hip region can cause a hamstring strain.

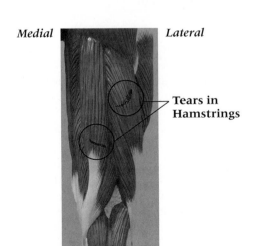

*Medial*     *Lateral*

→ **Tears in Hamstrings**

**Posterior view**

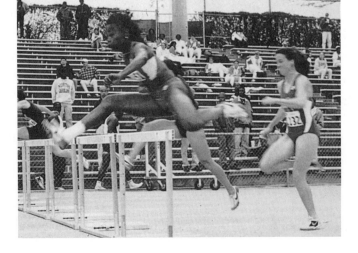

of knee flexion. It is possible to palpate a defect in the muscle with a grade 2 strain.

**Grade 3 hamstring strain**　A grade 3 hamstring strain is the rupturing of tendinous or muscular tissue, involving major hemorrhage and disability and a palpable and sometimes visual defect.

**Care**　Initially an ice pack and compression by an elastic wrap should be employed. Activity should be restricted until soreness has been minimized. Ballistic stretching and explosive sprinting should be avoided initially.[14]

Strains are always a problem to the athlete; they tend to recur because they sometimes heal with inelastic fibrous scar tissue.[12] The higher the incidence of strains at a particular muscle site, the greater the amount of scar tissue and the greater the likelihood of further injury.[31]

## Acute Femoral Fracture

**Cause of injury**　In sports, fractures of the femur occur most often in the shaft rather than at the bone ends and are almost always caused by a great force, such as falling from a height or being hit directly by another participant. A fracture of the shaft most often takes place in the middle third of the bone because of the anatomical curve at this point and because the majority of direct blows are sustained in this area.[15]

**Signs of injury**　Shock generally accompanies a fracture of the femur as a result of the extreme amount of pathology and pain associated with this injury. Bone displacement is usually present as a result of the great strength of the quadriceps muscle, which causes overriding of the bone fragments. Direct impact produces extensive soft-tissue injury with muscle lacerations, major internal bleeding, and muscle spasms.

An acute fractured femur is recognized by these classic signs:

- Deformity, with the thigh rotated outward
- A shortened thigh, caused by bone displacement
- Loss of thigh function
- Pain and point tenderness
- Swelling of the soft tissues

**Care**　Immediate emergency assistance and medical referral are necessary to prevent shock and a life threatening situation.[29]

## Femoral Stress Fractures

Femoral stress fractures most often result from repetitive, sustained activities such as distance running.

**Cause of injury**　Stress fractures of the femoral neck are fairly uncommon and femoral shaft stress fractures rarely occur. They occur most often in endurance athletes (for example, competitors in the triathlon or marathon) and thus the primary mechanism of injury is attributed to overuse. These injuries are more likely in females than males.[13]

**Signs of injury**　Onset of symptoms may occur several weeks after increasing the intensity of a training program. The athlete with a stress fracture complains of pain in the groin or anterior thigh, which increases during activity and may persist after activity. Pain may be referred to the knee. Pain is relieved with longer periods of rest. Eventually pain becomes constant even with no activity. The patient walks with a limp.[13]

**Care**  Initial treatment requires complete rest with no running. Stress fractures on the lateral side of the femoral neck are more likely to eventually displace and cause additional complications than those on the medial side. Stress fractures of the femoral shaft usually heal with conservative management but in rare cases can progress to failure of cortical bone. If a fracture does occur, surgery may be indicated, and the time required for fracture healing and remodeling can be as long as 12 months.

## RECOGNITION AND MANAGEMENT OF HIP AND GROIN INJURIES

The hip joint, the strongest and best-protected joint in the human body, is seldom seriously injured during sports activities. The hip joint is substantially supported by the ligamentous tissues and muscles that surround it, so any unusual movement that exceeds the normal range of motion may result in tearing of tissue.[34]

### Hip Sprain

**Cause of injury**  Hip sprains may occur as the result of a violent twist, either produced through an impact force delivered by another participant or by forceful contact with another object or sustained in a situation in which the foot is firmly planted and the trunk is forced in an opposing direction.[7]

**Signs of injury**  A hip sprain displays all the signs of a major acute injury but is best revealed through the athlete's inability to circumduct the thigh. Symptoms are similar to a stress fracture. There is significant pain in the hip region. Hip rotation increases pain.

**Care**  X-rays should be taken to rule out fracture; PRICE and analgesics are used as needed. Depending on the grade of sprain, weight bearing is restricted. Crutch walking is used for grade 2 and 3 sprains. Range-of-motion and progressive resistance exercises are delayed until the hip is pain free.

### Dislocated Hip Joint

**Cause of injury**  Dislocation of the hip joint rarely occurs in sports. The dislocated hip is caused by traumatic force along the long axis of the femur or by the athlete falling on his or her side. Such dislocations are produced when the knee is bent.[10]

**Signs of injury**  The incomplete dislocation or luxation presents a picture of a flexed, adducted, and internally rotated thigh (Figure 17-13).[36] Palpation reveals that the head of the femur has moved to a position posterior to the acetabulum. A hip dislocation causes serious pathology by tearing capsular and ligamentous tissue.[10] A fracture is often associated

**Figure 17-13**

Typical position for a hip dislocation: slightly flexed, adducted, and internally rotated.

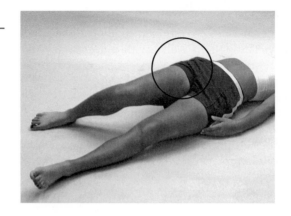

**avascular necrosis (necro sis)**
Death of an area caused by lack of circulation.

with this injury, accompanied by possible damage to the sciatic nerve and the nutrient artery, causing **avascular necrosis.**

**Care** Medical attention must be secured immediately after displacement, or muscle contractures may complicate the initial treatment. Immobilization usually consists of 2 weeks of bed rest and the use of a crutch for walking for a month or longer.[36]

**Complications** Complication of a posterior hip dislocation is likely. Such complications include muscle paralysis as a result of nerve injury in the area and later development of degeneration of the femoral head.

## Hip Labral Tear

**Cause of injury** The socket of the hip joint (acetabulum) is lined by articular cartilage called the labrum (Figure 17-14). This cartilage provides

**Figure 17-14**

**Tear within the labrum of the hip (lateral view)**

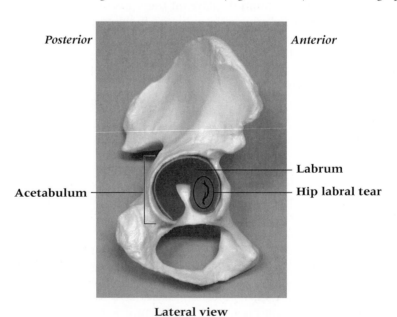

Lateral view

stability and cushioning for the hip joint, permitting the head of the femur to move smoothly and painlessly in the acetabulum. A hip labral tear most often results from repetitive movements such as running or pivoting of the hip that cause degeneration and breakdown of the labrum. It may also be caused by an acute injury such as a dislocation.[4]

**Signs of injury** Most commonly a hip labral tear can be asymptomatic. Occasionally, however, a hip labral tear may cause a catching, locking or clicking sensation in the hip joint; pain in the hip or groin; and a feeling of stiffness or limited motion.[4]

**Care** Treatment for a hip labral tear may consist of exercises to maximize hip range of motion, hip strengthening and stability exercises, and avoiding movements that place stress on the hip joint. Pain medications may also help and a physician may choose to inject a corticosteroid. If pain persists more than 4 weeks, surgery may be indicated to either remove a piece of the torn labrum or to repair the tear using sutures.

## Piriformis Syndrome

**Cause of condition** The sciatic nerve, which is located either under the piriformis muscle or actually piercing the piriformis muscle itself, is compressed or irritated by tightness or spasm of this muscle. This particular syndrome can often mimic another condition known as *sciatica*, and is often misdiagnosed as sciatica. The main difference between sciatica and piriformis syndrome is that sciatica is due to a herniated lumbar disc pressing on the sciatic nerve as it exits the lumbar spine.[14]

**Signs of condition** Compression of the sciatic nerve by the piriformis causes pain, numbness, and tingling in the butt that can extend below the knee and into the foot. The pain may worsen as a result of sitting for a long period of time, climbing stairs, walking, or running.

**Care** Generally, treatment for the syndrome begins with stretching exercises and massage. Anti-inflammatory drugs may be prescribed. Cessation of running, bicycling, or similar activities may be advised. A corticosteroid injection near where the piriformis muscle and the sciatic nerve meet may provide temporary relief. In some cases, surgery is recommended.

## Groin Strain

The groin is the depression between the thigh and the abdomen. The muscles in the groin region are responsible for adduction and internal rotation of the thigh.

**Cause of injury** Any one of the muscles in the groin region can be injured in sports activity and elicit a groin strain (Figure 17-15). In addition, overextension of the groin musculature may result in a strain.[25] Running, jumping, and twisting with external rotation can produce such injuries.[17] Groin injuries are very likely to occur in the early part of the season, particularly if an athlete has poor strength and flexibility in these muscles.[8]

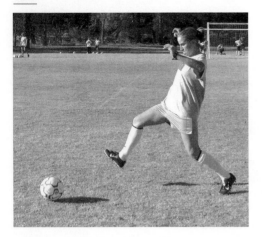

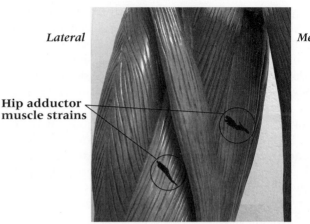

*Lateral*                                          *Medial*

**Hip adductor muscle strains**

**Figure 17-15**

Many sports that require stretch of the hip region can cause a groin strain.

**Signs of injury**   The strain can appear as a sudden twinge or feeling of tearing during a movement, or it may not be noticed until after termination of activity. As is characteristic of most tears, the groin strain also produces pain, weakness, and internal bleeding.[8]

**Care**   If it is detected immediately after it occurs, the strain should be treated by intermittent ice, pressure, and rest for 48 to 72 hours.[18]

Rest has been found to be the best treatment for groin strains. Until normal flexibility and strength return, a protective spica bandage should be applied. A groin wrap using an elastic bandage can help support the area (see Figure 10-4). Commercial restraints are also available to protect the injured groin (Figure 17-16). Note that a pelvic stress fracture may produce groin pain. Any athlete complaining of severe groin pain should be referred for medical attention.

**Figure 17-16**

Commercial restraints such as the SAWA groin and thigh braces are increasingly being used in athletic training.

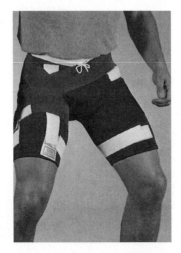

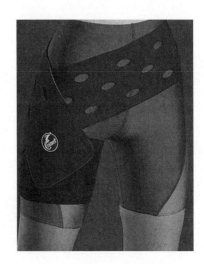

## Hip Joint Problems in the Adolescent Athlete

Two problems may occur in the hip joint in adolescent athletes: Legg-Perthes disease (coxa plana) and a slipped capital femoral epiphysis.[22]

### Legg-Perthes Disease (Coxa Plana)

**Cause of condition**   Legg-Perthes disease or coxa plana is due to a loss of blood circulation to the articular head of the femur (Figure 17-17). It occurs in children ages three to twelve and in boys more often than in girls. The reason for this condition is not clearly understood. Because of a disruption of circulation to the head of the femur, the articular cartilage dies and becomes flattened. This condition is referred to as avascular necrosis.

**Signs of condition**   The young athlete commonly complains of pain in the groin that sometimes is referred to the abdomen or knee. Limping is also typical. The condition can have a rapid onset, but more often it comes on slowly over a number of months. Examination may show limited hip movement and pain.[14]

**Care**   This condition can warrant complete bed rest to reduce the chances of a chronic hip condition. A special brace to avoid direct weight bearing on the hip may have to be worn. If treated in time, the head of the femur will revascularize and regain its original shape.

**Complications**   If the condition is not treated early enough, the head of the femur will become ill shaped, producing osteoarthritis in later life.

### Slipped Capital Femoral Epiphysis

**Cause of condition**   A slipped capital femoral epiphysis is an unusual disorder of the adolescent hip in which the epiphysis (growing end) of the femur slips from the femoral head in a backward direction.[22] This is due to weakness of the growth plate. Most often, it develops during periods of accelerated growth, shortly after the onset of puberty.[9] A slipped capital femoral epiphysis (Figure 17-18) is found mostly in boys between the ages of ten and seventeen who are very tall and thin or are obese. Although the cause is unknown, the slipped capital femoral

A young athlete who complains of pain in the groin, abdomen, or knee and who walks with a limp may display signs of coxa plana or a slipped capital femoral epiphysis.

**Figure 17-17**

Legg-Perthes disease. (A) Normal femoral head x-ray (B) Femoral head with avascular necrosis x-ray.

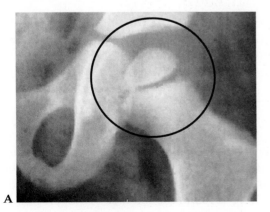

A

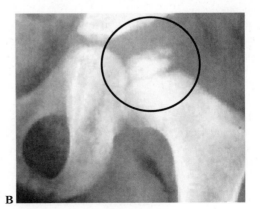

B

**Figure 17-18**

Slipped capital femoral epiphysis. The femoral head (proximal femoral epiphysis) slips posterior and inferior on the femoral neck (femoral metaphysis).

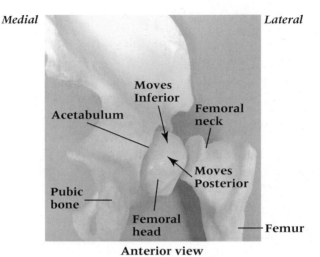

*Medial*   *Lateral*

Moves Inferior

Acetabulum

Femoral neck

Pubic bone

Moves Posterior

Femoral head

Femur

**Anterior view**

epiphysis may be related to the effects of a growth hormone. In one-quarter of the cases, both hips are affected.[20] The femoral head or proximal femoral epiphysis slips posterior and inferior relative to the femoral neck or femoral metaphysis.

**Signs of condition**   Symptoms of this condition are similar to those for Legg-Perthes disease. The athlete has a pain in the groin that arises suddenly as a result of trauma or over weeks or months as a result of prolonged stress. In the early stages of this condition, signs may be minimal; however, in its most advanced stage there is hip and knee pain and major limitations on movement together with a limp.

**Care**   In cases of minor displacement, rest and no weight bearing may prevent further slipping. Major displacement usually requires corrective surgery.

**Complications**   If the displacement goes undetected or if surgery fails to restore normal hip mechanics, severe hip problems may occur in later life.

## RECOGNITION AND MANAGEMENT OF INJURIES TO THE PELVIS

Athletes who perform activities involving violent jumping, running, and collisions can sustain serious acute and overuse injuries to the pelvic region (Figure 17-19).[34]

### Iliac Crest Contusion (Hip Pointer)

An iliac crest contusion, commonly known as a *hip pointer,* occurs most often in contact sports.

**Cause of injury**   The hip pointer results from a blow to the inadequately protected iliac crest (Figure 17-20). The hip pointer is one of the most handicapping injuries in sports. A direct impact to the unprotected iliac crest causes a severe pinching action to the soft tissue of that region.[21]

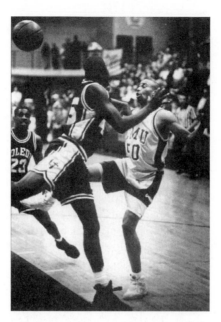

**Figure 17-19**

Athletes who perform activities involving jumping, running, and collisions can sustain serious acute and overuse injuries to the pelvic region.

**Signs of injury**   The hip pointer produces immediate pain, muscle guarding, and transitory paralysis of the soft structures. As a result, the athlete is unable to rotate the trunk or to flex the thigh without pain.[33]

**Care**   Cold and pressure should be applied immediately after injury and should be maintained intermittently for at least 48 hours. In severe cases bed rest for 1 to 2 days will speed recovery. Referral to a physician must be made and an x-ray examination given. When the athlete

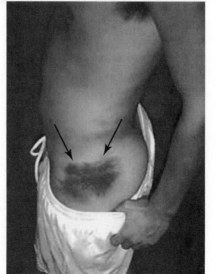

**Figure 17-20**

A blow to the pelvic rim can cause a bruise and hematoma known as a hip pointer.

A football player who is not wearing hip pads receives a hard compressive hit to his left iliac crest region.

**?** What injury has this athlete sustained? What are the expected symptoms and signs?

returns to play, a protective pad should be used to minimize the chances of additional injury. Protection is the key to recovery.

## Osteitis Pubis

**Cause of injury** Since the popularity of distance running has increased, a condition known as *osteitis pubis* has become more prevalent. It also occurs in soccer, football, and wrestling.[35] Repetitive stress on the *pubic symphysis* and adjacent bony structures by the pull of muscles in the area creates a chronic inflammatory condition.[28]

**Signs of injury** The athlete has pain in the groin region and in the bony projection under the pubic hair called the symphysis pubis. There is point tenderness on the pubic tubercle and pain when movements such as running, sit-ups, and squats are performed.[29] The pubic bones should be symmetrical from one side to the other.

**Care** Follow-up care usually consists of rest and an oral anti-inflammatory agent. A return to activity should be gradual.[11]

## Acute Fracture of the Pelvis

The pelvis is an extremely strong structure, and fractures stemming from sports are rare.

**Cause of injury** The acute pelvic fracture usually occurs as the result of a direct trauma.

**Signs of injury** The athlete responds to this injury with severe pain, loss of function, and shock.

**Care** If a pelvic fracture is suspected, the athlete should be immediately treated for shock and referred to a physician. The seriousness of this injury depends on the extent of shock and the possibility of internal injury.

## Stress Fractures of the Pelvis

**Cause of injury** As with other stress fractures, pelvic stress fractures can be produced by repetitive abnormal overuse forces. Pelvic stress fractures tend to occur during intensive training or competitive racing.[32]

**Signs of injury** Commonly the athlete complains of groin pain along with an aching sensation in the thigh that increases with activity and decreases with rest.

**Care** The athlete complains of pelvic pain following intense exercise. Referral to a physician for a detailed examination with an x-ray is a must. Once this injury is verified, rest is the treatment of choice for 2 to 5 months.

## Avulsion Fractures

**Cause of injury** An avulsion is the tearing away of a body part from its point of attachment. An avulsion fracture occurs when a tendon that attaches a muscle to a bone pulls part of the bone away after sudden, forceful contraction of that muscle. There are several muscles of the thigh that attach to various parts of the pelvis. Common sites for avulsion fractures in the pelvis include where the sartorius muscle attaches to the anterior superior iliac spine (ASIS), where the rectus femoris muscle attaches to the front anterior inferior iliac spine (AIIS), and where the hamstring muscle group attaches to the ischial tuberosity.[14]

**Signs of injury** The athlete complains of a sudden localized pain with limited movement. On inspection swelling and a point tenderness can be observed.

**Care** Early conditions require rest, limited activity, and graduated exercise.

## SUMMARY

- The thigh is composed of the femoral shaft, musculature, nerves and blood vessels, and the fascia that envelops the soft tissue. It is the part of the leg between the hip and the knee.
- The quadriceps contusion and hamstring strain are the most common sports injuries to the thigh, with the quadriceps contusion having the highest incidence.
- Of major importance in acute thigh contusion is early detection and the avoidance of internal bleeding.
- One major complication to repeated contusions is myositis ossificans.
- Hamstring strain occurs most often to the short head of the biceps femoris.
- The groin is the depression between the thigh and abdominal region. Groin strain can occur to any one of a number of muscles in this region. Running, jumping, or twisting can produce a groin strain.
- The hip joint, the strongest and best-protected joint in the human body, has a low incidence of acute sports injuries.
- Some young athletes develop conditions that stem from an immature hip joint. These conditions are coxa plana, or Legg-Perthes disease, and the slipped capital femoral epiphysis.
- A common problem in the pelvic region is the hip pointer, which results from a blow to the inadequately protected iliac crest. The contusion causes pain, spasm, and malfunction of the muscles in the area.

---

*Solutions to Critical Thinking* Exercises

---

**17-1** One of the best ways to determine the grade of a contusion to the quadriceps muscle is through the degree of restriction of knee flexion. With grade 1, there is a knee flexion of no more than 90 degrees; with grade 2, less than 90 degrees; and with grade 3, between 45 and 90 degrees.

**17-2** It is likely there is a moderate to severe hamstring strain.

**17-3** Because of the age of the athlete, consider the possibility of a growth problem. If it is a growth problem, it is most likely a slipped capital femoral epiphysis. This athlete should be immediately referred to a physician for x-ray examination.

**17-4** This athlete has sustained a hip pointer or contusion to the skin and musculature in the region of the iliac crest. The athlete most likely will experience severe pain, muscle spasm, and an inability to rotate his trunk or flex his hip without pain.

## REVIEW QUESTIONS AND CLASS ACTIVITIES

1. What signs and symptoms are seen in each of the three degrees of quadriceps contusions? How are they managed?
2. What complications can occur if a thigh contusion is mishandled?
3. Why do hamstring strains often become recurrent?
4. Where do fractures occur most often in the femur? How are they recognized? What emergency care must be given?
5. What muscles are most often injured in a groin strain? How is this type of injury managed?
6. What type of hip problems occur in the young athlete?
7. Describe hip pointer prevention and care.

### REFERENCES

1. Abraham, D: 2003. Young, M: Hamstring injuries—minimizing the risks, *Sports coach* 26(2):16–18.
2. Anderson, K: 2001. Hip and groin injuries in athletes, *American journal of sports medicine* 29(4):521–533.
3. Aronen, J, Garrick, J. 2006. Quadriceps contusions: clinical results of immediate immobilization in 120 degrees of knee flexion, *Clinical journal of sport medicine* 16(5):383–387.
4. Bharam, S, Philippon, M: 2008. Diagnosis and management of acetabular labral tears in the athlete, *International sportmed journal* 9(1):1.
5. Boyd KT, Peirce NS, Batt ME: 1997. Common hip injuries in sport, *Sports medicine* 24(4):273.
6. Brukner, P: 2002. Anterior thigh pain. In Brukner, P, editor, *Clinical sports medicine*, pp. 395–406, Sydney, McGraw-Hill.
7. Brukner, P: 2002. Hip and groin pain. In Brukner, P, editor, *Clinical sports medicine*, pp. 375–394, Sydney, McGraw-Hill.
8. Brumm, LF: 2001. Looking beyond the soft tissue: illustrative case studies of groin injuries, *Athletic therapy today* 6(4):24–27.
9. Choung, EW, Yang, F: 2003. Slipped capital femoral epiphysis in an obese teenager, *Physician and sports medicine* 31(7):39–41; 45.
10. Chudik, SC: 2002. Hip dislocations in athletes, *Sports medicine and arthroscopy review* 10(2):123–133.
11. Cibor, G: 2002. Osteitis pubis: a commonly overlooked cause of groin pain, *Sports medicine alert* 8(1):2–4.
12. Croisier, Jean Louis: 2004. Factors associated with recurrent hamstring injuries, *Sports medicine* 34(10):681–695.
13. DeFranco, M, Recht, M: 2006. Stress fractures of the femur in athletes. *Clinics in sports medicine* 25(1):89–103.
14. DePalma, B, Halverson, D: 2010. Rehabilitation of groin, hip, and thigh injuries. In Prentice, WE, editor: *Rehabilitation techniques in sports medicine, and athletic training*, 5th ed New York, McGraw-Hill.

15. Glorioso Jr, JE: 2002. Femoral supracondylar stress fractures: an unusual cause of knee pain, *Physician and sportsmedicine* 30(9):25–28.

16. Hacutt, JE: 2004. General types of injuries. In Birrer, RB, editor: *Sports medicine for the primary care physician*, 3rd ed Boca Raton, Fla, CRC Press.

17. Hagerstown, MT: 1996. Groin pain, *Sports medicine* 18:133.

18. Hasselman, CT, et al.: 1990. When groin pain signals an adductor strain, *Physician & sportsmedicine* 18(2):54.

19. Jackson, DL: 1991. Stress fracture of the femur, *Physician & sportsmedicine* 19:39.

20. Johnson, DL, Klabunde, LA: 1995. The elusive slipped capital femoral epiphysis, *Journal of athletic training* 20(2):124.

21. Kaeding, CC: 1995. Quadriceps strains and contusions, *Physician & sportsmedicine* 23(1):59.

22. Kocher, M, Tucker, R: 2006. Pediatric athlete hip disorders, *Clinics in sports medicine* 25(2):241–253.

23. Larson, CM: 2002. Evaluating and managing muscle contusions and myositis ossifans, *Physician and sportsmedicine* 30(2):41–44; 49–50.

24. Levandowski, R, Difliori, JP: 2004. Thigh injuries. In Birrer, RB, editor: *Sports medicine for the primary care physician,* 3rd ed Boca Raton, Fla, CRC Press.

25. Maffey, L, Emery, C: 2007. What are the risk factors for groin strain injury in sport? *Sports medicine* 37(10):881.

26. Melamed, H: 2002. Soft tissue problems of the hip in athletes. *Sports medicine and arthroscopy review* 10(2):168–175.

27. Robertson, K, Molloy, L: 2007. Hamstring muscle strains, *Modern athlete & coach* 45(2):10.

28. Rodriguez, C: 2001. Osteitis pubis syndrome in the professional soccer athlete: a case report, *Journal of athletic training* 36(4):437–440.

29. Roos, HP: 1997. Hip pain in sport, *Sports medicine arthroscopy review* 5(4):292.

30. Scopp, JM: 2001. The assessment of athletic hip injury, *Clinics in sports medicine* 20(4):647–659.

31. Sherry, MA, Best, TM: 2004. A comparison of 2 rehabilitation programs in the treatment of acute hamstring strains, *Journal of orthopaedic & sports physical therapy* 34(3):116–125.

32. Verrall, GM, Hamilton, IA, Slavotinek, JP: 2005. Hip joint range of motion reduction in sports-related chronic groin injury diagnosed as pubic bone stress injury. *Journal of science and medicine in sport* 8(1):77–84.

33. Weicker, GG, Munnings, F: 1993. How to manage hip and pelvis injuries in adolescents, *Physician and sportsmedicine* 21:72.

34. Weiss, J, Ramachandran, M: 2006. Hip and pelvic injuries in the young athlete, *Operative techniques in sports medicine* 14(3):212–217.

35. Wollin, M, Lovell, G: 2006. Osteitis pubis in four young football players: a case series demonstrating successful rehabilitation, *Physical therapy in sport* 7(3):153–160.

36. Yates, C, Bandy, W, Blasier, R: 2008. Traumatic dislocation of the hip in a high school football player, *Physical therapy* 88(6):780.

## ANNOTATED BIBLIOGRAPHY

Boyd, KT, Peirce, NS, Batt, ME: 1997. Common hip injuries in sports, *Sports medicine* 24(4):273.
   *Provides a detailed discussion of hip and pelvic anatomy and sports injuries.*

Brukner, P.: *Clinics in Sports Medicine,* 2nd ed, Sydney, 2002, McGraw-Hill.
   *Presents complete chapters on anterior thigh pain and hip and groin pain.*

Tile, M, Helfet, D, Kellum, J: *Fractures of
the Pelvis and Acetabulum*, Philadelphia,
2003, Lippincott Williams and Wilkins.
*This third edition of a book on
fractures of the pelvis and acetabulum* presents the current concepts in mechanism, biomechanics, and the most recent
methods in management of these
injuries.

## WEB SITES

World Ortho:
www.worldortho.com
*Use the search engine in this site to
locate relevant information.*
Wheeless' Textbook:
www.wheelessonline.com/
*An excellent page for injuries,
anatomy, and x-rays.*
Hip Pain
www.fpnotebook.com/Ortho/Hip/
index.htm

*Provides a detailed discussion of a
wide variety of thigh injuries and
conditions in an easy-to-follow outline
format.*
Sports Injury Bulletin/Groin injuries:
www.sportsinjurybulletin.com/
archive/groin.php
*Sports Injury Bulletin is funded by
private subscription and offers a free
archive of practical sports injury advice
for physios, coaches, and athletes*

# The Shoulder Complex

## CHAPTER 18

*When you finish this chapter you will be able to:*

- Identify the bones, articulations, stabilizing ligaments, and musculature of the shoulder complex.
- Explain how shoulder injuries may be prevented.
- Describe the process for assessing injuries to the shoulder.
- Recognize specific injuries that occur around the shoulder joint and describe plans for management.

The anatomy of the shoulder complex allows for a great degree of mobility. To achieve this mobility, stability of the complex is sometimes compromised and instability of the shoulder frequently leads to injury, particularly in those sports that involve overhead activity.[4] Sport activities such as throwing, swimming, or serving in tennis or volleyball place a great deal of stress on the supporting structures (Figure 18-1). Consequently, injuries related to overuse in the shoulder are commonplace in the athlete.[7]

Dynamic movement and stabilization of the shoulder complex require integrated function of the rotator cuff muscles, the joint capsule, and the muscles that stabilize and position the scapula.[31]

## ANATOMY

### Bones

The bones that comprise the shoulder complex and shoulder joint are the clavicle, scapula, and humerus (Figure 18-2). These three bones form the four major articulations associated with the shoulder complex: the sternoclavicular joint, the acromioclavicular joint, the glenohumeral joint, and the scapulothoracic joint.

Shoulder complex articulations:
- sternoclavicular
- acromioclavicular
- glenohumeral
- scapulothoracic

### Stabilizing Ligaments

Ligaments at each of the four articulations act collectively to provide stability to the shoulder complex (Figure 18-3).[36]

The clavicle articulates with the sternum to form the sternoclavicular joint, the only direct connection between the upper extremity and the trunk. The sternoclavicular joint is extremely weak because of its bony arrangement, but it is held securely by the sternoclavicular ligament that pulls the clavicle downward and toward the sternum, in effect

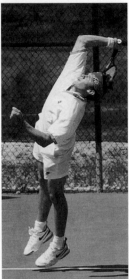

**Figure 18-1**

Overhead activities can produce a number of shoulder problems.

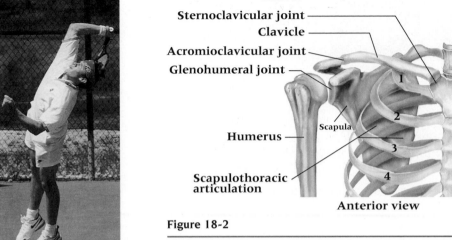

*Lateral*          *Medial*

Sternoclavicular joint
Clavicle
Acromioclavicular joint
Glenohumeral joint

1

2

Humerus — Scapula
3

Scapulothoracic
articulation
4

**Anterior view**

**Figure 18-2**

**Skeletal anatomy of the shoulder complex (anterior view)**

anchoring it. The clavicle is permitted to move up and down, forward and backward, and in rotation.[32]

The acromioclavicular joint is a gliding articulation of the lateral end of the clavicle with the acromion process of the scapula. This junction is rather weak. The acromioclavicular ligament along with the coracoclavicular ligament helps to maintain the position of the clavicle relative to the acromion. The coracoacromial ligament connects the coracoid to the acromion. This ligament along with the acromion forms the coracoacromial arch.

At the glenohumeral joint (the true shoulder joint), the round head of the humerus articulates with the shallow glenoid cavity of the scapula. The position of the glenohumeral joint is maintained by the surrounding glenohumeral ligaments that form the joint capsule and by the rotator cuff muscles.

The scapulothoracic joint is not a true joint; however, the movement of the scapula on the wall of the thoracic cage is critical to shoulder joint motion. Contraction of the scapular muscles that attach the scapula to

**Figure 18-3**

Shoulder complex articulations, ligaments, and bursae

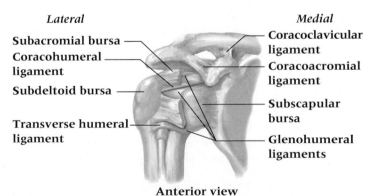

*Lateral*          *Medial*

Subacromial bursa
Coracohumeral ligament
Subdeltoid bursa

Transverse humeral ligament

Coracoclavicular ligament
Coracoacromial ligament
Subscapular bursa
Glenohumeral ligaments

**Anterior view**

the axial skeleton is critical in stabilizing the scapula, thus providing a base on which a highly mobile glenohumeral joint can function.[32]

## Muscles

The muscles that cross the glenohumeral joint produce dynamic motion and establish stability to compensate for a bony and ligamentous arrangement that allows for a great deal of mobility (Figure 18-4).[36] Movements at the glenohumeral joint include flexion, extension, abduction, adduction, and rotation. The muscles acting on the glenohumeral joint can be separated into three groups. The first group consists of muscles that originate on the axial skeleton and attach to the humerus, including the latissimus dorsi and the pectoralis major. The

Glenohumeral joint
movements:
• flexion
• extension
• abduction
• adduction
• external rotation
• internal rotation

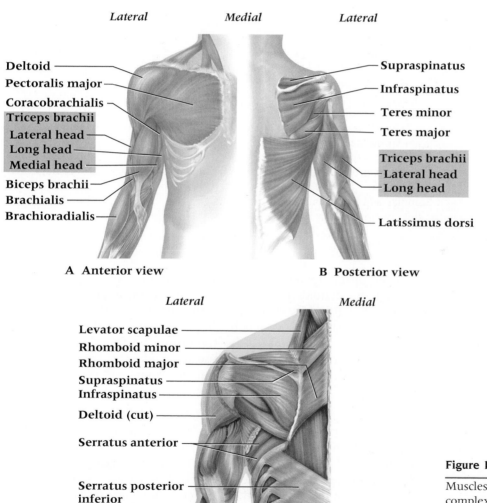

**Figure 18-4**

Muscles of the shoulder complex: (A) Anterior view. (B) Posterior view. (C) Scapular muscles (posterior view).

**TABLE 18-1** Muscles of the Shoulder Complex

| | |
|---|---|
| Flexion | Pectoralis major |
| | Anterior deltoid |
| | Biceps |
| Extension | Latissimus dorsi |
| | Teres major |
| | Posterior deltoid |
| Abduction | Supraspinatus |
| | Middle deltoid |
| Adduction | Pectoralis major |
| | Latissimus dorsi |
| Medial rotation | Pectoralis major |
| | Subscapularis |
| | Latissimus dorsi |
| | Teres major |
| Lateral rotation | Infraspinatus |
| | Teres minor |
| Scapular abduction and upward rotation | Serratus anterior |
| Scapular elevation | Trapezius |
| | Levator scapulae |
| Scapular adduction | Middle trapezius |
| | Rhomboid major |
| Scapular depression and adduction | Lower trapezius |
| Scapular adduction and downward rotation | Rhomboid major |
| | Rhomboid minor |

second group originates on the scapula and attaches to the humerus, including the deltoid, the teres major, the coracobrachialis, and the rotator cuff (subscapularis, supraspinatus, infraspinatus, teres minor). A third group of muscles attach the axial skeleton to the scapula and includes the levator scapula, the trapezius, the rhomboids, and the serratus anterior and posterior. The scapular muscles are important in providing dynamic stability to the shoulder complex[18] (Table 18-1).

## PREVENTION OF SHOULDER INJURIES

Ensuring proper physical conditioning is of major importance in preventing many shoulder injuries. As with all preventive conditioning, the program should be directed toward general body development and development of specific body areas for a given sport. If a sport places extreme, sustained demands on the arms and shoulders or if the shoulder is at risk for sudden traumatic injury, extensive conditioning must be used. All the muscles involved in movement of the shoulder complex should be strengthened through a full range of motion.

In particular, emphasis should be placed on strengthening the muscles of the rotator cuff in the cardinal movement planes to improve dynamic function and control in overhead activities. Likewise, attention should be given to strengthening the scapular stabilizers by incorporating exercises to resist scapular abduction, adduction, elevation, depression, upward rotation, and downward rotation. Strengthening the muscles that control the stability of the scapula helps provide a base for the function of the highly mobile glenohumeral joint.[25]

Proper warm-up must be performed gradually before dynamic arm movements are attempted. This warm-up causes a general increase in body temperature and is followed by sport-specific stretching of selected muscles.

All athletes in collision and contact sports should be instructed and drilled on how to fall properly. They must be taught not to try to catch themselves with an outstretched arm. Performing a shoulder roll is a safer way to absorb the shock of the fall. Specialized protective equipment such as shoulder pads must be properly fitted to avoid some shoulder injuries in tackle football.

## Using Correct Throwing Technique

**To prevent overuse shoulder injuries, it is essential that athletes be correctly taught the appropriate techniques of throwing a baseball or football, throwing a javelin, serving or spiking a volleyball, and serving or hitting an overhead smash in tennis.**[35] If the thrower uses faulty technique, the joints are affected by atypical stresses that result in trauma to the joint and its surrounding tissues.[4,25]

Relative to the shoulder complex, throwing involves five distinct phases: wind-up, cocking, arm acceleration, arm deceleration, and follow-through (Figure 18-5).

### Wind-up Phase

The wind-up or preparation phase lasts from the first movement until the ball leaves the gloved hand. During this phase the lead leg strides

Throwing phases:
- wind-up
- cocking
- acceleration
- deceleration
- follow-through

**Figure 18-5**

Phases of throwing from left to right: wind-up, cocking, acceleration, deceleration, follow-through

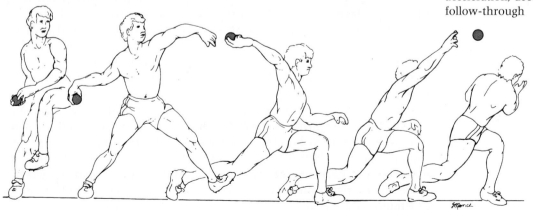

forward. Both shoulders abduct, externally rotate, and horizontally abduct.

### Cocking Phase

The cocking phase begins when the hands separate and ends when maximum external rotation of the humerus has occurred. During this phase the foot comes in contact with the ground.

### Acceleration Phase

The acceleration phase lasts from maximum external rotation until ball release. The humerus abducts, horizontally abducts, and internally rotates at velocities approaching 8000° per second. The scapula elevates, abducts, and upward rotates.

### Deceleration Phase

The deceleration phase lasts from ball release until maximum shoulder internal rotation. During this phase the external rotators of the rotator cuff contract eccentrically to decelerate the humerus. The rhomboids contract eccentrically to decelerate the scapula. Most throwing injuries occur during either the acceleration phase or the deceleration phase.

### Follow-through Phase

The follow-through phase lasts from maximum shoulder internal rotation until the end of the motion when there is a balanced position.

## ASSESSING THE SHOULDER COMPLEX

The shoulder complex is one of the most difficult regions of the body to evaluate.[33] One reason for this difficulty is that the biomechanical demands placed on these structures during overhand accelerations and decelerations are not yet clearly understood. It is essential to understand the athlete's major complaints and the possible mechanisms of the injury.

**Generally fitness professionals, coaches, and others working in areas related to exercise and sport science are not adequately trained to evaluate injuries. It is strongly recommended that injured athletes be referred to qualified medical personnel (i.e., physicians, athletic trainers, physical therapists) for injury evaluation.** Information on the following special tests has been included simply to give some idea about the different basic tests that nonmedical personnel may do to determine the nature and severity of the athlete's injury. The primary responsibility of those who are not health care personnel is to be able to recognize any potential "red flags" associated with the injury, provide appropriate first aid for the injury, and make correct decisions about how the injury should be managed initially, including immediate return to play or activity decisions. (Refer to Chapter 7.)

## History

The following questions in regard to the athlete's complaints can help determine the nature of the injury:

- What happened to cause this pain?
- Have you ever had this problem before?
- What is the duration and intensity of the pain?
- Where is the pain located?
- Is there crepitus during movement or numbness or distortion in temperature such as a cold or warm feeling?
- Is there a feeling of weakness or a sense of fatigue?
- What shoulder movements or positions seem to aggravate or relieve the pain?
- If therapy has been given before, what, if anything, offered pain relief (e.g., cold, heat, massage, or analgesic medication)?

## Observation

The athlete should be generally observed while walking and standing. Observation during walking can reveal asymmetry of arm swing or a lean toward the painful shoulder. The athlete is next observed from the front, side, and back while in a standing position. Observe for postural asymmetries, bony or joint deformities, or muscle spasm or guarding patterns.

### Anterior Observation

- Are both shoulder tips even with one another, or is one depressed?
- Is one shoulder held higher because of muscle spasm or guarding?
- Is the lateral end of the clavicle prominent (indicating acromioclavicular sprain or dislocation)?
- Is one lateral acromion process more prominent than the other (indicating a possible glenohumeral dislocation)?
- Does the clavicular shaft appear deformed (indicating possible fracture)?
- Is there loss of the normal lateral deltoid muscle contour (indicating glenohumeral dislocation)?
- Is there an indentation in the upper biceps region (indicating rupture of biceps tendon)?

### Lateral Observation

- Is there thoracic kyphosis or are the shoulders slumped forward (indicating weakness of the erector muscles of the spine and tightness in the pectoral region)?
- Is there forward or backward arm hang (indicating possible scoliosis)?

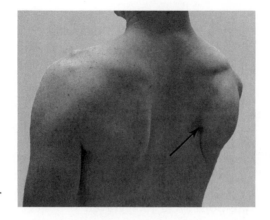

**Figure 18-6**

**Winged scapula**

### Posterior Observation

- Is there asymmetry such as a low shoulder, uneven scapulae, or winging of one scapula and not the other (indicating postural scoliosis)?
- Is the scapula protracted because of constricted pectoral muscles?
- Is there a distracted or winged scapula on one or both sides?
  A winged scapula on both sides could indicate a general weakness of the serratus anterior muscles; if only one side is winged, the long thoracic nerve may be injured (Figure 18-6).

### Palpation

Palpation of the bony structures should be done with the coach standing in front of and then behind the athlete. Both shoulders are palpated at the same time for pain sites and deformities. Palpation of the muscles around the shoulder detects point tenderness, abnormal swelling or lumps, muscle spasm or guarding, and trigger points. The shoulder is then also palpated anteriorly and posteriorly.

### Special Tests

A number of special tests can help to determine the nature of an injury to the shoulder complex.[33] The shoulder's active and passive range of motion should be noted and compared to the opposite side. Strength of the shoulder musculature should be assessed by resisted manual muscle testing. Both the muscles that act on the glenohumeral joint and those that act on the scapula should be tested.

Following are descriptions of other tests used to assess shoulder instability, shoulder impingement, and muscle weakness.

### Apprehension Test (Crank Test)

With the arm abducted 90 degrees, the shoulder is slowly and gently externally rotated as far as the athlete will allow. The athlete with a history of anterior glenohumeral instability shows great apprehension that is reflected by a facial grimace before an endpoint can be reached. At no time should this movement be forced (Figure 18-7).

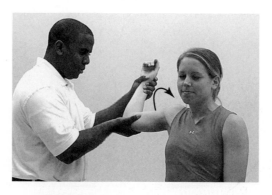

**Figure 18-7**

**Shoulder apprehension
test**

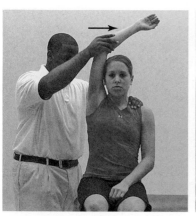

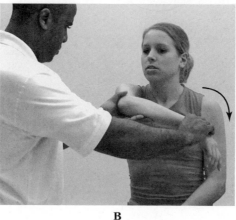

A                                              B

**Figure 18-8**

**Shoulder impingement
tests**

### Tests for Shoulder Impingement

Forced flexion and adduction of the humerus in the overhead position
may cause impingement of soft tissue structures between the humeral
head and the coracoacromial ligament. A second test involves horizontal adduction with forced internal rotation of the humerus that also produces impingement (Figure 18-8). A positive sign is indicated if the athlete feels pain and reacts with a grimace.[20]

### Test for Supraspinatus Muscle Weakness

The empty can test for supraspinatus muscle strength has the athlete
bring both arms into 90 degrees of forward flexion and 30 degrees of
horizontal adduction (Figure 18-9). In this position the arms are internally rotated as far as possible, thumbs pointing downward. A downward pressure is then applied. Weakness and pain can be detected as
well as comparative strength between the two arms.

One test for supraspinatus
weakness is the empty can
test.

### Test for Sternoclavicular Joint Instability

With the patient sitting, pressure is applied anteriorly, then superiorly, and
then inferiorly to the proximal clavicle to determine any instability or

**Figure 18-9**

Empty can test for supraspinatus muscle. Performed in 30° of horizontal adduction with the thumbs pointed down. The examiner applies pressure to force the arm downward.

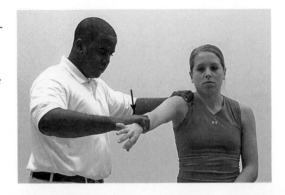

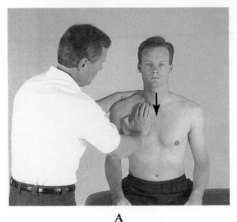

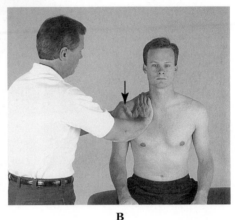

A B

**Figure 18-10**

(A) Assessing sternoclavicular joint stability. (B) Assessing acromioclavicular joint stability.

increased pain associated with a sprain (Figure 18-10A). Pressure applied to the tip of the shoulder in a medial direction may also increase pain.

### Test for Acromioclavicular Joint Instability

The acromioclavicular joint is first palpated to determine if there is any displacement of the acromion process and the distal head of the clavicle. Next, pressure is applied to the distal clavicle in all four directions to determine stability and any associated increase in pain (Figure 18-10B). Pressure is applied to the tip of the shoulder, which compresses the acromioclavicular joint and may also increase pain.[22]

## RECOGNITION AND MANAGEMENT OF SHOULDER INJURIES

### Clavicle Fractures

**Cause of injury** Clavicular fractures (Figure 18-11) are one of the most frequent fractures in sports. Fractures of the clavicle result from a fall on the outstretched arm, a fall on the tip of the shoulder, or a direct impact.[3]

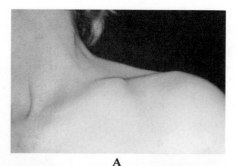

**A**

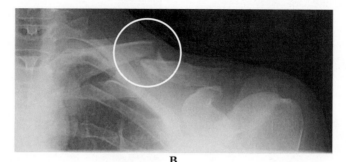

**B**

**Figure 18-11**

Clavicular fractures.
(A) Typical appearance of a
clavicle fracture, which
usually occurs in the middle
⅓ of the clavicle.
(B) X-ray of clavicle fracture.

**Signs of injury**   The athlete with a fractured clavicle usually supports the arm on the injured side and tilts his or her head toward that side, with the chin turned to the opposite side. During inspection the injured clavicle appears a little lower than the unaffected side. Palpation may also reveal swelling, point tenderness, and mild deformity.

**Care**   The clavicular fracture is cared for immediately by applying a shoulder immobilizer and by treating the athlete for shock, if necessary[15] (Figure 18-12). If x-ray examination reveals a fracture, a closed reduction should be attempted by the physician followed by immobilization with a clavicle strap[3] (Figure 18-13). Immobilization should be maintained for 6 to 8 weeks. Following this period of immobilization,

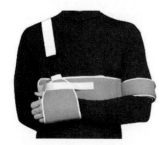

**Figure 18-12**

**Shoulder immobilizer**

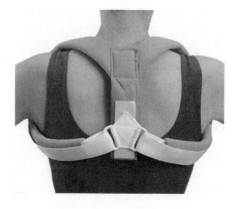

**Figure 18-13**

**Protective sling for
clavicular fracture**

*Lateral*                        *Medial*

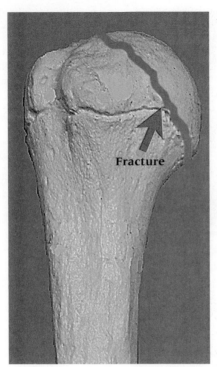

A

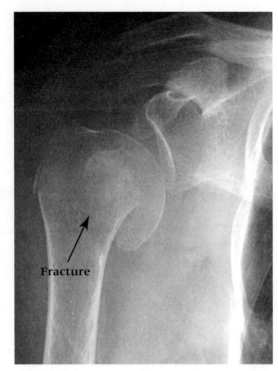

B

**Figure 18-14**

Humeral fracture
(A) Upper humerus fracture
diagram. (B) X-ray view.

gentle isometric and mobilization exercises should begin with the athlete using a sling for an additional 3 to 4 weeks to provide protection. Occasionally, clavicle fractures may require operative management.[10]

## Fractures of the Humerus

**Cause of injury** Fractures of the humerus (Figure 18-14) happen occasionally in sports, usually as the result of a direct blow, a dislocation, or the impact of falling onto the outstretched arm.

**Signs of injury** A fracture of the humerus is difficult to recognize by visual inspection alone; x-ray examination gives the only positive proof. Some of the more prevalent signs that may be present are pain, inability to move the arm, swelling, point tenderness, and discoloration of the superficial tissue.

**Care** Recognition of humeral shaft fractures requires immediate application of a splint or immediate support with a sling, treatment for shock, and referral to a physician. The athlete with a fracture to the humerus will be out of competition for approximately 2 to 6 months depending on the location and severity of the fracture.[4]

## Sternoclavicular Joint Sprain

**Cause of injury** A sternoclavicular sprain (Figure 18-15) is a relatively uncommon occurrence in sports. The mechanism of the injury is

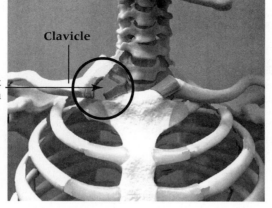

Clavicle

Sternoclavicular ligament
sprain and dislocation

**Figure 18-15**

**Sternoclavicular sprain
and dislocation**

either an indirect force transmitted through the humerus, the shoulder joint, and the clavicle, or a direct impact to the clavicle. Usually the clavicle is displaced upward and forward.

**Signs of injury** A sprain to the sternoclavicular joint can be described in three degrees. A grade 1 sprain is characterized by little pain and disability, with some point tenderness but no joint deformity. A grade 2 sprain displays subluxation of the sternoclavicular joint with visible deformity, pain, swelling, point tenderness, and an inability to abduct the shoulder through a full range of motion or to bring the arm across the chest, indicating disruption of the stabilizing ligaments. The grade 3 sprain, which is the most severe, presents a picture of complete dislocation with gross displacement of the clavicle at its sternal junction, swelling, and disability, indicating complete rupture of the sternoclavicular ligament.[11] A posterior or "retro-sternal" dislocation of the clavicle is rare but has the potential to be a life-threatening injury due to hemorrhage and compromise of the nearby trachea.[6]

**Care** PRICE should be used immediately, followed by immobilization (refer to Figure 18-13). Immobilization is usually maintained for 3 to 5 weeks, followed by graded reconditioning exercises.[17] There is a high incidence of recurrence of sternoclavicular sprains.

## Acromioclavicular Joint Sprain

**Cause of injury** The acromioclavicular joint is extremely vulnerable to sprains, especially in collision sports.[12] The primary mechanisms are a fall on an outstretched arm or direct impact to the tip of the shoulder that forces the acromion process downward, backward, and inward while the clavicle is pushed down against the rib cage[5,8] (Figure 18-16A).

**Signs of injury** In a grade 1 acromioclavicular sprain, there is point tenderness and discomfort during movement at the junction between the acromion process and the outer end of the clavicle. There is no deformity, indicating only mild stretching of the acromioclavicular ligaments (Figure 18-16B).

**18-1 *Critical Thinking***
Exercise

A soccer player is tripped to the ground on a hard tackle and lands on the tip of her left shoulder. She complains of pain both in the tip of her shoulder and in her chest. She has difficulty lifting her arm above her shoulder because of the pain.

**?** What injury diagnosis might result from this mechanism of injury?

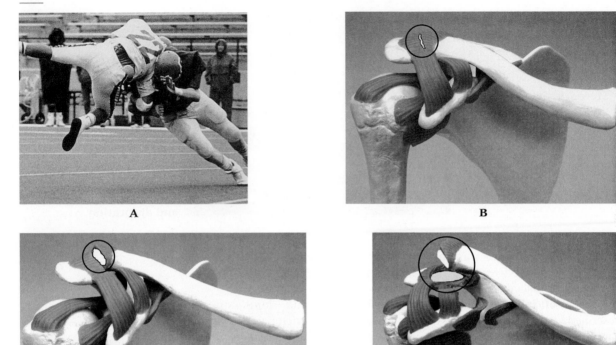

**Figure 18-16**

(A) Mechanism of AC injury
(B) Grade 1 AC sprain
(C) Grade 2 AC sprain
(D) Grade 3 AC sprain

A grade 2 sprain shows definite displacement and prominence of the lateral end of the clavicle when compared to the unaffected side. There is point tenderness during palpation of the injury site, and the athlete is unable to fully abduct through a full range of motion or to bring the arm completely across the chest (Figure 18-16C).

A grade 3 sprain involves rupture of the acromioclavicular and coracoclavicular ligaments with dislocation of the clavicle. Such an injury has gross deformity and prominence of the distal clavicle, severe pain, loss of movement, and instability of the shoulder complex (Figure 18-16D).

**Care** Immediate care of the acromioclavicular sprain involves three basic procedures: (1) application of cold and pressure to control local hemorrhage, (2) stabilization of the joint by a shoulder immobilizer (refer to Figure 18-12), and (3) referral to a physician for definitive diagnosis and treatment.[22] Immobilization ranges from 3 to 4 days with a grade 1 to approximately 2 weeks with a grade 3. With all grades, an aggressive rehabilitation program involving joint mobilization, flexibility exercises, and strengthening exercises should begin immediately following the recommended period of protection.[22] Progression should be as rapid as the athlete can tolerate without increased pain or swelling.

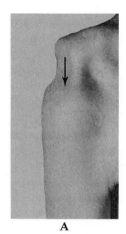 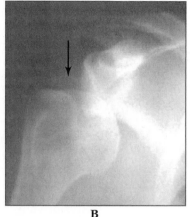

A      B

**Figure 18-17**

(A) Anterior shoulder dislocation appearance. (B) X-ray of anterior/inferior shoulder dislocation.

## Glenohumeral Dislocations

**Cause of injury** The most common glenohumeral dislocation is one in which the head of the humerus is forced out of its joint capsule in an anterior direction past the glenoid labrum and then downward to rest under the coracoid process (Figure 18-17). The mechanism for an anterior dislocation is abduction, external rotation, and extension that forces the humeral head out of the glenoid cavity (see Figure 18-7).[23] An arm tackle in football or rugby or abnormal forces created in executing a throw can produce a sequence of events resulting in dislocation. On a rare occasion the humerus dislocates in an inferior direction.

Once an athlete has suffered a glenohumeral dislocation, he or she faces a high probability of recurrence because of chronic instability.[14,28]

**Signs of injury** The athlete with an anterior dislocation displays a flattened deltoid contour. Palpation of the axilla reveals prominence of the humeral head. The athlete carries the affected arm in slight abduction and external rotation and is unable to touch the opposite shoulder with the hand of the affected arm. There is often moderate to severe pain and disability.[29]

**Care** Initial management of the shoulder dislocation requires immediate immobilization in a position of comfort using a sling; immediate reduction by a physician; and control of the hemorrhage by cold packs. After the dislocation has been reduced and immobilized, muscle reconditioning should be initiated as soon as possible.[14] Protective sling immobilization should continue for approximately 1 week after reduction (refer to Figure 18-11). The athlete is instructed to begin a strengthening program, progressing as quickly as pain allows. Protective shoulder braces may help limit shoulder motion (Figure 18-18).[11]

## Shoulder Impingement Syndrome

**Cause of injury** Shoulder impingement involves a mechanical compression of the supraspinatus tendon, the subacromial bursa, and the long head of the biceps tendon, all of which are located under the

**18-2 Critical Thinking**
Exercise

A gymnast has a recurrent anterior dislocation of the glenohumeral joint. He is extremely worried that his shoulder will dislocate again.

**?** What types of activities should he concentrate on during rehabilitation to help reduce the likelihood of a subsequent dislocation?

One test for glenohumeral instability is the apprehension test.

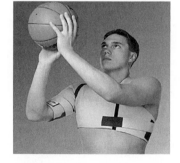

**Figure 18-18**

Protective brace for the shoulder prevents overhead motion.

**Figure 18-19**

As the arm flexes into an overhead position, shoulder impingement compresses soft tissue structures under the coracoacromial arch.

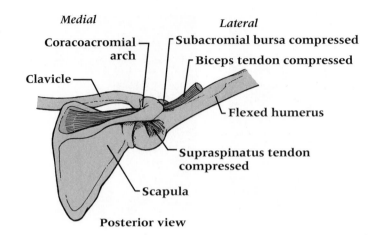

*Medial*                                    *Lateral*

Coracoacromial —
arch

Clavicle —

⌐ Subacromial bursa compressed

⌐ Biceps tendon compressed

└ Flexed humerus

Supraspinatus tendon
compressed

└ Scapula

**Posterior view**

Shoulder impingement involves a mechanical compression of the supraspinatus tendon, the subacromial bursa, and the long head of the biceps tendon under the coracoacromial arch.

Rotator cuff muscles:
• subscapularis
• supraspinatus
• infraspinatus
• teres minor

coracoacromial arch (Figure 18-19).[24] Repetitive compression eventually leads to irritation and inflammation of these structures. Impingement most often occurs in repetitive overhead activities such as throwing, swimming, serving a tennis ball, or spiking a volleyball.[26]

**Signs of injury**   The athlete complains of diffuse pain around the acromion whenever the arm is in an overhead position. There may be a painful arc in the range of motion between 70 and 120 degrees of abduction.[24] The external rotators are generally weaker than the internal rotators. There may be some tightness in the posterior and inferior joint capsule. There usually is a positive impingement test, and the empty can test may increase pain.[34]

**Care**   Management of impingement involves restoring normal biomechanics to the shoulder joint in an effort to maintain space under the coracoacromial arch during overhead activities.[2] PRICE can be used to modulate pain initially. Exercises should concentrate on strengthening the rotator cuff muscles, on strengthening those muscles that produce movement of the scapula, and on stretching the posterior and inferior joint capsule.[21] The activity that caused the problem in the first place should be modified so that the athlete has initial control over the frequency and the level of the activity with a gradual and progressive increase in intensity.[13]

## Rotator Cuff Strains

**Cause of injury**   The most common rotator cuff tendon strain involves the supraspinatus muscle, although any of the rotator cuff tendons are subject to injury[1] (Figure 18-20). The mechanism of rotator cuff strains involves dynamic rotation of the arm at a high velocity as occurs during overhead throwing or any other activity in which there is rotation of the humerus.[19,25,37] Most rotator cuff tears occur in the supraspinatus in individuals with a long history of shoulder impingement or instability and are relatively uncommon in athletes under the age of 40.[9] Tears of the rotator cuff muscles are almost always near their insertion on the humerus.

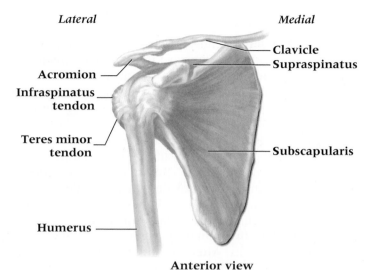

*Lateral*                    *Medial*

Clavicle
Supraspinatus
Acromion
Infraspinatus tendon
Teres minor tendon
Subscapularis
Humerus

**Anterior view**

**Figure 18-20**

Medial rotator cuff muscles (anterior view)

**Signs of injury**   Like other muscle strains, rotator cuff strains present pain with muscle contraction, some tenderness on palpation, and loss of strength because of pain. A tear or complete rupture of one of the rotator cuff tendons produces an extremely disabling condition in which pain, loss of function, swelling, and point tenderness are symptoms.[27] In the case of a complete tear of the supraspinatus tendon, both the impingement test and the empty can test are positive.[34,37]

**Care**   PRICE can be used to modulate pain initially. Exercises should concentrate on progressive strengthening of the rotator cuff muscles. The frequency and level of the activity should be reduced initially with a gradual and progressive increase in intensity.[17]

## Shoulder Bursitis

**Cause of injury**   The shoulder joint is subject to chronic inflammatory conditions resulting from trauma or from overuse.[3] Bursitis may develop from a direct impact, from a fall on the tip of the shoulder, or as a result of shoulder impingement. The bursa that is most often inflamed is the subacromial bursa (see Figure 18-3).

**Signs of injury**   The athlete has pain when trying to move the shoulder, especially in abduction or with flexion, adduction, and internal rotation. There is also tenderness to palpation in the area just under the acromion. Impingement tests are positive.

**Care**   The use of cold packs and anti-inflammatory medications to reduce inflammation is necessary. If impingement is the primary mechanism precipitating bursitis, then, as previously discussed, measures should be taken to correct this activity.[16] The athlete must maintain a consistent program of exercise, with emphasis placed on maintaining a full range of motion, so that muscle contractures and adhesions do not immobilize the joint.

## Biceps Tenosynovitis

**Cause of injury**   Tenosynovitis of the long biceps muscle tendon is common among athletes engaged in overhead activities. Biceps tenosynovitis is prevalent among pitchers, tennis players, volleyball players, and javelin throwers.[30] The repeated stretching of the biceps in these highly ballistic activities may eventually cause an inflammation of both the tendon and its synovial sheath.[4]

**Signs of injury**   There is tenderness in the anterior upper arm. There may also be some swelling, increased warmth, and crepitus caused by the inflammation. The athlete may complain of pain when performing dynamic overhead throwing activities.[12]

**Care**   Biceps tenosynovitis is best cared for by complete rest for several days, combined with daily applications of cold to reduce inflammation. Anti-inflammatory medications are also beneficial in reducing inflammation. After the inflammation is controlled, a gradual program of strengthening and stretching the biceps muscle should be initiated.[32]

## Contusions of the Upper Arm

**Cause of injury**   Contusions of the upper arm are frequent in contact sports. Although any muscle of the upper arm is subject to bruising, the area most often affected is the lateral aspect, primarily the brachialis muscle and portions of the triceps and biceps muscles. Repeated contusions to the lateral aspect of the upper arm can lead to myositis ossificans, more commonly known as linebacker's arm or blocker's exostosis. In myositis ossificans, abnormal calcification or bone growth occurs in a muscle or in soft tissues adjacent to bone.[28]

**Signs of injury**   Bruises to the upper arm area can be particularly handicapping, causing pain and tenderness, increased warmth, discoloration, and difficulty in achieving full extension and flexion of the elbow.

**Care**   PRICE should be applied for a minimum of 24 hours after injury. In most cases this condition responds rapidly to treatment, usually within a few days. The key to treatment is to provide protection to the contused area to prevent repeated episodes that increase the likelihood of myositis ossificans.[28] It is also important for the athlete to maintain a full range of motion through stretching of the contused muscle.

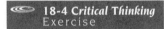

**18-4 Critical Thinking**
Exercise

A football offensive lineman contuses his upper arm while blocking.

**?** What should the coach be mainly concerned about and how can this be avoided?

## SUMMARY

- For the shoulder complex to have such a great degree of mobility, some compromise in stability had to be made; thus, the shoulder is highly susceptible to injury. Many sport activities that involve repetitive overhead movements place a great deal of stress on the shoulder joint.

- Four major articulations are associated with the shoulder complex: the sternoclavicular joint and ligament, the acromioclavicular joint and ligament, the glenohumeral joint and ligament, and the scapulothoracic joint.

- The muscles acting on the shoulder joint consist of those that originate on the axial skeleton and attach to the humerus, those that originate on the scapula and attach to the humerus, and a third group that attaches the axial skeleton to the scapula.

- When evaluating injuries to the shoulder complex, the coach must take into consideration all four joints. A number of special tests can provide insight relative to the nature of a particular injury.

- Fractures may occur to the clavicle or humerus, whereas sprains may occur at the sternoclavicular, acromioclavicular, or glenohumeral joints.

- Shoulder dislocations are relatively common, with an anterior dislocation the most likely to occur. After a dislocation has been reduced and immobilized, muscle reconditioning should be initiated as soon as possible.

- Shoulder impingement most often occurs in athletes involved with overhead activities. Shoulder impingement involves a mechanical compression of the supraspinatus tendon, the subacromial bursa, and the long head of the biceps tendon under the coracoacromial ligament.

- A number of injuries, including rotator cuff strain, bursitis, contusions, and biceps tenosynovitis, are all common injuries to the shoulder complex in athletes.

---

## *Solutions to Critical Thinking* Exercises

**18-1** Falling on the tip of the shoulder is a typical mechanism of injury for a sprain of the acromioclavicular joint, the sternoclavicular joint, or both. It is also possible that a clavicular fracture has occurred.

**18-2** Exercises should be designed to strengthen the muscles of the rotator cuff in particular and the muscles that allow the scapula to provide a stable base of support. Exercises that stress neuromuscular control should begin immediately in the rehabilitation program.

**18-3** This athlete's pain is likely caused by mechanical impingement or compression of the supraspinatus tendon, the subacromial bursa, or the long head of the biceps under the coracoacromial arch as the arm moves into a fully abducted or flexed position. The space under the arch becomes even more compressed as the humerus is internally rotated, which occurs during the follow-through.

**18-4** The biggest concern is that following repeated contusions myositis ossificans may develop in the biceps or brachialis. This can be prevented by having the athlete wear a protective pad to prevent subsequent contusion.

## REVIEW QUESTIONS AND CLASS ACTIVITIES

1. What are the bony and soft-tissue structures associated with the shoulder complex?
2. What four major joints make up the shoulder complex?
3. How can shoulder injuries be prevented?
4. Discuss the throwing motion and the injuries that can occur in each phase.
5. What causes clavicular fractures? How are they cared for?
6. Discuss the mechanism of injury of sternoclavicular and acromioclavicular ligament sprains.
7. What is the common mechanism of an anterior glenohumeral dislocation? How is it cared for?
8. What structural anatomic problems need to be addressed when treating shoulder impingement?
9. Briefly describe the history of a rotator cuff tear.
10. How does an athlete develop bursitis in the shoulder?
11. What is myositis ossificans and how can you prevent its development?
12. How may an athlete develop biceps tenosynovitis?

**REFERENCES**

1. Allen, AA: 2001. Shoulder impingement and rotator cuff disease—an overview, in Chan, M, Chang, K: *Controversies in orthopedic sports medicine,* Champaign, IL, Human Kinetics, pp. 337–345.
2. Almekinders, LC: 2001. Impingement syndrome, *Clinics in sports medicine* 20(3):491–504.
3. Anderson, K: 2003. Evaluation and treatment of distal clavicle fractures, *Clinics in sports medicine* 22(2):319–326.
4. Andrews J, Wilk K: 1994. *The athlete's shoulder,* New York, Churchill Livingstone.
5. Axe, MJ: 2000. Acromioclavicular joint injuries in the athlete, *Sports medicine and arthroscopy review* 8(2): 182–191.
6. Bicos, J: 2003. Treatment and results of sternoclavicular joint injuries, *Clinics in sports medicine* 22(2):359–370.
7. Burkhart SS, Morgan CD, Kibler B: 2000. Shoulder injuries in overhead athletes: the "dead arm" revisited, *Clinics in sports medicine* 19(1):125.
8. Buss, DD, Watts, JD: 2003. Acromioclavicular injuries in the throwing athlete, *Clinics in sports medicine* 22(2):327–341.
9. Cavallo RJ, Speer KP: 1998. Shoulder instability and impingement in throwing athletes, *Medicine & science in sports & exercise* 30(4 suppl):S18.
10. Craig E: 2004. Fractures of the clavicle. In Rockwood C, Masten F, Wirth M, editors: *The shoulder,* Philadelphia, Elsevier Health Sciences.
11. DeCarlo, M. et al.: 1996. Evaluation of shoulder instability braces, *Journal of sport rehabilitation* 5(2):143.
12. Edwards, TB, Walch, G: 2003. Biceps tendinitis: classification and treatment with tenotomy, *Operative techniques in sports medicine* 11(1):2–5.
13. Garretson III, RB: 2003. Clinical evaluation of injuries to the acromioclavicular and sternoclavicular joints, *Clinics in sports medicine* 22(2): 239–254.
14. Hayes, K: 2002. Shoulder instability: management and rehabilitation, *The journal of orthopaedic & sports physical therapy* 32(10):497–509.
15. Housner, JA, Kuhn, JE: 2003. Clavicle fractures: individualizing treatment for fracture type, *Physician and sportsmedicine* 31(12): 30–36.

16. Kesson, M, Atkins, E: 1999. Subacromial bursitis, *SportEX medicine* 2:38–39.

17. Kibler, WB: 1998. Shoulder rehabilitation: principles and practice, *Medicine and science in sports and exercise* 30(4 suppl):S40.

18. Kibler WB: 1998. The role of the scapula in athletic shoulder function, *American journal of sports medicine* 26(2):325.

19. Krabak, BJ, Sugar, R, McFarland, EG: 2003. Practical nonoperative management of rotator cuff injuries, *Clinical journal of sport medicine* 13(2):102–105.

20. Masten F, Arntz C: 1998. Subacromial impingement. In Rockwood C, Masten F, Wirth M, editors: *The shoulder*, Philadelphia, WB Saunders.

21. Matthews, I, Burgess, J: 2006. Rehabilitation of shoulder impingement syndrome, *SportEX medicine* 28:18.

22. Mazzocca, A, Arciero, R: 2007. Evaluation and treatment of acromioclavicular joint injuries. *American journal of sports medicine* 35(2):316–329.

23. McCarty, EC, Ritchie, P, Gill, HS: 2004. Shoulder instability: return to play, *Clinics in sports medicine* 23(3):335–351.

24. McFarland, E, Selhi, H: 2006. Clinical evaluation of impingement: what to do and what works, *Journal of bone & joint surgery, American* 88(2):432.

25. Molloy, L, Robertson, K: 2007. The throwing shoulder: common injuries and management, *Modern athlete & coach* 45(4):15.

26. Myers JB: 1999. Conservative management of shoulder impingement syndrome in the athletic population, *Journal of sport rehabilitation* 8(3):230.

27. Myers, J, 2007: Rotator cuff tear. *Sports physiotherapy* 2:8–9.

28. Pagnani M, Warren R: 1995. Instability of the shoulder. In Nicholas JA, Hershman EB, editors: *The upper extremity in sports medicine*, St Louis, Mosby.

29. Park, MC: 2002. Shoulder dislocation in young athletes: current concepts in management, *Physician and sportsmedicine* 30(12): 41–48.

30. Patton, WC: 2001. Biceps tendinitis and subluxation, *Clinics in sports medicine* 20(3):505–529.

31. Peterson, L: 2001. Shoulder and upper arm, in *Sports injuries: their prevention and treatment*, 3rd ed, Champaign, IL, Human Kinetics, pp. 111–156.

32. Schneider, R, Myers, J, Ruemski, T, Prentice, W: 2010. Rehabilitation of shoulder injuries. In Prentice, W, editor: *Rehabilitation techniques in sports medicine and athletic training*, New York, McGraw-Hill.

33. Tennent, TD, Beach, WR, Meyers, JF: 2003. A review of the special tests associated with shoulder examination, *American journal of sports medicine* 31(1):154–160.

34. Tong, C, Ho, H, Chan, K: 2003. Shoulder impingement and rotator cuff disorders in the athletic shoulder, *International sportmed journal* 4(2):57–62.

35. Whiteley, R: 2007. Baseball throwing mechanics as they relate to pathology and performance—a review, *Journal of sports science & medicine* 6(1):1.

36. Wilk KE, Arrigo CA, Andrews JR: 1997. Current concepts: the stabilizing structures of the glenohumeral joint, *Journal of Orthopedic & Sports Physical Therapy* 25(6):364.

37. Wolin PM, Tarbet JA: 1997. Rotator cuff injury: addressing overhead overuse, *Physician and Sportsmedicine* 25(6):54.

**ANNOTATED BIBLIOGRAPHY**

Andrews J, Wilk K: 1994. *The athlete's shoulder,* New York, Churchill Livingstone.

*Concentrates on both conservative and surgical treatment of shoulder injuries occurring specifically in the athletic population.*

Donatelli, R: 2003. *Physical therapy of the shoulder,* Philadelphia, Churchill Livingstone.

*Clinical reference on shoulder rehabilitation, for physical therapists and rehabilitation professionals.*

Iannotti, J, Williams, G: 2006. *Disorders of the shoulder*, volumes 1 and 2: *Diagnosis and Management,* Baltimore, Lippincott, Williams, and Wilkins.

*A complete two-volume set that covers essentially every subject relative to the shoulder complex.*

Krishnan, S, Hawkins, R: 2004. *The Shoulder and the Overhead Athlete,* Baltimore, Lippincott, Williams & Wilkins.

*This text delivers comprehensive and up-to-date information on the evaluation, treatment, rehabilition, and prevention of shoulder injuries in throwing and other overhead activities.*

**WEB SITES**

Wheeless' Textbook of Orthopaedics: www.wheelessonline.com/

*An excellent page for injuries, anatomy, and x rays.*

Karolinska Institute Library: Musculoskeletal Disease: www.mic.ki.se/Diseases/ c05.html

MEDLINEplus: Shoulder Injuries and Disorders: www.nlm.nih.gov.medlineplus/ shoulderinjuriesanddisorders.html

*Search MEDLINE for recent research articles on shoulder injuries and disorders.*

AAOS Online Service Fact Sheet: The Shoulder http://orthoinfo.aaos.org/fact/ thr_report.cfm?Thread_ID= 121&topcategory=Shoulder

*Information on causes and management of shoulder injuries from the American Academy of Orthopedic Surgeons.*

# The Elbow, Forearm, Wrist, and Hand

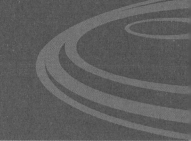

*When you finish this chapter you will be able to:*

- Describe the bony, ligamentous, and muscular anatomy of the elbow, forearm, wrist, and hand.
- List considerations for preventing injuries to the elbow, forearm, wrist, and hand.
- Describe assessment of common elbow, forearm, wrist, and hand injuries.
- Discuss the possible causes and signs of various injuries that can occur in the elbow, forearm, wrist, and hand.
- Explain the procedures that can be used in caring for elbow, forearm, wrist, and hand injuries.

## ANATOMY OF THE ELBOW JOINT

### Bones

The elbow complex is composed of three bones: the humerus, the radius, and the ulna (Figure 19-1). The distal end of the humerus forms the medial and lateral epicondyles. The olecranon process of the ulna (see Figure 19-10) articulates with the trochlea and olecranon fossa on the posterior humerus. The radial head articulates with the capitellum of the ulna. Three separate joints collectively form the elbow complex: the humeroulnar joint, the humeroradial joint, and the radioulnar joint. Flexion and extension occur at the humeroulnar and humeroradial joints. Pronation (rotating the forearm inward) and supination (rotating the forearm outward) occur at the radioulnar joint.

### Ligaments

The ulnar (medial) collateral ligament is most important for stability to a valgus force of the elbow and extends from the medial epicondyle to the proximal ulna. The annular ligament extends from the ulna, forming a sling around the radial head and thus allowing free rotation of the radius. The radial (lateral) collateral ligament, which provides stability to a varus force, extends from the lateral epicondyle and attaches primarily to the annular ligament[18] (refer to Figure 19-1).

### Muscles

The muscles of the elbow consist of the biceps brachii and the brachialis and the brachioradialis muscles, all of which are flexors of the elbow.

**Figure 19-1**

Bones and ligaments of the elbow joint (anterior view)

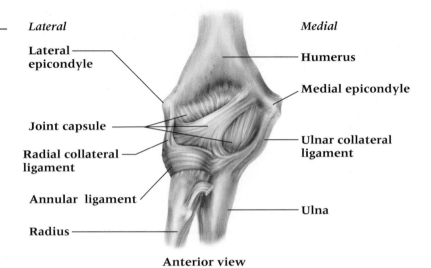

Anterior view

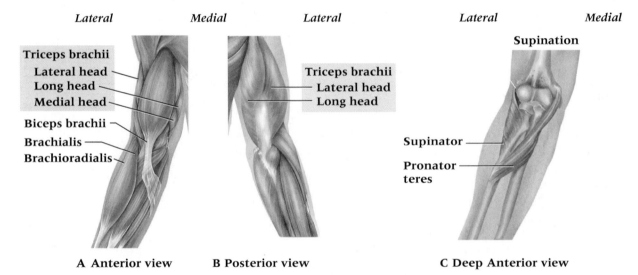

**A Anterior view**  **B Posterior view**  **C Deep Anterior view**

**Figure 19-2**

**Muscles of the elbow joint:**
(A) Anterior view.
(B) Posterior view.
(C) Deep pronator teres and supinator muscles (anterior view).

The brachialis is the primary elbow flexor. Extension is controlled by the triceps brachii muscle. The biceps brachii and supinator muscles allow supination of the forearm; the pronator teres and pronator quadratus act as pronators[21] (Figure 19-2) (Table 19-1).

| **TABLE 19-1** Muscles of the Elbow | |
| --- | --- |
| Elbow flexion | Biceps brachii |
| | Brachialis |
| | Brachioradialis |
| Elbow extension | Triceps brachii |

## ASSESSING ELBOW INJURIES

**Generally fitness professionals, coaches, and others working in areas related to exercise and sport science are not adequately trained to evaluate injuries. It is strongly recommended that injured athletes be referred to qualified medical personnel (i.e., physicians, athletic trainers, physical therapists) for injury evaluation.** Information on the following special tests has been included simply to give some idea about the different basic tests that nonmedical personnel may do to determine the nature and severity of the athlete's injury. The primary responsibility of those who are not health care personnel is to be able to recognize any potential "red flags" associated with the injury, provide appropriate first aid for the injury, and make correct decisions about how the injury should be managed initially, including immediate return to play or activity decisions (refer to Chapter 7).

### History

As with all sports injuries, it is important to understand how the injury occurred. The following questions aid in evaluation of the elbow:

- Is this a new injury or is this a chronic problem that has existed for some time?
- Is the pain or discomfort caused by a direct trauma such as falling on an outstretched arm or landing on the tip of a bent elbow?
- Can the problem be attributed to sudden overextension of the elbow or to repeated overuse of a throwing-type motion?
- Are there movements or positions of the arm that increase or decrease the pain?
- Has a previous elbow injury been diagnosed or treated?
- Is there a feeling of locking or a grating during movement?
- Is there any tingling or numbness radiating down the forearm or in the hand and fingers?

The location and duration should be ascertained. Like shoulder pain, elbow pain or discomfort may be from internal organ dysfunction or referred from a nerve root irritation or nerve impingement.

NOTE: Elbow pain may not be directly associated with an elbow injury but rather may be referred pain from the neck or shoulder.

### Observation

The athlete's elbow should be observed for obvious deformities and swelling. Flexion, extensibility, and the carrying angle of the elbow should be observed:

- An abnormally increased or abnormally decreased carrying angle may indicate an injury (Figure 19-3). A normal carrying angle is 5 to 15°.
- A carrying angle that is too great or too little may indicate a bony or growth plate fracture.

**Figure 19-3**

Testing for elbow carrying angle and the extent of cubitus valgus and cubitus varus. Normal is 5–15°.

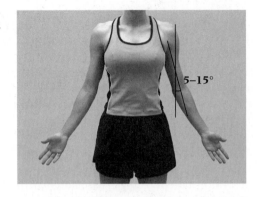

5–15°

**Figure 19-4**

Testing for elbow flexion and extension

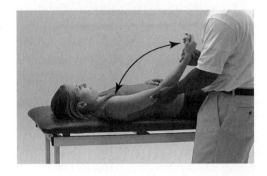

**Figure 19-5**

Observing elbow hyperextension

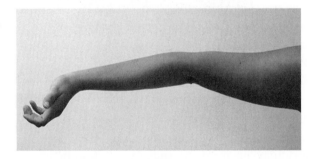

■ A decrease in normal flexion, an inability to extend fully, or a beyond-normal extension on one side more than the other (Figure 19-4) may be a sign of joint problems. Elbow hyperextension (Figure 19-5) is more common in females than in males.

## Palpation

Pain sites and deformities are determined through careful palpation of the epicondyles, olecranon process, distal aspect of the humerus, the proximal aspect of the ulna and the proximal radial head.

Soft tissue to be palpated includes the muscles and muscle tendons, joint capsule, and ligaments surrounding the joint.

## PREVENTION OF ELBOW, FOREARM, AND WRIST INJURIES

The elbow, forearm, and wrist are vulnerable to a variety of both acute traumatic injuries as well as chronic overuse type injuries. Acute injuries usually occur from either a direct blow or falling on an outstretched hand. In contact sports such as football or in high impact collision sports like baseball, wearing appropriate protective padding can reduce the force of the impact thus minimizing both the likelihood and the severity of the injury. Learning how to fall correctly by landing and rolling without putting the hand out to break the fall can help to prevent many of the injuries that would normally occur in either the wrist, forearm, or elbow.

The chances of developing chronic overuse injuries that typically occur in the elbow or in the wrist may be reduced by using several strategies. Limit the number of repetitions in throwing a baseball or in hitting a tennis ball. Make certain that the mechanics of the throwing or hitting techniques being used are correct and are not creating unnecessary stresses and strains. Select and use equipment (e.g., tennis racket, with the appropriate grip size, baseball bat) that is appropriate for a specific skill level. Maintain appropriate levels of strength and endurance in the muscles surrounding these joints by engaging in strength training. Routinely stretch the muscles in the elbow, forearm, and wrist to make certain that they have the necessary flexibility to allow movement through a full range of motion. If a chronic overuse problem seems to be developing, take some time off and give the injury a chance to heal before it gets worse.

## RECOGNITION AND MANAGEMENT OF INJURIES TO THE ELBOW

### Olecranon Bursitis

**Cause of injury** The olecranon bursa (Figure 19-6), lying between the end of the olecranon process and the skin, is the most frequently injured bursa in the elbow. The superficial location of the olecranon

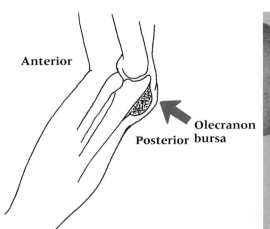

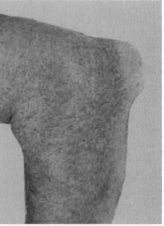

**Figure 19-6**

Olecranon bursitis

bursa makes it prone to acute or chronic injury, particularly as the result of direct blows or falling on the tip of the elbow.[44]

**Signs of injury**   The inflamed bursa produces pain, marked swelling, and point tenderness. Occasionally, swelling will appear almost spontaneously and will occur without the usual pain and heat.

**Care**   If the condition is acute, ice and compression should be applied for 20 minutes. Chronic olecranon bursitis requires a program of protective therapy. In rare cases aspiration by a physician hastens healing. Although seldom serious, olecranon bursitis can be annoying and should be well protected by padding while the athlete is engaged in competition.

## Elbow Sprains

**Cause of injury**   Sprains to the elbow are usually caused by hyperextension or a force that bends or twists the lower arm outward (valgus force) causing injury to the medial collateral ligament as occurs during the cocking phase of throwing[13] (see Figure 18-5).

**Signs of injury**   The athlete complains of pain and the inability to throw or grasp an object. There is a point tenderness over the medial collateral ligament.

**Care**   Immediate care for an elbow sprain consists of cold and a pressure bandage for at least 24 hours with sling support fixed at 90 degrees of flexion. A main concern should be to progressively aid the elbow in regaining a full range of motion, followed by active exercises. During rehabilitation, throwing activities should be controlled by limiting and gradually progressing the number of throws until full mobility and strength have returned.[29] If the elbow is unstable, a surgical procedure that has been called a "Tommy John" procedure is often used to repair the medial collateral ligament and joint capsule.

## Lateral Epicondylitis

**Cause of injury**   *Lateral epicondylitis* is one of the most common problems of the elbow occurring in sports. Tennis elbow is another name for lateral epicondylitis stemming from a backhand stroke involving overextending the wrist.[10] The cause of lateral epicondylitis is repetitive extension of the wrist, which eventually causes irritation and inflammation to the insertion of the extensor muscle of the lateral epicondyle.[19]

**Signs of injury**   The athlete complains of an aching pain in the region of the lateral epicondyle during and after activity (Figure 19-7). The pain gradually becomes worse with weakness in the hand and wrist. Inspection reveals tenderness at the lateral epicondyle and pain on resisted extension of the wrist and full extension of the elbow.[11]

**Care**   Treatment includes immediate use of PRICE, nonsteroidal anti-inflammatory drugs (NSAIDs), and analgesics as needed.[22] Rehabilitation includes range-of-motion exercises, progressive resistance exercises, deep friction massage, hand grasping while in supination (palm up), and avoiding pronation (palm down) movements. Mobilization and stretching may be used within pain-free limits.[32] The athlete may wear

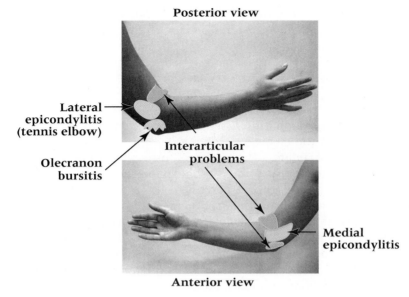

Posterior view

Lateral
epicondylitis
(tennis elbow)

Olecranon
bursitis

Interarticular
problems

Medial
epicondylitis

Anterior view

**Figure 19-7**

Typical pain sites in the elbow region

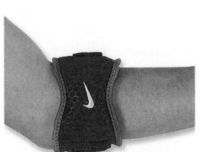

**Figure 19-8**

Counterforce brace for treatment of elbow and epicondylitis

a counterforce brace or neoprene elbow sleeve for 1 to 3 months (Figure 19-8). The athlete must be taught proper skill techniques and the proper use of equipment to avoid recurrence of the injury.[11]

## Medial Epicondylitis

**Cause of injury**  Irritation and inflammation of the medial epicondyle may result from a number of different sport activities that require repeated forceful flexions of the elbow. It has also been referred to as Little League elbow,[20] pitcher's elbow, racquetball elbow, golfer's elbow, and javelin-thrower's elbow.[18]

**Signs of injury**  Pain occurs around the medial epicondyle of the humerus during forceful wrist flexion and may radiate down the arm. There is usually point tenderness and in some cases mild swelling. Passive movement of the wrist seldom elicits pain, although active movement does.[9]

**Care**  Conservative management of moderate to severe medial epicondylitis usually includes use of rest, cryotherapy, or heat through the application of ultrasound.[9] Analgesics and anti-inflammatory agents may be prescribed by a physician. A counterforce brace applied just below the bend of the elbow is highly beneficial in reducing elbow stress (refer to Figure 19-8). For more severe cases elbow splinting and complete rest for 7 to 10 days may be warranted.[20]

### Elbow Osteochondritis Dissecans

Although osteochondritis dissecans is more common in the knees it can also occur in the elbow.

**Cause of injury**  The cause of osteochondritis dissecans is unknown; however, impairment of the blood supply can lead to fragmentation and separation of a portion of the articular cartilage and bone, creating loose bodies within the joint.[14,17]

**Signs of injury**  The adolescent athlete usually complains of sudden pain and locking of the elbow joint. Range of motion returns slowly over a few days. Swelling, pain, and crepitation may also occur.[17,18]

**Care**  Repeated episodes of locking may warrant surgical removal of the loose bodies. If they are not removed, traumatic arthritis can eventually occur.[36]

### Ulnar Nerve Injuries

**Cause of injury**  Because of the exposed position of the medial humeral condyle, the ulnar nerve is subject to a variety of problems. The athlete with a pronounced outward angle (cubitus valgus) of the elbow may develop a nerve friction problem.[35] The ulnar nerve can also become recurrently dislocated because of a structural deformity or can become impinged by a ligament during flexion-type activities.[7]

Athletes with a pronounced cubitus valgus are prone to injuring the ulnar nerve.

**Signs of injury**  Rather than being painful, ulnar nerve injuries usually respond with a **paresthesia** to the fourth and fifth fingers.[35] The athlete complains of burning and tingling in the fourth and fifth fingers.[7]

**paresthesia**
Lack of sensation.

**Care**  The management of ulnar nerve injuries is conservative; aggravation of the nerve, such as placing direct pressure on it, is avoided. When stress on the nerve cannot be avoided, surgery may be performed to transpose it anteriorly to the elbow.[44]

### Dislocation of the Elbow

**Cause of injury**  Dislocation of the elbow has a high incidence in sports activity and most often is caused either by a fall on the outstretched hand with the elbow in a position of hyperextension or by a severe twist while the elbow is in a flexed position (Figure 19-9).[37]

**19-1 Critical Thinking**
Exercise

A female javelin thrower complains of pain on the medial aspect of her elbow that is also referred distally to the forearm. The athlete senses an intermittent numbness, a burning sensation, and tingling in the fingers.

**?** What condition does this athlete have, and how could it have occurred?

**Signs of injury**  The bones of the forearm (ulna and radius) may be displaced backward, forward, or laterally. The appearance of the most common dislocation is a deformity of the olecranon process wherein it extends backward, well beyond its normal alignment with the upper arm.

Elbow dislocations involve rupturing and tearing of most of the stabilizing ligamentous tissue accompanied by profuse internal bleeding and subsequent swelling.[27] There is severe pain and disability. The

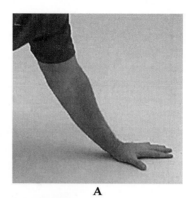

A

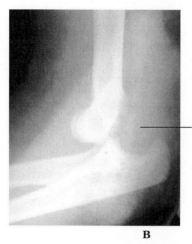

Posterior elbow
dislocation

B

**Figure 19-9**

(A) A fall on the outstretched
hand can produce an elbow
dislocation and/or fracture.
(B) Posterior dislocation X-ray.

complications of such a trauma may include injury to the major nerves
and blood vessels.[23] Check to see if there is a pulse present in the wrist
following elbow dislocation. The absence of a pulse creates a more
emergent situation.

**Care**   The primary responsibility is to provide the athlete with an im-
mobilizing splint and to refer the athlete immediately to a physician for
reduction as soon as possible. In most cases the physician administers an
anesthetic before reduction to relax the muscles. After reduction, the
physician often immobilizes the elbow in a position of flexion and applies
a splint, which should be used for approximately 3 weeks. A dislocated
elbow, like a fracture, may also have possible neurovascular problems.[37]

Neurovascular problems are a
possibility when an elbow is
dislocated or fractured.

### Fractures of the Elbow

**Cause of injury**   An elbow fracture can occur in almost any sporting event and is usually caused by a fall on the outstretched hand or
the flexed elbow or by a direct blow to the elbow.[5] Children and young
athletes have a much higher rate of this injury than do adults. A fracture can take place in any one or more of the bones that comprise the
elbow. A fall on the outstretched hand quite often fractures the humerus
above the condyles or the bones of the forearm or wrist.

**Signs of injury**   An elbow fracture may or may not result in visible deformity. There usually is hemorrhage, swelling, and muscle spasm in the injured area.

**Care**   Because of the seriousness of an elbow fracture, careful immediate care must be rendered. Following the application of ice and a sling support, the athlete must be referred immediately for medical attention. A fractured elbow is associated with rapid swelling that may cause a condition called Volkmann's contracture, an extremely serious and often irreversible condition.[5]

## ANATOMY OF THE FOREARM

### Bones

The bones of the forearm are the ulna and the radius (Figure 19-10). The ulna, which may be thought of as a direct extension of the humerus, is long, straight, and larger at its upper end than at its lower end. The radius, considered an extension of the hand, is thicker at its lower end than at its upper end.

### Joints

The forearm has three articulations: the superior, middle, and distal radioulnar joints.

**Figure 19-10**

Bones of the forearm with interosseous membrane

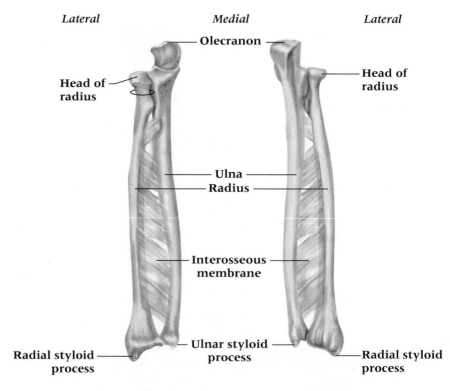

A  Anterior view          B  Posterior view

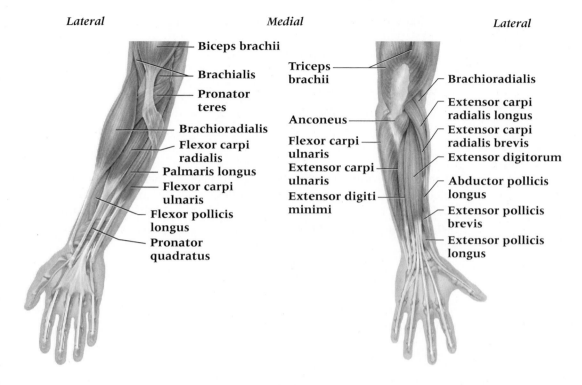

*Lateral*  ·  *Medial*  ·  *Lateral*

- Biceps brachii
- Brachialis
- Pronator teres
- Brachioradialis
- Flexor carpi radialis
- Palmaris longus
- Flexor carpi ulnaris
- Flexor pollicis longus
- Pronator quadratus

- Triceps brachii
- Anconeus
- Flexor carpi ulnaris
- Extensor carpi ulnaris
- Extensor digiti minimi

- Brachioradialis
- Extensor carpi radialis longus
- Extensor carpi radialis brevis
- Extensor digitorum
- Abductor pollicis longus
- Extensor pollicis brevis
- Extensor pollicis longus

**A Anterior view**

**B Posterior view**

**Figure 19-11**

**Muscles of the forearm:**
(A) Anterior view.
(B) Posterior view.

## Muscles

The forearm muscles consist of flexors and pronators, positioned anteriorly and attached to the medial epicondyle, and of extensors and supinators, which lie posteriorly and are attached to the lateral epicondyle (Figure 19-11). The flexors of the wrist and fingers are separated into superficial muscles and deep muscles (Table 19-2).

## ASSESSING FOREARM INJURIES

### History

The following questions are asked in the evaluation of forearm injuries:

- What caused the injury (e.g., blunt trauma, throwing, or chronic overuse)?

**TABLE 19-2** Muscles of the Forearm

| | |
|---|---|
| Forearm pronation | Pronator teres |
| | Pronator quadratus |
| Forearm supination | Supinator |
| | Biceps brachii |

- What were the symptoms at the time of injury? Did symptoms occur later?
- Were symptoms localized or diffuse?
- Was there swelling or discoloration?
- Was there immediate loss of function?
- What treatment was given?
- Did this injury occur immediately or has it occurred gradually?

## Observation

The entire forearm is first visually inspected, including the wrist and elbow, looking for obvious deformities, swelling, and skin defects. If a deformity is not present, the athlete is then observed pronating and supinating the forearm.

## Palpation

The injured forearm is palpated at the point of injury and in areas distant to that site and the point of injury. Palpation can reveal tenderness, edema, fracture deformity, change in skin temperature, bone fragments, or a lack of continuity between bones.

## RECOGNITION AND MANAGEMENT OF INJURIES TO THE FOREARM

### Contusion

**Cause of injury**   The forearm is constantly exposed to bruising in contact sports such as football. The ulnar side receives the majority of blows in arm blocks and consequently the greater amount of bruising. Bruises to this area may be classified as acute or chronic. The acute contusion can, on rare occasions, result in a fracture.[34] The chronic contusion develops from repeated blows to the forearm with attendant multiple irritations.

**Signs of injury**   Most often muscles or bones develop varying degrees of pain, swelling, and accumulation of blood (hematoma). Extensive scar tissue may replace the hematoma, and in some cases, a bony callus replaces the scar tissue.

**Care**   Care of the contused forearm requires proper attention in the acute stages by application of PRICE for 20 minutes every 1½ waking hours, followed the next day by cold and exercise. Protection of the forearm is important for athletes who are prone to this condition. The best protection consists of a full-length sponge rubber pad for the forearm early in the season.

### Forearm Splints and Other Strains

Forearm splints, like shin splints, commonly occur early and late in the sports season.

**Cause of injury**   Forearm strains occur in a variety of sports most often from repeated static contractions. Forearm splints occur often in gymnastics. The reason for this problem is probably static muscle contractions of the forearm, such as those that occur when an athlete performs

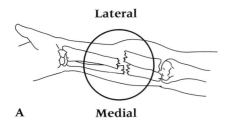

Lateral

A       Medial

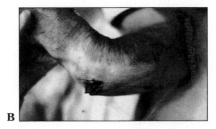

B

**Figure 19-12**

(A) Fracture of the radius and ulna (B) Open fracture of the ulna

on the side horse. Constant static muscle contraction causes minute tears in the deep connective tissues of the forearm.

**Signs of injury** The main symptom of forearm splints is a dull ache of the extensor muscles crossing the back of the forearm. Muscle weakness may accompany the dull ache. Palpation reveals an irritation of the deep tissue between the muscles. The cause of this condition is uncertain; like shin splints, forearm splints usually appear either early or late in the season, indicating poor conditioning or chronic fatigue.

**Care** Care of forearm splints is symptomatic. The athlete should concentrate on increasing the strength of the forearm through resistance exercises. Emphasis should also be placed on rest, cold, or heat and on use of a supportive wrap during activity.

### Forearm Fractures

**Cause of injury** Fractures of the forearm (Figure 19-12) are particularly common among active children and youths. Forearm fractures occur as the result of a blow or a fall on the outstretched hand. Fractures to the ulna or the radius singly are much rarer than simultaneous fractures to both.[22]

**Signs of injury** The break usually presents all the features of a long-bone fracture: pain, swelling, deformity, and a false joint. The older the athlete, the greater the danger of extensive damage to soft tissue and the greater the possibility of paralysis.[34]

**Care** To prevent complications, a cold pack must be applied immediately to the fracture site, the arm splinted and put in a sling, and the athlete referred to a physician. The athlete usually is incapacitated for about 8 weeks.[15]

### Colles' Fracture

**Cause of injury** Colles' fracture (Figure 19-13), among the most common forearm fractures, involves the lower (distal) end of the radius.[34] The cause of a Colles' fracture is usually a fall on the outstretched hand with extended wrist, forcing the forearm backward and upward into hyperextension. A Smith's fracture occurs when the athlete falls on a flexed wrist and is much less common.

**Signs of injury** In most cases there is a visible deformity to the wrist. Sometimes no deformity is present, and the injury may be passed

**Figure 19-13**

**Common appearance of the forearm in Colles' fracture**

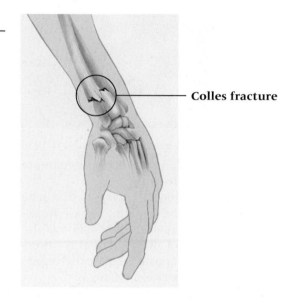

Colles fracture

off as a bad sprain. Bleeding is profuse in this area, with the accumulated fluids causing extensive swelling in the wrist and, if unchecked, in the fingers and forearm. Ligamentous tissue is usually unharmed, but tendons may be torn away from their attachment, and there may possibly be median nerve damage.

**Care**  The main responsibility is to apply ice, splint the wrist, put the limb in a sling, and then refer the athlete to a physician for x-ray examination and immobilization. Lacking complications, Colles' fracture will keep an athlete out of sports for 1 to 2 months.

## ANATOMY OF THE WRIST, HAND, AND FINGERS

### Bones

The wrist is formed by the distal aspect of the radius and the ulna with a proximal row of four carpal bones and a distal row of four carpal bones that articulate with five metacarpals. The metacarpal bones join the carpal bones above and the phalanges below, forming metacarpophalangeal (MCP) articulations. The four fingers each have a proximal, middle, and distal phalanx, whereas the thumb has only two phalanges (Figure 19-14).

### Ligaments

The wrist is composed of a complex series of multiple ligaments that bind the carpal bones to one another, to the ulna and radius, and to the proximal metacarpal bones. Of major interest in wrist injuries are the ulnar collateral ligament and radial collateral ligament. Crossing the volar aspect of the carpal bones is the flexor retinaculum. This ligament

**《◯》 19-2 *Critical Thinking***
Exercise

A young athlete falls off the parallel bars onto his outstretched left hand, forcing the wrist into hyperextension. There is a visible deformity to the wrist.

? Describe the deformity presented and the actions that should be taken.

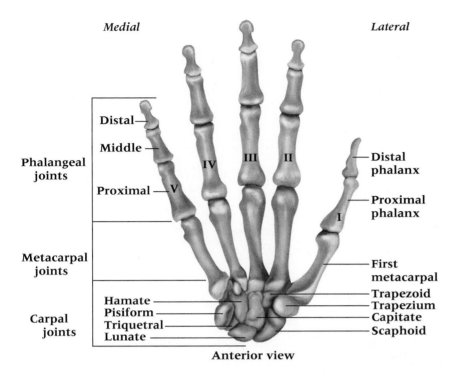

**Figure 19-14**

Bones of the wrist, hand, and fingers (anterior view)

Medial      Lateral

Phalangeal joints
- Distal
- Middle
- Proximal

IV  III  II

Distal phalanx

Proximal phalanx

I

Metacarpal joints

First metacarpal

Carpal joints
- Hamate
- Pisiform
- Triquetral
- Lunate

Trapezoid
Trapezium
Capitate
Scaphoid

**Anterior view**

serves as the roof of the carpal tunnel, in which the median nerve is often compressed (Figure 19-15A). The interphalangeal joints have medial and lateral collateral ligaments and a thickened joint capsule on the palmar surface that is referred to as the *volar plate*.

## Muscles

The wrist and hand are a complex of extrinsic muscles (which originate outside of the hand) and intrinsic muscles (which originate in the hand) muscles. In general both the extrinsic and intrinsic muscles located on the medial aspect and front of the wrist and hand flex the wrist and fingers. The muscles on the posterior and lateral aspect of the wrist and hand extend the wrist and fingers (Figure 19-15). Intrinsic muscles of the hand also abduct, adduct, and in the thumb create opposition, of the metacarpals (Table 19-3).

## ASSESSMENT OF THE WRIST, HAND, AND FINGERS

### History

As with other conditions, the evaluator asks about the location and type of pain:

- What increases or decreases the pain?
- Has there been a history of trauma or overuse?
- What therapy or medications, if any, have been given?

**Figure 19-15**

Muscles of the hand:
(A) Palmar aspect (anterior view).
(B) Dorsal aspect (posterior view).

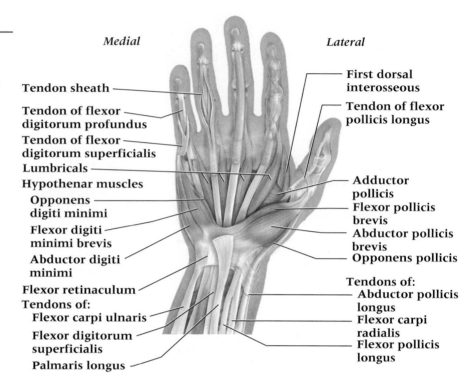

*Medial*

*Lateral*

Tendon sheath

Tendon of flexor digitorum profundus

Tendon of flexor digitorum superficialis

Lumbricals

Hypothenar muscles

Opponens digiti minimi

Flexor digiti minimi brevis

Abductor digiti minimi

Flexor retinaculum

Tendons of:
  Flexor carpi ulnaris

  Flexor digitorum superficialis

  Palmaris longus

First dorsal interosseous

Tendon of flexor pollicis longus

Adductor pollicis

Flexor pollicis brevis

Abductor pollicis brevis

Opponens pollicis

Tendons of:
  Abductor pollicis longus

  Flexor carpi radialis

  Flexor pollicis longus

**A  Palmar aspect (anterior)**

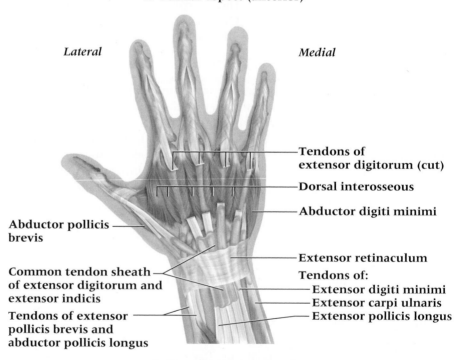

*Lateral*

*Medial*

Abductor pollicis brevis

Common tendon sheath of extensor digitorum and extensor indicis

Tendons of extensor pollicis brevis and abductor pollicis longus

Tendons of extensor digitorum (cut)

Dorsal interosseous

Abductor digiti minimi

Extensor retinaculum

Tendons of:
  Extensor digiti minimi
  Extensor carpi ulnaris
  Extensor pollicis longus

**B  Dorsal aspect (posterior)**

**TABLE 19-3** Muscles of the Wrist, Hand, and Fingers

| | |
|---|---|
| Wrist flexion | Flexor carpi radialis |
| | Flexor carpi ulnaris |
| Wrist extension | Extensor carpi radialis longus |
| | Extensor carpi radialis brevis |
| | Extensor carpi ulnaris |
| Finger flexion | Flexor digitorum profundus |
| | Flexor digitorum superficialis |
| Finger extension | Extensor digitorum communis |
| | Extensor digiti minimi |
| | Extensor indicis |
| Thumb flexor | Flexor pollicis longus |
| Thumb extension | Extensor pollicis longus |
| | Extensor pollicis brevis |
| Thumb abductor | Abductor pollicis longus |

## Observation

As the athlete is observed, arm and hand asymmetries are noted:

- Are there any postural deviations?
- Does the athlete hold the part in a stiff or protected manner?
- Is the wrist or hand swollen?

Hand usage such as writing or unbuttoning a shirt is noted. The general attitude of the hand is observed. When the athlete is asked to open and close the hand, the evaluator notes whether this movement can be performed fully and rhythmically. Another general functional activity is to have the athlete touch the tip of the thumb to each fingertip several times. The last factor to be observed is the color of the fingernails. Nails that are very pale instead of pink may indicate a problem with blood circulation.

## Palpation

The bones of the wrist region are palpated for pain and deformity. The examiner palpates each carpal bone, metacarpal bone, MCP joint, and each phalanx, starting with the PIP joint and progressing to the distal interphalangeal (DIP) joint. Each tendon is palpated as it crosses the wrist region. The examiner palpates the flexor muscles of the fingers and thumb. On the dorsal aspect, the examiner palpates the extensor tendons and phalanges.

## RECOGNITION AND MANAGEMENT OF WRIST AND HAND INJURIES

### Wrist Sprain

**Cause of injury** It is often very difficult to distinguish between a wrist sprain and a tendon strain in the carpal region. A sprain is by far the most common wrist injury.[2] It can occur from any abnormal, forced

Sprains are the most common wrist injury in sports and often the worst managed.

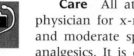

movement of the wrist. Falling on the hyperextended wrist is the most common cause of wrist sprain, but violent flexion or torsion can also cause injury (see Figure 19-9).[33]

**Signs of injury**  The athlete complains of pain, swelling, and difficulty moving the wrist. On examination there is tenderness, swelling, and limited range of motion.

**Care**  All athletes having severe sprains should be referred to a physician for x-ray examination to determine possible fractures. Mild and moderate sprains should initially be given PRICE, splinting, and analgesics. It is desirable to have the athlete start wrist-strengthening exercises almost immediately after the injury has occurred. Taping for support can benefit healing and help prevent further injury.

## Wrist Tendinitis

**Cause of injury**  Wrist tendinitis occurs in weight lifters, rowers, and participants in other sports that require the athlete to perform repetitive wrist accelerations and decelerations.[43]

**Signs of injury**  The athlete complains of pain with use or pain in passive stretching. There is tenderness and swelling over the tendon.

**Care**  Acute pain and inflammation are managed by ice massage for 10 minutes four times a day for the first 48 to 72 hours, anti-inflammatory medication, and rest. A wrist splint may protect the injured tendon. When swelling has subsided range of motion is stressed. When pain and swelling have subsided, progressive resistance exercise can be instituted.

## Carpal Tunnel Syndrome

**Cause of injury**  The carpal tunnel is located on the anterior aspect of the wrist. The floor of the carpal tunnel is formed by the carpal bones and the roof by the flexor retinaculum (see Figure 19-15A). A number of anatomical structures course through this limited space, including eight long finger flexor tendons, their synovial sheaths, and the median nerve. Carpal tunnel syndrome results from an inflammation of the tendons and synovial sheaths within this space, which ultimately leads to compression of the median nerve.[30] Carpal tunnel syndrome most often occurs in athletes who engage in activities that require repeated wrist flexion, although it can also result from direct trauma to the anterior aspect of the wrist.[24]

**Signs of injury**  Compression of the median nerve usually results in both sensory and motor deficits. Sensory changes can result in tingling, numbness, and paresthesia in the arc of median nerve innervation over the thumb, index and middle fingers, and palm of the hand. The median nerve innervates the lumbrical muscles of the index and middle fingers and three of the thenar muscles. Thus weakness in thumb movement is associated with this condition.

**Care**  Initially, conservative treatment involving rest, immobilization in slight wrist extension, and nonsteroidal anti-inflammatory medication is recommended. If the syndrome persists, injection with a corticosteroid

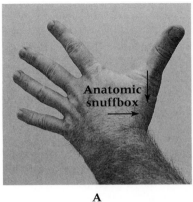
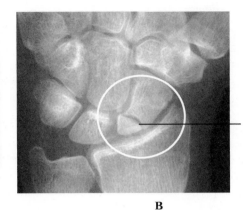

A            B

Scaphoid
fracture

and possible surgical decompression of the transverse carpal ligament may be necessary.[24]

## Scaphoid Fracture

**Cause of injury** The scaphoid bone is the most frequently fractured carpal bone.[31] The injury is usually caused by a fall on an outstretched hand, which compresses the scaphoid bone between the radius and the second row of carpal bones.[33]

**Signs of injury** The signs of a recent scaphoid fracture include swelling in the area of the carpal bones and severe point tenderness over the scaphoid bone in the anatomic snuffbox[3] (Figure 19-16).

**Care** In an athlete with these signs, cold should be applied, the area should be splinted, and the athlete should be referred to a physician for an x-ray study and casting.[31] It is not uncommon for a scaphoid fracture to be missed on an initial x-ray. In most cases, cast immobilization lasts for approximately 6 weeks and is followed by strengthening exercises coupled with protective taping. Immobilization is discontinued for rehabilitation.[3] The wrist needs protection against impact loading for an additional 3 months. In many cases the scaphoid does not heal properly, and surgery is often necessary.[39]

## Hamate Fracture

**Cause of injury** A fracture of the hamate bone, and in particular the hook of the hamate, can occur from a fall but more commonly occurs from contact when holding a sports implement such as the handle of a tennis racket, a baseball bat, a lacrosse stick, a hockey stick, or a golf club.[2,10]

**Signs of injury** Wrist pain and weakness and point tenderness are experienced. There is possibly tingling, numbness, and weakness in the little and ring fingers because the ulnar nerve may be compromised because of its close proximity to the hamate.

**Care** Casting of the wrist is usually the treatment of choice. The hook of the hamate can be protected by wearing a doughnut pad to take pressure off the area.[10]

**Figure 19-16**

(A) A fracture of the scaphoid results in point tenderness in the anatomic snuffbox. (B) X-ray of a fractured scaphoid.

**19-3 *Critical Thinking***
Exercise

A basketball player stumbles and falls on an outstretched hand. She complains of pain at the base of the thumb at the wrist. She is very point tender.

**?** What specific injury might be causing her pain and what should be done?

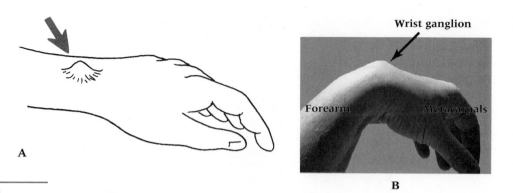

**A**

**Figure 19-17**

Dorsal wrist ganglion

**19-4 Critical Thinking**
Exercise

A football player gets into a fistfight on the field and injures his right hand.

? What type of injury should be suspected?

## Wrist Ganglion

**Cause of injury**   A wrist ganglion (Figure 19-17) is considered by many to be either a herniation of the joint capsule, of the synovial sheath of a tendon, or a cystic structure. It usually appears slowly, after repeated forced hyperextension of the wrist, and contains a clear, mucinous fluid. The ganglion most often appears on the back of the wrist.[28]

**Signs of injury**   The athlete complains of occasional pain with a lump at the site. Pain increases with wrist extension. There is a cystic structure that may feel soft, rubbery, or very hard.

**Care**   An old method of treatment was first to break down the swelling through digital pressure and then apply a felt pressure pad for a time to encourage healing. A newer approach is the use of a combination of aspiration and chemical cauterization, with subsequent application of a pressure pad.[4] Neither of these methods prevents the ganglion from recurring. Surgical removal is the best of the various methods of treatment.

## Metacarpal Fracture

**Cause of injury**   Fractures of the fifth metacarpal are associated with boxing and the martial arts and are usually called a *boxer's fracture* (Figure 19-18). The cause of metacarpal fractures is commonly a direct axial force caused by punching the wall or another person.[8]

**Figure 19-18**

Boxer's fracture of the fifth metacarpal

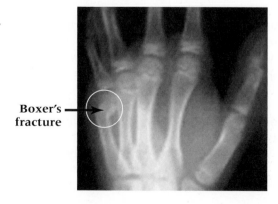

Boxer's fracture

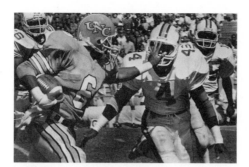

**Figure 19-19**

Injuries to the wrist and fingers are very common in contact sports.

**Signs of injury**   There is point tenderness and likely a palpable defect in the shaft of the fifth metacarpal. When the athlete makes a fist, the knuckle will appear depressed or sunken. Swelling is rapid.

**Care**   An athlete with a suspected boxer's fracture should be referred to a physician for reduction and immobilization for a period lasting 3 to 4 weeks.

## RECOGNITION AND MANAGEMENT OF FINGER INJURIES

The fingers are extremely vulnerable to injury in contact sports (Figure 19-19). While finger injuries are very often not considered to be serious by most people, they can create serious long-term dysfunction in many cases. Thus it is imperative that these injuries be correctly managed.

### Mallet Finger

**Cause of injury**   The mallet finger is sometimes called *baseball finger* or *basketball finger*. It is caused by a blow from a thrown ball that strikes the tip of the finger, jamming and avulsing the extensor tendon from its insertion along with a piece of bone.[1]

**Signs of injury**   The athlete complains of pain at the distal interphalangeal joint. X-ray examination may show a bony avulsion from the dorsal proximal distal phalanx. The athlete is unable to extend the finger, carrying it at approximately a 30-degree angle. There is also point tenderness at the site of the injury, and the avulsed bone often can be palpated (Figure 19-20).

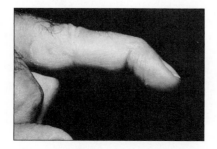
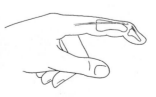

**Figure 19-20**

Mallet finger

**Figure 19-21**

Splinting of a mallet finger

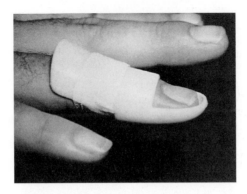

**Care** PRICE is given for the pain and swelling. If there is no fracture the distal phalanx should immediately be splinted in a position of extension 24 hours a day for a period of 6 to 8 weeks (Figure 19-21).

### Boutonnière Deformity

**Cause of injury** The boutonnière, or buttonhole, deformity is caused by a rupture of the extensor tendon over the middle phalanx. Trauma occurs to the tip of the finger, which forces the DIP joint into extension and the PIP joint into flexion.[1]

**Signs of injury** The athlete complains of severe pain and inability to extend the DIP joint. There is swelling, point tenderness, and an obvious deformity.[35]

**Care** Care of the boutonnière deformity includes cold application followed by splinting of the PIP joint in extension.[42] NOTE: If this condition is inadequately splinted, the classic boutonnière deformity will develop (Figure 19-22). Splinting is continued for 5 to 8 weeks. While splinted, the athlete is encouraged to flex the distal phalanx.[41]

### Jersey Finger

**Cause of injury** Jersey finger is a rupture of the flexor digitorum profundus tendon from its insertion on the distal phalanx. It most often

**Figure 19-22**

(A) Boutonnière deformity
(B) Oval-8 Splint

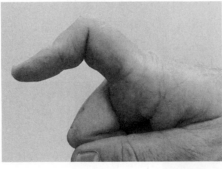

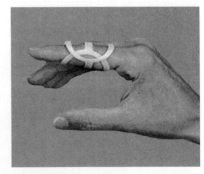

A                                              B

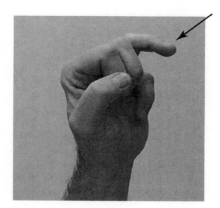

**Figure 19-23**

A Jersey finger involves ruture of the flexor tendon and loss of ability to flex the finger.

occurs in the ring finger when the athlete tries to grab a jersey of an opponent, either rupturing the tendon or avulsing a small piece of bone[28] (Figure 19-23).

**Signs of injury**  Because the tendon is no longer attached to the distal phalanx the DIP joint cannot be flexed and the finger is in an extended position. There is pain and point tenderness over the distal phalanx.

**Care**  If the tendon is not surgically repaired the athlete will never be able to flex the DIP joint, causing weakness in grip strength; otherwise function is relatively normal. If surgery is done the course of rehabilitation requires about 12 weeks and there is often poor gliding of the tendon with the possibility of rerupture.

## Gamekeeper's Thumb

**Cause of injury**  A sprain of the ulnar collateral ligament of the MCP joint of the thumb is common among athletes, especially skiers and tackle football players. It can also occur in baseball and softball players when the thumb is hit by a ball exerting torque on the joint.[26] The mechanism of injury is usually a forceful abduction of the proximal phalanx, which is occasionally combined with hyperextension.[28]

**Signs of injury**  The athlete complains of pain over the ulnar collateral ligament with a weak and painful pinch. Inspection demonstrates tenderness and swelling over the medial aspect of the thumb.

**Care**  Because the stability of pinching can be severely reduced, proper immediate and follow-up care must be performed. If there is instability in the joints, the athlete should be immediately referred to an orthopedist. If the joint is stable, x-ray examination should be performed to rule out fracture. Splinting of the thumb should be applied for protection over a 3-week period or until it is pain free.[38]

## Collateral Ligament Sprain

**Cause of injury**  A collateral ligament sprain of a finger is very common in sports such as basketball, volleyball, and football. A common cause

**480**

Figure 19-24

Open dislocation of the
thumb

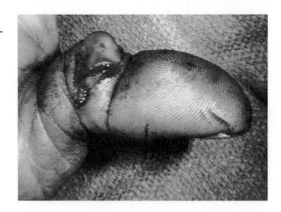

of collateral sprains is an axial force to the tip of the finger, producing the "jammed" effect.[26]

**Signs of injury** Severe point tenderness exists at the joint site, especially in the region of the collateral ligaments. There may be a lateral or medial joint instability when the joint is in 150 degrees of flexion.

**Care** Care of a collateral sprain includes ice packs for the acute stage, x-ray examination, and splinting.

## Dislocations of the Phalanges

**Cause of injury** Dislocations of the phalanges (Figure 19-24) occur frequently in sports and are caused mainly by a blow to the tip of the finger by a ball. The force of injury is usually directed upward from the palmar side, displacing either the first or second joint dorsally.[16] The resultant problem is primarily a tearing of the supporting capsular tissue, accompanied by hemorrhaging. However, there may be a rupture of the flexor or extensor tendon and chip fractures in and around the dislocated joint.[8]

**Care** Reduction of the dislocated thumb should be performed by a physician. To ensure the most complete healing of dislocated finger joints, splinting should be maintained for about 3 weeks in 30 degrees of flexion.[37] Inadequate immobilization can cause an unstable joint and/or excessive scar tissue and possibly a permanent deformity. When the athlete returns to activity, the dislocated finger can be "buddy-taped" to the adjacent finger for additional support.

Special consideration must be given to dislocations of the thumb and second or third joints of the fingers.[9] A properly functioning thumb is necessary for hand dexterity; consequently, *any injury to the thumb should be considered serious.*[16] Thumb dislocations occur frequently at the second joint, resulting from a sharp blow to its tip with the trauma forcing the thumb into hyperextension and dislocating the second joint downward. Any dislocation of the third joint of the finger can lead to complications and requires the immediate care of an orthopedist. *All hand dislocations must be x-rayed to rule out fracture.*

## Phalanx Fractures

**Cause of injury** Phalanx fractures can occur from a variety of actions: The fingers are stepped on, hit by a ball, or twisted.[8]

**Signs of injury** The athlete complains of pain and swelling in a finger. Tenderness is felt at the point of fracture.

**Care** The finger suspected of fracture should be splinted in flexion around a gauze roll or a curved splint to avoid full extension. Flexion splinting reduces the deformity by relaxing the flexor tendons. Fracture of the distal phalanx is less complicated than fracture of the middle or proximal phalanx.

## Subungual Hematoma

**Cause of injury** A contusion or a crushing injury to the distal finger can cause blood to accumulate in the nail bed under the fingernail. Blood that accumulates in a confined space underneath the nail is likely to produce extreme pain and can ultimately cause loss of the nail.[13]

**Signs of injury** Bleeding into the nail bed may be either immediate or slow, producing considerable pain. The area under the fingernail assumes a bluish-purple color and gentle pressure on the nail greatly exacerbates pain.

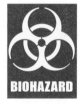

**Care** An ice pack should be applied immediately, and the hand should be elevated to decrease bleeding. Within the next 12 to 24 hours, the pressure of the blood under the nail should be released by drilling a small hole through the nail into the nail bed. This drilling must be done under sterile conditions and is best done by either a physician or an athletic trainer. It is not uncommon to have to drill the nail a second time because more blood is likely to accumulate.

## SUMMARY

- The humeroradial and humeroulnar joints of the elbow allow the movements of flexion and extension, and the radioulnar joint allows forearm pronation and supination.

- Olecranon bursitis occurs from falling on the tip of the elbow.

- The ulnar collateral ligament of the elbow is injured as a result of a valgus force from repetitive overhead throwing.

- Medial epicondylitis is also called golfer's elbow, raquetball elbow, or pitcher's elbow and occurs because of repetitive forced flexion of the wrist.

- Lateral epicondylitis or tennis elbow occurs with repetitive wrist extension.

- Elbow dislocations result from elbow hyperextension from a fall on an extended arm, with the radius and ulna dislocating posteriorly. The degree of stability present determines the course of rehabilitation.

If the elbow is stable, a brief period of immobilization is followed
by rehabilitation.

- Fractures in the elbow may occur from a direct blow or from falling
  on an outstretched hand. They may be treated by casting or in
  some cases by surgical reduction and fixation.

- The forearm is composed of two bones, the ulna and the radius,
  and the flexors and extensors of the wrist. Sports injuries to the
  region commonly consist of contusions, chronic forearm splints,
  acute strains, and fractures.

- Injuries to the wrist usually occur as the result of a fall on an
  outstretched hand or repeated movements of flexion, extension,
  and/or rotation. Common injuries are sprains, tendinitis, carpal
  tunnel syndrome, scaphoid fracture, hamate fracture, and wrist
  ganglion.

- Injuries to the hand and fingers occur frequently in sports activities.
  Common injuries include a boxer's fracture, mallet finger,
  boutonnière deformity, jersey finger, gamekeeper's thumb, sprains,
  dislocations and fractures of the phalanges, and subungual
  hematoma.

---

### Solutions to Critical Thinking Exercises

**19-1** This javelin thrower has sustained an ulnar nerve injury. Because of a pronounced elbow cubitus valgus, the ulnar nerve recurrently subluxates. Because of ligamentous laxity, there is nerve impingement and compression.

**19-2** This injury is a Colles' fracture, which is caused by the fracture displacement of the distal radius. An ice compress, a splint, and a sling should be applied. The athlete is then referred to a physician for an x-ray and definitive treatment.

**19-3** This is likely a scaphoid fracture. The wrist and thumb should be immobilized in a splint and she should be sent to a physician for an x-ray.

**19-4** Suspect a fracture of a metacarpal bone. The injury may appear as an angular or rotational deformity. PRICE and analgesics are given along with an x-ray examination. The injury is splinted for about 4 weeks, and early range-of-motion exercises are prescribed.

## REVIEW QUESTIONS AND CLASS ACTIVITIES

1. Describe the procedures for assessing an elbow injury.
2. Describe the mechanism and management of elbow sprains.
3. How does the elbow develop medial and lateral epicondylitis?
4. What are the symptoms and signs of elbow osteochondritis dissecans?
5. Describe a dislocated elbow—its cause, appearance, and care.
6. Compare forearm splints and shin splints. How does each occur?
7. What is the difference between a wrist strain and a wrist sprain?
8. Describe the Colles' fracture of the forearm—its cause, appearance, and care.

9. How does carpal tunnel syndrome develop and how would you care for it?
10. Discuss injuries that can occur to the lunate, scaphoid, and hamate bones in the wrist.
11. What is the difference between a mallet finger, a boutonnière deformity, and jersey finger?
12. What is the gamekeeper's thumb and how should it be treated?
13. Should a dislocated finger be reduced by an athletic trainer?
14. How should a subungual hematoma be managed?

## REFERENCES

1. Bach AW: 1999. Finger joint injuries in active patients: pointers for acute and late-phase management, *Physician and sportsmedicine* 27(3):89.

2. Birkbeck DP: 2001. Overview of common hand and wrist injuries in athletics, *Athletic therapy today* 6(2): 6–12.

3. Brooks, S, Wluka, AE, Stuckey, S: 2005. The management of scaphoid fractures, *Journal of science and medicine in sport* 8(2):181–189.

4. Brukner P: 2002. Wrist and hand pain. In Brukner, P, editor: *Clinical sports medicine*, 2nd ed, Sydney, McGraw Hill, pp. 292–320.

5. Brukner P: 2002. Elbow and forearm pain. In Brukner, P, editor: *Clinical sports medicine*, 2nd ed, Sydney, McGraw Hill, pp. 274–291.

6. Buettner CM, Leaver-Dunn D: 2000. Prevention and treatment of elbow injuries in adolescent pitchers, *Athletic therapy today* 5(3):19.

7. Cain, Jr., EL, Dugas, JR, Andrews, JR: 2003. Ulnar nerve injury in the throwing athlete, *Sports medicine and arthroscopy review* 11(1):40–46.

8. Caso JT, Hastings H: 1998. Metacarpal and phalangeal fractures in athletics. In Rettig AC, editor: *Hand and wrist. Clinics in sports medicine*, vol 17, no 3, Philadelphia, WB Saunders.

9. Ciccotti, MC: 2004. Diagnosis and treatment of medial epicondylitis of the elbow, *Clinics in sports medicine* 23(4):693–705.

10. David, TS; Zemel, NP; Mathews, PV: 2003. Symptomatic, partial union of the hook of the hamate fracture in athletes, *American journal of sports medicine* 31(1):106–111.

11. De Smedt, T, de Jong, A, Van Leemput, W: 2007. Lateral epicondylitis in tennis: update on aetiology, biomechanics and treatment, *British journal of sports medicine* 41(11):816–819.

12. Field LD, Savoie FH: 2000. Surgical treatment of ulnar collateral ligament injuries, *Athletic therapy today* 5(3):25.

13. Fincher AL: 1999. Taking finger injuries seriously, *Athletic therapy today* 4(3):45.

14. Hall TL, Galea AM: 1999. Osteochondritis dissecans of the elbow: diagnosis, treatment, and prevention, *Physician and sportsmedicine* 27(2):75.

15. Hanker GJ: 2001. Radius fractures in the athlete, *Clinics in sports medicine* 20(1):189–201.

16. Haugstvedt, J: 2004. Finger injuries, In Bahr, R, editor: *Clinical guide to sports injuries,* Champaign, IL, Human Kinetics.

17. Hennrikus, W: 2006. Elbow disorders in the young athlete, *Operative techniques in sports medicine* 14(3): 165–172.

18. Hughes, PE, Paletta, Jr., GA: 2003. Little Leaguer's elbow, medial epicondyle injury, and osteochondritis dissecans, *Sports medicine and arthroscopy review* 11(1):30–39.

19. Kaminsky, SB, Baker, Jr., CL: 2003. Lateral epicondylitis of the elbow, *Sports medicine and arthroscopy review* 11(1):63–70.

20. Klingele, KE: 2002. Little League elbow: valgus overload injury in the paediatric athlete, *Sports medicine* 32(15):1005–1015.

21. Loftice, J, Fleisig, GS, Zheng, N: 2004. Biomechanics of the elbow in sports, *Clinics in sports medicine* 23(4):519–530.

22. McCambridge TM: 2001. Pain relief for lateral epicondylitis, *Clinical journal of sport medicine* 11(4): 293–294.

23. Mehta, JA, Bain, GI: 2004. Elbow dislocations in adults and children, *Clinics in sports medicine* 23(4): 609–627.

24. Michlovitz, SL: 2004. Conservative interventions for carpal tunnel syndrome, *Journal of orthopaedic & sports physical therapy* 34(10): 589–600.

25. Peterson L: 2001. Forearm, wrist and hand. In Peterson, L, editor: *Sports injuries: their prevention and treatment*, 3rd ed, Champaign, IL, Human Kinetics, pp. 182–200.

26. Peterson, J, Bancroft, L: 2006. Injuries of the fingers and thumb in the athlete, *Clinics in sports medicine* 25(3):527–542.

27. Plancher KD: 2001. Fracture dislocations of the elbow in athletes, *Clinics in sports medicine* 20(1): 59–76.

28. Rettig, AC: 2003. Athletic injuries of the wrist and hand. Part I. Traumatic injuries of the wrist, *American journal of sports medicine* 31(6):1038–1048.

29. Rettig AC: 2001. Nonoperative treatment of ulnar collateral ligament injuries in throwing athletes, *American journal of sports medicine* 29(1): 15–17.

30. Rettig AC: 2001. Wrist and hand overuse syndromes, *Clinics in sports medicine* 20(3):591–611.

31. Rizzo, M, Shin, A: 2006. Treatment of acute scaphoid fractures in the athlete. *Current sports medicine reports* 5(5):242.

32. Safran M: 2002. Simplified tennis elbow treatment. *Physician and sportsmedicine* 30(12):51.

33. Schneider AM: 2010. Rehabilitation of wrist, hand, and finger injuries. In Prentice WE, editor, *Rehabilitation techniques in sports medicine and athletic training*, ed 5, New York, McGraw-Hill.

34. Schnirring, L: 2003. A rise in kids' distal forearm fractures: what's the cause? *Physician and sportsmedicine* 3(11):11;14–15.

35. Shin, R, Ring, D: 2007. The ulnar nerve in elbow trauma, *Journal of bone & joint surgery, American* 89(5):1108.

36. Stubbs MJ: 2001. Osteochondritis dissecans of the elbow, *Clinics in sports medicine* 20(1):1–9.

37. Uhl TL: 2000. Uncomplicated elbow dislocation rehabilitation, *Athletic therapy today* 5(3):31.

38. Walsh K: 2001. Rehabilitation of postsurgical hand and finger injuries in the athlete, *Athletic therapy today* 6(2):13–18.

39. Westkaemper JG: 2000. Common sports injuries of the hand and wrist, in *Controversies in orthopedic sports medicine*, Champaign, IL, Human Kinetics, pp. 413–424.

40. Whaley, AL, Baker, CL: 2004. Lateral epicondylitis, *Clinics in sports medicine* 23(4): 677–691.

41. Wharam, P: 2003. Boutoniere deformity, *New Zealand journal of sports medicine* 31(1):20–21.

42. Williams MS: 2001. Quick splint for acute boutonniere injuries. *Physician and sportsmedicine* 29(8): 69–70.

43. Youngman, J: 2003. What exactly is wrist tendinitis in athletes, and what are the most effective ways to treat it?, *Sports injury bulletin* (30): 1–4.

44. Zulia P, Prentice W: 2010. Rehabilitation of elbow injuries. In Prentice W, editor: *Rehabilitation techniques in sports medicine and athletic training*, 5th ed., New York, McGraw-Hill.

**ANNOTATED BIBLIOGRAPHY**

Altchek D, Andrews J: 2001. *The Athlete's Elbow,* Baltimore, Lippincott, Williams & Wilkins.

*Text provides information on the biomechanics and anatomy of the elbow, as well as guidelines for the evaluation and treatment of injury to the joint. Based on the work of leading authorities on elbow injuries in athletes.*

Burke, S, Saunders, R, McClinton, M: 2005. *Hand and upper extremity rehabilitation: A practical guide,* Philadelphia, Churchill Livingston.

# The Spine

*When you finish this chapter you will be able to:*

- Describe the anatomy of the cervical, thoracic, and lumbar spine.
- Explain how the nerve roots from the spinal cord combine to form specific peripheral nerves.
- Formulate measures to prevent injury to the spine.
- Describe a process to assess injuries of the cervical and lumbar spine.
- Recognize specific injuries that can occur to the various regions of the spine.

Regions of the spinal column:
- cervical
- thoracic
- lumbar
- sacrum
- coccyx

T he spine is one of the most complex regions of the body. It contains a multitude of bones, joints, ligaments, and muscles, all of which are collectively involved in spinal movement. The relationship of the spinal cord and the peripheral nerves and their proximity to the vertebral column add to the complexity of this region. Injury to the cervical spine has potentially life-threatening implications. Low back pain is one of the most common ailments known to humans. Thus some understanding of the anatomy, assessment techniques, and specific injuries of the spine is essential.

## ANATOMY OF THE SPINE

### Bones

Movements of the vertebral column:
- flexion
- extension
- lateral flexion
- rotation

The spine, or vertebral column, is composed of thirty-three individual bones called *vertebrae* (Figure 20-1). Twenty-four are classified as movable, or true, and nine are classified as immovable, or false. The movable vertebrae are the cervical vertebrae, thoracic vertebrae, and lumbar vertebrae. The false vertebrae, which are fixed by fusion, form the sacrum and the coccyx. The design of the spine allows a high degree of flexibility forward and laterally and limited mobility backward. Rotation around a central axis in the areas of the neck and the lower back is also permitted.

#### The Cervical Spine

Because of the vulnerability of the cervical spine to sports injuries, coaches should have a general knowledge of the cervical spine anatomy and its susceptibility to sports injuries.[1,28] The cervical spine consists of seven vertebrae, with the first two differing from the other true

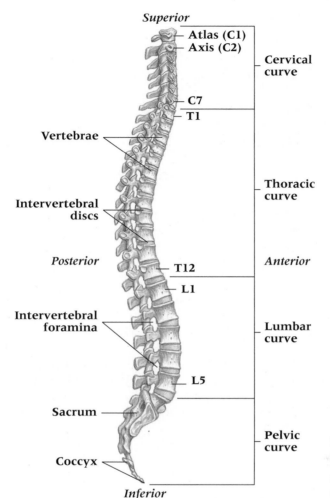

*Superior*

— Atlas (C1)
— Axis (C2)

Cervical
curve

— C7
— T1

Vertebrae

Intervertebral
discs

*Posterior*

— T12

*Anterior*

Thoracic
curve

— L1

Intervertebral
foramina

Lumbar
curve

— L5

Sacrum

Pelvic
curve

Coccyx

*Inferior*

**Figure 20-1**

Vertebrae and curves of the
different regions of the spinal
column

vertebrae (Figure 20-2). These first two are called the *atlas* and the *axis*, respectively, and they function together to support the head on the spinal column and to permit cervical rotation.

### The Thoracic Spine

The thoracic spine consists of twelve vertebrae (Figure 20-3). Thoracic vertebrae have long transverse processes and prominent but thin spinous processes. Thoracic vertebrae 1 through 10 articulate with the ribs. There is very little movement in the thoracic vertebrae.

### The Lumbar Spine

The lumbar spine is composed of five vertebrae (Figure 20-4). They are the major support of the low back and are the largest and thickest of

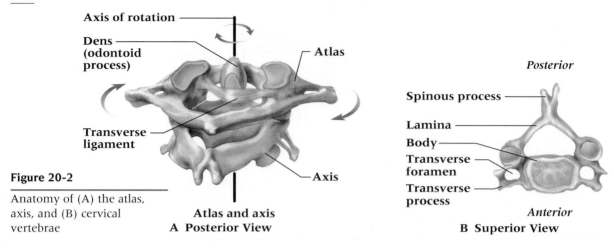

Axis of rotation

Dens
(odontoid
process)

Atlas

Transverse
ligament

Axis

**Figure 20-2**

Anatomy of (A) the atlas,
axis, and (B) cervical
vertebrae

**Atlas and axis
A  Posterior View**

*Posterior*

Spinous process

Lamina

Body

Transverse
foramen

Transverse
process

*Anterior*

**B  Superior View**

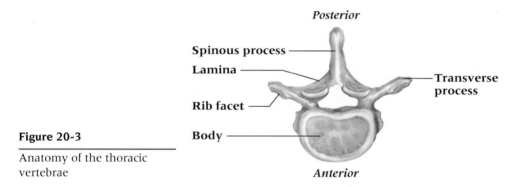

*Posterior*

Spinous process

Lamina

Rib facet

Body

Transverse
process

**Figure 20-3**

Anatomy of the thoracic
vertebrae

*Anterior*

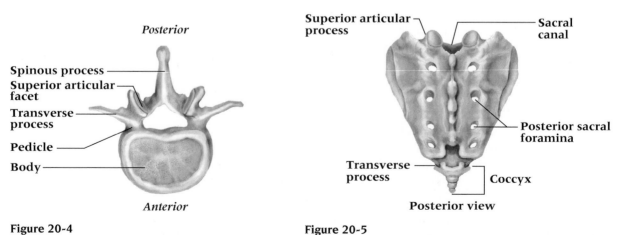

*Posterior*

Spinous process

Superior articular
facet

Transverse
process

Pedicle

Body

*Anterior*

**Figure 20-4**

Anatomy of the lumbar vertebrae

Superior articular
process

Sacral
canal

Posterior sacral
foramina

Transverse
process

Coccyx

**Posterior view**

**Figure 20-5**

Anatomy of the sacrum and coccyx

the vertebrae, with large spinous and transverse processes. Movement occurs in all the lumbar vertebrae; however, there is much less flexion than extension. Rotation is important in the lumbar region.

### The Sacrum

The sacrum is formed by the fusion of five vertebrae and, with the two hip bones, constitutes the pelvis (Figure 20-5). The sacrum articulates with the ilium to form the sacroiliac joints. During both sitting and standing the body's weight is transmitted through these joints. A complex of ligaments serves to make these joints very stable.[6]

### The Coccyx

The coccyx, or tailbone, is the most inferior part of the vertebral column and consists of four or more fused vertebrae (refer to Figure 20-5). The gluteus maximus muscle attaches to the coccyx posteriorly.

## Intervertebral Articulations and Discs

Intervertebral articulations are between vertebral bodies. Between each of the cervical, thoracic, and lumbar vertebrae lie fibrocartilaginous intervertebral discs (Figure 20-6). Each disc is composed of the annulus fibrosus and the nucleus pulposus. The annulus fibrosus forms the periphery of the intervertebral disk and is composed of strong, fibrous tissue. In the center is the semifluid nucleus pulposus, compressed under pressure. The discs act as important shock absorbers for the spine.

## Ligaments

The major ligaments that join the various vertebral parts are the anterior longitudinal ligament, the posterior longitudinal ligament, and the supraspinous ligament (Figure 20-7). The interspinous, supraspinous, and intertransverse ligaments stabilize the transverse and spinous processes, extending between adjacent vertebrae. The sacroiliac joint is maintained by the extremely strong dorsal sacral ligaments. The sacrotuberous and the sacrospinous ligaments maintain the position of the sacrum relative to the ischium.

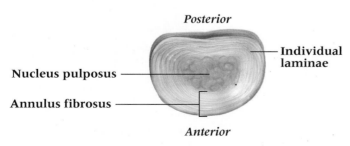

*Posterior*

Individual laminae

Nucleus pulposus

Annulus fibrosus

*Anterior*

**Figure 20-6**

Intervertebral disc

**Figure 20-7**

Ligaments of the vertebral
column (dorsolateral view)

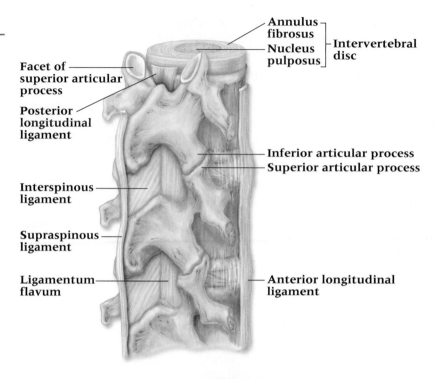

Facet of
superior articular
process

Posterior
longitudinal
ligament

Interspinous
ligament

Supraspinous
ligament

Ligamentum
flavum

Annulus
fibrosus

Nucleus
pulposus

Intervertebral
disc

Inferior articular process

Superior articular process

Anterior longitudinal
ligament

**Figure 20-8**

Muscles of the vertebral
column

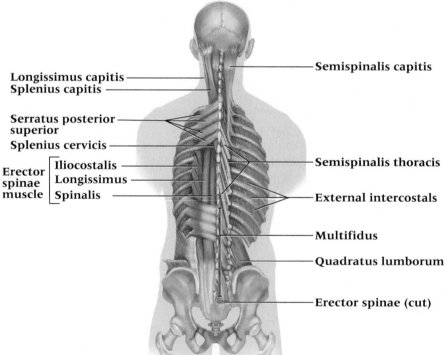

Longissimus capitis

Splenius capitis

Serratus posterior
superior

Splenius cervicis

Erector
spinae
muscle

Iliocostalis

Longissimus

Spinalis

Semispinalis capitis

Semispinalis thoracis

External intercostals

Multifidus

Quadratus lumborum

Erector spinae (cut)

**Posterior view**

## Muscles

The muscles that extend the spine and rotate the vertebral column can be classified as either superficial or deep (Figure 20-8). The superficial muscles, or erector spinae, extend from the vertebrae to ribs. The erector spinae are a group of paired muscles made up of three columns, or bands: the longissimus group, the iliocostalis group, and the spinalis group. Each of these groups is further divided into regions: the cervicis region in the neck, the thoracis region in the middle back, and the lumborum region in the low back. Generally the erector spinae muscles extend the spine.

The deep muscles extend from one vertebra to another. The deep muscles include the interspinals, multifidus, rotatores, thoracis, and the semispinalis cervicis. These muscles extend and rotate the spine (Table 20-1).

## Spinal Cord and Spinal Nerves

The spinal cord is that portion of the central nervous system that is contained within the vertebral canal of the spinal column. It extends from the cranium to the first or second lumbar vertebra. The lumbar roots and the sacral nerves form a horselike tail called the cauda equina.

Thirty-one pairs of spinal nerves extend from the sides of the spinal cord: eight cervical, twelve thoracic, five lumbar, five sacral, and one coccygeal (Figure 20-9).

---

**TABLE 20-1** Muscles of the Spine

| | |
|---|---|
| Extend the spine (Superficial muscles) | Erector spinae |
| |   Longissimus group |
| |     Cervicis |
| |     Thoracis |
| |     Lumborum |
| |   Iliocostalis |
| |     Cervicis |
| |     Thoracis |
| |     Lumborum |
| |   Spinalis |
| |     Cervicis |
| |     Thoracis |
| |     Lumborum |
| Extend and rotate the spine (Deep muscles) | Interspinalis |
| | Multifidus |
| | Rotatores |
| | Thoracis |
| | Semispinalis cervicis |

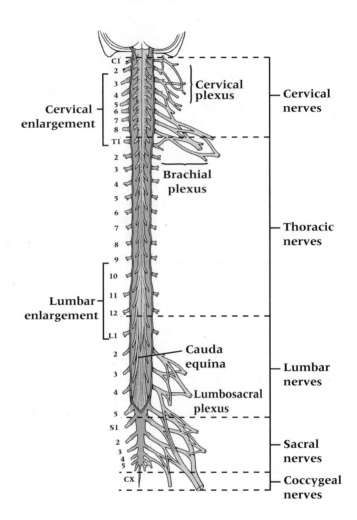

**Figure 20-9**

The regions of the spinal cord
and its nerve roots

## PREVENTING INJURIES TO THE SPINE

### Cervical Spine

#### Strength

**Acute traumatic injuries to the spine can be potentially life threatening,** particularly if the cervical region of the spinal cord is involved.[10] Thus the athlete must do everything possible to minimize the chance of injury. Strengthening the musculature of the neck is critical. The neck muscles can function to protect the cervical spine by resisting excessive hyperflexion, hyperextension, or rotational forces. During participation the athlete should be in a constant state of readiness to "bull" the neck when making contact with an opponent. This protection is accomplished by elevating both shoulders and isometrically contracting the muscles surrounding the neck. Protective cervical collars can also help limit movement of the cervical spine. Athletes with long, weak necks are especially at risk. Tackle football players and wrestlers must have highly stable necks. Specific strengthening exercises are essential for the development of stability. A variety of different exercises that incorporate isotonic, isometric, or isokinetic contractions can be used.

### Flexibility

In addition to strong muscles, the athlete's neck should have a full range of motion. Ideally the athlete should be able to place the chin on the chest and to extend the head back until the face is parallel with the ceiling. There should be at least 40 to 45 degrees of lateral flexion and enough rotation to allow the chin to reach a level even with the tip of the shoulder. Flexibility is increased through stretching exercises and strength exercises that are in full range of motion. When flexibility is restricted, manual static stretching can be beneficial.

### Using Proper Technique

Athletes involved in collision sports—in particular football and rugby, which involve tackling an opponent—must be taught and required to use techniques that reduce the likelihood of cervical injury.[11] The head, especially one in a helmet, should not be used as a weapon. Football helmets do not protect players against neck injury. In the illegal spearing situation, the athlete uses the helmet as a weapon by striking the opponent with its top.[11] Most serious cervical injuries in football result from deliberate axial loading while spearing.[19] **It cannot be stressed enough to the athlete the importance of using appropriate tackling techniques.** In other sports, such as diving, wrestling, and bouncing on a trampoline, the athlete's neck can be flexed at the time of contact. Energy of the forward-moving body mass cannot be fully absorbed, and fracture or dislocation or both can occur. Diving into shallow water causes many catastrophic neck injuries. Many of the same forces are applied in wrestling. In such trauma, paraplegia, quadriplegia, or death can result.

## Lumbar Spine

Low back pain is caused by many factors, many of which can be prevented by using proper body mechanics when sitting, lying, standing, or bending (Focus Box 20-1).[2]

### Strength and Flexibility

It is important to be aware of any postural anomalies that the athletes possess (see Figure 20-9). With this knowledge, individual corrective programs can be established. Basic conditioning should include an emphasis on trunk flexibility. Every effort should be made to produce maximum range of motion in rotation and in both lateral and forward flexion. Both strength and flexibility should be developed in the spinal extensors (erector spinae). Abdominal strength is essential to ensure

20-1  *Focus Box*

**Recommended Postures and Practices for Preventing Low Back Pain**

*Sitting*

1. Do not sit for long periods.
2. Avoid sitting forward on a chair with back arched.
3. Sit on a firm, straight-backed chair.
4. The low back should be slightly rounded or positioned firmly against the back of the chair.
5. The feet should be flat on the floor with knees above the level of the hips (if unable to adequately raise the knees, the feet should be placed on a stool).
6. Avoid sitting with legs straight and raised on a stool.

*Standing*

1. If standing for long periods:
   a. Shift position from one foot to the other.
   b. Place one foot on a stool.
2. Stand tall, flatten low back, and relax knees.
3. Avoid arching back.

*Lifting and carrying*

1. To pick up an object:
   a. Bend at knees and not the waist.
   b. Do not twist to pick up an object—face it squarely.
   c. Tuck in buttocks and tighten abdomen.
2. To carry an object:
   a. Hold object close to body.
   b. Hold object at waist level.
   c. Do not carry object on one side of the body—if it must be carried unbalanced, change from one side to the other.

*Sleeping*

1. Do not stay in one position too long.
2. The bed should be flat and firm yet comfortable.
3. Do not sleep on the abdomen.
4. Do not sleep on the back with legs fully extended.
5. If sleeping on the back, a pillow should be placed under the knees.
6. Ideally, sleep on the side with the knees drawn up.
7. Arms should never be extended overhead.
8. The least strain on the back is in the fully recumbent position with the hips and knees at angles of 90 degrees. In the case of a chronic or a subacute low back condition, a firm mattress affords better rest and relaxation of the lower back. Placing a ¾-inch plywood board underneath the mattress gives a firm, stable surface for the injured back. Sleeping on a water bed often relieves low back pain. The value of a water bed is that it supports the body curves equally, decreasing abnormal pressures to any one body area.

proper postural alignment.[2] Muscle strength imbalances between the abdominals and the erectors can very often be the cause of low back pain. It is also essential to incorporate exercises to improve core stability (see Chapter 4). The core is composed of the muscles of the lumbar, pelvic, and hip regions. It has been clearly demonstrated that strengthening of the core muscles is extremely critical for normal function of the spine.[18]

### Using Proper Technique

In weight lifters, the chance of injury to the lumbar spine can be minimized by using proper lifting techniques. Incorporating appropriate breathing techniques that involve inhaling and exhaling deeply during lifting can help stabilize the spine. Weight belts can also help stabilize the lumbar spine. Spotters can greatly enhance safety by helping lift and lower the weight.

## ASSESSMENT OF THE SPINE

**Generally fitness professionals, coaches, and others working in areas related to exercise and sport science are not adequately trained to evaluate injuries. It is strongly recommended that injured athletes be referred to qualified medical personnel (i.e., physicians, athletic trainers, physical therapists) for injury evaluation.**

Assessment of injuries to the spine is somewhat more complex than assessment of the joints of the extremities because of the number of articulations involved in spinal movement.[15] It is also true that injury to the spine, or in particular the spinal cord, may have life-threatening or life-altering implications. Thus the coach must be able to rule out spinal injury by asking the appropriate questions.[1]

### History

The most critical part of the evaluation is to rule out the possibility of spinal cord injury.[5] Questions that address this possibility should first establish the mechanism of injury:

- What do you think happened?
- Did you hit someone with or land directly on the top of your head?
- Were you knocked out or unconscious? Any time an impact is sufficient to cause unconsciousness, the potential for injury to the spine exists.
- Do you have any pain in your neck?
- Do you have tingling, numbness, or burning in your shoulders, arms, or hands?
- Do you have equal muscle strength in both hands?
- Are you able to move your ankles and toes? Any sensory or motor changes bilaterally may indicate some spinal cord injury.
- Any changes in bowel or bladder routines?

*A yes response to any of these questions necessitates that the athlete not be moved at all until the rescue squad arrives.* Emergency care of the athlete with suspected cervical spine injury was discussed in detail in Chapter 7.

Once cervical spine injury has been ruled out, other general questions may provide some indication as to the nature of the problem:

- Where is the pain located?
- What kind of pain do you have?
- What were you doing when the pain began?
- Were you standing, sitting, bending, or twisting?
- Did the pain begin immediately?
- How long have you had this pain?
- Do certain movements or positions cause more pain?
- Can you assume a position that gets rid of the pain?
- Is there any tingling or numbness in the arms or legs?
- Is there any pain in the buttocks or the back of the legs?
- Have you ever had any back pain before?
- What position do you usually sleep in? How do you prefer to sit?

It is important to remember that pain in the back may be caused by many different conditions. The source may be musculoskeletal or visceral, or it may be referred.

## Observation

Observing the posture and movement capabilities of the athlete during the evaluation can help clarify the nature and extent of the injury. General observations relative to posture include the following:

- Does posture exhibit signs of kyphosis, lordosis, or scoliosis (Figure 20-10)?
- Is the athlete willing to move the head and neck freely?
- Are the shoulders level and symmetrical?
- Is the head tilted to one side?
- Is one scapula lower or more prominent than the other?
- Is the trunk bent or curved to one side?
- Is the space between the body and arm greater on one side?
- Is one hip more prominent than the other?
- Are the hips tilted to one side?
- Are the ribs more pronounced on one side?
- Does one arm hang longer than the other?
- Does one arm hang farther forward than the other?
- Is one patella lower than the other?

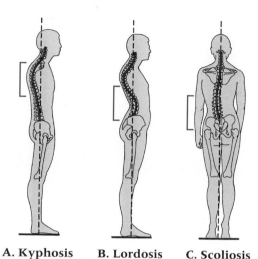

**Figure 20-10**

**Abnormal postures:**
(A) Kyphosis (B) Lordosis
(C) Scoliosis.

**A. Kyphosis    B. Lordosis    C. Scoliosis**

## Palpation

Palpation should be performed with the athlete lying prone and the spine as straight as possible. The head and neck should be slightly flexed. In cases of low back pain, a pillow placed under the hips might make the athlete more comfortable. The spinous processes and transverse process of each vertebra along with the sacrum and coccyx should be palpated for spots of tenderness or increases in pain. The musculature on each side of the spine should also be palpated for tenderness or guarding. Palpation should progress from proximal to distal. It should be remembered that referred pain can produce tender areas away from the site of injury.

## Special Tests

Information on the following special tests has been included simply to give some idea about the different basic tests that nonmedical personnel may do to determine the nature and severity of the athlete's injury. The primary responsibility of those who are not health care personnel is to be able to recognize any potential "red flags" associated with the injury, provide appropriate first aid for the injury, and make correct decisions about how the injury should be managed initially, including immediate return to play or activity decisions (refer to Chapter 7).

Special tests for the lumbar spine should be performed in standing, sitting, supine, side-lying, and prone positions.[13] Special tests include testing both the cervical and lumbar spines in forward bending, backward bending, side bending, and rotation. Any increase in pain or restriction in movement indicates the existence of some condition or injury that should be referred for further evaluation.[13]

**Figure 20-11**

Straight leg raising test: pain in SLR test may indicate a problem in the sciatic nerve, sacroiliac joint, or lumbar spine.

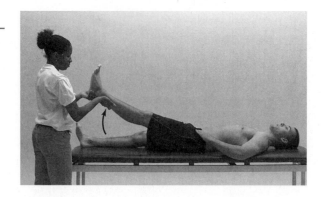

### Straight Leg Raises

Straight leg raising applies pressure to the sacroiliac joint and may indicate a problem either in the sciatic nerve, the sacroiliac joint, or the lumbar spine (Figure 20-11).

### Compression and Distraction Tests

Sacroiliac compression and distraction tests are useful in determining if there is a problem in the sacroiliac joint (Figure 20-12).

## RECOGNITION AND MANAGEMENT OF CERVICAL SPINE INJURIES AND CONDITIONS

Because the neck is so mobile, it is extremely vulnerable to a wide range of sports injuries.[29] Although relatively uncommon, severe sports injury to the neck can produce catastrophic impairment of the spinal cord.[13] The neck is also prone to subtle injuries stemming from stress, tension, and postural malalignments.[3]

### Cervical Fractures

**Cause of injury**  Fortunately, neck fractures are relatively uncommon in athletics. Nevertheless, be prepared to handle such a situation

**Figure 20-12**

(A) Sacral compression; (B) Sacral distraction; both tests can help determine if there is a problem in the sacroiliac joint.

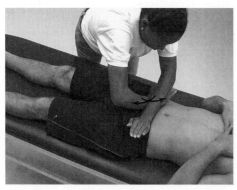

A

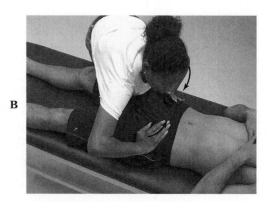

B

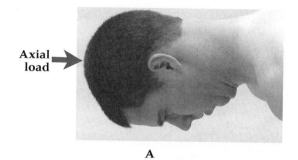

Axial load →

**A**

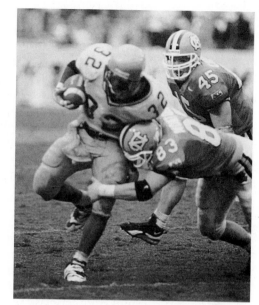

**B**

**Figure 20-13**

In axial loading, contact is made with the top of the head with the neck in a flexed position.

should it arise. **Axial loading** of the cervical vertebrae from a force to the top of the head combined with flexion of the neck can result in an anterior compression[33] (Figure 20-13). In axial loading, the normal anterior curve in the cervical spine flattens out. If the head is also rotated when making contact, a dislocation may occur along with the fracture.[22] Those sports having the highest incidence of neck fractures are gymnastics, ice hockey, diving, football, and rugby.[33]

**Signs of injury**   The athlete may have one or more of the following signs of cervical fracture: neck point tenderness and restricted movement, cervical muscle spasm, cervical pain and pain in the chest and extremities, numbness in trunk and/or limbs, weakness or paralysis in limbs and/or trunk, a loss of bladder and/or bowel control.

**Care**   An unconscious athlete should be treated as if a serious neck injury is present until a physician rules out this possibility.[14] In cases of suspected cervical fracture, the athlete should not be moved except by the rescue squad.[7] Always be aware that an athlete can sustain a catastrophic spinal injury from improper handling and transportation[3] (see Chapter 7 for a detailed description of the emergency care of spinal injuries).

> **axial loading**
> A blow to the top of the athlete's head while in flexion.

## Cervical Dislocations

**Cause of injury**   Cervical dislocations are not common, but they do occur much more frequently in sports than do fractures. Dislocations usually result from violent flexion and rotation of the head, as occurs in pool diving accidents.[33]

A unilateral cervical dislocation can cause the neck to tilt toward the dislocated side, with tight muscles on the elongated side and relaxed muscles on the tilted side.

**Signs of injury**   For the most part, a cervical dislocation produces many of the same signs as a fracture. Both can result in considerable pain, numbness, and muscle weakness or paralysis. The most easily discernible difference is the position of the neck in a dislocation: a unilateral dislocation causes the neck to be tilted toward the dislocated side with extreme muscle tightness on the elongated side and a relaxed muscle state on the tilted side.

**Care**   Because a dislocation of a cervical vertebra has a greater likelihood of causing injury to the spinal cord, even greater care must be exercised when moving the patient. The procedures described in Chapter 7 should be applied to cervical dislocations.

### Acute Muscle Strains of the Neck and Upper Back

**Cause of injury**   In a strain of the neck or upper back, the athlete has usually turned the head suddenly or has forced flexion, extension, or rotation. Muscles involved are typically the upper trapezius, sternocleidomastoid, the scalenes on the front of the neck, and the splenius capitis and cervicis.

**Signs of injury**   Localized pain, point tenderness, and restricted motion are present. Muscle guarding resulting from pain is common, and there is a reluctance to move the neck in any direction.

**Care**   Care usually includes use of PRICE immediately after the strain occurs and use of a cervical collar for protection (Figure 20-14). Follow-up management may include range-of-motion exercises followed by isometric exercises progressing to full-range isotonic strengthening exercises. In addition, cold or superficial heat and analgesic medications are used as prescribed by the physician.

### Cervical Sprain (Whiplash)

**Cause of injury**   A cervical sprain can occur from the same mechanism as the strain but usually results from a more violent motion. More

**Figure 20-14**

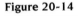

Wearing a soft cervical collar helps reduce pain and spasm in an athlete with an injured neck.

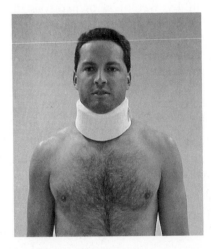

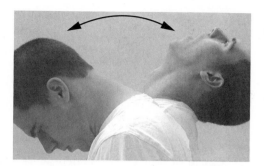

**Figure 20-15**

Whiplash injury involves a sudden forward or backward acceleration of the head relating to the vertebral column.

commonly, a cervical sprain occurs when the head snaps suddenly, such as when the athlete is tackled or blocked while unprepared (Figure 20-15). Frequently muscle strains occur with ligament sprains. A sprain of the neck produces tears in the supporting tissue of the anterior or posterior longitudinal ligaments, the interspinous ligament, or the supraspinous ligament.[9]

**Signs of injury**  The sprain displays all the signs of the strained neck but the symptoms persist longer. There may also be tenderness over the transverse and spinous processes that serve as sites of attachment for the ligaments. Pain may not be experienced initially but always appears the day after the trauma.

**Care**  As soon as possible, the athlete should have a physician evaluation to rule out the possibility of fracture, dislocation, or disk injury. A soft cervical collar may be applied to reduce muscle spasm. PRICE is used for 48 to 72 hours while the injury is in the acute stage of healing. In an athlete with a severe injury, the physician may prescribe 2 to 3 days of bed rest along with analgesics and anti-inflammation agents. Therapy might include cold or heat and massage. Mechanical traction may also be prescribed to relieve pain and muscle spasm.

## Acute Torticollis

**Cause of injury**  Acute torticollis is a very common condition in which the athlete usually complains of pain on one side of the neck when awakening. This stiff neck happens when a small piece of synovial membrane lining the joint capsule is impinged or trapped between the cervical vertebrae. This problem can also occasionally follow exposure to a cold draft of air or holding the head in an unusual position over time.

**Signs of injury**  During inspection, there is palpable point tenderness and muscle spasm. Head movement is restricted to the side opposite the irritation with marked muscle guarding. X-ray examination rules out a more serious injury.

**Care**  Cold or heat and massage may be used to modulate pain in an attempt to break a pain-spasm-pain cycle. Gentle traction, rotation, and lateral bending, first in the pain-free direction then in the direction of pain, can help reduce the guarding. The athlete should gradually engage in strengthening and stretching exercises, not only for the neck but also for the shoulder complex to help prevent recurrence. The athlete may find it helpful to wear a soft cervical collar for comfort (refer to Figure 20-14). This muscle guarding generally lasts for 2 to 3 days, during which the athlete progressively regains motion. The athlete should not return to activity until full range of motion has been regained.

### Pinched Nerve (Brachial Plexus Injury)

**20-1 Critical Thinking**
Exercise

When making a tackle a football player experiences burning and tingling with a loss of strength in his left arm.

**?** What condition has most likely occurred and how should the coach manage this problem?

**Cause of injury**   A pinched nerve resulting from stretching or compression of the brachial plexus is the most common of all cervical neurological injuries in the athlete.[21] Other terms commonly used to indicate this condition are *stinger* or *burner*.[30] The primary mechanism of injury is the stretching of the brachial plexus of nerves when the neck is forced laterally to the opposite side while the shoulder is depressed, as occurs with a shoulder block in football.[23]

**Signs of injury**   The athlete complains of a burning sensation, numbness and tingling, and pain extending from the shoulder down to the hand, with some loss of function of the arm and hand that lasts for several minutes. Rarely, symptoms may persist for several days. Neck range of motion is usually normal. Repeated brachial plexus nerve stretch injuries may result in permanent damage.[23]

**Care**   Once the symptoms have completely resolved and there are no associated neurological symptoms, the athlete may return to full activity.[26] Thereafter the athlete should begin strengthening and stretching exercises for the neck musculature. A football player should be fitted with shoulder pads and a cervical neck roll to limit neck range of motion during impact.

## RECOGNITION AND MANAGEMENT OF LUMBAR SPINE INJURIES AND CONDITIONS

### Low Back Pain

**Cause of injury**   Low back pain is one of the most common and disabling ailments known to humans. In sports, back problems are common and are most often the result of either congenital anomalies, mechanical back defects caused mainly by faulty posture, or trauma to the back including sprains, strains, or contusions.

**Signs of injury**   With repeated episodes of injury, the athlete may develop recurrent or chronic low back pain. Gradually this problem can lead to muscular weakness and impairment of sensation and reflex responses. The older the athlete, the more prone he or she is to developing chronic low back pain. The incidence of this condition at the high school level is low, but it becomes progressively greater with increasing age.

**Care**   The athlete, like everyone else in the population, can prevent low back pain by avoiding unnecessary stresses and strains associated with standing, sitting, lying, working, or exercising.[4] Care should be taken to avoid postures and positions that can cause injuries (refer to Focus Box 20-1).

## Lumbar Vertebrae Fracture and Dislocation

**Cause of injury** Fractures in the lumbar region of the vertebral column are not serious in terms of bone injury, but they pose dangers when related to spinal cord damage. Lumbar vertebrae fractures of the greatest concern in sports are compression fractures and fractures of the transverse and spinous processes.

The compression fracture may occur as a result of hyperflexion of the trunk. Falling from a height and landing on the feet or buttocks may also produce a compression fracture. Fractures of the transverse and spinous processes result most often from a kick or other direct impact to the back. Dislocations of the lumbar vertebrae in sports are rare, occurring only when there is an associated fracture.

**Signs of injury** Recognition of the compression fracture is difficult without an x-ray examination. A basic evaluation may be made with a knowledge of the history and point tenderness over the affected vertebrae. Fractures of the transverse and spinous processes may be directly palpable. There will be point tenderness and some localized swelling along with muscle guarding to protect the area.

**Care** If the symptoms and signs associated with a fracture are present, the injured athlete should be x-rayed. Transporting and moving the athlete should be done on a spine board as described in Chapter 7 to minimize movement of the fractured segment.

## Low Back Muscle Strains

**Cause of injury** There are two mechanisms of the typical low back strain in sports activities.[29] The first happens from a sudden extension, usually in combination with trunk rotation. The second is the chronic strain commonly associated with faulty posture.

**Signs of injury** Evaluation should be performed immediately after injury to rule out the possibility of fracture. Discomfort in the low back may be diffused or localized in one area. Pain is present on active extension and with passive flexion.

**Care** Initially, cold packs and/or ice massage should be used to decrease muscle guarding. An elastic wrap or an abdominal support corset-type brace helps compress the area (Figure 20-16). A graduated program of stretching and strengthening begins slowly during the acute stage. Injuries of moderate-to-severe intensity may require complete bed rest to help break the pain–muscle spasm cycle.

## Lumbar Sprains

**Cause of injury** Sprains may occur in any of the ligaments in the lumbar spine. The most common sprain occurs when the athlete is bending forward and twisting while lifting or moving some object. Lumbar

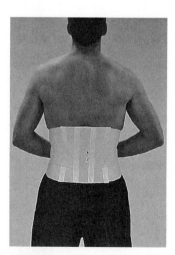

**Figure 20-16**

An abdominal brace helps support the lumbar area.

sprain can occur with a single episode or with chronic repetitive stress that becomes progressively worse with activity.

**Signs of injury**   The pain is localized and located just lateral to the spinous process. Pain becomes sharper with certain movements or postures, and the athlete limits movement in painful ranges. Flexion, extension, and rotational movements of the vertebrae can increase pain.

**Care**   Initial treatment should include PRICE to reduce pain. Strengthening exercises for abdominals and back extensors and stretching in all directions should be limited to a pain-free range. An abdominal brace or support should be worn to limit movement during early return to activity. As with sprains to other joints in the body, some time is required for healing.

### Back Contusions

**Cause of injury**   Back contusions rank third to strains and sprains in incidence. Because of its surface area, the back is quite vulnerable to bruises in sports. Football produces the greatest number of these injuries. A significant impact to the back can cause serious injury to the kidneys leading to the presence of some blood in the urine (see Chapter 21). Contusion of the back must be distinguished from a vertebral fracture. In some instances this distinction is possible only through an x-ray examination.

**Signs of injury**   The bruise causes local pain, muscle spasm, and point tenderness. A swollen, discolored area may be visible also.

**Care**   Cold and pressure should be applied intermittently for approximately the first 72 hours or longer with rest. Ice massage combined with gradual stretching benefits soft-tissue contusion in the region of the low back. Recovery usually ranges from 2 days to 2 weeks.

### Sciatica

**Cause of injury**   The term *sciatica* has been incorrectly used as a general term to describe all low back pain without reference to exact causes. **Sciatica** is an inflammatory condition of the sciatic nerve that can accompany recurrent or chronic low back pain.[26] This nerve is particularly vulnerable to torsion or direct blows that tend to impose abnormal stretching and pressure on it as it emerges from the spine[12] (Figure 20-17).

**Signs of injury**   Sciatica may begin either abruptly or gradually. It produces a sharp shooting pain that follows the nerve pathway along the posterior and medial thigh. There may also be some tingling and numbness along its path. The nerve may be extremely sensitive to palpation. Straight leg raising usually intensifies the pain.

**Care**   In the acute stage, rest is essential. The cause of the inflammation must be identified and treated. If there is a disk protrusion, lumbar traction may be appropriate. Because recovery from sciatia usually occurs within 2 to 3 weeks, surgery should be delayed to see if symptoms resolve. Oral anti-inflammatory medication may help reduce inflammation.

> **sciatica** (sigh **at** tika)
> Inflammatory condition of the sciatic nerve; commonly associated with peripheral nerve root compression.

*Medial*          *Lateral*

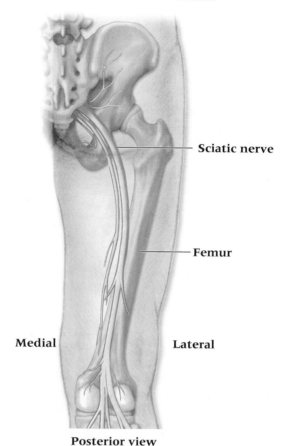

Sciatic nerve

Femur

**Medial**          **Lateral**

**Posterior view**

**Figure 20-17**

Sciatic nerve (posterior view) in the posterior hip and thigh

## Herniated Lumbar Disk

**Cause of injury**   The mechanism of a disk injury is the same as that of the lumbar sprain—forward bending and twisting that places abnormal strain on the lumbar region. This movement produces herniation of the nucleus pulposus of a disk, which can impinge on a nerve root (Figure 20-18).[13] The pain associated with disk herniation is substantial. The disk most often injured lies between the L4 and the L5 vertebrae.[29]

**Signs of injury**   A herniated lumbar disk usually creates centrally located pain that radiates on one side to the buttocks and down the back of the leg or pain that spreads across the back.[13] Symptoms are worse on rising in the morning. Onset may be sudden or gradual, with pain increasing after the athlete sits and then tries to resume activity. Posture exhibits a slight forward bend with side bending away from the side of pain. Straight leg raising increases pain.[29]

**Care**   Initially, rest and ice should be used to help modulate pain. In many cases but certainly not all, backward bending or extension

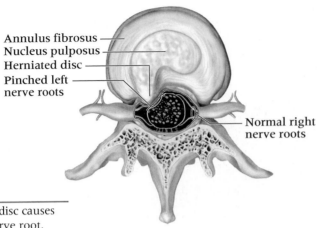

Annulus fibrosus
Nucleus pulposus
Herniated disc
Pinched left nerve roots

Normal right nerve roots

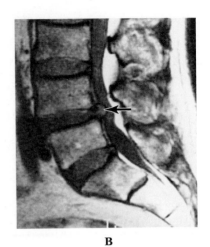

**Figure 20-18**

(A) A herniated disc causes pressure on a nerve root.
(B) MRI of herniated disc.

A                                                    B

makes the athlete more comfortable. As pain and posture return to normal, back extensor and abdominal stabilization exercises should be used.[25] Sometimes the symptoms resolve with time. But signs of nerve damage may necessitate surgery.

## Spondylolysis and Spondylolisthesis

Spondylolisthesis is considered to be a complication of a spondylolysis.

**Cause of condition** Spondylolysis refers to a degeneration of the vertebrae and, more commonly, a defect in the articular processes of the vertebrae (Figure 20-19A).[24] It is often attributed to a congenital weakness with the defect occurring as a stress fracture. It is more common among boys.[27] Sports movements that characteristically hyperextend the spine, such as arching the back in gymnastics, lifting weights, blocking in football, kicking in football, serving in tennis, spiking in volleyball, and using the butterfly stroke in swimming, are most likely to cause this condition.[24]

Spondylolisthesis is a complication of spondylolysis often resulting in hypermobility of a vertebral segment.[12] Spondylolisthesis has the highest incidence with L5 slipping on S1 (Figure 20-19B).[31] A direct blow or sudden twist or chronic low back strain may cause the defective vertebra to displace itself forward on the sacrum[32] (Figure 20-20).

**Signs of condition** The athlete complains of persistent aching pain or stiffness across the low back, with increased pain after, not usually during, physical activity. The athlete feels the need to change positions frequently or "pop" the low back to reduce the pain. There may be tenderness localized to one segment.[19]

**Care** Initially, bracing and occasionally bed rest for 1 to 3 days helps to reduce pain. The major focus in rehabilitation should be directed toward exercises that control or stabilize the hypermobile lumbar segment.[25] Progressive trunk-stabilization strengthening exercises,

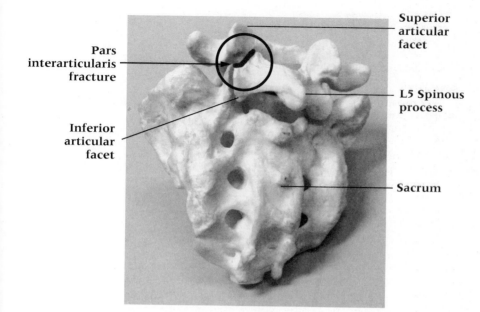

Pars interarticularis fracture

Superior articular facet

Inferior articular facet

L5 Spinous process

Sacrum

**A Posterior Oblique View**

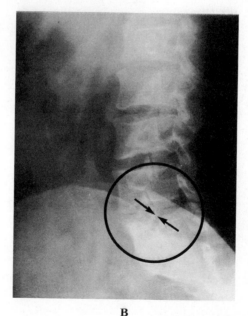

B

**Figure 20-19**

**Spondylolysis:**

(A) Fracture of the pars interarticularis between superior and inferior articular facets.
(B) X-ray view of fracture.

especially through the midrange, should be incorporated. Braces are most helpful during high-level activities. It may be necessary for the athlete to avoid vigorous activity.[31]

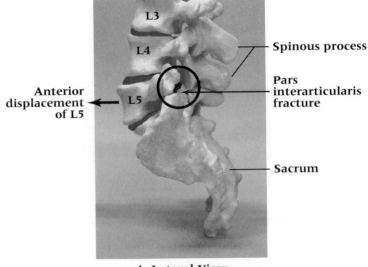

**A  Lateral View**

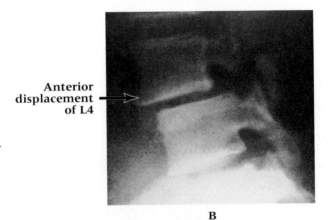

**B**

**Figure 20-20**

**Spondylolisthesis:**

(A) Anterior displacement of
L5 with pars articularis
fracture

(B) X-ray view.

## RECOGNITION AND MANAGEMENT OF SACROILIAC JOINT AND COCCYX INJURIES

The sacroiliac is the junction formed by the ilium and the sacrum, and it is fortified by strong ligaments that allow little motion to take place. Because the sacroiliac joint is a synovial joint, disorders can include sprain, inflammation, hypermobility, and hypomobility.[20]

### Sacroiliac Sprain

**Cause of injury**   A sprain of the sacroiliac joint may result from twisting with both feet on the ground, stumbling forward, falling backward, stepping too far down and landing heavily on one leg, or forward bending with the knees locked during lifting.[20]

**⪦ 20-3 Critical Thinking**
Exercise

During a takedown move a wrestler falls down hard on his buttocks in a sitting position. He complains of intense localized pain at the tip of his spine.

**?** What has most likely been injured?

**Signs of injury**   A sprain of the sacroiliac joint may have palpable pain and tenderness directly over the joint with some associated muscle guarding. Hip levels may appear to be asymmetrical.[5,8]

**Care**   Ice can be used to reduce pain. A supportive brace is also helpful in an acute sprain. Core strengthening exercises for the lumbo-pelvic-hip complex should be incorporated to improve stability to a hypermobile joint.[8]

### Coccyx Injuries

**Cause of injury**   Coccygeal injuries in sports are prevalent and occur primarily from direct impact, which may result from forcibly sitting down, falling, or being kicked by an opponent. Injuries to the coccyx may include sprains, contusions, or fractures.

**Signs of injury**   Pain in the coccygeal region is often prolonged and at times chronic. There is tenderness over the bone, and the athlete has difficulty sitting.

**Care**   Treatment consists of analgesics and a ring seat to relieve the pressure on the coccyx while sitting. It should be noted that pain from a fractured coccyx may last for many months. Once a coccygeal injury has healed, the athlete should be protected against reinjury by appropriately applied padding.

## SUMMARY

- The spine, or vertebral column, is composed of thirty-three individual vertebrae. The design of the spine allows for flexion, extension, lateral flexion, and rotation. The movable vertebrae are separated by intervertebral disks, and position is maintained by a series of muscular and ligamentous supports. The spine can be divided into three different regions: the cervical, thoracic, and lumbar regions. The sacrum and coccyx are fused vertebrae within the vertebral column.

- The spinal cord is that portion of the central nervous system that is contained within the vertebral canal of the spinal column. Thirty-one pairs of spinal nerves extend from the sides of the spinal cord.

- Acute traumatic injuries to the spine can be potentially life threatening, particularly if the cervical region of the spinal cord is involved. Thus the athlete must do everything possible to minimize injury. Strengthening of the musculature of the neck is critical. In addition to strong muscles, the athlete's neck should have a full range of motion. Athletes involved in collision sports must be taught and required to use techniques that reduce the likelihood of cervical injury.

- Low back pain is one of the most common and disabling ailments known to humans. The athlete, like everyone else in the population, can prevent low back pain by avoiding unnecessary stresses and strains associated with standing, sitting, lying, working, or exercising. Care should be taken to avoid postures and positions that can cause injuries.

- The most critical part of assessment of the spine is to rule out the possibility of spinal cord injury. Observing the posture and movement capabilities of the athlete during the evaluation can help clarify the nature and extent of the injury.

- Because the cervical and lumbar regions of the spine are so mobile, they are extremely vulnerable to a wide range of sports injuries, including fractures, dislocations, strains, sprains, contusions, lesions of the intervertebral disks, herniations, injuries to spinal nerves, and degenerative conditions.

---

## *Solutions to Critical Thinking* Exercises

---

**20-1** It is most likely that the athlete has a brachial plexus injury that is sometimes called a stinger or burner. Normally the symptoms resolve on their own over several minutes. Consider having the athlete wear a cervical collar.

**20-2** The gymnast likely has a spondylolisthesis that has resulted in hypermobility of a vertebral segment. Initially, rest will help to reduce pain. The major focus in rehabilitation should be directed toward exercises that control or stabilize the hypermobile segment. Progressive trunk-strengthening exercises, especially to the abdominal muscles through the midrange, should be incorporated. A brace can be helpful during practice.

**20-3** The wrestler has most likely contused his coccyx. Fractures of this bone are relatively uncommon. It may be necessary to apply a protective pad over the injured area.

## REVIEW QUESTIONS

1. Identify the various regions of the spine.
2. What is the relationship between the spinal cord and the nerve roots?
3. Discuss the various considerations in prevention of cervical injuries.
4. Describe the special tests used in evaluating the lumbar and sacroiliac portions of the spine.
5. What can be done to minimize the incidence of low back pain?
6. Describe the mechanism of injury for a herniated disk.
7. How does a spondylolysis become a spondylolisthesis?
8. What is the usual mechanism for injury to the sacroiliac joint?

## REFERENCES

1. Anderson C: 1993. Neck injuries, backboard, bench, or return to play, *Physician and sportsmedicine* 21(8):23.
2. Brukner, P: 2002. Low back pain. In Brukner, P, editor: *Clinical sports medicine*, 2nd rev. ed, Sydney, McGraw-Hill, pp. 330–361.
3. Brukner, P: 2002. Neck pain. In Brukner, P, editor: *Clinical sports medicine*, 2nd rev. ed, Sydney, McGraw-Hill, pp. 215–228.
4. Carpenter DM, Nelson BW: 1999. Low back strengthening for the prevention and treatment of low back pain, *Medicine and science in sports & exercise* 31(1):18.
5. Chen, YC: 2002. Sacroiliac joint pain syndrome in active patients: a look behind the pain, *Physician and sportsmedicine* 30(11):30–37.
6. Cuppett, M: 2001. The anatomy and pathomechanics of the sacroiliac

joint, *Athletic therapy today* 6(4): 6–14.

7. Del Rossi, G: 2002. Management of cervical-spine injuries, *Athletic therapy today* 7(2):46–51.

8. Foley, B, Buschbacher, R: 2006. Sacroiliac joint pain anatomy, biomechanics, diagnosis, and treatment. *American journal of physical medicine & rehabilitation* 85(12): 997–1006.

9. Halperin, JS: 2002. Whiplash, *American journal of physical medicine & rehabilitation* 81(11):856.

10. Hammann L: 2000. Functional back rehabilitation, *Athletic therapy today* 5(2): 22.

11. Heck, JF, Clarke, KS, Peterson, TR: 2004. National Athletic Trainers' Association position statement: head-down contact and spearing in tackle football, *Journal of athletic training* 39(1):101–111.

12. Herring S, Weinstein S: 1995. Assessment and neurological management of athletic low back injury. In Nicholas J, Herschman E, editors: *The lower extremity and spine in sports medicine*, St Louis, Mosby.

13. Hooker D: 2010. Back rehabilitation. In Prentice W, editor: *Rehabilitation techniques in sports medicine and athletic training*, New York, McGraw-Hill.

14. Kim, DH,Vaccaro, AR, Berta, SC: 2003. Acute sports-related spinal cord injury: contemporary management principles, *Clinics in sports medicine* 22(3):501–512.

15. King, MA: 2000. Core stability: creating a foundation for functional rehabilitation, *Athletic therapy today* 5(2):6–13.

16. Langer, P, Fadale, P: 2008. Catastrophic neck injuries in the collision sport athlete. *Sports medicine & arthroscopy review* 16(1):7.

17. Magee, DJ: 2003. Evaluating tests for SIJ dysfunction, *Physician and sportsmedicine* 31(12):9; 12.

18. May, S, Johnson, R: 2008. Stabilisation exercises for low back pain: a systematic review. *Physiotherapy* 94(3):179.

19. Nyska, M: 2000. Spondylolysis as a cause of low back pain in swimmers, *International journal of sports medicine* 21(5):375–379.

20. Prather, H: 2003. Sacroiliac joint pain: practical management, *Clinical journal of sport medicine* 13(4): 252–255.

21. Rapport L, O'Leary P, Cammisa F: 1995. Diagnosis and treatment of cervical spine injuries. In Nicholas J, Herschman, E, editors: *The lower extremity and spine in sports medicine*, St Louis, Mosby.

22. Schimelpfenig, S: 2008. Acute neck injury. *Clinical journal of sport medicine* 18(2):218.

23. Shannon, B: 2002. Cervical burners in the athlete, *Clinics in sports medicine*, 21(1):29–35.

24. Standaert, CJ: 2002. Spondylosysis in the adolescent athlete, *Clinical journal of sport medicine* 12(2): 119–122.

25. Stone JA: 1999. Back stabilization exercises, *Athletic therapy today* 4(3):23.

26. Sustained pain relief for experimental sciatica treatment, 2003. *Sports medicine digest* 25(11):125.

27. Thein-Nissenbaum, J, Boissonnault, W: 2005. Differential diagnosis of spondylolysis in a patient with chronic low back pain, *Journal of orthopaedic & sports physical therapy* 35(5):319.

28. Vaccaro, AR, Harrop, JS, Daffiner, SD: 2003. Acute cervical spine injuries in the athlete, *International sportmed journal* 4(1):34–40.

29. Watkins, RG: 2002. Lumbar disc injury in the athlete, *Clinics in sports medicine* 21(1):147–165.

30. Weinberg, J, Rokito, S, Silber, JS: 2003. Etiology, treatment, and prevention of athletic "stingers," *Clinics in sports medicine* 22(3): 493–500.

31. Wicker, A: 2008. Spondylolysis and spondylolisthesis in sports. *International sportmed journal* 9(2):74.

32. Wimberly, RL: 2002. Spondylolis-thesis in the athlete, *Clinics in sports medicine* 21(1):133–145.
33. Zmurko, MG; Tannoury, TY, Tan-noury, CA: 2003. Cervical sprains, disc herniations, minor fractures, and other cervical injuries in the athlete, *Clinics in sports medicine* 22(3): 513–521.

### ANNOTATED BIBLIOGRAPHY

Braggins S: 2000. *Back care: a clinical approach,* Philadelphia, Churchill Livingstone.
 *A comprehensive text that focuses on all aspects of treatment and rehabilita-tion of the spine.*
Malanga, GA: 2002. *Whiplash,* Philadel-phia, Hanley & Belfus.
 *Offers current scientific information on the repercussions of, and treatment for, whiplash.*
McKenzie, R: 2003. *The lumbar spine: mechanical diagnosis & therapy.* 2nd ed, Wellington, NZ, Spinal Publications New Zealand.
 *Written by a world authority on back pain, the text explains how back pain occurs and how it is best treated.*

McGill, S, editor: 2002. Low back disor-ders: evidence-based prevention and rehabilitation, Champaign, IL, Human Kinetics.
 *Prevention and rehabilitation ap-proaches are presented to help profes-sionals make clinical decisions for building prevention and rehabilitation programs.*
White A, Schofferman J: 1995. *Spine care: diagnosis and conservative treat-ment,* vol. 1, St Louis, Mosby.
 *A two-volume set that looks at both conservative and surgical management of back injuries.*

### WEB SITES

MEDLINEplus: Back Pain
 www.nlm.nih.gov/medlineplus/
 backpain.html
 *Information on back pain from the Mayo Foundation for Medical Education and Research.*
*Physician and Sportsmedicine*:
 Low-Back Pain Relief
 www.physsportsmed.com/
 index.php?art=psm_01_1997?article
 =1100
 *Discusses causes and relief for low back pain.*
Back Pain
 http://orthopedics.about.com/od/
 backneck/Back_Spine_Neck_
 Information.htm
 *Discusses the many causes of low back pain.*

AAFP-Diagnosis and Management
 of Acute Low Back Pain
 www.aafp.org/afp/20000315/
 1779.html
 *Information on managing low back pain from the American Academy of Family Practice.*
The Cleveland Clinic Foundation:
 Spinal Cord Trauma:
 http://my.clevelandclinic.org/
 disorders/spinal_cord_injury/hic_the
 _spinal_cord_and_injury.aspx
Spine-Health:
www.spine-health.com
 *Written and updated by a multispecialty team of medical professionals. It provides a comprehensive overview of causes and treatments for low back pain, and a variety of services and in-depth features.*

# The Thorax and Abdomen

*When you finish this chapter you will be able to:*

- Describe the anatomy of the thorax and abdomen.
- Identify the location and function of the heart and lungs.
- Indicate the location and function of the abdominal viscera.
- Explain the techniques for assessing thoracic and abdominal injuries.
- Differentiate between various injuries to the structures of the thorax.
- Recognize various injuries and conditions in structures of the abdomen.

This chapter covers injuries to the thorax and abdomen. In an athletic environment, injuries to the thorax and abdomen have a lower incidence than injuries to the extremities and the spine. However, unlike the musculoskeletal injuries to the extremities discussed to this point, injuries to the heart, lungs, and abdominal viscera can be potentially serious and even life threatening if not recognized and managed appropriately. It is essential to be familiar with anatomy and the more common injuries seen in the abdomen and thorax (Figure 21-1).

## ANATOMY OF THE THORAX

The thorax is that portion of the body commonly known as the chest, which lies between the base of the neck and the diaphragm. It is contained within the thoracic vertebrae and the twelve pairs of ribs that give it its shape (Figure 21-2). Its main function is to protect the vital respiratory and circulatory organs and to assist the lungs in inspiration and expiration during the breathing process.[21]

The ribs are flat bones that are attached to the thoracic vertebrae in the back and to the sternum in the front. The upper seven ribs are called sternal or true ribs, and each rib is joined to the sternum by a separate costal cartilage. The eighth, ninth, and tenth ribs (false ribs) have cartilages that join each other and the seventh rib before uniting with the sternum. The eleventh and twelfth ribs (floating ribs) remain unattached to the sternum but do have muscle attachments. The intercostal muscles, which lie between the ribs, and the diaphragm muscle, which separates the thoracic cavity from the abdominal cavity, function in inspiration and expiration (Figure 21-3) (Table 21-1).

The thoracic cage protects the heart and lungs.

**Figure 21-1**

Collision sports can produce serious trunk injuries.

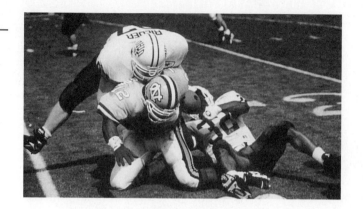

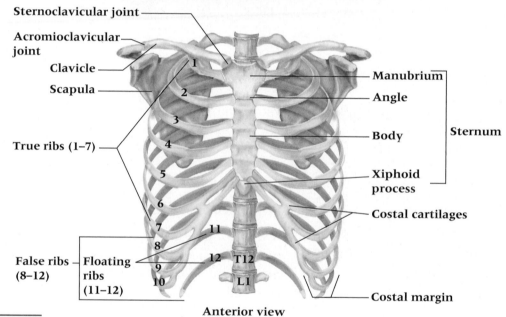

Sternoclavicular joint

Acromioclavicular joint

Clavicle

Scapula

True ribs (1–7)

1

2

3

4

5

6

7

8

9

10

11

12

T12

L1

Manubrium

Angle

Body

Xiphoid process

Costal cartilages

Costal margin

Sternum

False ribs (8–12)

Floating ribs (11–12)

Anterior view

**Figure 21-2**

Bony anatomy of the thoracic cage

## ANATOMY OF THE ABDOMEN

The abdominal cavity lies between the diaphragm and the pelvis and is bounded by the margin of the lower ribs, the abdominal muscles, and the vertebral column. The abdominal muscles—the rectus abdominis, the external and internal obliques, and the transverse abdominis—collectively produce trunk flexion and rotation, but more importantly, they function to protect the underlying abdominal viscera (Figure 21-4) (Table 21-1).[21]

Solid internal organs are more at risk for injury than are hollow organs.

The abdominal viscera are composed of both hollow and solid organs. The solid organs are the kidneys, spleen, liver, pancreas, and adrenal glands. The hollow organs include the stomach, intestines,

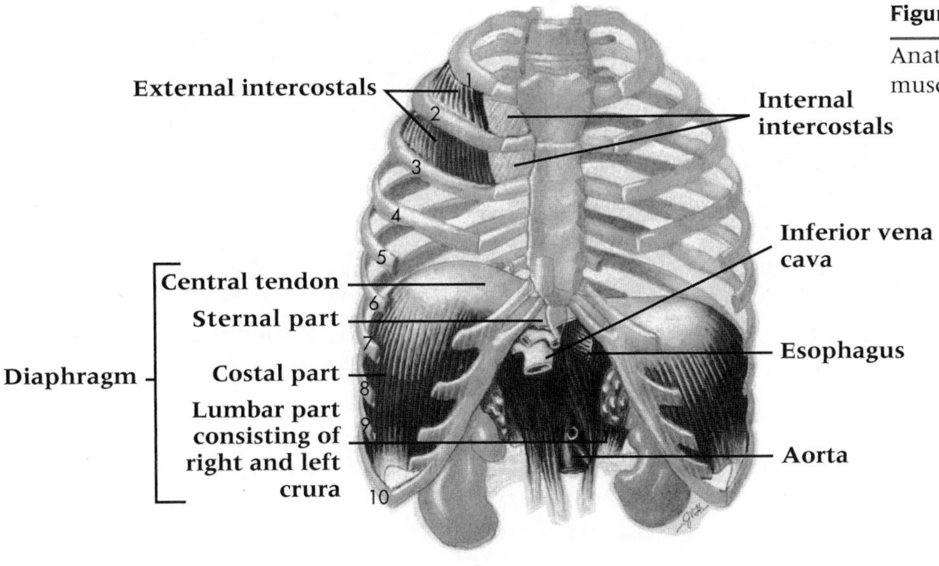

Figure 21-3

Anatomy of the thoracic muscles

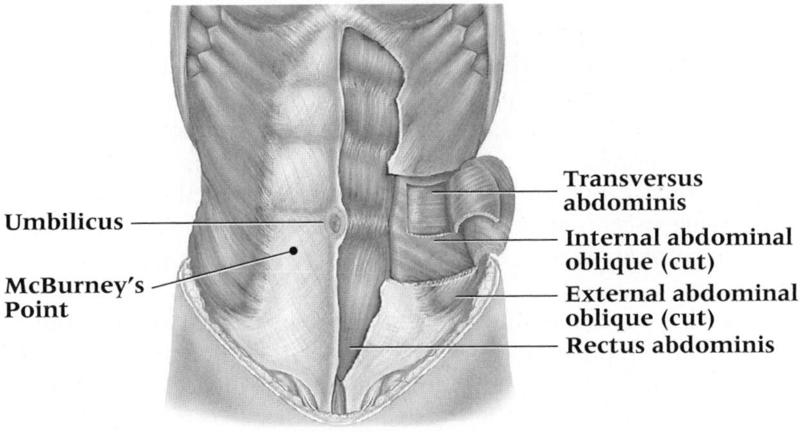

Anterior view

Figure 21-4

Muscles of the abdominal wall (anterior view)

Anterior view

**TABLE 21-1** Muscles of the Abdomen and Thorax

| | |
|---|---|
| Trunk rotation | Rectus abdominis |
| | External oblique |
| | Internal oblique |
| Trunk flexion | Internal oblique |
| | External oblique |
| | Transverse abdominis |
| | Rectus abdominis |
| Muscles of respiration | Intercostals |
| | Diaphragm |

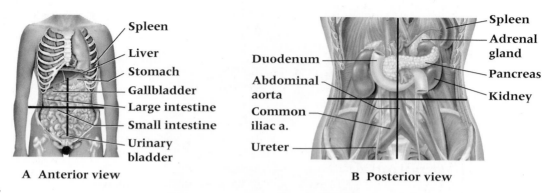

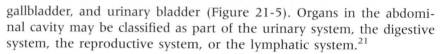

**A  Anterior view**

**B  Posterior view**

**Figure 21-5**

**Abdominal viscera:**

(A) Anterior abdominal viscera divided into four quadrants. (B) Posterior abdominal viscera.

Abdominal viscera are part of the urinary, digestive, reproductive, and lymphatic systems.

gallbladder, and urinary bladder (Figure 21-5). Organs in the abdominal cavity may be classified as part of the urinary system, the digestive system, the reproductive system, or the lymphatic system.[21]

## PREVENTING INJURIES TO THE THORAX AND ABDOMEN

Injuries to the thorax may be prevented by wearing appropriate protective equipment, particularly in collision sport activities. In football, for example, shoulder pads are usually designed to extend to at least below the level of the sternum. Rib protectors may be worn to cover the entire thoracic cage if necessary (Figure 21-6).

The muscles of the abdomen should be strengthened to protect the underlying viscera. A consistent regimen of sit-up exercises done in various positions can markedly increase the strength and size of the abdominal musculature.

Making sure that the hollow organs, in particular the stomach and bladder, are emptied before competition can reduce the chance of injury to those structures. Meals should be eaten at least 3 to 4 hours before competition to allow foods to clear the stomach. Urinating immediately before stepping onto the field or court protects the bladder from injury.

## ASSESSMENT OF THE THORAX AND ABDOMEN

**Generally fitness professionals, coaches, and others working in areas related to exercise and sport science are not adequately trained to evaluate injuries. It is strongly recommended that injured athletes be referred to qualified medical personnel (i.e., physicians, athletic trainers, physical therapists) for injury evaluation.** Information on the following special tests has been included simply to give some idea about the different basic tests that nonmedical personnel may do to determine the nature and severity of the athlete's injury. The primary responsibility of those who are not health care personnel is to be able to recognize any potential "red flags" associated with the injury, provide appropriate first aid for the injury, and make correct

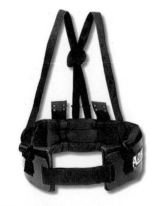

**Figure 21-6**

Protective rib belt

decisions about how the injury should be managed initially, including immediate return to play or activity decisions (refer to Chapter 7).

Injuries to the thorax and abdomen can produce potentially life-threatening situations. An injury that may seem relatively insignificant at first may rapidly develop into one that requires immediate and appropriate medical attention.[22] The initial primary survey should focus on those signs and symptoms that indicate some life-threatening condition. The injured athlete should be continually monitored to identify any disruption of normal breathing or circulation or any indication of internal hemorrhage that could precipitate shock. Most injuries to the thorax and abdomen require immediate referral to a physician.

## History

The questions asked to determine a history in the case of thoracic and abdominal injuries are somewhat different from those questions pertinent to musculoskeletal injuries of the extremities.[12] The primary mechanism of injury should be determined first:

- What happened to cause this injury?
- Was there direct contact or a direct blow?
- What position were you in?
- What type of pain is there (sharp, dull, localized, etc.)?
- Was there immediate or gradual pain?
- Do you feel any pain other than in the area where the injury occurred? (See Figure 21-9.)
- Have you had any difficulty breathing?
- Are certain positions more comfortable than others?
- Do you feel faint, lightheaded, or nauseous?
- Do you feel any pain in your chest?
- Did you hear or feel a pop or crack in your chest?
- Have you had any muscle spasms?
- Have you noticed any blood in your urine?
- Is there any difficulty or pain in urinating?
- Was the bladder full or empty?
- How long has it been since you have eaten?

## Observation

If the athlete is observed immediately following injury, check for normal breathing and respiratory patterns:

- Most important, is the athlete breathing at all?
- Is the athlete having difficulty breathing deeply, or is the athlete struggling to catch his or her breath?
- Does breathing cause pain?
- Is the athlete holding the chest wall?

- Is there symmetry in movement of the chest during breathing?
- If the wind was knocked out, did normal breathing return rapidly or was there prolonged difficulty? This difficulty may indicate a more severe injury.
- What is the body position of the athlete?
- Is there protrusion or swelling of any portion of the abdomen? This may indicate internal bleeding.
- Does the thorax appear to be symmetrical? Rib fractures can cause one side to appear different.
- Are the abdominal muscles tight and guarding?
- Is the athlete holding or splinting a specific part of the abdomen?

It is important to monitor vital signs, including pulse, respiration, and blood pressure (see Table 7-1). A rapid, weak pulse and/or a significant drop in blood pressure is an indication of some potentially serious internal injury often involving loss of blood. Other signs of abdominal injury might include blood in the urine, abdominal splinting, rapid weak pulse, and signs of shock.

### Palpation

#### Thorax

The hands should first be placed on either side of the chest wall to check for symmetry in chest wall movement during deep inspiration and expiration and to begin to isolate areas of tenderness (Figure 21-7). Once a tender area is identified, palpate along the rib and in the space between the ribs to locate a specific point of tenderness.

#### Abdomen

To palpate the abdominal structures, the athlete should be supine with the arms at the sides and the abdominal muscles relaxed (Figure 21-8). Uninjured areas should be palpated first with the tips of the fingers to feel for any tightness or rigidity. An athlete with an abdominal injury voluntarily contracts the abdominal muscles to guard or protect the tender

In acute abdominal injury, boardlike rigidity is likely.

**Figure 21-7**

Checking asymmetry of chest wall during breathing

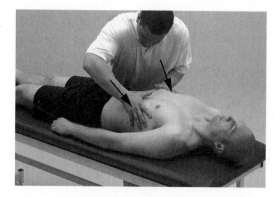

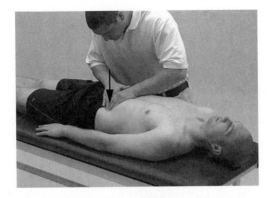

**Figure 21-8**

Palpating the abdomen for
guarding or rigidity

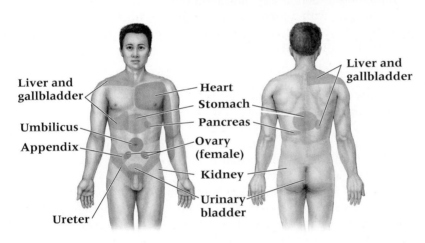

**Figure 21-9**

Patterns of pain referred from
abdominal structures

area. If there is bleeding or irritation inside the abdominal cavity, the abdomen will exhibit what is referred to as "boardlike rigidity" and cannot be voluntarily relaxed.[12] Pressure on the abdominal organs may elicit referred pain in predictable patterns away from the source[22] (Figure 21-9).

# RECOGNITION AND MANAGEMENT OF THORACIC INJURIES

## Rib Contusions

**Cause of injury**  A blow to the rib cage can contuse intercostal muscles between the ribs or, if severe enough, produce a fracture. Because the intercostal muscles are essential for breathing, when they are bruised, both expiration and inspiration become very painful.

**Signs of injury**  Characteristically the pain is sharp during breathing, there is point tenderness, and pain is elicited when the rib cage is compressed. X-ray examination should be routine in such an injury.

**Care**  PRICE and anti-inflammatory agents are commonly used. As with most rib injuries, contusions to the thorax are self-limiting, responding best to rest and cessation of sports activities.

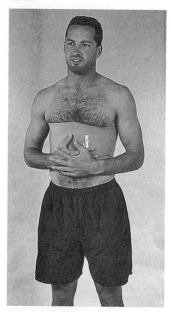

**Figure 21-10**

A commercial rib brace can provide moderate support to the thorax.

A rib fracture may be indicated by a severe, sharp pain during breathing.

## Rib Fractures

**Cause of injury**  Rib fractures are not uncommon in sports and have their highest incidence in collision sports.[15] Fractures can be caused either by direct impact, as by a kick, or by compression of the rib cage, as may occur in football or wrestling. Ribs five through nine are the most commonly fractured. There is always the possibility that a rib fracture can cause damage to or puncture the underlying lung.

**Signs of injury**  The rib fracture is usually quite easily detected. The athlete complains of severe pain during inspiration and point tenderness with sharp pain during palpation.

**Care**  The athlete should be referred to the team physician for x-ray examination if there is any indication of fracture. The rib fracture is usually managed with support and rest. Simple fractures heal within 3 to 4 weeks. A rib brace can offer the athlete some rib cage stabilization and comfort (Figure 21-10).

## Costal Cartilage Injury

**Cause of injury**  Costal cartilage injuries have a higher incidence than do fractures. This injury can occur from a direct blow to the thorax or indirectly from a sudden twist or a fall on a ball, compressing the rib cage. A costal cartilage injury displays signs similar to the rib fracture, with the exception that pain is localized in the junction of the rib cartilage and rib (Figure 21-11).

**Signs of injury**  The athlete complains of sharp pain during sudden movement of the trunk and of difficulty in breathing deeply. Palpation reveals point tenderness with swelling. In some cases there is a rib deformity and a complaint that the rib makes a crackling noise (crepitus) as it moves in and out of place.

**Care**  As with a rib fracture, the costal cartilage injury is managed by rest and immobilization by a rib brace. Healing takes anywhere from 1 to 2 months, precluding any sports activities until the athlete is symptom free.

## Intercostal Muscle Injuries

**Cause of injury**  The muscles of the thorax are all subject to contusions and strains in sports. The intercostals are especially vulnerable.

**Figure 21-11**

A costal cartilage injury involves separation of the rib and costal cartilage.

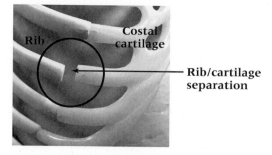

Traumatic injuries occur most often from direct blows or sudden torsion of the athlete's trunk.

**Signs of injury**   Like other muscle strains, pain occurs on active motion. However, injuries to muscles in this region are particularly painful during inspiration and expiration, laughing, coughing, or sneezing.

**Care**   Care requires immediate application of cold and compression for approximately 20 minutes. After hemorrhaging has been controlled, immobilization should be used to make the athlete more comfortable (refer to Figure 21-10).

## Injuries to the Lungs

**Cause of injury**   Fortunately, injuries to the lungs resulting from sports trauma are rare.[17] However, because of the seriousness of this type of injury, the coach must be able to recognize the basic signs. The most serious of the conditions are pneumothorax, tension pneumothorax, hemothorax, and traumatic asphyxia.

*Pneumothorax* is a condition in which the pleural cavity surrounding the lung becomes filled with air that has entered through an opening in the chest (Figure 21-12A).[2] As the pleural cavity fills with air, the lung on that side collapses.

A *tension pneumothorax* occurs when the pleural cavity on one side fills with air and displaces the lung and the heart toward the opposite side, thus compressing the opposite lung (Figure 21-12B).

*Hemothorax* is the presence of blood within the pleural cavity (Figure 21-12C). It results from the tearing or puncturing of the lung or pleural tissue, involving the blood vessels in the area.

*Traumatic asphyxia* occurs as the result of a violent blow to or compression of the rib cage, causing a cessation of breathing.[19] A condition of this type demands immediate mouth-to-mouth resuscitation and immediate medical attention.

**Signs of injury**   Signs may include difficulty breathing or shortness of breath, chest pain on the side of the injury, coughed up blood,

Lung injuries can result in:
- pneumothorax
- tension pneumothorax
- hemothorax
- traumatic asphyxia

**Figure 21-12**

(A) Pneumothorax.
(B) Tension pneumothorax.
(C) Hemothorax.

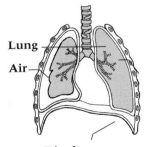

Lung
Air
Diaphragm

**(A) Pneumothorax**

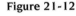

Collapsed lung
Compressed lung
Wound

**(B) Tension pneumothorax**

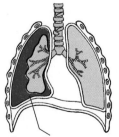

Pleural space filled with blood

**(C) Hemothorax**

Common causes of sudden
death syndrome:
- hypertrophic
  cardiomyopathy
- anomalous origin of the
  coronary artery
- Marfan's syndrome

cyanosis (bluish skin), and potentially shock. With a total collapse of the lung, medical attention is required immediately.[3]

**Care**   Each of these conditions is a medical emergency requiring immediate physician attention. Thus the athlete must be transported to the emergency room as quickly as possible.

## Sudden Death Syndrome in Athletes

**Cause of condition**   In athletes 35 years old and younger, the most common cause of exercise-induced sudden death is some congenital cardiovascular abnormality. The three most prevalent causes are hypertrophic cardiomyopathy, anomalous origin of the coronary artery, and Marfan's syndrome.[18] Hypertrophic cardiomyopathy is a condition in which there is thickened cardiac muscle with no evidence of chamber enlargement, and extensive myocardial scarring.[11] In an anomalous origin of the coronary artery, one of the two coronary vessels originates in a different site than normal, thus compromising or obstructing that artery because of its unusual course. In people with Marfan's syndrome, there is an abnormality of the connective tissue resulting in weakening of the aorta and cardiac valves, which can lead to a rupture of either a valve or of the aorta itself. Another potential cause of sudden death in athletes is coronary artery disease (CAD) resulting from atherosclerosis, in which there is a narrowing of the coronary arteries usually due to hypercholesterolemia in the young athlete.[17]

Noncardiac causes of sudden death have also been attributed to the use of certain drugs including alcohol, cocaine, amphetamines, and erythropoietin (which stimulates red blood cell production).[17] A vascular event due to bleeding in the brain caused by a cerebral aneurysm or head trauma that causes intracranial bleeding may also result in sudden death. Obstructive respiratory diseases such as asthma can result in sudden death because of drug toxicity or undertreatment.

**Signs of condition**   Common symptoms and signs associated with cardiac causes of sudden death may include chest pain or discomfort during exertion, heart palpitations or flutters, syncope, nausea, profuse sweating, heart murmurs, shortness of breath, general malaise, and fever.[8]

**Care**   This condition is a life-threatening emergency situation that requires immediate access of the rescue squad.[19] Be prepared to perform CPR until the rescue squad arrives (see Chapter 7).

**Prevention**   It has been suggested that a major number of deaths could be avoided by counseling, screening, and early identification of preventable causes of sudden death.[19] Initial screening should include the following questions:

Has a physician ever told you that you have a heart murmur?

Have you had chest pain during exercise?

Have you fainted during exercise?

Has anyone in your family under 35 ever died suddenly?

Has anyone in your family been diagnosed with a thickened heart?
Does anyone in your family have Marfan's syndrome?

If the answer is yes to any of these questions, a more in-depth medical
examination should be performed. Resting and exercise electrocardio-
grams and echocardiograms may be necessary to determine existing
pathology.[19]

### Breast Problems

**Cause of injury**  Violent up-and-down and lateral movements of
the breasts, such as are encountered in running and jumping, can bruise
and strain the breast, especially in large-breasted women. Constant un-
controlled movements of the breast over time can stretch the Cooper's
ligament, which supports the breast at the chest wall, leading to premature sagging of the breasts. *"Runner's nipples,"* in which the shirt rubs
the nipples and causes an abrasion, can be prevented by placing an adhesive bandage over each nipple before participation. *"Bicyclist's nipples"*
can also occur as the result of a combination of cold and evaporation
of sweat, causing the nipples to become painful. Wearing a windbreaker
can prevent this problem.

**Care**  Wearing a well-designed bra that has minimum elasticity and
allows little vertical or horizontal breast movement is most desirable
(refer to Figure 6-17).[16] Breast injuries usually occur during physical
contact with either an opponent or equipment. In sports such as fencing
or field hockey, female athletes should protect themselves by wearing
plastic cup protectors.

## RECOGNITION AND MANAGEMENT
## OF ABDOMINAL INJURIES

Although abdominal injuries comprise only about 10 percent of sports
injuries, they can require long recovery periods and can be life threatening.[12] The abdominal area is particularly vulnerable to injury in all contact sports. A blow can produce superficial or even deep internal injuries,
depending on its location and intensity.[22] In internal injuries of the abdomen that occur in sports, the solid organs are most often affected.
Strong abdominal muscles give good protection when they are tensed,
but when relaxed, the underlying organs may be easily injured. It is very
important to protect the trunk region properly against the traumatic
forces of collision sports. Good conditioning is essential, as is the use of
proper protective equipment and the application of safety rules.

### Abdominal Strains and Contusions

**Cause of injury**  Abdominal muscle strains occur with sudden
twisting of the trunk or reaching overhead. The rectus abdominus is the
most commonly strained abdominal muscle. Potentially these types of
injuries can be incapacitating.[7]

Contusions to the abdominal wall occur because of compressive forces. Although not very common, when they do happen, they are more likely to occur in collision sports such as football or ice hockey; however, any sports implement or high-velocity projectile can cause injury. Hockey goalies and baseball catchers are vulnerable to injury without their protective torso pads. The extent and type of injury varies depending on whether the force is blunt or penetrating.

**Signs of injury** An abdominal muscle strain or contusion of the rectus abdominis muscle can be disabling. A severe blow may cause a hematoma that develops under the fascial tissue surrounding this muscle. The pressure that results from hemorrhage causes pain and tightness in the region of the injury.[7]

**Care** Initially, ice and an elastic compression wrap should be used. Also look for signs of possible internal injury. Treatment should be conservative, and exercise should be kept within pain-free limits.

### Hernia

Inguinal hernias occur in males; femoral hernias occur in females.

**Cause of injury** The term *hernia,* sometimes referred to as a *sports hernia,* refers to the protrusion of abdominal viscera through a portion of the abdominal wall. Hernias resulting from sports most often occur in the groin area.[13] Inguinal hernias, which occur in men (more than 75 percent), and femoral hernias, most often occurring in women, are the most prevalent types. The inguinal hernia results from an abnormal enlargement of the opening of the inguinal canal through which the vessels and nerves of the male reproductive system pass (Figure 21-13A). In contrast, the femoral hernia arises in the canal that transports the vessels and nerves that go to the thigh and lower limb[26] (Figure 12-13B).

When intra-abdominal tension is produced in these areas, muscles produce contraction around these canal openings. If the muscles fail to react, abdominal contents may be pushed through the opening.

**Signs of injury** A hernia may be recognized by the following: previous history of a blow or strain to the groin area that produced pain and prolonged discomfort, superficial protrusion in the groin area that is increased by coughing, or reported feeling of weakness and pulling sensation in the groin area.[9]

**Care** Most physicians think that any athlete who has a hernia should be prohibited from engaging in hard physical activity until surgical repair has been made. Mechanical devices, designed to prevent hernial protrusion, are for the most part unsuitable in sports because of the friction and irritation they produce. Exercise has been thought by many to be beneficial to a mild hernia, but such is not the case. Exercise will not affect the stretched inguinal or femoral canals positively.[26]

### Blow to the Solar Plexus

A blow to the solar plexus can lead to transitory paralysis of the diaphragm and to unconsciousness.

**Cause of injury** A blow to the middle portion of the abdomen, or solar plexus, produces a transitory paralysis of the diaphragm (having

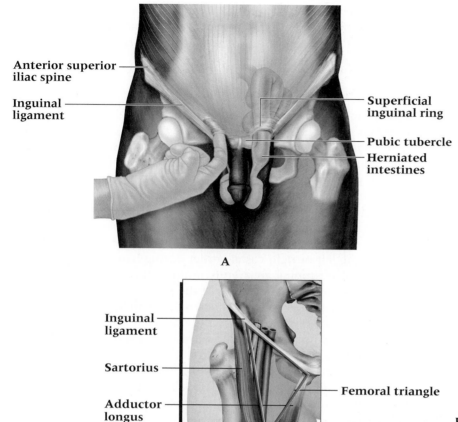

**A**

**B**

**Figure 21-13**

(A) Inguinal canal where
inguinal hernias appear.
(B) Femoral hernias are
found in the femoral triangle.

the wind knocked out). There should always be some concern that a blow hard enough to knock out the wind could also cause internal organ injury.

**Signs of injury**   Paralysis of the diaphragm stops respiration and leads to anoxia. When the athlete is unable to inhale, short-term panic may result. These symptoms are usually transitory. It is necessary to allay such fears and instill confidence in the athlete.[14]

**Care**   In dealing with an athlete who has had the wind knocked out of him or her, adhere to the following procedures: help the athlete overcome apprehension by talking in a confident manner; loosen the athlete's belt and the clothing around the abdomen; have the athlete bend the knees; and encourage the athlete to relax by initiating short inspirations and long expirations.

Because of the fear of not being able to breathe, the athlete may hyperventilate. Hyperventilation is an increased rate of ventilation that

**21-1 Critical Thinking**
Exercise

A wrestler is engaged in a strenuous off-season weight-lifting program. Recently he has begun to experience pain in his groin. Whenever he strains hard to lift a weight, and especially if he holds his breath, the pain appears. He is concerned that he has developed a hernia.

**?** What symptoms and signs indicate that the athlete does have a hernia?

results in increased levels of oxygen. It causes a variety of physical re-actions such as dizziness, a lump in the throat, pounding heart, or faint-ing. Have the athlete breathe slowly into a paper bag to increase levels of carbon dioxide.

### Stitch in the Side

**Cause of injury**   A stitch in the side is the name given an idiopathic condition that occurs in some athletes.[14] The cause is obscure, although several hypotheses have been advanced. Among these causes are the following: constipation, intestinal gas, overeating, diaphragmatic spasm as a result of poor conditioning, lack of visceral support because of weak abdominal muscles, distended spleen, breathing techniques that lead to a lack of oxygen in the diaphragm, and ischemia of either the diaphragm or the intercostal muscles.[17]

**Signs of injury**   A stitch in the side is a cramplike pain that devel-ops on either the left or right costal border during hard physical activity. Sports that involve running apparently produce this condition.

**Care**   Immediate care of a stitch in the side demands relaxation of the spasm, for which two methods have proved beneficial. First, the ath-lete is instructed to stretch the arm on the affected side as high as pos-sible. If this is inadequate, flexing the trunk forward on the thighs may prove of some benefit.[14]

Athletes with recurrent abdominal spasms may need special study. Identification of poor eating habits, poor elimination habits, or an in-adequate athletic training program may explain the athlete's particular problem. A stitch in the side, although not considered serious, may re-quire further evaluation by a physician if abdominal pains persist.

### Injury of the Spleen

**Cause of injury**   Injuries to the spleen are uncommon but occur most often because of a fall or a direct blow to the left upper quadrant of the abdomen when some existing medical condition has caused en-largement of the spleen.[5] Infectious mononucleosis is the most likely cause of spleen enlargement.

**Signs of injury**   The gross indications of a ruptured spleen must be recognized so that an immediate medical referral can be made.[25] Indi-cations include a history of a severe blow to the abdomen and possibly signs of shock, abdominal rigidity, nausea, and vomiting. There may be a reflex pain occurring approximately 30 minutes after injury, called Kehr's sign, which radiates to the left shoulder and one-third of the way down the left arm.[25] A ruptured spleen can hemorrhage profusely into the abdominal cavity, causing the athlete to die of internal bleeding days or weeks after the injury.

**Care**   Conservative nonoperative treatment is recommended ini-tially along with a week of hospitalization.[25] At 3 weeks, the athlete can engage in light conditioning activities and at 4 weeks can fully return

Infectious mononucleosis can cause spleen enlargement.

Athletes who complain of external pain in the shoulders, trunk, or pelvis after a severe blow to the abdomen or back may be describing referred pain from an injury to an internal organ.

to activity as long as no symptoms appear. If surgical repair is necessary, the athlete will require 3 months to recover, whereas removal of the spleen will require 6 months before the athlete can return to activity. If the spleen is enlarged due to mononucleosis, the athlete may resume training 3 weeks after the onset if the spleen is not enlarged or painful and if there is no fever.

## Kidney Contusion

**Cause of injury** The kidneys are seemingly well protected within the abdominal cavity. However, on occasion, contusions and even ruptures of these organs occur.[22] The kidney may be susceptible to injury because of its normal distention by blood. An external force applied to the back of the athlete causes abnormal extension of an engorged kidney, resulting in injury.[27]

**Signs of injury** An athlete who has received a contusion of the kidney may display signs of shock, nausea, vomiting, rigidity of the back muscles, and hematuria (blood in the urine). As with injuries to other internal organs, kidney injury may cause referred pain. Pain may radiate forward around the trunk into the lower abdominal region.

**Care** Any athlete who reports having received a severe blow to the abdomen or back region should be instructed to urinate two or three times and to look for the appearance of blood in the urine.[27] If there is any sign of hematuria, immediate referral to a physician must be made.[2] Medical care of the contused kidney usually consists of a 24-hour hospital observation, with a gradual increase of fluid intake. If the hemorrhage fails to stop, surgery may be indicated. Controllable contusions usually require 2 weeks of bed rest and close surveillance after activity is resumed. In questionable cases, complete withdrawal from one active playing season may be required.

*Kidney and bladder contusions can cause hematuria.*

> **21-3 Critical Thinking**
> Exercise
>
> A football receiver jumps to catch a high pass thrown over the middle. A defensive back hits the receiver in the low back. The athlete does not seem to have a specific injury. After the game he notices blood in his urine and becomes worried.
>
> ? Is blood in the urine a cause for concern, and what should be done to manage it?

## Liver Contusion

**Cause of injury** In sports activities, liver injury is very rare. A hard blow to the right side of the rib cage can tear or seriously contuse the liver, especially if it is enlarged as a result of some disease such as hepatitis.[24]

**Signs of injury** An injury to the liver can cause hemorrhage and shock, requiring immediate surgical intervention. Liver injury commonly produces a referred pain that is just below the right scapula, right shoulder, substernal area, and on occasion, the anterior left side of the chest.

**Care** A liver contusion requires immediate referral to a physician for diagnosis and treatment.

*Hepatitis can cause enlargement of the liver.*

## Appendicitis

**Cause of injury** Inflammation of the appendix can be chronic or acute. It is caused by a variety of factors, for example, a fecal obstruction. Its highest incidence is in males between the ages of fifteen and twenty-five. Appendicitis can be mistaken for a common gastric complaint.

Appendicitis is often mistaken for a common gastric problem.

In its early stages, the appendix becomes red and swollen; in later stages it may become gangrenous, rupturing into the bowels and causing peritonitis. Bacterial infection is a complication of rupture of the inflamed appendix.[24]

**Signs of injury**   The athlete may complain of a mild-to-severe pain in the lower abdomen, associated with nausea, vomiting, and a low-grade fever ranging from 99° to 100° F (37° to 38° C). Later, the cramps may localize into a pain in the lower right side, and palpation may reveal abdominal rigidity and tenderness at a point between the anterior superior spine of the ilium and the umbilicus (McBurney's point)[24] (see Figure 21-4).

**Care**   Surgical removal of the inflamed appendix is often necessary. If the bowel is not obstructed, there is no need to rush surgery. However, an obstructed bowel with an acute rupture is a life-threatening condition.

### Injuries to the Bladder

**Cause of injury**   On rare occasions a blunt force to the lower abdominal region may injure the urinary bladder particularly if it is distended by urine. The appearance of red blood cells within the urine (hematuria) is often associated with contusion of the bladder during running and has been referred to as a "runner's bladder."[24]

**Signs of injury**   With any impact to the abdominal region, the possibility of internal damage must be considered, and after such trauma the athlete should be instructed to check periodically for blood in the urine. Bladder injury commonly causes referred pain to the lower trunk, including the upper thigh anteriorly. With a bladder rupture, the athlete will be unable to urinate.

### Scrotal/Testicular Contusion

**Cause of injury**   As the result of their considerable sensitivity and particular vulnerability, the scrotum and the testicles may sustain a contusion that causes a very painful, nauseating, and disabling condition.

**Signs of injury**   As is characteristic of any contusion or bruise, there is hemorrhage, fluid effusion, and muscle spasm, the degree of which depends on the intensity of the impact to the tissue.[9]

**Care**   Immediately following a testicular contusion, the athlete is placed on his side and instructed to flex his thighs to his chest (Figure 21-14). As the pain diminishes, a cold pack is applied to the scrotum. Increasing or unresolved pain after 15 to 20 minutes requires prompt referral to a physician for evaluation.

### Gynecological Injuries

In general the female reproductive organs have a low incidence of injury in sports.[18] By far the most common gynecological injury in the female athlete involves a contusion to the external genitalia, or vulva, which includes the labia, clitoris, and the vestibule of the vagina.[6] A

Injuries to the reproductive organs in sports are much more likely to occur in the male because the male genitalia are more exposed.

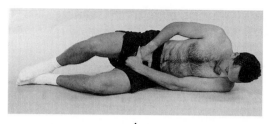

A

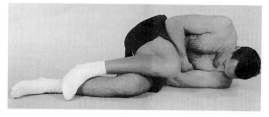

B

**Figure 21-14**

Body position following scrotum contusion

hematoma results from the contusion, which most often occurs with a direct impact to this area. A contusion of this area may also injure the pubic symphisis, producing ostitis pubis[1] (see Chapter 17).

## SUMMARY

- The thorax is that portion of the body commonly known as the chest, which lies between the base of the neck and the diaphragm. Its main functions are to protect the vital respiratory and circulatory organs and to assist the lungs in inspiration and expiration during the breathing process. Within the thoracic cage lie the lungs and the heart.

- The abdominal cavity lies between the diaphragm and the bones of the pelvis and is bounded by the margin of the lower ribs, the abdominal muscles, and the vertebral column. The abdominal viscera are composed of both hollow and solid organs. Organs in the abdominal cavity may be classified as part of the urinary system, the digestive system, the reproductive system, or the lymphatic system.

- Injuries to the heart, lungs, and abdominal viscera can be potentially serious and even life threatening if not recognized and managed appropriately.

- When evaluating an injury to the abdomen or thorax, the initial primary survey should focus on those signs and symptoms that indicate some life-threatening condition. Asking pertinent questions, observing body positioning, and palpation of the injured structures are critical in assessing the nature of the injury.

- Rib fractures and contusions, costal border injuries, muscle strains, and breast injuries are all common injuries to the chest wall.

- Injuries involving the lungs include pneumothorax, tension pneumothorax, hemothorax, and traumatic asphyxia.

- The most common cause of exercise-induced sudden death is some congenital cardiovascular abnormality. The three most prevalent conditions are hypertrophic cardiomyopathy, anomalous origin of the coronary artery, and Marfan's syndrome.

- Injuries to the abdominal wall include muscle strains, getting the wind knocked out, and the development of an inguinal or femoral hernia.

- With any injury to the abdominal region, internal injury to the abdominal viscera must be considered. Injuries to the liver, spleen, and kidneys are among the more common athletic injuries associated with the abdominal viscera.

- Injuries to the reproductive organs in sports are much more likely to occur in the male because the male genitalia are more exposed.

---

*Solutions to Critical Thinking* Exercises

---

**21-1** Most often an athlete with a hernia has some previous history of a blow or strain to the groin area that produced pain and prolonged discomfort. There may be a superficial protrusion in the groin area that is increased by coughing, or the athlete may have a feeling of weakness and a pulling sensation in the groin area. An inguinal hernia results from an abnormal enlargement of the opening of the inguinal canal through which the abdominal contents may be pushed.

**21-2** Try to modify this athlete's eating habits, which might be producing constipation or gas. Cramps can be caused by improper breathing techniques that may cause a lack of oxygen in the diaphragm and ischemia of either the diaphragm or the intercostal muscles. Cramps may also be caused by a diaphragmatic spasm that results from poor conditioning or a lack of visceral support because of weak abdominal muscles. Athletes with recurrent abdominal spasms should have further evaluation by a physician if the abdominal pains persist.

**21-3** Any time blood appears in the urine there is cause for concern. In this case it is likely that the kidneys have been contused and the blood that appears in the urine will disappear over the next couple of days. Nevertheless, the athlete should be referred to the team physician for diagnosis.

**21-4** Be concerned about the possibility of injury to an organ that can potentially lead to internal blood loss and eventually result in shock. It is possible that the spleen, liver, stomach, small intestine, pancreas, or gallbladder may be injured. It is also possible that there may be a contusion to the muscles of the abdominal wall that is causing muscle guarding.

## REVIEW QUESTIONS AND CLASS ACTIVITIES

1. Describe the anatomy of the thorax.
2. Differentiate among rib contusions, rib fractures, and costal border injuries.
3. Compare the signs of pneumothorax, tension pneumothorax, hemothorax, and traumatic asphyxia.
4. Identify the possible causes of sudden death syndrome among athletes.

5. List the abdominal viscera and other structures associated with the urinary system, the digestive system, the lymphatic system, and the reproductive system.
6. What muscles protect the abdominal viscera?
7. What conditions of the abdominal viscera produce pain in the abdominal region?
8. Contrast the signs of a ruptured spleen with signs of a severely contused kidney.
9. How do you manage an athlete who has had his or her wind knocked out?
10. Distinguish an inguinal hernia or a femoral hernia from a groin strain.
11. Describe the signs of a stitch in the side.

## REFERENCES

1. Cibor, G: 2002. Osteitis pubis: a commonly overlooked cause of groin pain, *Sports medicine alert* 8(1):2–4.
2. Ciocca M: 2000. Pneumothorax in a weight lifter: the importance of vigilance, *Physician sportsmedicine* 28(4):97.
3. Davis, PF: 2002. Primary spontaneous pneumothorax in a track athlete, *Clinical journal of sport medicine* 12(5):318–319.
4. Evans, C, Schwarz, L, Masihi, M: 2008. Screening for heart disease in athletes by athletic trainers and sports physical therapists, *Journal of Sport Rehabilitation* 17(2):171.
5. Fait, PE: 2003. Third-degree spleen laceration in a male varsity athlete, *Athletic therapy today* 8(3):32–33.
6. Finch, CF: 2002. The risk of abdominal injury to women during sport, *Journal of science and medicine in sport* 5(1):46–54.
7. Gregory, PL: 2002. Musculoskeletal problems of the chest wall in athletes, *Sports medicine* 32(4): 235–250.
8. Hosey, RG, Armsey, TD: 2003. Sudden cardiac death, *Clinics in sports medicine* 22(1):51–66.
9. Lacroix VJ: 2000. A complete approach to groin pain, *Physician sportsmedicine* 28(1):66.
10. Managing a traumatic pneumothorax: 2006. *Athletic therapy today* 11(5):51.
11. Maron, BJ: 2002. Hypertrophic cardiomyopathy: practical steps for preventing sudden death, *Physician and sportsmedicine* 30(1):19–24.
12. McGown, A: 2004. Blunt abdominal and chest trauma, *Athletic therapy today* 9(1):40.
13. Meyers WC et al.: 2000. Management of severe lower abdominal or inguinal pain in high-performance athletes, *American journal of sports medicine* 28(1):2.
14. Morton, DP: 2003. Exercise related transient abdominal pain, *British journal of sports medicine* 37(4): 287–288.
15. O'Kane J, O'Kane E, Marquet J: 1998. Delayed complication of a rib fracture, *Physician Sportsmed* 26(4):69.
16. Page KA, Steele JR: 1999. Breast motion and sports brassiere design: implications for future research, *Sports Medicine* 27(4):205.
17. Perron, AD: 2003. Chest pain in athletes, *Clinics in sports medicine* 22(1): 37–50.
18. Pfeifer, S, Patrizio, P: 2002. The female athlete: some gynecologic considerations, *Sports medicine and arthroscopy review* 10(1).
19. Pigozzi, F, Rizzo, M: 2008. Sudden death in competitive athletes. *Clinics in sports medicine* 27(1):153.
20. Puffer, JC: 2002. The athletic heart syndrome: ruling out cardiac

pathologies, *Physician and sportsmedicine* 30(7):41–47.

21. Saladin K: 2006. *Anatomy and Physiology,* Boston, McGraw-Hill.

22. Shultz, SJ: 2000. Thorax and abdomen. In Shultz, SJ, editor: *Assessment of athletic injuries,* Champaign, IL, Human Kinetics, pp. 380–405.

23. Stopka, CB, Zambito, KL: 1999. Referred visceral pain: what every sports medicine professional needs to know, *Athletic therapy today* 4(1):29.

24. *Tabor's cyclopedic medical dictionary:* 2005. Philadelphia, FA Davis.

25. Terrell, TR: 2002. Management of splenic rupture and return-to-play decisions in a college football player, *Clinical journal of sport medicine* 12(6):400–402.

26. Unverzagt, C, Schuemann, T, Mathisen, J: 2008. Differential diagnosis of a sports hernia in a high-school athlete. *Journal of orthopaedic & sports physical therapy* 38(2):63.

27. Wexler, RK: 2003. Renal laceration in a high school football player, *Physician and sportsmedicine* 31(2): 43–46.

## ANNOTATED BIBLIOGRAPHY

*Tabor's cyclopedic medical dictionary:* 2005. Philadelphia, FA Davis.

> *Despite the dictionary format, this is an excellent guide for the athletic trainer searching for clear, concise descriptions of various injuries and illnesses accompanied by brief recommendations for management and treatment.*

Saladin K: 2006. *Anatomy and physiology,* Boston, McGraw-Hill.

> *This anatomy text helps to clarify anatomy of the various systems of the abdomen and thorax.*

## WEB SITES

Acute Appendicitis:
http://emedicine.medscape.com/article/773895-overview

Anatomy of the Human Body:
www.bartleby.com/107/

Chest Trauma:
www.madsci.com/manu/trau_che.htm#30

National Heart, Lung, and Blood Institute: www.nhlbi.nih.gov/

TRAUMA.ORG:
www.trauma.org/index.php/main/category/c13/

*Abdominal trauma and goals of management*

American Thoracic Society—About ATS:
www.thoracic.org/

Sports Injury Clinic: abdominal injuries
www.sportsinjuryclinic.net/cybertherapist/front/stomach.htm

# The Head, Face, Eyes, Ears, Nose, and Throat

*When you finish this chapter you will be able to:*

- Describe the anatomy of the head, face, eyes, ears, nose, and throat.
- Explain how injuries to the head, face, eyes, ears, nose, and throat can be prevented.
- Discuss the assessment process in dealing with injuries to the head and face.
- Discuss recognition and management of concussions and mild head injuries.
- Recognize common injuries to the face, eyes, ears, nose, and throat.

Injuries to the region of the head, face, eyes, ears, nose, and throat are common in sports. The severity of injuries to this region can vary from something as benign as a nosebleed to a severe concussion.

Sports injuries to the head can be life threatening.

## PREVENTING INJURIES TO THE HEAD, FACE, EYES, EARS, NOSE, AND THROAT

Although injuries to the head and face are more prevalent in collision and contact sports, the potential for head injuries exists in all sports.[20] Wearing a helmet or protective headgear and in some instances a face mask in sports like football, ice hockey, lacrosse, wrestling, and baseball has dramatically reduced the incidence of injuries to the head, face, eyes, ears, and nose. Some have argued that if the face mask were eliminated in a sport like football, the number of cervical spine and head injuries would likely be reduced because the athlete would be less likely to use the head when making contact. However, it is certain that the incidence of injuries to the face, eyes, ears, and nose would significantly increase. A helmet can only do so much in preventing injury to the brain.

Unquestionably, the single most important consideration in reducing injuries to this region is teaching athletes to use correct techniques when initiating contact. All football helmets have written warnings that discourage the use of the head as a weapon. **It is imperative to make certain that athletes are taught and are using correct and safe techniques.**

## ANATOMY OF THE HEAD

### Bones

The skull is composed of twenty-two bones. With the single exception of the mandible, all of the bones are joined together in immovable joints called *sutures*. The cranial vault, which houses the brain, is enclosed by the cranium or skull and is made up of the frontal, ethmoid, sphenoid, two parietal, two temporal, and the occipital bones (Figure 22-1).

### The Brain

The brain is the part of the central nervous system that is contained within the bony cavity of the cranium and is divided into four sections. The *cerebrum* or *cortex* coordinates all voluntary muscle activities and interprets sensory impulses in addition to controlling higher mental functions including memory, reasoning, intelligence, learning, judgment, and emotions. The *cerebellum* controls movements of skeletal muscle and plays a critical role in the coordination of voluntary muscular movements. The *pons* controls sleep, posture, respiration, swallowing, and the bladder. The *medulla oblongata* is the lowest part of the brainstem and regulates heart rate, breathing (in conjunction with the pons), blood pressure, coughing, sneezing, and vomiting.[35]

#### Meninges

The *meninges* are three membranes that protect the brain and the spinal cord. Outermost is the *dura mater*. A layer of fat that contains vital arteries and veins separates this membrane from the bony wall and forms the epidural space. The *arachnoid* lines the dura mater. The space between the arachnoid and the *pia mater*, the membrane that helps contain the spinal fluid, is called the subarachnoid space (Figure 22-2).[35]

**Figure 22-1**

Bones of the skull and face
(lateral view)

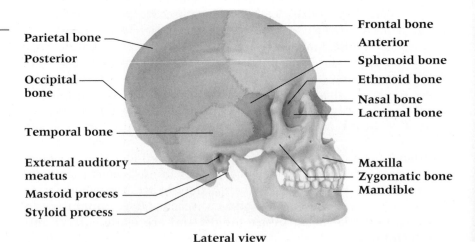

Parietal bone

Posterior

Occipital bone

Temporal bone

External auditory meatus

Mastoid process

Styloid process

Frontal bone

Anterior

Sphenoid bone

Ethmoid bone

Nasal bone

Lacrimal bone

Maxilla

Zygomatic bone

Mandible

**Lateral view**

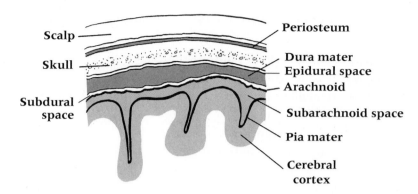

**Figure 22-2**

Cross-section of the meningal membranes

*Cerebrospinal fluid* is contained between the arachnoid and the pia mater membrane and completely surrounds and suspends the brain. Its main function is to act as a cushion, helping to diminish the transmission of shocking forces.

## ASSESSING HEAD INJURIES

An athlete who receives either a direct blow to the head or body contact that causes the head to snap forward, backward, or rotate to the side must be carefully evaluated for injury to the brain. Injuries to the brain may or may not result in unconsciousness; disorientation or amnesia; motor, coordination, or balance deficits; and cognitive deficits.[1]

### Dealing with an Unconscious Athlete

It must be emphasized that the majority of head injuries do not result in a loss of consciousness.

On-the-field management of the unconscious athlete was discussed in detail in Chapter 7. It is essential to be able to recognize and interpret the signs that an unconscious athlete presents. Priority first aid for any head injury must always deal with any life-threatening condition, but in particular loss of breathing.[12] When dealing with an unconscious athlete, always suspect a cervical neck injury and manage the situation accordingly as described in Chapter 7.[9] It is recommended that an athlete who has been unconscious be removed from the field on a spine board by the rescue squad.

If no life-threatening conditions exist, note the length of time that the athlete is unconscious, and do not attempt to move the athlete until consciousness is regained and the rescue squad has arrived. Once the athlete regains consciousness, or in cases in which the athlete may never have lost consciousness, try to obtain a history from the athlete.

### History

An athlete who has sustained a head injury may or may not be able to respond to questions about exactly what happened to cause the

All unconscious athletes should be handled as if they have a serious neck injury.

loss of consciousness. Nevertheless the following questions should be asked:

- Do you know where you are?
- Can you tell me what happened to you?
- Can you remember if you have ever been knocked out before?
- Does your head hurt?
- Do you have any pain in your neck?
- Can you move your hands and feet?

### Observation

The following observations should be made:

- Is the athlete disoriented and unable to tell where he or she is, what time it is, what date it is, who the opponent is?
- Is there a blank or vacant stare? Does the athlete have difficulty keeping the eyes open?
- Is there slurred or incoherent speech?
- Are there delayed verbal and motor responses (slow to answer questions or follow instructions)?
- Is there gross disturbance to coordination (i.e., stumbling, inability to walk a straight line, can't touch finger to nose)?
- Is there an inability to focus attention, and is the athlete easily distracted?
- Does there appear to be a memory deficit exhibited by repeated asking of the same questions or not knowing what happened?
- Does the athlete have normal cognitive function (serial 7s, assignment on a particular play)?
- Is there a normal emotional response from the athlete?
- How long was the athlete's affect abnormal?
- Is there a clear, straw-colored fluid in the ear canal (cerebrospinal fluid leakage that occurs with skull fracture)?

### Palpation

Palpation of the skull should be performed in a systematic manner to identify areas of point tenderness or deformity of the skull that may indicate the presence of a skull fracture.

### Special Tests

#### Neurological Exam

A neurological exam consists of testing five major areas: cerebral testing to assess cognitive function, cranial nerve testing, cerebellar testing to assess coordination and motor function, sensory testing, and reflex testing. The neurological exam should be done by a trained health care professional.

## Eye Function

Abnormal function of the eyes is often related to head injuries and the following observations should be made:[17]

1. Pupils should be equal, accommodate, round, and reactive to light (PEARL).
2. Eyes should track smoothly. A constant involuntary back and forth, up and down, or rotary movement of the eyeball is called *nystagmus.*[9]
3. Blurred vision is determined by difficulty or inability to read a game program or the scoreboard.

Checking for eye signs can yield important information about possible brain injury.

## Balance Tests

If the athlete is capable of standing, a modified Romberg test can be used to assess static balance. The best on-the-field balance test uses a tandem stance (Figure 22-3).[21] A positive sign is seen when the athlete begins to sway, cannot keep the eyes closed, or obviously loses balance.

## Coordination Tests

A number of tests have been used to determine whether the head injury has affected coordination. These tests include the finger-to-nose test, heel-to-toe walking, and the standing heel-to-knee test. Inability to perform any of these tests may be indicative of injury to the cerebellum.

## Cognitive Tests

The purpose of cognitive testing is to establish the effects of head trauma on various cognitive functions and obtain an objective measure to assess the athlete's status and improvement.[13] Two commonly used on-the-field cognitive tests are serial 7s, in which the athlete counts backward from 100 by 7, and naming the months in reverse order. Recently other cognitive tests also referred to as *neuropsychological assessments,* such as the Standardized Assessment of Concussion (SAC) test, have been developed for use in both on- and off-the-field evaluation.[22] (See Focus Box 22-1.)

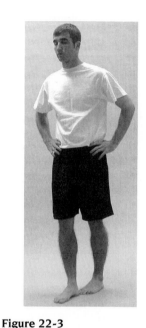

**Figure 22-3**

A modified Romberg test using a tandem stance

**22-1 *Critical Thinking***
Exercise

A soccer player is attempting to head a ball and collides with another player. He does not have a loss of consciousness but appears dazed and confused.

? What questions should be asked to determine his cognitive function?

# RECOGNITION AND MANAGEMENT OF SPECIFIC HEAD INJURIES

Head injuries occur from direct and blunt forces to the skull. It is estimated that at least thirty to forty major head injuries and occasionally a death occur during sport-related activities each year.[14]

## Skull Fracture

**Cause of injury**  Skull fractures occur most often from a blunt trauma, such as a baseball to the head, a shot to the head, or a fall from a height.

Standardized Assessment of Concussion (SAC) Form[21]

### 1) ORIENTATION:

| | | |
|---|---|---|
| Month: _____ | 0 | 1 |
| Date: _____ | 0 | 1 |
| Day of week: _____ | 0 | 1 |
| Year: _____ | 0 | 1 |
| Time (within 1 hr.): _____ | 0 | 1 |
| Orientation Total Score _____ / | 5 | |

### 2) IMMEDIATE MEMORY: (all 3 trials are completed regardless of score on trial 1 & 2; total score equals sum across all 3 trials)

| List | Trial 1 | Trial 2 | Trial 3 |
|---|---|---|---|
| Word 1 | 0   1 | 0   1 | 0   1 |
| Word 2 | 0   1 | 0   1 | 0   1 |
| Word 3 | 0   1 | 0   1 | 0   1 |
| Word 4 | 0   1 | 0   1 | 0   1 |
| Word 5 | 0   1 | 0   1 | 0   1 |
| Total | | | |

Immediate Memory Total Score ___/    15
(Note: Subject is not informed of Delayed Recall testing of memory)

### NEUROLOGICAL SCREENING:

Loss of Consciousness: (occurrence, duration)
Pre- & Post-Traumatic Amnesia: (recollection of events pre- and post-injury)
Strength:
Sensation:
Coordination:

### 3) CONCENTRATION:

*Digits Backward* (If correct, go to next string length. If incorrect, read trial 2. Stop after incorrect on both trials.)

| | | | |
|---|---|---|---|
| 4-9-3 | 6-2-9 _____ | 0 | 1 |
| 3-8-1-4 | 3-2-7-9 _____ | 0 | 1 |
| 6-2-9-7-1 | 1-5-2-8-6 _____ | 0 | 1 |
| 7-1-8-4-6-2 | 5-3-9-1-4-8 _____ | 0 | 1 |

*Months in reverse order*: (entire sequence correct for 1 point)
Dec-Nov-Oct-Sep-Aug-Jul
Jun-May-Apr-Mar-Feb-Jan _____    0        1
Concentration Total Score _____ /       5

#### EXERTIONAL MANEUVERS
(when appropriate)

| | |
|---|---|
| 5 jumping jacks | 5 push-ups |
| 5 sit-ups | 5 knee-bends |

### 4) DELAYED RECALL

| | | |
|---|---|---|
| Word 1 | 0 | 1 |
| Word 2 | 0 | 1 |
| Word 3 | 0 | 1 |
| Word 4 | 0 | 1 |
| Word 5 | 0 | 1 |
| Delayed Recall Total Score _____ | / | 5 |

### Summary of Total Scores:

| | | |
|---|---|---|
| *Orientation* _____ | / | 5 |
| *Immediate Memory* _____ | / | 15 |
| *Concentration* _____ | / | 5 |
| *Delayed Recall* _____ | / | 5 |
| **Overall Total Score** _____ | / | 30 |

McCrea, 2001[21]

---

**Signs of injury**   The athlete complains of severe headache and nausea. Palpation may infrequently reveal a defect such as a skull indention. There may be blood in the middle ear, blood in the ear canal, bleeding through the nose, discoloration around the eyes called "raccoon eyes," or behind the ear called "Battle's sign." Cerebrospinal fluid (straw colored) may appear in the ear canal and nose.[2]

    **Care**   It must be noted that it is not the skull fracture itself that causes the most serious problem but complications that stem from intracranial bleeding, bone fragments embedded in the brain, and infection.[18] Such an injury requires immediate hospitalization and referral to a neurosurgeon.

## Cerebral Concussion (Mild Traumatic Brain Injury)

**Cause of injury** Concussion has been traditionally defined as a clinical syndrome characterized by immediate and transient posttraumatic impairment of neural functions, such as alterations of consciousness, disturbance of vision, loss of equilibrium, etc.[14] It is important to realize that in the athletic population, the majority of concussions do not involve loss of consciousness.[14]

Direct blows occur when the athlete is struck in the head by some object (i.e., a ball, a baseball bat, a lacrosse stick, or contact with another player). A direct blow may also occur when the athlete's moving head strikes some fixed object (i.e., the floor, a goal post), resulting in impact deceleration of the brain. A blow to the head can produce an injury to the brain either at the point of contact (coup injury) or on the opposite side, which is referred to as a *contrecoup* injury. Acceleration, deceleration, and particularly rotational forces produce shaking of the brain within the skull.[7]

Recently the term *mild traumatic brain injury* (MTBI) has gained popularity in the sports medicine community and is broadly defined as immediate, transient impairment of cerebral function[1,2] with no focal lesions found on neuroimaging.

**Signs of injury** Altered consciousness and **posttraumatic amnesia** represent two important parameters that must be considered following a concussion. Posttraumatic amnesia can present as either *anterograde amnesia* (can't remember things that occurred after the injury) or *retrograde amnesia* (can't remember things that occurred before injury).[10] Additional signs and symptoms of concussion are highly variable but generally may include headache, tinnitus (ringing in ears), nausea, irritability, confusion, disorientation, dizziness, loss of consciousness, difficulty concentrating, blurred vision, photophobia (sensitivity to light), and sleep disturbance.[10,12]

For many years the Glasgow Coma Scale was used to determine the level of consciousness after head injury. However, because of decreased severity typically associated with sports activity, this scale is rarely used by physicians for classifying head injuries that occur in athletes.

In recent years, considerable debate has raged over a variety of classification and grading systems that have been proposed for determining severity of concussion. To date no single system of classification has been universally endorsed.[3] Table 22-1 provides a recommended guide for classifying three grades of cerebral concussion.[5] There may be too much emphasis placed on these grading scales.[10] *It appears that the most logical approach is to grade the concussion based on the presence and overall duration of symptoms only after all concussion signs and symptoms have resolved.*

**Care** Returning an athlete to competition following concussion often creates a difficult dilemma for the sports medicine team.[1] Certainly there is a difference between injuries with or without loss of consciousness or amnesia; however, the other signs and symptoms

> Most concussions do not involve loss of consciousness.

> **posttraumatic amnesia**
> Inability of athlete to recall events

**TABLE 22-1** Cantu Evidence-Based Grading System for Concussion[10]

| Grade 1 (mild) | Grade 2 (moderate) | Grade 3 (severe) |
| --- | --- | --- |
| No loss of consciousness; posttraumatic amnesia lasting less than 30 minutes; postconcussion signs and symptoms other than amnesia lasting less than 24 hours. | Loss of consciousness lasting less than 1 minute; posttraumatic amnesia lasting longer than 30 minutes but less than 24 hours; postconcussion signs and symptoms lasting longer than 24 hours but less than 7 days. | Loss of consciousness lasting more than 1 minute or posttraumatic amnesia lasting longer than 24 hours; postconcussion signs or symptoms lasting longer than 7 days. |

should also be monitored closely. Returning an athlete who has experienced any type of injury to the brain to competition too early has the potential to become a very costly decision, one that could lead to death.[5]

**Any time an athlete loses consciousness for any reason, the athlete must be removed from further activity immediately.** If the athlete has sustained a concussion that causes unconsciousness, it must always be suspected that the athlete may also have a cervical neck injury. In this case the rescue squad should be called and must remove the athlete from the field using a spine board.[9]

The decision to allow an athlete with a concussion to return to play is more difficult and to date has been based primarily on the subjective judgment of the team physician and athletic trainer if one is available. The coach or athletic trainer should always consult with a physician in these cases and the physician should clear the athlete for returning to participation.[36] Recent studies have indicated that the recovery period following even a mild concussion may be longer than has been thought.[5] **Athletes who have sustained a concussion should not be permitted to return to activity until ALL postconcussive symptoms including visual, motor, or sensory changes and difficulty with thought or memory have resolved.**[23] Permitting an athlete, particularly one in a contact sport, to return before symptoms resolve may place the athlete at risk.[24] It appears that following even a mild concussion, symptoms may take at least 3–5 days to resolve.[23] Table 22-2 provides guidelines that a physician can use in decision making for return to play following head injury.

Even after postconcussive symptoms have disappeared and the athlete has returned to play, there is still a danger of recurrent concussions, which can produce cumulative traumatic injury to the brain.[4] If more than one concussion occurs during a season, decisions must be made in consultation with the athlete, his or her family, the physician, and possibly the coach as to whether the athlete should continue to compete. Table 22-2 provides some recommendations for return to play after recurrent concussion.

**TABLE 22-2** Guidelines for Returning to Play after Repeated or Recurrent Concussions[5,6]

| Grade | First Concussion | Second Concussion | Third Concussion |
|---|---|---|---|
| 1 (mild) | May return to play if asymptomatic* for 1 week; terminate season if CT or MRI abnormality. | Return to play in 2 weeks if asymptomatic* at the time for 1 week. | Terminate season; may return to play next season if asymptomatic. |
| 2 (moderate) | Return to play after asymptomatic* for 2 weeks; terminate season if CT or MRI abnormality. | Minimum of 1 month out of play; may return to play then if asymptomatic* for 1 week; consider terminating season. | Terminate season; may return to play next season if asymptomatic. |
| 3 (severe) | Minimum of 1 month out of play; may then return to play if asymptomatic* for 1 week. | Terminate season; may return to play next season if asymptomatic. | Consider no further contact sports. |

*Asymptomatic in all cases means no postconcussive symptoms exist.

## Postconcussion Syndrome

**Cause of condition**  Postconcussion syndrome is a poorly understood condition that occurs following concussion. It may occur in cases of concussion that do not involve loss of consciousness or amnesia, or in severe concussions.[26]

**Signs of condition**  The athlete complains of a range of postconcussion problems including persistent headache, impaired memory, lack of concentration, anxiety and irritability, giddiness, fatigue, depression, and visual disturbances. These symptoms can begin immediately or within several days following the initial trauma and may last for weeks or even months before resolving.[26]

**Care**  Unfortunately, there is no clear-cut treatment for postconcussion syndrome. The athlete should not be allowed to return to play until all of the symptoms of this condition have resolved. Once symptoms have resolved, a gradual return to activity is recommended while continuing to monitor signs and symptoms that could return in consultation with the athlete, his or her family, the physician, and the coach.

## Second Impact Syndrome

**Cause of injury**  Second impact syndrome occurs as a result of rapid swelling of the brain following a second head impact occurring before the symptoms of a previous concussion have resolved.[7] This second impact may be relatively minor and in some cases may not even involve a blow to the head. A blow to the chest or back may create enough force to snap the athlete's head and create acceleration and deceleration

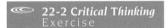
**22-2 Critical Thinking**
Exercise

A football player receives a grade 2 concussion. It is his second concussion this season.

**?** What guidelines should be followed regarding his return to play?

Second impact syndrome is a life-threatening emergency that must be dealt with immediately.

542

**22-3 *Critical Thinking***
Exercise

A volleyball player is knocked to the ground and hits the back of her head on the court, briefly losing consciousness. A few minutes after regaining consciousness she appears to be absolutely normal with no residual signs of concussion.

? Should she be allowed to return to the game?

forces upon an already compromised brain. Second impact syndrome is most likely to occur in athletes less than 18 years of age.

**Signs of injury** Often athletes do not even lose consciousness and may look "stunned." They may remain on their feet and be able to leave the playing field under their own power. However, within 15 seconds to several minutes, their condition worsens rapidly with loss of consciousness leading to coma, dilated pupils, loss of eye movement, and respiratory failure.[7] This is a life-threatening situation that has a mortality rate of approximately 50 percent.

**Care** Second impact syndrome is a life-threatening emergency that must be dealt with within a matter of approximately 5 minutes by dramatic life-saving measures performed in an emergency care facility.[1] The best way to manage second impact syndrome is to prevent it from occurring. Thus decisions to allow an athlete to return to play following an initial head injury must be carefully made based on the absence of postconcussive symptoms.

## Cerebral Contusion

**Cause of injury** A contusion of the cerebrum is a focal injury to the brain that involves small hemorrhages or *intracerebral bleeding* within either the cortex, the brainstem, or the cerebellum (Figure 22-4).[2] Brain contusions usually result from an impact injury in which the head strikes a stationary immovable object such as the floor.

**Signs of injury** Depending on the extent of trauma and the injury site, signs of injury may vary significantly. In most instances there is a loss of consciousness in an athlete who subsequently becomes very alert and talkative. A neurological exam is normal; however, symptoms such as headaches, dizziness, and nausea persist.

**Care** Hospitalization with a variety of imaging tests is standard for a cerebral contusion. Treatment varies according to the clinical status of the athlete.[2] A decision to return to play can only be made by the physician when the athlete is asymptomatic and a computed tomography (CT) scan is normal.

## Epidural Hematoma

**Cause of injury** A blow to the head, often resulting from a skull fracture, can cause a tear of the meningeal arteries that are embedded in bony grooves in the skull (Figure 22-5). Because of arterial blood pressure, blood accumulation and the creation of an *epidural hematoma* are extremely fast.[13]

**Figure 22-4**

Intracerebral bleeding

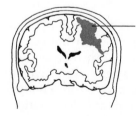

Intracerebral bleeding

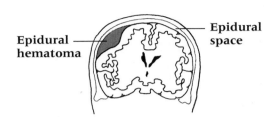

**Signs of injury**  In most cases initially there is a loss of consciousness. In some cases, once consciousness is regained, the athlete may be lucid, with few or none of the symptoms of serious head injury. Gradually symptoms begin to worsen with severe head pains, dizziness, nausea, dilation of one pupil usually on the same side as the injury, or sleepiness. Later stages of cerebral hemorrhage are characterized by deteriorating consciousness, neck rigidity, depression of pulse and respiration, and convulsions. This is a life-threatening situation, necessitating urgent neurosurgical care.

**Care**  A CT scan is necessary to diagnose an epidural hematoma. The pressure of an epidural hematoma must be surgically relieved as soon as possible to avoid the possibility of death or permanent disability.

## Subdural Hematoma

**Cause of injury**  Acute *subdural hematomas* occur much more frequently than epidural hematomas. Subdural hematomas result from acceleration and deceleration forces that tear vessels that bridge the dura mater and the brain.[13] Subdural hematomas usually involve venous bleeding and thus signs of injury tend to appear more slowly, maybe even after several hours (Figure 22-6).

**Signs of injury**  With subdural hematoma, the athlete may be unconscious with dilation of one pupil, usually on the same side as the injury. There may also be signs of headache, dizziness, nausea, or sleepiness.[20]

**Care**  An acute subdural hematoma is a life-threatening situation that requires immediate medical attention. A diagnostic CT scan or magnetic resonance imaging (MRI) is necessary to determine the extent and location of the hemorrhage.[20]

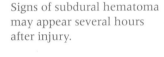

Signs of subdural hematoma may appear several hours after injury.

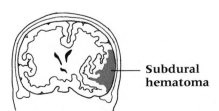

## Migraine Headaches

**Cause of condition**  Migraine is a disorder characterized by recurrent attacks of severe headache with sudden onset, with or without visual or gastrointestinal problems. The athlete who has a history of repeated minor blows to the head such as those that may occur in soccer or who has sustained a major cerebral injury may, over time, develop migraine headaches. The exact cause is unknown, but it is believed by many to be a vascular disorder.[28]

**Signs of condition**  Flashes of light, blindness in half the field of vision (hemianopia), and paresthesia are thought to be caused by vasoconstriction of intercerebral vessels. Headache is believed to be caused by dilation of scalp arteries. The athlete complains of a severe headache that is diffused throughout the head and often accompanied by nausea and vomiting. There is evidence of a familial predisposition for those athletes who experience migraine headaches after head injury.[28]

**Care**  The best management is prevention. Prophylactic medications are available to help reduce the recurrence of migraines. For severe attacks, administration of a prescription drug called Triptan has a high success rate.

## Scalp Injuries

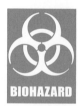

**Cause of injury**  The scalp can receive lacerations, abrasions, contusions, and hematomas. The cause of scalp injury is usually blunt or penetrating trauma. A scalp laceration can exist in conjunction with a serious skull or cerebral injury.

**Signs of injury**  The athlete complains of being hit in the head. Bleeding is often extensive, making it difficult to pinpoint the exact site. Matted hair and dirt can also disguise the actual point of injury.

**Care**  The treatment of a scalp laceration poses a special problem because of its general inaccessibility. Wounds that are more than ½ inch (1.25 cm) long and ⅛ inch (0.3 cm) deep should be referred to a physician for treatment. In less severe wounds the bleeding should be controlled and an antiseptic applied, followed by the application of a protective coating such as collodion and a sterile gauze pad. A tape adherent is then painted over the skin area to ensure that the tape sticks to the skin.

## ANATOMY OF THE FACE

The facial skin covers primarily subcutaneous bone with very little protective muscle, fascia, or fat. The supraorbital ridges house the frontal sinuses. In general the facial skeleton is composed of dense bony buttresses combined with thin sheets of bone. The middle third of the face consists of the maxillary bone, which supports the nose and nasal passages. The lower aspect of the face consists of the lower jaw or mandible. Besides supporting teeth, the mandible also supports the larynx, trachea, upper airway, and upper digestive tract (refer to Figure 22-1).

# RECOGNITION AND MANAGEMENT OF SPECIFIC FACIAL INJURIES

## Mandible Fracture

**Cause of injury** Fractures of the lower jaw or mandible (Figure 22-7) occur most often in collision sports. They are second in incidence of all facial fractures. Because it has relatively little padding and sharp contours, the lower jaw is prone to injury from a direct blow. The most frequently fractured area is near the jaw's frontal angle.[33]

**Signs of injury** The main indications of a fractured mandible are deformity, loss of normal occlusion of the teeth, pain when biting down, bleeding around teeth, and lower lip anesthesia.

**Care** Fracture of the mandible requires temporary immobilization with an elastic bandage followed by reduction and fixation of the jaw by the physician. Mild repetitive activities can be carried out, such as light weight lifting, swimming, or cycling during recovery. Fixation is from 4 to 6 weeks. Full activity is resumed in 2 to 3 months with appropriate special headgear and customized mouth guard.

## Zygomatic Complex (Cheekbone) Fracture

**Cause of injury** A fracture of the zygoma represents the third most common facial fracture. The mechanism of injury is a direct blow to the cheekbone.[33]

**Signs of injury** An obvious deformity occurs in the cheek region, or a bony discrepancy can be felt during palpation. There is usually a nosebleed *(epistaxis)*, and the athlete commonly complains of seeing double *(diplopia)*. There is also numbness of the cheek.

**Care** Care usually involves cold application for the control of edema and immediate referral to a physician. Healing takes from 6 to 8 weeks. Proper protective gear must be worn when returning to activity.

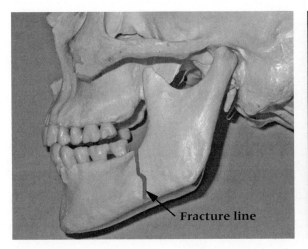

**Fracture line**

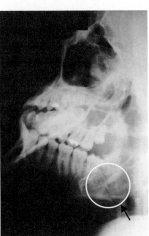

**Figure 22-7**

Mandible fracture

## Facial Lacerations

**Cause of injury**   Facial lacerations are common in contact and collision sports. Lacerations about the face are caused by a direct impact to the face with a sharp object or by an indirect compressive force.[29]

**Signs of injury**   The athlete feels pain and there is substantial bleeding and obvious tearing of the epidermis, dermis, and often the subcutaneous layer of skin (Figure 22-8).

**Care**   Refer to the physician for definitive care, such as suturing. In cases of *eyebrow lacerations,* do not shave the eyebrow because it may not regrow, or if it does it may do so in an irregular pattern. Lip, oral, ear, cheek, and nasal lacerations, as with all facial lacerations, are grossly contaminated and must be carefully cleaned before suturing can be successful. Infection must be avoided. Systemic antibiotics and tetanus prophylaxis may be necessary.[29]

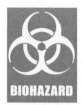

**Figure 22-8**

Facial lacerations can be a
medical emergency.

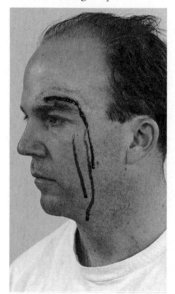

## DENTAL ANATOMY

The tooth is a composite of mineral salts of which calcium and phosphorus are most abundant. The portion protruding from the gum, called the *crown,* is covered by the hardest substance within the body, enamel. The portion that extends into the alveolar bone of the mouth is called the *root* and is covered by a thin, bony substance known as *cementum.* Underneath the enamel and cementum lies the bulk of the tooth, a hard material known as *dentin.* Within the dentin is a central canal and chamber containing the *pulp,* which is composed of nerves, lymphatics, and blood vessels that supply the entire tooth (Figure 22-9). With the use of face guards and properly fitting mouthguards most dental injuries can be prevented (see Chapter 6).

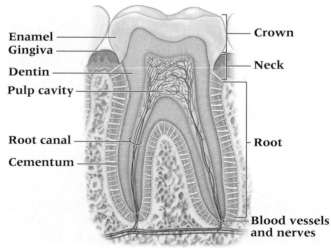

Enamel — Crown
Gingiva —
Dentin — — Neck
Pulp cavity —
Root canal — — Root
Cementum —
Blood vessels
and nerves

**Figure 22-9**

Normal tooth anatomy

## PREVENTING DENTAL INJURIES

**There is universal agreement within the dental community that all athletes, but particularly those in contact and collision sports, should routinely wear mouthguards to prevent injuries to the teeth**[15] (see Chapter 6). Without question the mandatory use of mouthguards by both high school and collegiate football players has significantly reduced the incidence of oral injuries in those sports. However, there is still a high incidence of dental injuries in those sports that do not require mouthguards to be worn.[13,25]

Athletes should practice good dental hygiene that includes regular brushing, rinsing, and flossing. Like everyone else, athletes should have dental screenings at least once each year to prevent the development of dental caries (cavities) in which the soft or bony tissue of a tooth gradually decays and degenerates. If this decay progresses, the tissue surrounding the tooth can become inflamed and an *abscess* forms from a bacterial infection of the tooth. Poor dental hygiene can also lead to *gingivitis,* which is an inflammation of the gums with swelling, redness, tenderness, and a tendency to bleed easily. Chronic gingivitis can lead to *periodontitis,* which involves an inflammation and/or a degeneration of the dental periosteum, the surrounding bone, and the cementum; loosening of the teeth; a recession of the gingiva; and infection.[16]

## RECOGNITION AND MANAGEMENT OF SPECIFIC DENTAL INJURIES

### Tooth Fractures

**Cause of injury** Any impact to the upper or lower jaw or direct trauma can potentially fracture the teeth.[16] There are essentially three types of fractures that can occur to the teeth: an uncomplicated crown fracture, a complicated crown fracture, and a root fracture (Figure 22-10).

**Signs of injury** In an uncomplicated crown fracture a small portion of the tooth is broken but there is no bleeding from the fracture and the pulp chamber is not exposed. In a complicated crown fracture a portion of the tooth is broken and there is bleeding from the fracture. The pulp chamber is exposed and there is a great deal of pain. Because a root fracture occurs below the gum line diagnosis is difficult and may require x-ray. Root fractures account for only 10 to 15 percent of all fractures. The tooth may appear to be in the normal position but there is bleeding from the gum around the tooth and the crown of the tooth may be pushed back or loose. Any impact great enough to cause a fracture of a tooth can also produce a fracture of the mandible or even a concussion.[31]

**Care** Neither uncomplicated nor complicated crown fractures require immediate treatment by a dentist. The fractured piece of tooth can simply be placed in a plastic bag, and if the fractured tooth is not extremely sensitive to air or cold, the athlete can continue to play and see the dentist within 24 to 48 hours after the game. If there is bleeding, a

Tooth fractures:
* uncomplicated crown fracture
* complicated fracture
* root fracture

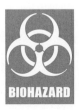

Dentist

**Figure 22-10**

Tooth fractures:

(A) Uncomplicated crown fracture; (B) Complicated crown fracture; (C) Root fracture.

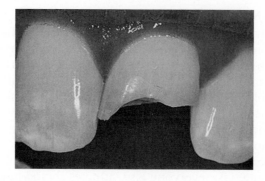

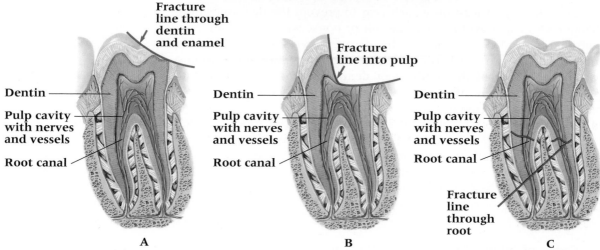

**Fracture line through dentin and enamel**

**Fracture line into pulp**

Dentin

Pulp cavity with nerves and vessels

Root canal

Dentin

Pulp cavity with nerves and vessels

Root canal

Dentin

Pulp cavity with nerves and vessels

Root canal

**Fracture line through root**

A

B

C

piece of gauze can be placed over the fracture. For the sake of appearance the fractured piece of tooth can either be glued in place or capped using a synthetic composite material.

In the case of a root fracture the athlete may continue to play but should see the dentist as soon as possible after the game. If the tooth is pushed back do not try to force it forward because doing so is likely to make the fracture worse. The dentist will reposition the tooth and apply a brace to be worn for 3 to 4 months.[31] A mouthguard should be worn while competing.

### Tooth Subluxation, Luxation, and Avulsion

**Cause of injury**  The same mechanisms that cause fractures of the teeth may also cause loosening or dislocation of the tooth.[31] Loosening of the tooth can result in concussion or subluxation, luxation, or avulsion.

**Signs of injury**  A tooth may be slightly loosened or totally dislodged. In the case of a concussion or subluxation the tooth is still in its normal place and only slightly loose. There is little if any pain; however, the tooth just feels different. In a luxation there is no fracture but the tooth is very loose and has moved either forward to an extruded

**22-4 Critical Thinking**
Exercise

A field hockey player is accidentally hit in the mouth with a stick. One of her front teeth is knocked completely out and she spits the tooth out into her hand.

? How should this situation be handled?

position, or backward to an intruded position. In an avulsion, the tooth is knocked completely out of the mouth.

**Care** For a subluxation, no immediate treatment is required and the athlete should be referred to a dentist within 48 hours for evaluation only. In a luxation, the tooth should only be moved back into its normal position if it is easy to move. The athlete should be referred to a dentist as soon as possible, especially if it is not possible to reposition the tooth to its normal position. With an avulsion, the coach can safely and easily try to reimplant the tooth. The avulsed tooth can be rinsed off but should never be scraped or scrubbed to get dirt off. If it is not possible to reimplant the tooth, it should be stored in a "Save a Tooth" kit, which contains Hank's Balanced Salt Solution (HBSS), or in milk or saline.[31] The athlete should be referred to the dentist immediately. The sooner the tooth can be reimplanted the better the prognosis.

An avulsed tooth should be reimplanted immediately.

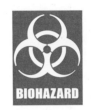

Dentist

## ANATOMY OF THE NOSE

The nose functions to clean, warm, and humidify inhaled air. The external portion of the nose is formed by a combination of bone in the superior portion and fibrocartilage inferiorly that spreads laterally to form the ala. The nasal cavity extends from the nostrils posteriorly to the choane. A nasal septum divides the nasal cavity into right and left chambers.

## RECOGNITION AND MANAGEMENT OF SPECIFIC NASAL INJURIES

### Nasal Fractures and Chondral Separation

**Cause of injury** A fracture of the nose is one of the most common fractures of the face. The force of the blow to the nose may come either from the side or from a straight frontal force. A lateral force causes greater deformity than a straight-on blow.[4]

**Signs of injury** Nasal fractures appear frequently as a separation of the frontal processes of the maxilla, a separation of the lateral cartilages, or a combination of the two (Figure 22-11). In nasal fractures hemorrhage is profuse because of laceration of the mucous lining. Swelling is immediate. Deformity is usually present if the nose has received a lateral blow. Gentle palpation may reveal abnormal mobility and emit a grating sound (crepitus).[32]

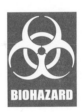

**Care** Control the bleeding and then refer the athlete to a physician for x-ray examination and reduction of the fracture.[32] Simple and uncomplicated fractures of the nose do not hinder and are not unsafe for the athlete, and he or she can return to competition within a few days. Fracture deformity reduction must be performed by a trained person.[3] Adequate protection can be provided through splinting.

### Deviated Septum

**Cause of injury** As with fracture, the mechanism of injury to the septum is by compression or lateral trauma.

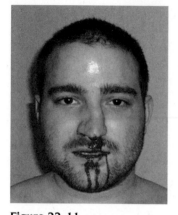

**Figure 22-11**

A serious nose fracture may
be a medical emergency.

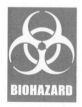

**Signs of injury** A careful evaluation of the nose must be made after the trauma. Injury commonly produces bleeding and in some cases a septal hematoma. The athlete complains of nasal pain.

**Care** At the site where a hematoma may occur, compression is applied. When a hematoma is present, it must be drained immediately through a surgical incision through the nasal septal mucosa. After surgical drainage, a small wick is inserted for continued drainage, and the nose is firmly packed to prevent the hematoma from re-forming. If a hematoma is neglected, an abscess will form, causing bone and cartilage loss and ultimately a difficult deformity to correct.[32]

### Nosebleed (Epistaxis)

**Cause of injury** Nosebleeds in sports are usually the result of direct blows that cause varying degrees of contusion to the septum. *Epistaxis* can be classified as either anterior or posterior. Anterior epistaxis originates from the nasal septum and posterior epistaxis from the lateral wall. Anterior epistaxis is by far the more common and may result from a direct blow, a sinus infection, high humidity, allergies, a foreign body lodged in the nose, or some other serious facial or head injury.[37]

**Signs of injury** Hemorrhages arise most often from the highly vascular anterior aspect of the nasal septum. In most situations the nosebleed presents only a minor problem and stops spontaneously after a short time. However, there are persistent types that require medical attention and possibly cauterization. As always when dealing with blood, universal precautions must be used.

**Care** An athlete with an acute nosebleed should sit upright with a cold compress placed both over the nose and the ipsilateral carotid artery while applying finger pressure to the affected nostril for 5 minutes. It has also been suggested that a piece of rolled-up gauze be placed between the upper lip and gum, thus placing direct pressure on the arteries that supply the nasal mucosa.[37]

If this procedure fails to stop the bleeding within 5 minutes, more extensive measures should be taken. The application of gauze or a felt plug provides corking action and encourages blood clotting. If a plug is used, the ends should protrude from the nostrils at least ½ inch to facilitate removal. After bleeding has ceased, the athlete may resume activity but should be reminded not to blow the nose under any circumstances for at least 2 hours after the initial insult.

### ANATOMY OF THE EAR

The ear (Figure 22-12) is responsible for the sense of hearing and equilibrium. It is composed of three parts: the external ear; the middle ear (tympanic membrane) lying just inside the skull; and the internal ear (labyrinth), which is formed in part by the temporal bone of the skull. The middle ear and internal ear are structured to transport auditory impulses to the brain. Aiding the organs of hearing and equalizing pressure

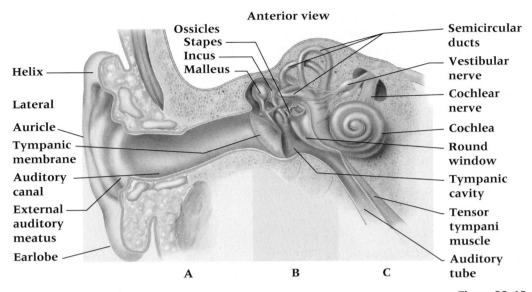

**Anterior view**

Ossicles
Stapes
Incus
Malleus

Helix

Lateral

Auricle

Tympanic
membrane

Auditory
canal

External
auditory
meatus

Earlobe

A          B          C

Semicircular
ducts

Vestibular
nerve

Cochlear
nerve

Cochlea

Round
window

Tympanic
cavity

Tensor
tympani
muscle

Auditory
tube

**Figure 22-12**

**Ear anatomy:**

(A) External ear. (B) Middle ear. (C) Inner ear.

between the middle and the internal ear is the eustachian tube, a canal that joins the nose and the middle ear.[35]

Sports injuries to the ear occur most often to the external portion. The external ear is separated into the auricle (pinna) and the external auditory canal (meatus). The auricle, which is shaped like a shell, collects and directs waves of sound into the auditory canal. It is composed of flexible yellow cartilage, muscles, and fat padding and is covered by a closely adhering, thin layer of skin. Most of the blood vessels and nerves of the auricle turn around its borders, with just a few penetrating the cartilage proper.

## RECOGNITION AND MANAGEMENT OF SPECIFIC INJURIES TO THE EAR

### Auricular Hematoma (cauliflower ear)

**Cause of injury** Hematoma of the ear is common in boxing, rugby, and wrestling. Hematomas are most common in athletes who do not wear protective headgear. This condition usually occurs from either compression or a shearing injury (single or repeated) to the auricle that causes subcutaneous bleeding into the auricular cartilage.[35]

**Signs of injury** Trauma may tear the overlying tissue away from the cartilaginous plate, resulting in hemorrhage and fluid accumulation. A hematoma usually forms before the limited circulation can absorb the fluid. If the hematoma goes unattached, a sequence of coagulation, organization, and fibrosis results in a keloid (excessive scar) that appears elevated, rounded, white, nodular, and firm, resembling a cauliflower (Figure 22-13). Often it forms in the region of the helix fossa or concha; once developed, the keloid can be removed only through surgery.[35]

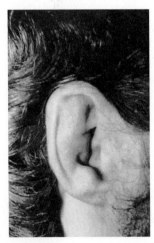

**Figure 22-13**

Cauliflower ear

**Care** To prevent this disfiguring condition, some friction-reducing agent such as petroleum jelly should be applied to the ears of athletes susceptible to this condition. They should also routinely wear ear guards in practice and in competition.

If an ear becomes "hot" because of excessive rubbing or twisting, the immediate application of a cold pack to the affected spot alleviates hemorrhage. Once swelling is present in the ear, special care should be taken to prevent the fluid from solidifying; a cold pack should be placed immediately over the ear and held tightly by an elastic bandage for at least 20 minutes. If the swelling is still present at the end of this time, aspiration by a physician is required.[4] After drainage, pressure is applied to the area to prevent return of the hematoma.

## Rupture of the Tympanic Membrane

**Cause of injury** Rupture of the tympanic membrane is commonly seen in contact and collision sports, and in water polo and diving.[18] A fall or slap to the unprotected ear or sudden underwater pressure variation can rupture the tympanic membrane.

**Signs of injury** The athlete complains of a loud pop followed by pain in the ear, nausea, vomiting, and dizziness. The athlete demonstrates hearing loss and a physician can see a visible rupture of the tympanic membrane through an otoscope.

Rupture of the tympanic membrane can cause temporary hearing loss.

**Care** Small to moderate perforations of the tympanic membrane usually heal spontaneously in 1 to 2 weeks.[18] Infection can occur and must be continually monitored. Individuals with a ruptured tympanic membrane should not fly until the condition has resolved.

## Swimmer's Ear (Otitis Externa)

**Cause of injury** A common condition in athletes engaged in water sports is *swimmer's ear,* or external otitis. Swimmer's ear is a general term for infection of the ear canal.[27] Contrary to current thought among swimming coaches, swimmer's ear is not usually associated with a fungal infection. Water can become trapped in the ear canal as a result of obstructions created by cysts, bone growths, ear wax plugs, or swelling caused by allergies.[35]

**Signs of injury** The athlete may complain of itching, discharge, or even a partial hearing loss. The athlete also complains of pain and dizziness.

**Care** Prevention of ear infection can best be attained by drying the ears thoroughly with a soft towel, using ear drops containing a mild acid (3 percent boric acid) and alcohol solution before and after each swim, and avoiding situations that can cause ear infections such as overexposure to cold wind or sticking foreign objects into the ear.[27]

When the swimmer displays symptoms of external otitis, immediate referral to a physician must be made. Tympanic membrane rupture should be ruled out. Antibiotics may be used in athletes with a mild ear infection.[35] In the event of a perforated ear drum, custom-made ear plugs must be used.

## Middle Ear Infection (Otitis Media)

**Cause of injury**  Otitis media is an accumulation of fluid in the middle ear caused by local and systemic inflammation and infection.

**Signs of injury**  There usually is intense pain in the ear, fluid draining from the ear canal, and a transient loss of hearing. In addition, the systemic infection may also cause fever, headache, irritability, loss of appetite, and nausea.[35]

**Care**  A physician may choose to draw a small amount of fluid from the middle ear to determine the most appropriate antibiotic therapy. Analgesics can be used to help reduce pain. The problem generally begins to resolve within 24 hours, although pain may last for 72 hours.

## Impacted Cerumen

**Cause of condition**  *Cerumen* or ear wax is secreted by glands in the outer portion of the ear canal. Occasionally an excessive amount of ear wax may accumulate, clogging the ear canal.[8]

**Signs of condition**  When cerumen becomes impacted there is some degree of hearing loss that is usually muffled. However, there generally is little or no pain because no infection is involved.[8]

**Care**  Initially an attempt can be made to remove excess cerumen by irrigating the ear canal with warm water. The athlete should not attempt to remove the cerumen with a cotton tip applicator because that may increase the degree of impaction. If irrigation fails, the impacted cerumen must be physically removed by a physician using a curette.[8]

## ANATOMY OF THE EYE

The eye has many anatomical protective features. It is firmly retained within an oval socket formed by the bones of the head. A cushion of soft fatty tissue surrounds it, and a thin skin flap (the eyelid), which functions by reflex action, covers the eye for protection. The lashes and eyebrows, which act as a filtering system, prevent foreign particles from entering the eye. A soft mucous lining that covers the inner conjunctiva transports and spreads tears, which are secreted by many accessory lacrimal glands. A larger lubricating organ is located above the eye and secretes quantities of fluid through the lacrimal duct to help wash away foreign particles. The eye proper is well protected by the sclera, a tough white outer layer possessing a transparent center portion called the *cornea*.

The cornea covers the pupil, which is the central opening of the eye. Light passes through the cornea, then through the anterior chamber past the iris to the lens, and finally through the vitreous body, all of which function collectively to focus an image on the retina that the optic nerve detects (Figure 22-14).

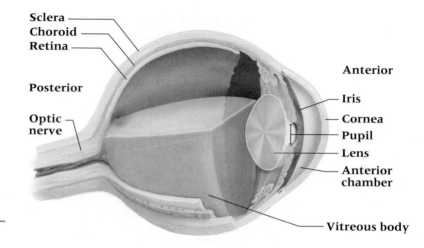

**Figure 22-14**

Eye anatomy

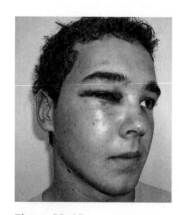

**Figure 22-15**

A blow to the orbit can cause
a black eye.

## RECOGNITION AND MANAGEMENT OF SPECIFIC EYE INJURIES

It should be strongly recommended that athletes wear appropriate eye guards to reduce the likelihood of injury to the eye (see Chapter 6). This is particularly true in sports that involve the use of some projectile object (i.e., raquetball, lacrosse, baseball, etc.).

### Orbital Hematoma (Black Eye)

**Cause of injury**  Although well protected, the eye may be bruised during sports activity. The severity of eye injuries varies from a mild bruise, to an extremely serious condition affecting vision, to fracture of the orbital cavity. Fortunately, most of the eye injuries sustained in sports are mild. A blow to the eye may initially injure the surrounding tissue and produce capillary bleeding into the tissue spaces. If the hemorrhage goes unchecked, the result may be a classic "black eye" (Figure 22-15).[38]

**Signs of injury**  The signs of a more serious contusion may be displayed as a subconjunctival hemorrhage or as faulty vision.

**Care**  Care of an eye contusion requires cold application for at least half an hour, plus a 24-hour rest period if the athlete has distorted vision. Under no circumstances should an athlete blow the nose after an acute eye injury. To do so might increase hemorrhaging.

### Orbital Fractures

**Cause of injury**  A fracture of the bony framework of the orbit surrounding the eye can occur when a blow to the eyeball forces it backwards, compressing the orbital fat until a blow-out or rupture occurs to the floor of the orbit. Both fat and the inferior extraocular muscles can bulge through this fracture.[30]

**Signs of injury**   The athlete with a fracture of the orbit often exhibits *diplopia* (double vision), restricted movement of the eye, a downward displacement of the eye, and pain accompanied by soft tissue swelling and hemorrhage. There may be numbness associated with injury to the infraorbital nerve on the floor of the orbit. An x-ray must be taken to confirm the fracture.[30]

**Care**   A physician should administer antibiotics prophylactically to decrease the likelihood of infection. A fracture in the orbital floor allows communication with the maxillary sinus, which may contain potentially infectious bacteria. Most orbital fractures are treated surgically although some physicians prefer to wait and see if the symptoms resolve on their own.

### Foreign Body in the Eye

**Cause of injury**   Foreign bodies in the eye are a frequent occurrence in sports and are potentially dangerous.[38]

**Signs of injury**   A foreign object produces considerable pain and disability. No attempt should be made to remove the body by rubbing or by using the fingers.

**Care**   Have the athlete close the eye until the initial pain has subsided, and then attempt to determine if the object is in the vicinity of the upper or lower lid. Foreign bodies in the lower lid are relatively easy to remove by depressing the tissue and then wiping it with a sterile cotton applicator. Foreign bodies in the area of the upper lid are usually much more difficult to localize. Gently pull the upper eyelid over the lower lid while the subject looks downward. This causes tears to be produced, which may flush the object down onto the lower lid. If this method is unsuccessful, gently pull the eyelid down and place an applicator stick crosswise at its base; have the athlete look down; then grasp the lashes and turn the lid back over the stick. Holding the lid and the stick in place with one hand, use the sterile cotton swab to lift out the foreign body (Figure 22-16). After the foreign particle is removed, the affected eye should be washed with saline solution. Often there is residual soreness after removal of the foreign body, which may be alleviated by the application of petroleum jelly or some other mild ointment. If there is extreme difficulty in removing the foreign body or if it has become embedded in the eye itself, the eye should be closed and "patched" with a gauze pad, which is held in place by strips of tape. The athlete is referred to a physician as soon as possible.

### Corneal Abrasions

**Cause of injury**   An athlete who gets a foreign object in his or her eye usually tries to rub it away. In doing so, the cornea can become abraded.[17]

**Signs of injury**   The athlete complains of severe pain and watering of the eye, photophobia, and spasm of the orbicular muscle of the eyelid.

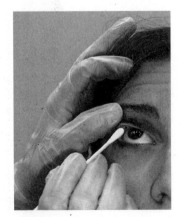

**Figure 22-16**

Removing a foreign object from the eye

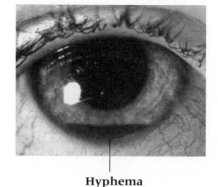

**Figure 22-17**

A hyphema is a collection of
blood in the anterior
chamber of the eye.

**Hyphema**

**Care**   The eye should be patched, and the athlete should be sent
to a physician. Antibiotic ointment prescribed by the physician is applied and a semipressure patch placed over the closed eyelid.[25]

### Hyphema

**Cause of injury**   A blunt blow to the anterior aspect of the eye can
produce a *hyphema,* which is a collection of blood within the anterior
chamber[34] (Figure 22-17). This injury is often caused by being struck
in the eye with a racquetball or squash ball when not wearing appropriate protective eyewear.

**Signs of injury**   Initially there is a reddish tinge in the anterior
chamber and within the first 2 hours the blood settles inferiorly or may
fill the entire chamber. The blood may turn pea green. Vision is partially or completely blocked. A hyphema is a major eye injury that can
lead to serious problems of the lens, choroid, or retina.

**Care**   Athletes with a hyphema should be immediately referred to
a physician. Conventional treatment involves hospitalization and bed
rest with the head elevated 30 to 45 degrees, patching of both eyes,
sedation, and medication to reduce pressure in the anterior chamber.
The initial hemorrhage resorbs in a few days, although occasionally
there is rebleeding. If not managed properly, irreversible vision damage
can occur.

### Retinal Detachment

**Cause of injury**   A blow to the athlete's eye can partially or completely separate the retina from its underlying attachment. Retinal
detachment is more common among athletes who have myopia (near-
sightedness).[17]

**Signs of injury**   Detachment is painless; however, early signs include seeing specks floating before the eye, flashes of light, or blurred
vision. As the detachment progresses, the athlete complains of a "curtain" falling over the field of vision. Any athlete with symptoms of
detachment must be immediately referred to an ophthalmologist.

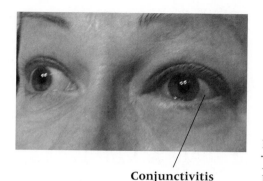

Conjunctivitis

**Figure 22-18**

Acute conjunctivitis in the
left eye

**Care** Initial treatment is bed rest with patches on both eyes. The athlete should immediately be referred to an ophthalmologist to determine if surgery is required.

### Acute Conjunctivitis

**Cause of injury** The conjunctiva is the tissue that lines the back of the eyelid, moves into the space between the eyelid and eye globe, and spreads up over the sclera to the cornea.[17] Acute conjunctivitis is usually caused by various bacteria or allergens. It may begin with conjunctival irritation from wind, dust, smoke, or air pollution. It may also be associated with the common cold or other upper respiratory conditions.

**Signs of injury** The athlete complains of eyelid swelling, sometimes with a purulent discharge. Itching is associated with allergy. Eyes may burn or itch (Figure 22-18).

**Care** Acute conjunctivitis can be highly infectious. The athlete should be referred to a physician for treatment.

## RECOGNITION AND MANAGEMENT OF INJURIES TO THE THROAT

### Contusions

**Cause of injury** Blows to the throat do not occur frequently in sports, but occasionally an athlete may receive a kick or blow to the throat. One type of trauma is known as "clotheslining," in which the athlete is struck in the throat region. Such a force can conceivably injure the carotid artery, causing a clot to form that occludes the blood flow to the brain. This same clot can become dislodged and migrate to the brain. In either case, serious brain injury may result.

**Signs of injury** Immediately after throat trauma the athlete may experience severe pain and spasmodic coughing, speak with a hoarse voice, and complain of difficulty in swallowing. A fracture of the larynx is rare, but it is possible and may be indicated by an inability to breathe and expectoration of frothy blood.[4] Cyanosis may be present. Throat contusions are extremely uncomfortable and are often frightening to the athlete.

**Care** The most immediate concern is the integrity of the airway. If the athlete is experiencing difficulty in breathing he or she should be sent to an emergency care facility immediately. In most situations cold may be applied intermittently to control superficial hemorrhage and swelling, and after a 24-hour rest period moist hot packs may be applied. For the most severe neck contusions, stabilization with a well-padded collar is beneficial.

## SUMMARY

- An athlete who receives either a direct blow to the head or body contact that causes the head to snap forward, backward, or rotate to the side must be carefully evaluated for injury to the brain. Injuries to the brain may or may not result in unconsciousness; disorientation or amnesia; motor, coordination, or balance deficits; or cognitive deficits.

- It is important to realize that in the athletic population, the majority of concussions do not involve loss of consciousness.

- Concussions usually occur as a result of a direct impact or through a combination of rotational acceleration and deceleration forces.

- A variety of classification systems have been proposed for determining severity of concussion. To date, none of these classification systems has been universally endorsed and thus debate continues.

- Returning an athlete to competition following concussion often creates a difficult dilemma for the sports medicine team. There must be ongoing concern about second impact syndrome and epidural and subdural hematomas.

- Injuries to the face can involve fractures of the mandible, maxilla, or zygoma, dislocations of the mandible, and facial lacerations.

- Any impact to the upper or lower jaw or direct trauma can cause one of three types of fractures to the teeth: an uncomplicated crown fracture, a complicated crown fracture, or a root fracture. A tooth may also be subluxated, luxated, or avulsed. Be aware of when to refer an athlete for dental care.

- Most injuries to the ear involve the auricle; cauliflower ear is the most common injury. Rupture of the tympanic membrane, swimmer's ear, and middle ear infections are also common in the athletic population.

- For the most part, injuries to the eye should be treated by physicians who are specifically trained. Orbital fractures, a foreign body in the eye, a hyphema, and retinal detachments are all considered serious injuries to the eye.

- The most serious consequence of a throat contusion is airway interference.

*Solutions to Critical Thinking* Exercises

**22-1** Ask him or her to count backwards from 100 by 7s and to name the months in reverse order. Both of these tests assess cognitive function.

**22-2** The athlete should be out of play for at least 1 month. After this period he or she may return to play if asymptomatic for 1 week. The physician may consider terminating the athlete for the rest of the season.

**22-3** Absolutely not. Whenever an athlete suffers a loss of consciousness, they are automatically finished for that day and should be cleared by a physician before being allowed to return to play.

**22-4** Take the tooth and, without trying to clean it off, attempt to reimplant the tooth. The athlete should then be immediately referred to a dentist.

## REVIEW QUESTIONS AND CLASS ACTIVITIES

1. What is the difference between the terms *concussion* and *mild head injury?*
2. Identify a classification system for determining grades of concussion.
3. How is second impact syndrome related to concussion?
4. What immediate care procedures should be performed for athletes with facial lacerations?
5. Describe the immediate care procedures that should be performed when a tooth is fractured and when it is dislocated.
6. Describe the procedures that should be performed for an athlete with a nosebleed.
7. How can cauliflower ear be prevented?
8. How should a foreign body in the eye be treated?

**REFERENCES**

1. Almquist J: 2001. Assessment of mild head injuries, *Athletic therapy today* 6(1):13–17.
2. Bailes JE: 2001. Classification of sport-related head trauma: a spectrum of mild to severe injury, *Journal of athletic training* 36(3): 236–243.
3. Boden, B, Tacchetti, R, Cantu, R: 2007. Catastrophic head injuries in high school and college football players. *American journal of sports medicine* 35(7):1075–1081.
4. Brukner P: 2002. Facial injuries. In Brukner, P, editor: *Clinical sports medicine,* 2nd rev. ed, Sydney, McGraw-Hill, pp. 203–214.
5. Cantu RC: 2001. Posttraumatic retrograde and antegrade amnesia: pathophysiology and implications in grading and safe return to play, *Journal of athletic training* 36(3):244.
6. Cantu, RC: 2003. Recurrent athletic head injury: risks and when to retire, *Clinics in sports medicine* 22(3):593–603.
7. Cantu RC: 1998. Second impact syndrome. In Cantu RC, *Clinical Sports Medicine* 17(1):37.
8. Daniels J: 2002. Easy ear wax removal, *Physician and sportsmedicine* 30(9):50.
9. Del Rossi G: 2002. Management of cervical-spine injuries, *Athletic therapy today* 7(2):46–51.
10. Guskiewicz, KM; Bruce, SL; Cantu, RC: 2004. National Athletic Trainers' Association position statement: Management of sport-related concussion, *Journal of athletic training* 39(3):280–297.
11. Guskiewicz K, Cantu RC: 2004. The concussion puzzle: the evaluation of sport-related concussion,

*American journal of medicine and sport,* 6(1):13–19.

12. Guskiewicz K, Ross S, Marshall S: 2001. Postural stability and neuropsychological deficits after concussion in college athletes, *Journal of athletic training* 36(3): 263.

13. Jordan BD: 1999. Management of concussion in sports, *Neurology* 53(4):892.

14. Kelly JP: 1999. Traumatic brain injury and concussion in sports, *JAMA* 282(10):989.

15. Knapik, J, Marshall, S, Lee, R: 2007. Mouthguards in sport activities, *Sports medicine* 37(2): 117.

16. Kumamoto DP et al.: 1995. Oral trauma, *Physician and Sportsmedicine* 23(5):53.

17. Laio J, Zagelbaum BM: 1999. Eye injuries in sports, *Athletic therapy today* 4(5):36.

18. Lenker C: 2000. Traumatic tympanic membrane perforation in a collegiate football player, *Athletic therapy today* 5(1):43.

19. Lindley TR: 2000. Concussion management on the field: the recognition and treatment of head injuries in athletes, *Rehab management* 13(3): 20.

20. Logan SM: 2001. Acute subdural hematoma in a high school football player after 2 unreported episodes of head trauma: a case report, *Journal of athletic training* 36(4):433–436.

21. Majerske, C, Mihalik, J: 2008. Concussion in sports: postconcussive activity levels, symptoms, and neurocognitive performance, *Journal of athletic training* 43(3): 265.

22. McCrae M: 2001. Standardized mental status testing on the sideline after sport related concussion, *Journal of athletic training* 36(3):274.

23. McCrea, M, Guskiewicz, KM, Marshall, KM: 2004. Acute effects and recovery time following concussion in collegiate football players (Abstract), *British journal of sports medicine* 38(3):369.

24. Mitchko, J, Huitric, M: 2007. CDC's approach to educating coach about sport-related concussion, *American journal of health education* 38(2):99–103.

25. Moeller, JL, Rifat, SF: 2003. Identifying and treating uncomplicated corneal abrasions, *Physician and sportsmedicine* 31(8):15–17.

26. Moss RI: 2001. Preventing post-concussion sequelae, *Athletic therapy today* 6(2):28–29.

27. Moylan, F: 2003. Swimmer's ear mystery, *Physician and sportsmedicine* 31(9): 48.

28. Nadelson, C: 2006. Sport and exercise-induced migraines. *Current sports medicine reports* 5(1):29.

29. Nelson, B, Huchun, A, Tuzman, J: 2007. Facial injuries in sport. *Sports medicine update:* 2–5.

30. Petrigliana FA: 2003. Orbital fractures in sport: a review, *Sports medicine* 33(4):317–322.

31. Roberts WO: 2000. Field care of the injured tooth, *Physician and sportsmedicine* 28(1):101.

32. Romeo, S, Hawley, C: 2005. What to do for nasal injuries, *Physician and sportsmedicine* 33(4):54.

33. Romeo, S, Hawley, C: 2005. Facial injuries in sports: A team physician's guide to diagnosis and treatment, *Physician and sportsmedicine* 33(4):45–53

34. Stilger VG, Alt JM, Robinson TW: 1999. Traumatic hyphema in an intercollegiate baseball player: a case report, *Journal of athletic training* 34(1):25.

35. *Tabers cyclopedic medical dictionary,* 2005. Philadelphia, FA Davis.

36. Valovich-McLeod, T, Schwartz, C: 2007. Sport-related concussion misunderstandings among youth coaches, *Clinical journal of sport medicine* 17(2):140–142.

37. Weir J: 1997. Effective management of epistaxis in athletes, *Journal of athletic training* 32(3): 254.

38. Young, J, Sallis, R, Smith, G: 2008. Ocular injury rates in college sports, *Medicine & science in sports & exercise* 40(3):428.

### ANNOTATED BIBLIOGRAPHY

Cantu RI: 2000. *Neurologic athletic head and spine injuries,* Philadelphia, WB Saunders.

*The text addresses topics related to neurologic athletic head and spine injuries such as injury epidemiology, prevention, on-the-field management, diagnosis, treatment, rehabilitation, and return-to-play decisions.*

Currie D, Ritchie E, Scott S: 2000. *The management of head injuries,* London, Oxford University Press.

*Chapters cover initial assessment, resuscitation, neurological deterioration, scalp and skull injuries, cervical spine injuries, children's injuries, and more.*

Special Issue: 2001. Concussion in athletes, *Journal of Athletic Training* 36(3): July–September.

*This issue contains a variety of data-based research articles dealing with sport-related concussion.*

**WEB SITES**

American Academy of Neurology www.aan.com

American Academy of Ophthalmology: www.aao.org

American Academy of Otolaryngology Head and Neck Surgery: www.entnet.org

American Dental Association Online: www.ada.org/

SPORTS DENTISTRY ON LINE: www.sportsdentistry.com/

# General Medical Conditions and Additional Health Concerns

CHAPTER 23

*When you finish this chapter you will be able to:*

- Explain the causes, prevention, and care of the most common skin infections in sports.
- Describe respiratory tract illnesses common to athletes.
- Identify disorders of the gastrointestinal tract.
- Describe how to avoid problems with the diabetic athlete.
- Describe the dangers that hypertension presents to an athlete.
- Describe the adverse effects that various anemias have on the athlete.
- Explain what a coach should do with an athlete who is having a grand mal seizure.
- Identify contagious viral diseases that may be seen in athletes.
- Explain the concerns of the female athlete in terms of menstruation, osteoporosis, and reproduction.
- Identify specific sexually transmitted infections.

In addition to the injuries that have been discussed in previous chapters, a variety of additional medical and health-related conditions can potentially affect athletes and their ability to compete or practice. Like everyone else, athletes inevitably become ill. When illnesses occur, it becomes important to recognize these conditions and to follow up with referral to appropriate care.[9] With the illnesses and conditions discussed in this chapter, appropriate care usually means referring the athlete to a physician to provide medical care. **The majority of illnesses and conditions discussed in this chapter require referral to a physician for care.** The information provided in this chapter serves as a reference for making appropriate decisions regarding care of the sick athlete.

## SKIN INFECTIONS

The skin is the largest organ of the human body. It is composed of three layers—epidermis, dermis, and subcutis. The most common skin infections in sports are caused by viruses, bacteria, and fungi.[1] Focus Box 23-1 lists the most common skin infections. To some extent these viral, bacterial, and fungal infections can be prevented by taking appropriate measures such as using universal precautions, avoiding direct contact with infected individuals, and washing your hands.

**Common Viral, Bacterial, and Fungal Skin Infections Found in Athletes***

Viral infections

    Herpes simplex type 1—cold sore, fever blister

    Herpes simplex type 2—genital herpes

    Herpes gladiatorum (back or shoulders)

    Herpes zoster

    Verruca virus (warts)

Bacterial infections

    Staphylococcus

      Boils

    Streptococcus

      Impetigo

      Infected hair follicles (boil)

      Infected sweat glands (folliculitis)

      Methicillin-resistant staphylococcus aureus (MRSA)

Fungal infections

    Ringworm (tinea)

      Tinea capitis (head)

      Tinea corporis (body)

      Tinea unguium (toenails and fingernails)

      Tinea cruris (jock rash)

      Tinea pedis (athlete's foot)

*All of these conditions should be referred to a physician or dermatologist for treatment.

## Viral Infections

A virus is the smallest of the microorganisms that can live only inside a cell. When the virus enters a cell it may immediately trigger a disease (influenza) or it can remain dormant for years (herpes). A virus can damage the host cell by blocking its normal function and using the metabolism of the host cell for its own reproduction. Eventually the virus destroys the host cell and progressively invades other cells.

Viral infections most likely to affect the skin are herpes simplex and herpes zoster.

### Herpes

**Cause of condition**　Herpes simplex is a viral infection that results in a skin eruption of vesicles that tend to recur in the same place, usually at sites at which mucous membranes join the skin. Herpes simplex is further classified as either type 1 or type 2. Type 1 occurs as a cold sore or fever blister around the lips and type 2 usually occurs around the

*Herpes is a common virus that attacks the skin of athletes.*

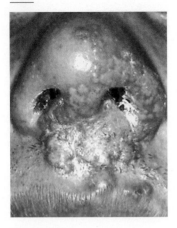

**Figure 23-1**

Herpes simplex type 1 on the upper lip and nose

BIOHAZARD

genitals and is classified as a sexually transmitted infection (Figure 23-1). Herpes simplex that appears on the back or shoulders is called *herpes gladiatorum* and occurs most often in wrestlers.[18,38]

*Herpes zoster* appears in a specific pattern on the body in an area that is innervated by a specific nerve root. It may appear on the face or anywhere on the trunk. Herpes zoster is the reappearance of the chicken pox virus that has remained dormant for many years. It is most likely to appear when the immune system is compromised.

**Symptoms of condition**   Athletes about to experience an outbreak of herpes usually feel a tingling, itching soreness immediately before a small area of redness appears. The athlete also reports feeling ill, particularly with first episode outbreaks. These symptoms are followed by the appearance of painful, fluid-filled vesicles that take on a crusty appearance. These vesicles usually heal in about 10 days.[38]

**Care**   Athletes with active lesions should be held out of any contact activity until the fluid-filled vesicles have disappeared.[13] It is important to take universal precautions when dealing with the herpes virus. Herpes may spread by contact with the fluid inside the vesicles. Outbreaks of herpes must run their course. Acyclovir, an over-the-counter medication taken orally and applied topically, has been effective in treating the symptoms. However, athletes must realize that the virus is not destroyed and that the herpes will probably reappear in the same area.

### Verruca Virus and Warts

**Cause of condition**   Numerous forms of verruca exist, including the verruca plana (flat wart), verruca plantaris (plantar wart), and the condyloma acuminatum (venereal wart). Different isotypes of human papilloma virus have been identified.[34] The human papilloma virus uses the skin's epidermal layer for reproduction and growth. The verruca wart enters the skin through a lesion that has been exposed to contaminated fields, floors, or clothing. Contamination can also occur from exposure to other warts.

**Symptoms of condition**   This wart appears as a small, round, elevated lesion with rough, dry surfaces. It may be painful if pressure is applied. These warts are subject to secondary bacterial infection, particularly if they are located on the hands or feet, where they may be constantly irritated (Figure 23-2).

**Care**   Vulnerable warts must be protected until they can be treated by a physician. The application of a topical salicylic acid preparation or liquid nitrogen and electrocautery are the most common ways of managing this condition.

### Bacterial Infections

**Cause of condition**   Bacteria are one-celled plantlike microorganisms that are capable of multiplying in an environment that supports their reproduction. Bacteria that cause disease are called *pathogens*.

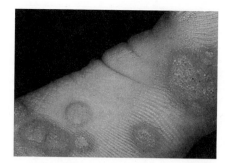

**Figure 23-2**

Common warts on the thumb

Millions of nonpathogenic bacteria normally live on the skin and mucous membranes of the body. Development of a disease involves entry of the bacterial pathogen into a host, growth of bacteria and production of toxic substances, and the response of the host to fight that infection. Many different types of bacterial pathogens can produce infection in the body. The two types of bacteria most likely to infect the skin are *streptococcus* (strep) and *staphylococcus* (staph).[1] **Impetigo** contagiosa is a common skin disease, primarily observed in children, with the greatest number of cases occurring in late summer and early fall. It is caused by streptococci and spreads rapidly when athletes are in close contact with one another. It is characterized by the eruption of small vesicles that form into pustules and later yellow crustations (Figure 23-3A). A **boil** or furuncle is a localized, pus-forming infection of staphylococcus bacteria that originates in a hair follicle (Figure 23-3B). Boils can become large and very painful. They commonly occur in athletes wearing protective equipment, such as where football shoulder pads come in contact with the skin. **Folliculitis** is an inflammatory reaction of the hair follicles, usually around the face or neck or in the groin area (Figure 23-3C).

**Symptoms of condition** The symptoms of localized infection are similar to the signs of inflammation, including tenderness, warmth,

**impetigo**
A bacterial strep infection.

**boil (furuncle)**
A staph infection originating in a hair follicle.

**folliculitis**
Inflammation of hair follicles.

**Figure 23-3**

**Bacterial infections:**

(A) Impetigo contagiosa on the face.

(B) Boil on the chest.

(C) Folliculitis on the neck.

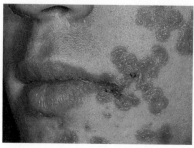

**A**

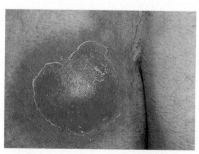

**B**

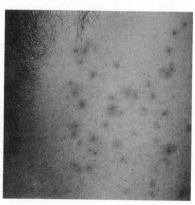

**C**

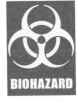

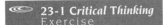

redness, and swelling. Pus may form in an infected area from either staph or strep.

**Care** Bacterial infections should be treated with specific antibiotic medications that inhibit the growth and proliferation of a particular bacterium. The area should also be treated with warm compresses. If an open, pus-filled lesion develops, it should be drained. Every precaution should be taken to minimize the spread of infection and transmission to another person.

### Methicillin-Resistant Staphylococcus Aureus (MRSA)

**Cause of condition** MRSA stands for methicillin-resistant staphylococcus aureus. In recent years some strains of staphylococcus bacteria have become resistant to some antibiotics.[37] MRSA strains are not only resistant to the antibiotic called methicillin, but also to many other types of antibiotics.[32] MRSA occurs most commonly in people who are already in the hospital and ill or have wounds or open sores such as bedsores or burns. The wounds or sores may become infected with MRSA and the infection is then difficult to treat. MRSA can also cause infections in people outside a hospital.

**Symptoms of condition** MRSA infections can cause a broad range of symptoms depending on the part of the body that is infected. Infection often results in redness, swelling, and tenderness at the site of infection (Figure 23-4). Sometimes, people may carry MRSA without having any symptoms.[37]

**Care** Antibiotics are not completely powerless against MRSA, but those infected with this bacteria may require a much higher dose over a much longer period, or the use of an alternative antibiotic. Many MRSA infections can only be treated with antibiotics that need to be given directly into a vein. The course of treatment is often for several weeks.[32]

### Fungal Infections

**Cause of condition** The most common fungal infection found in athletes is *ringworm* (Figure 23-5). Ringworm fungi are the cause of

**Figure 23-4**

Methacillin-Resistant
Staphylococcus Aureus
(MRSA) on the Forearm

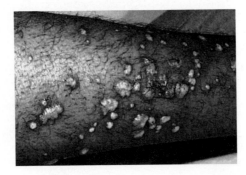

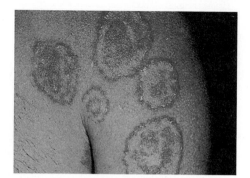

**Figure 23-5**

Tinea of the shoulder and upper chest

most skin, nail, and hair fungal infections. Ringworm can be found all over the body and is more appropriately referred to by the term *tinea* plus the Latin term for whatever body part is affected. The two most common sites for ringworm are in the groin (tinea cruris) and in the foot (tinea pedis).[38]

**Symptoms of tinea of the groin (tinea cruris)**   Tinea of the groin (tinea cruris), more commonly called "jock rash," appears as a bilateral and often symmetrical brownish or reddish lesion resembling the outline of a butterfly in the groin area.[29]

The athlete complains of mild to moderate itching, which can lead to scratching and the possibility of a secondary bacterial infection.

**Care**   Conditions of this type must be treated until cured. Infection not responding to normal management must be referred to the physician. Most ringworm infections respond to the many nonprescription medications that are available as aerosol sprays, liquids, powders, or ointments. Medications that are irritating or tend to mask the symptoms of a groin infection must be avoided.

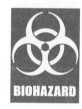

**Symptoms of athlete's foot (tinea pedis)**   The foot is the area of the body most commonly infected by dermatophytes, usually by tinea pedis, or athlete's foot (Figure 23-6). The fungus is usually found in the space between the third and fourth digits and on the plantar surface of the arch. The same organism attacks toenails. This fungus causes scaling and thickening of the soles. The athlete wearing shoes that are enclosed sweats, encouraging fungal growth. However, the likelihood of getting athlete's foot is based mainly on the athlete's individual susceptibility. Other conditions that may be thought to be athlete's foot include a dermatitis caused by allergy or an eczema-type skin infection.[29]

Athlete's foot can reveal itself in many ways but appears most often as an extreme itching on the soles of the feet and between and on top of the toes. It appears as a rash, with small pimples or minute blisters that break and exude a yellowish serum. Scratching because of itchiness can cause the tissue to become inflamed and infected, manifesting a red, white, or gray scaling of the affected area.[1]

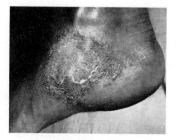

**Figure 23-6**

Athlete's foot (tinea pedis)

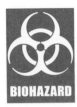

**Basic Care of Athlete's Foot**

- Keep the feet as dry as possible through frequent use of talcum powder.
- Wear clean white socks to avoid reinfection, changing them daily.
- Use a standard fungicide for specific medication. Over-the-counter medications such as Desenex and Tinactin are useful in the early stages of the infection. For stubborn cases see the team physician; a dermatologist may need to make a culture from foot scrapings to determine the best combatant to be used.

The best cure for athlete's foot is prevention. To keep the condition from spreading to other athletes, the following steps should be faithfully followed by individuals in the sports program:

- Powder the feet daily.
- Dry the feet thoroughly, especially between and under the toes, after every shower.
- Keep sports shoes and street shoes dry by dusting them with powder daily.
- Wear clean sports socks and street socks daily.
- Clean and disinfect the shower and dressing rooms daily.

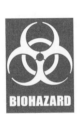

**Care**   Griseofulvin is the most effective medication for management of tinea pedis. Of major importance is good foot hygiene. Topical medications used for tinea corporis can be beneficial (Focus Box 23-2).[1]

## RESPIRATORY CONDITIONS

The respiratory tract is an organ system through which various communicable diseases can be transmitted.[26] It is commonly the port of entry for acute infectious diseases that are spread from person to person or by direct contact. Some of the more prevalent conditions affecting athletes are the common cold, sore throat, asthma, hay fever, and air pollution.

### The Common Cold

**Cause of condition**   Upper respiratory tract infections, especially colds and associated conditions, are common in the sports program and can play havoc with entire teams. The common cold is attributed to a filterable virus, which produces an infection of the upper respiratory tract of a susceptible individual.[21] The susceptible person is believed to be one who has, singly or in combination, any of the following characteristics:[41]

- Physical debilitation from overwork or lack of sleep.
- Chronic inflammation from a local infection.

- Inflammation of the nasal mucosa from an allergy.
- Inflammation of the nasal mucosa from breathing foreign substances such as dust.
- Sensitivity to stress.

**Symptoms of condition**    The onset of the common cold is usually rapid; symptoms vary among individuals. The typical effects are a general feeling of **malaise** with an accompanying headache, sneezing, and nasal discharge. Some individuals may register a fever of 100° to 102°F (38° to 39°C) and have chills. Various aches and pains may also accompany the symptoms. The nasal discharge starts as a watery secretion and gradually becomes thick and discolored from the inflammation.[21]

**Care**    Care of the cold is usually symptomatic, with emphasis on isolation, bed rest, and light eating. Medications include acetaminophen for relieving general discomfort, rhinitis tablets for drying the secreting mucosa, and nasal drops to relieve nasal congestion.[41] If a cough is present, various syrups may be given to afford relief. The athlete should avoid intense training while experiencing a severe respiratory infection. Intense training can suppress the immune system.[26]

| |
|---|
| **malaise** (muh **laze**) Discomfort and uneasiness caused by an illness. |

## Sinusitis

**Cause of condition**    Sinusitis is an inflammation of the nasal sinuses. Sinusitis can stem from an upper respiratory infection caused by a variety of bacteria. As a result, nasal mucous membranes swell and block the sinuses. A painful pressure occurs from an accumulation of mucus.

**Symptoms of condition**    The skin area over the sinus may be swollen and painful to the touch. The athlete may experience a headache and a feeling of being out of sorts.

**Care**    If an infection is present, antibiotics may be warranted. Nasal vasoconstrictors may be helpful in nasal drainage.

## Sore Throat (Pharyngitis)

**Cause of condition**    A sore throat, or pharyngitis, usually is the result of postnasal drip associated with a common cold or sinusitis. It may also be an indication of a more serious condition, including either viral or bacterial infection.

**Symptoms of condition**    Frequently the condition starts as a dryness in the throat and progresses to soreness with pain and swelling. It is sometimes accompanied by a headache, a fever of 101° to 102° F (38° to 39°C), chills, coughing, and a general feeling of fatigue. On examination the throat may appear dark red and swollen, and mucous membranes may be coated.

**Care**    In most cases bed rest is considered the best treatment, combined with symptomatic medications such as aspirin and a hot saltwater gargle. A physician may prescribe antibiotics if other measures are inadequate.

## Tonsillitis

**Etiology**   The tonsils are pieces of lymphatic tissue covered by epithelium that are found at the entrance of the pharynx. Within each tonsil are deep clefts, or pits, lined by lymphatic nodules. Ingested or inhaled pathogens collect in the pits and penetrate the epithelium, where they come in contact with lymphocytes and cause an acute inflammation and bacterial infection.[40] Complications include sinusitis, middle ear infections (otitis media), or tonsillar abcesses.

**Symptoms and signs**   The tonsils appear inflamed, red, and swollen with yellowish exudate in the pits. The athlete has difficulty swallowing and may have a relatively high fever with chills. Headache and pain in the neck and back may also be present.[26]

**Management**   The throat should be cultured to look for streptococcal bacteria, and if the culture is positive, antibiotics should be used for 10 days. Gargling with warm saline solution, a liquid diet, and antipyretic medication should all be recommended. Frequent bouts of tonsillitis may eventually necessitate surgical removal of the tonsils.

## Influenza

**Cause of condition**   Influenza, or the flu, is one of the most persistent and debilitating diseases. It usually occurs in various forms as an annual epidemic, causing severe illness among the populace.[36]

Influenza is caused by a virus that enters the tissue's cell through its genetic material. Within the tissue, the virus multiplies and is released from the cell by a budding process and is spread throughout the body. Not all athletes need influenza vaccines; however, athletes engaging in winter sports, basketball, wrestling, and swimming may require them.[25]

**Symptoms of condition**   The athlete with the flu has the following symptoms: fever, cough, headache, malaise, and inflamed respiratory mucous membranes with coryza. It should be noted that certain viruses can increase the body's core temperature. Flu generally has an incubation period of 48 hours and comes on suddenly, accompanied by chills and a fever of 102° to 103°F (39° to 39.5°C), which develop over a 24-hour period. The athlete complains of a headache and general aches and pains—mainly in the back and legs. The headache increases in intensity, along with photophobia and aching at the back of the skull. There is often a sore throat, burning in the chest, and in the beginning, a nonproductive cough, which later may develop into bronchitis. The skin is flushed, and the eyes are inflamed and watery. The acute stage of the disease usually lasts up to 5 days. Weakness, sweating, and fatigue may persist for many days.[27]

**Care**   Flu prevention includes staying away from infected persons, maintaining good resistance through healthy living, and annual vaccines. If the flu is uncomplicated, its management consists of bed rest. During the acute stage, the temperature often returns to normal. Symptomatic care such as acetaminophen, steam inhalation, cough medicines, and gargles may be given.[36]

## Seasonal Allergies (Rhinitis)

**Cause of condition** Hay fever is an acute seasonal allergic condition that results from airborne pollens. Hay fever can occur during the spring as a reaction to tree pollens such as oak, elm, maple, alder, birch, and cottonwood. During the summer, grass and weed pollens can be the culprits. In the fall, ragweed pollen is the prevalent cause. Airborne fungal spores also have been known to cause hay fever.[3]

**Symptoms of condition** In the early stages, the athlete's eyes, throat, mouth, and nose begin to itch, followed by watering of the eyes, sneezing, and a clear, watery, nasal discharge. In the later stages, the athlete may complain of a sinus-type headache, emotional irritability, difficulty in sleeping, red and swollen eyes and nasal mucous membranes, and a wheezing cough. It should be noted that other common adverse allergic conditions are asthma, **anaphylaxis**, **urticaria**, and **angioedema**.[3]

**Care** Most athletes obtain relief from hay fever through over-the-counter oral antihistamines. To avoid the problem of sedation stemming from these drugs, the athlete may ingest a decongestant during the day and a long-acting antihistamine before going to bed.[20]

## Acute Bronchitis

**Cause of condition** Bronchitis is an inflammation of the mucous membranes of the bronchial tubes. It occurs in both acute and chronic forms. Bronchitis in an athlete is more likely to be in the acute form. Acute bronchitis usually occurs as an infectious winter disease that follows a common cold or other viral infection of the upper respiratory region. Secondary to this inflammation is a bacterial infection that may follow overexposure to air pollution. Fatigue, malnutrition, and/or chills could be predisposing factors.[27]

**Symptoms of condition** The symptoms of an athlete with acute bronchitis usually start with an upper respiratory tract infection, nasal inflammation and profuse discharge, slight fever, sore throat, and back and muscle pains. A cough signals the beginning of bronchitis. In the beginning, the cough is dry, but in a few hours or days, a clear mucous secretion begins, becoming yellowish, indicating an infection. In most cases, the fever lasts 3 to 5 days, and the cough lasts 2 to 3 weeks or longer. The athlete may wheeze and rale when auscultation of the chest is performed. Pneumonia can complicate bronchitis.[27]

**Care** To avoid bronchitis, an athlete should not sleep in an area that is extremely cold or exercise in extremely cold air without wearing a face mask to warm inhaled air. Management of acute bronchitis involves rest until fever subsides, drinking three to four glasses of water per day, and taking an antifever medication, a cough suppressor, and an antibiotic (when severe lung infection is present) daily.

---

**anaphylaxis**
An immediate transcient allergic reaction resulting in swelling of tissues and dilation of capillaries.

**urticaria**
Sudden vascular reaction of skin resulting in wheals or papules and itching.

**angioedema**
A well defined area of swelling, occurring as a result of an allergic response.

**rhinitis** (rye **nye** tis)
Inflammation of the nasal mucous lining.

The athlete undergoing a
sudden asthma attack should
• be relaxed and reassured.
• use a previously specified
  medication.
• drink water.
• perform controlled
  breathing.
• be removed from what
  might be triggering the
  attack.

## Bronchial Asthma

**Cause of condition**   As one of the most common respiratory diseases, bronchial asthma can be produced from a number of stressors, such as a viral respiratory tract infection, emotional upset, changes in barometric pressure or temperature, exercise, inhalation of a noxious odor, or exposure to a specific allergen.[31]

**Symptoms of condition**   Bronchial asthma is characterized by a spasm of the bronchial smooth muscles, edema, and inflammation of the mucous lining. In addition to asthma's narrowing of the airway, copious amounts of mucus are produced. Difficulty in breathing may cause the athlete to hyperventilate, resulting in dizziness. The attack may begin with coughing, wheezing, shortness of breath, and fatigue[31] (Focus Box 23-3).

**Care**   Prevention should include efforts to identify and control the causative factors. Acute attacks can be managed by using physician-prescribed medications administered through inhalers. Relief from an inhaler usually occurs in a matter of minutes. If breathing difficulty persists, the athlete should be taken to an emergency care facility.

## Exercise-Induced Asthma (EIA)

**Cause of condition**   Exercise-induced asthma (EIA) is also known as exercise-induced bronchial obstruction.[33] It is a disease that occurs almost exclusively in asthmatic persons. An asthmatic attack can be stimulated by exercise in some individuals and can be provoked in others, only on rare occasions, during moderate exercise.[12] The exact cause of EIA is not clear. Loss of heat and water causes the greatest loss of airway reactivity. Eating certain foods such as shrimp, celery, and peanuts can cause EIA. Sinusitis can also trigger an attack in an individual with chronic asthma.[42]

**Symptoms of condition**   The athlete with EIA may show signs of swelling of the face, swelling of the palms and soles of the feet, chest tightness, shortness of breath, coughing, nausea, hypertension, diarrhea, fatigue, itching, respiratory stridor (high-pitched noise on respiration), headaches, and redness of the skin.[42]

**Care**   Long, continuous running causes the most severe bronchospasm. Swimming is the least bronchospasm producing, which may be because of the moist, warm air environment. A regular exercise program can benefit asthmatics and nonasthmatics.[12] Fewer symptoms occur with short, intense work followed by rest than occur with sustained exercise. There should be a gradual warm-up and cooldown. The duration of exercise should build slowly to 30 to 40 minutes four or five times a week. Exercise intensity and loading also should be graduated slowly. An example is 10 to 30 seconds of work followed by 30 to 90 seconds of rest.[33] Many athletes with chronic asthma and/or EIA use an inhaled bronchodilator (Figure 23-7). Metered-dose inhalers are preferred for administration. It has also been found that prophylactic use

23-3 *Focus Box*

### Management of the Acute Asthmatic Attack

Athletes who have a history of asthma usually know how to care for themselves when an attack occurs. However, the athletic trainer must be aware of what to look for and what to do if called on.

Early symptoms and signs

- Anxious appearance
- Sweating and paleness
- Flared nostrils
- Breathing with pursed lips
- Fast breathing
- Vomiting
- Hunched-over body posture
- Physical fatigue unrelated to activity
- Indentation in the notch below the Adam's apple
- Sinking in of rib spaces as the athlete inhales
- Coughing for no apparent reason
- Excess throat clearing
- Irregular, labored breathing or wheezing

Actions to take

- Attempt to relax and reassure the athlete.
- If medication has been cleared by the team physician, have the athlete use it.
- Encourage the athlete to drink water.
- Place in a semireclining position to make breathing easier.
- Have the athlete perform controlled breathing along with relaxation exercises.
- If an environmental factor triggering the attack is known, remove it or the athlete from the area.
- If these procedures do not help, immediate medical attention may be necessary.

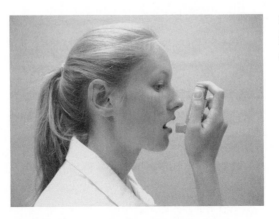

**Figure 23-7**

Position for using a metered-dose inhaler

**Using a Metered-Dose Inhaler**

A metered-dose inhaler includes a pressurized canister with measured doses of medication inside. The athlete squeezes the top of the canister. The pressure within the canister converts the medication into a fine powder. The athlete places his or her lips on or near the inhaler's mouthpiece to inhale the mist. Using a metered-dose inhaler calls for coordinating two actions: squeezing the canister and inhaling the medication (Figure 23-7). Many individuals who use the metered-dose inhaler use it improperly; however, with careful and repeated instruction, more than 90 percent of people can use it correctly. Metered dose inhalers can use a spacer, which is a tube four to eight inches long that attaches to the inhaler that allows time to inhale more slowly. The spacer acts as a holding chamber that keeps medication from escaping into the air.

People with asthma can rely too much on inhaled bronchodilators. Because these fast-acting medications can relieve symptoms quickly, there is a tendency particularly among athletes to use them too often, leading to an overdose.[33]

of the bronchodilator 15 minutes before exercise delays the symptoms by 2 to 4 hours.[42] Focus Box 23-4 discusses using a metered-dose inhaler. Asthmatic athletes who receive medication for their condition should make sure that what they take is legal for competition. They should also be certain that they always have their inhaler with them in case of an emergency. *Remind the athletes who have asthma that they need to be responsible for having their inhalers with them or at least accessible at all times.*[12]

## GASTROINTESTINAL DISORDERS

Like any other individual, the athlete may develop various complaints associated with the digestive system. The athlete may display various disorders of the gastrointestinal tract as a result of poor eating habits or the stress related to competition.[5] It is important to recognize the more severe conditions so that early referrals to a physician can be made. It is also essential to make certain that with all of these gastrointestinal problems, the athlete replaces fluids and electrolytes to prevent dehydration.

### Indigestion

A balanced diet is as important as brushing the teeth in preventing gum disease.

**Cause of condition**    Indigestion (dyspepsia) can be caused by any number of conditions, including food idiosyncrasies, emotional stress before competition, esophageal and stomach spasms, and/or inflammation of the mucous lining of the esophagus and stomach.[14]

**Symptoms of condition**    Indigestion can cause sour stomach, nausea, and flatulence (gas).

**Care**  Care of acute dyspepsia involves the elimination of irritating foods from the diet, development of regular eating habits, and avoidance of anxieties that may lead to gastric distress.

## Vomiting

**Cause of condition**  Vomiting results from some type of irritation, most often in the stomach, that stimulates the vomiting center in the brain to cause a series of forceful contractions of the diaphragm and abdominal muscles, compressing the stomach and forcefully expelling the contents.[14]

**Care**  Antinausea medications should be administered. Fluids to prevent dehydration should be administered by mouth if possible. If vomiting persists, fluids and electrolytes must be administered intravenously.

## Diarrhea

**Cause of condition**  Diarrhea can be caused by problems in diet, inflammation of the intestinal lining, gastrointestinal infection, ingestion of certain drugs, and psychogenic factors.

**Symptoms of condition**  Diarrhea is characterized by abdominal cramps, nausea, and possibly vomiting coupled with frequent elimination of stools. Extreme weakness caused by fluid dehydration is usually present. The cause of diarrhea is often difficult to establish.

**Care**  Less severe cases can be cared for by omitting foods that cause irritation, eating bland food until symptoms have ceased, and using over-the-counter medications to control intestinal activity. The BRAT diet, which consists of bananas, rice, apples, and toast, has been recommended.

*Indigestion, vomiting, diarrhea, and constipation are common problems in the athlete.*

## Constipation

**Cause of condition**  Constipation can be caused by insufficient moisture in the feces, causing it to be hard and dry, lack of sufficient roughage and bulk in the diet, poor bowel habits, nervousness and anxiety, or overuse of laxatives and enemas.[14]

**Symptoms of condition**  There is occasional intense cramping and pain in the lower abdomen, with difficulty eliminating hard-packed stools.

**Care**  Athletes can eliminate constipation by eating cereals, fruits, vegetables, and fats that stimulate bowel movement. Laxatives or enemas should be avoided unless prescribed by a physician.

## Food Poisoning

**Cause of condition**  Food poisoning (gastroenteritis), which may range from mild to severe, results from infectious organisms (bacteria) that enter the body in either food or drink. Foods become contaminated by improper food refrigeration or from an infected food handler.

**Symptoms of condition**  Infection results in nausea, vomiting, cramps, and diarrhea that usually subside in 3 to 6 hours.

**Care**   The athlete should be referred to a physician. Management requires rapid replacement of lost fluids and electrolytes, which in severe cases may need to be replaced intravenously. If tolerated, light fluids or foods such as clear, strained broth, bouillon, or bland cereals may be given.

### Gastrointestinal Bleeding

**Cause of condition**   Gastrointestinal bleeding that is reflected in bloody stools can be caused by gastritis, iron-deficiency anemia, ingestion of aspirin or other anti-inflammatory agents, colitis, or even stress and bowel irritation. Distance runners often have blood in their stools during and following a race.

**Care**   Athletes with gastrointestinal bleeding must be referred immediately to a physician.

## OTHER CONDITIONS THAT CAN AFFECT THE ATHLETE

### Infectious Mononucleosis

**Cause of condition**   Infectious mononucleosis is an acute viral disease that affects mainly young adults and children. It has major significance to athletes because it can produce severe fatigue and raise the risk of spleen rupture.[30] Incubation is 4 to 6 weeks. The virus is carried in the throat and transmitted to another person by saliva. It has been called the "kissing disease."[30]

**Symptoms of condition**   The disease usually starts with a 3- to 5-day period of headache, fatigue, loss of appetite, and general muscle ache. From the fifth to the fifteenth day, there is fever, swollen lymph glands, and a sore throat.[30] By the second week, 50 to 70 percent of those infected have an enlarged spleen, 10 to 15 percent have jaundice, and 5 to 15 percent have a skin rash, a pinkish flush to the cheeks, and puffy eyelids.[21]

The spleen should not be
enlarged when the athlete
returns to practice and
competition.

**Care**   Care of mononucleosis is supportive and symptomatic. In many cases the athlete with this disease may resume easy training in 3 weeks after the onset of illness if (1) the spleen is not markedly enlarged or painful; (2) the athlete is without a fever; (3) liver function tests are normal; and (4) the sore throat and any other complications have been resolved.[30]

### Anemia in Athletes

#### Iron-Deficiency Anemia

**Cause of condition**   Iron deficiency is the most common form of true anemia among athletes.[10] It occurs as the result of low levels of **hemoglobin** (the oxygen-carrying molecules in blood) and also of red blood cells (hematocrit). For men, iron deficiency is usually caused by blood loss in the gastrointestinal tract. For women, the most common

**hemoglobin**
Molecules that carry oxygen
in blood.

causes are menstruation and not taking in enough iron in the diet. Athletes who are vegetarians might lack iron.

**Symptoms of condition** In the first stages of iron deficiency, the athlete's performance begins to decline. The athlete may complain of feeling tired and lethargic. During training there may also be complaints of muscle fatigue and nausea. Athletes with mild iron-deficiency anemia may display some mild impairment in their maximum performance.

**Care** The athlete with symptoms of anemia should be sent to a physician for blood work to determine the level of hemoglobin and the hematocrit. It is important to differentiate anemia from mononucleosis because symptoms are similar. Some ways that athletes can manage iron deficiency are to (1) follow a proper diet, including more red meat or dark chicken; (2) avoid coffee or tea, which hamper iron absorption from grains; (3) ingest vitamin C sources, which enhance iron absorption; and (4) take an iron supplement.

### Sickle-Cell Anemia

**Cause of condition** Sickle-cell anemia is a chronic hereditary anemia. The red blood cell with an abnormal sickle shape has less potential for transporting oxygen and is more fragile than normal cells. A sickle cell's life span is 15 to 25 days, compared to the 120-day life span of a normal red cell; this short life of the sickle cell can produce severe anemia in individuals with acute sickle-cell anemia. Approximately 35 percent of the black population in the United States has this condition; 8 to 13 percent are not anemic but carry this trait in their genes (sicklemia).[11] The person with the sickle-cell trait may participate in sports and never encounter problems until symptoms are brought on by some unusual circumstance.[11]

**Symptoms of condition** An athlete may never experience any complications from having the sickle-cell trait. However, a sickle-cell crisis can be brought on by exposure to high altitudes or by elevated body temperature. Crisis symptoms include fever, severe fatigue, skin pallor, muscle weakness, and severe pain in the limbs and abdomen. Abdominal pain in the right upper quadrant is somewhat common. The athlete may also experience headache and convulsions.[11]

**Care** Treatment of a sickle-cell crisis is usually symptomatic. The physician may elect to give anticoagulants and analgesics for pain.

### Diabetes Mellitus

**Cause of condition** Diabetes mellitus is a complex hereditary or developmental disease involving some imbalance between blood sugar and the hormone insulin, which is produced by the pancreas. Decreased effectiveness of insulin or an insufficient amount is responsible for most cases of diabetes. Until recently diabetics were usually discouraged from or forbidden competitive sports participation. Today an ever-increasing number of diabetics are active sports participants, functioning effectively in almost all sports. Because the key to the control of diabetes is the control of blood sugar, the insulin-dependent athlete must constantly juggle food intake, insulin, and exercise to maintain blood sugar in its proper range if he or she is to perform at maximum levels. Diet, exercise, and insulin are the major factors in the everyday lifestyle of the diabetic athlete, who out of necessity must develop an ordered and specific living pattern to cope with the demands of daily existence and strenuous physical activity.[8]

Diabetic athletes engaging in vigorous physical activity should eat before exercising and, if the exercise is protracted, should have hourly glucose supplementation. As a rule the insulin dosage is not changed, but food intake is increased. The response of diabetics varies among individuals and depends on many variables. Although there are some hazards, with proper medical evaluation and planning by a consultant in metabolic diseases, diabetics can feel free to engage in most physical activities.[40]

Problems in the diabetic athlete result either in insulin shock, in which there is too little blood sugar relative to insulin, or in diabetic coma, in which there is too much blood sugar and not enough insulin. Those who work with athletes who have diabetes mellitus must be aware of the major symptoms of diabetic coma and insulin shock and of the proper actions to take when either one occurs.[8]

**Symptoms of insulin shock** Insulin shock occurs when there is too little blood sugar, resulting in hypoglycemia and shock. It is characterized by physical weakness, moist and pale skin, drooping eyelids, and normal or shallow respirations.

**Care for insulin shock** The diabetic athlete who either forgets to eat or who engages in intense exercise and metabolizes large amounts of glycogen is more likely to experience insulin shock.[8] To avoid this problem, the athlete must adhere to a carefully planned diet that includes a snack before exercise.[2] The snack should contain a combination of a complex carbohydrate and a protein, for example, cheese and crackers. Activities that last for more than 30 to 40 minutes should be accompanied by snacks and simple carbohydrates. Some diabetics carry with them a lump of sugar or have candy or orange juice readily available in the event that an insulin reaction seems imminent.[40]

Key questions to ask a diabetic athlete are:

- Have you eaten today and when?
- Have you taken your insulin today and when?

**Symptoms of diabetic coma** The signs of a diabetic coma develop slowly over a 24 hour period and include labored breathing or gasping for air, fruity-smelling breath (caused by acetone), nausea and vomiting, extreme thirst, dry mucous lining of the mouth, flushed skin, and mental confusion or unconsciousness followed by coma.

**Care for diabetic coma** Because the diabetic coma threatens life, early detection is essential. The only way to correct the insulin–blood sugar imbalance of a diabetic coma is to inject insulin. An injection of insulin into the athlete normally prevents coma. If the athlete does not respond within minutes following injection, emergency care is needed.[2]

## Epilepsy

**Cause of condition**   Epilepsy is not a disease but is a symptom manifested by a large number of underlying disorders.[6] Some types of epilepsy involve a genetic predisposition and a low threshold to having seizures. In others, altered brain metabolism or a history of injury may be the cause.

Each person with epilepsy must individually consider whether he or she should engage in competitive sports.[6] The general recommendation is that an individual who has daily or even weekly major seizures should not participate in collision sports. This prohibition is not because a hit in the head necessarily triggers a seizure, but because unconsciousness during participation could result in a serious injury.[15] If the seizures are properly controlled by medication or only occur during sleep, little if any sports restriction should be imposed except for scuba diving, swimming alone, or participation in activities at some height.[39]

**Symptoms of condition**   Epilepsy is defined as "a recurrent disorder of cerebral function characterized by a sudden, brief attack of altered consciousness, motor activity, sensory phenomena, or inappropriate behavior." A seizure can range from extremely brief episodes (petit mal seizures) to major episodes (grand mal seizures), unconsciousness, and tonic-clonic muscle contractions.[39]

**Care**   The athlete commonly takes an anticonvulsant medication that is specific for the type and degree of seizures that occur. On occasion an athlete may experience some undesirable side effects from drug therapy, such as drowsiness, restlessness, nystagmus, nausea, vomiting, problems with balance, skin rash, or other adverse reactions.[39]

When an athlete with epilepsy becomes aware of an impending seizure, he or she should immediately sit or lie down to avoid injury. When a seizure occurs without warning, the following steps should be taken:[15]

- Be emotionally composed.
- If possible, cushion the athlete's fall.
- Keep the athlete away from surrounding objects that may cause injury.
- Loosen restricting clothing.
- Do not try to force anything between the athlete's teeth.
- Allow the athlete to awaken normally after the seizure.

## Meningitis

**Cause of condition**   Meningitis is an inflammation of the meninges, or membranes, that surround the spinal cord and brain that

*Individuals who have major daily or weekly seizures may be prohibited from collision sports.*

Athletes should not share
water bottles because of the
chances of transmitting
meningitis.

is caused by infection, usually from the meningococcus bacteria. Bacteria may enter the central nervous system through the nose or throat following infections of the ear, throat, or respiratory tract. The bacteria get into the meninges, and inflammation spreads to the adjacent nervous tissue, causing swelling of the brain, enlargement of the ventricles, and hemorrhage of the brain stem. Meningitis is a serious disease in children; it usually occurs between the ages of three months and two years.

**Symptoms of condition**   Symptoms include a high fever, stiff neck, intense headache, and sensitivity to light and sound, and they progress to vomiting, convulsions, and coma.

**Care**   If the symptoms of meningitis appear, immediately get the athlete to a physician. The cerebrospinal fluid (CSF) must be analyzed for bacteria and the presence of white blood cells. CSF is taken through a puncture in the lumbar area, or spinal tap. If meningococcus bacteria are identified, isolation is necessary for at least 24 hours due to their highly contagious nature. Intravenous antibiotics must begin immediately. Because of the severity of this condition, the patient should be monitored and treated in an intensive care unit.

## Hypertension (High Blood Pressure)

Hypertension may be a factor
that excludes players from
sports participation.

**Cause of condition**   Hypertension is classified as primary, or essential, and secondary.[7] Primary hypertension accounts for 90 percent of all cases and has no disease associated with it. Secondary hypertension is related to a specific underlying cause, such as kidney disorder, overactive adrenal glands (increased blood volume), hormone-producing tumor, narrowing of the aorta, pregnancy, and medications (oral contraceptives, cold remedies, etc.). The presence of prolonged high blood pressure increases the chances of premature mortality and morbidity due to such causes as coronary artery disease, congestive heart failure, and stroke.[7]

**Symptoms of condition**   Primary hypertension is usually asymptomatic until complications occur.[28] High blood pressure may cause dizziness, flushed appearance, headache, fatigue, epistaxis, and nervousness.

**Care**   The upper range of normal blood pressure is a systolic pressure of 120 mm/Hg and a diastolic pressure of 80 mm/Hg. The risk of death from heart disease and stroke begins to rise at blood pressures as low as 115 over 75, and it doubles for each 20 over 10 mm/Hg increase. Blood pressure is classified as follows: normal—less than 120/less than 80 mm/Hg; prehypertension—120–139/80–89 mm/Hg; stage 1 hypertension—140–159/90–99 mm/Hg; stage 2 hypertension—at or greater than 160/at or greater than 100 mm/Hg (Table 23-1).[28] Medication is not recommended for those with prehypertension unless it is required by another condition, such as diabetes or chronic kidney disease. However, those with prehypertension should make any needed lifestyle changes, including losing excess weight, becoming physically

**TABLE 23-1** Classifying Blood Pressure

| Blood Pressure Classification | Systolic (mm/Hg) | | Diastolic (mm/Hg) |
|---|---|---|---|
| Normal | less than 120 | and | less than 80 |
| Prehypertension | 120–139 | or | 80–89 |
| **High** | | | |
| Stage 1 | 140–159 | or | 90–99 |
| Stage 2 | 160 or higher | or | 100 or higher |

active, limiting alcoholic beverages, quitting smoking, and following a heart-healthy eating plan. It is recommended that those who have Stage 1 or 2 hypertension should also be on medication.[28]

## Common Contagious Viral Diseases

It is not within the scope of this text to describe in detail all the various infectious diseases to which athletes may be prone. However, on occasion the athlete may exhibit recognizable manifestations of such a disease; a coach should be aware of certain signs that might indicate a contagious viral disease (Table 23-2). When indications of a contagious disease are present, the athlete should be referred to a physician without delay.[13]

## CANCER

### Testicular Cancer

**Cause of condition**   Testicular cancer is the most common cancer in American males between the ages of 15 and 34. Although the exact cause of testicular cancer is unknown, several factors seem to increase risk including a past medical history of undescended testicle(s), abnormal testicular development, low levels of male hormones, sterility, development or previous testicular cancer, or family history of testicular cancer. Cancer usually affects only one testicle.[35]

**Symptoms of condition**   Testicular cancer can result in pain or discomfort in a testicle or the scrotum, a lump or enlargement in either testicle, swelling or sudden collection of fluid in the scrotum, a feeling of heaviness in the scrotum, a dull ache in the abdomen or groin, unexplained fatigue, and/or enlargement or tenderness of the breasts.[35]

**Care**   Testicular cancer is highly treatable when diagnosed early. Depending on the type and stage of testicular cancer, a patient may receive one of several treatments, including surgical removal of the testicle, chemotherapy or radiation therapy, or a combination. Regular testicular self-examinations can help identify dangerous growths early, when the chance for successful treatment of testicular cancer is highest.

**TABLE 23-2** Some Infectious Viral Diseases

| Disease | Sites Involved | Signs of Conditions | Care | Prevention |
|---|---|---|---|---|
| Measles (rubeola) | Skin, respiratory tract, and conjunctivae | Appearance—like common cold with fever, cough, conjunctivitis, photophobia, and spots in throat, followed by skin rash | Bed rest and use of smoked glasses; symptomatic | Vaccine available |
| German measles (rubella) | Skin, respiratory tract, and conjunctivae | Cold symptoms, skin rash, and swollen lymph nodes behind ear | Symptomatic | Vaccine available; gamma globulin given in postexposure situations |
| Chicken pox (varicella) | Trunk; then face, neck, and limbs | Mild cold symptoms followed by appearance of vesicles | Symptomatic | Vaccine available, including zoster immune globulin (ZIG) or varicell-zoster immune globulin (VZIG) |
| Mumps (epidemic parotiditis) | Salivary glands | Headache, drowsiness, fever, abdominal pain, pain during chewing and swallowing, swelling of neck under jaw | Symptomatic | Temporary immunization by virus vaccine |
| Influenza (flu) | Respiratory tract | Aching of low back, generalized aching, chills, headache, fever, and bronchitis | Symptomatic | Moderate temporary protection from polyvalent influenza virus |
| Cold (coryza) | Respiratory tract | Mild fever, headache, chills, and nasal discharge | Symptomatic | Possible help from vitamins and/or cold vaccine; avoid exposure |
| Infectious mononucleosis | Trunk | Sore throat, fever, skin rash, general aching, and swelling of lymph glands | Symptomatic | None; avoid extreme fatigue |

## Breast Cancer

**Cause of condition**   Breast cancer is the most common type of cancer in women and is the second leading cause of death by cancer in women. Breast cancer may occur at any age, though the risk of breast cancer increases with age. Family history has long been known to be a risk factor for breast cancer. The risk is highest if the affected relative developed breast cancer at a young age, had cancer in both breasts, or if she is a close relative. Hormonal influences play a role in the development of breast cancer. The most common place for breast cancer to metastasize is into the lymph nodes under the arm or to the brain, the bones, and the liver.[35]

**Symptoms of condition**   In the early stages breast cancer usually has no symptoms and is not painful. Quite often breast cancer is discovered before symptoms are present, either by feeling a lump on the breast or in the armpit or by finding an abnormality on mammography.[35]

**Care** Self breast exams should be done frequently. Not all lumps are malignant but all should be evaluated by a physician who may use mammogram, MRI, ultrasound, or biopsy. If a malignancy is found, surgery is the primary treatment for breast cancer. Additional treatments may include radiation therapy, chemotherapy, or hormonal therapy.

## MENSTRUAL IRREGULARITIES AND THE FEMALE REPRODUCTIVE SYSTEM

During the prepubertal period, girls are the equal of, and are often superior to, boys of the same age in activities requiring speed, strength, and endurance. The difference between males and females is not readily apparent until after puberty. At puberty males begin to exhibit a slow, gradual increase in strength, speed, and endurance.

Menarche, the onset of the menses, normally occurs between the tenth and the seventeenth year, and the majority of girls enter it between 13 and 15 years of age. There is some indication that strenuous training and competition may delay the onset of menarche. The greatest delay is related to higher caliber competition. The late-maturing girl commonly has longer legs, narrower hips, and less adiposity and body weight for her height, all of which are more conducive to sports.[22]

As interest and participation in girls' and women's sports grow, the various myths that have surrounded female participation and the effects of participation on menarche, menstruation, and childbirth are gradually being dispelled. The effects of sustained and strenuous training and competition on the menstrual cycle and the effects of menstruation on performance, however, still cannot be fully explained.

> During the prepubertal period, girls are the equal of, and are often superior to, boys of the same age in activities requiring speed, strength, and endurance.

> The onset of menarche may be delayed by strenuous training and competition.

### Menstrual Irregularities

Menarche may be delayed in highly physically active women. **Amenorrhea** (absence of menses) and *oligomenorrhea* (diminished flow) have been common in professional female ballet dancers, gymnasts, and long-distance runners.[17] Runners who decrease training, because of an injury for example, often report a return of regular menses. Weight gain together with less intense exercise also is reported to reverse amenorrhea and oligomenorrhea. Because these irregularities may or may not be normal aspects of thinness and hard physical training, it is advisable that a physician be consulted. To date, there is no indication that these conditions adversely affect reproduction. Almost any type of menstrual disorder can be caused by overly stressful and demanding sports activity—amenorrhea, dysmenorrhea, menorrhagia (excessive menstruation), oligomenorrhea, polymenorrhea (abnormal frequent menstruation), irregular periods, or any combination of these.[17]

> **amenorrhea**
> (amen oh **ree** ah)
> Absence or suppression of menstruation.

Women who have moderate
to severe dysmenorrhea
require examination by a
physician.

## Dysmenorrhea

Dysmenorrhea (painful menstruation) apparently is prevalent among more active women; however, it is inconclusive whether specific sports participation can alleviate or produce dysmenorrhea. For women with moderate to severe dysmenorrhea, gynecological consultation is warranted to rule out a pathological condition.[22]

Dysmenorrhea is caused by ischemia (a lack of normal blood flow to the pelvic organs) or by a possible hormonal imbalance. This syndrome, which is identified by cramps, nausea, lower abdominal pain, headache, and, on occasion, emotional lability, is the most common menstrual disorder. Physicians usually prescribe mild to vigorous exercises that help ameliorate dysmenorrhea. Physicians also generally advise a continuance of the usual sports participation during the menstrual period, provided the performance level of the individual does not drop below her customary level of ability. Among athletes, swimmers have the highest incidence of dysmenorrhea; it occurs most often, quite probably, as the result of strenuous sports participation during the menses. Generally, oligomenorrhea, amenorrhea, and irregular or scanty flow are more common in sports that require strenuous exertion over a long period. A great deal of variability exists among female athletes with regard to the menstrual pattern and its effect on physical performance. Each individual must learn to make adjustments to her lifestyle that permits her to function effectively and efficiently with a minimum of discomfort or restriction.

**23-3 Critical Thinking**
Exercise

A female athlete has been diagnosed as having both an eating disorder and amenorrhea.

? Why may these two medical disorders eventually be associated with osteoporosis?

## The Female Athletic Triad

A young female athlete, driven to excel in her chosen sport and pressured to fit a specific athletic image to reach her goals, is at risk for the development of the *female athletic triad*.[15] It is a combination of three medical disorders including *disordered eating*, *amenorrhea*, and *osteoporosis*, a bone disease marked by softening and decreased density.[19] Focus Box 23-5 identifies lifestyle habits that may place a woman at risk for female athletic triad.

---

**23-5** **Focus Box**

**Identifying a Woman at Risk for Female Athletic Triad**

- Compulsive exercise for more than 1 hour a day beyond that normally required as part of practice and competition.
- Cannot skip a day of exercise.
- Restricts the amounts and kind of foods consumed.
- Eats alone most of the time.
- Thinks and talks a lot about food and body weight.
- Seems depressed.
- Has excessive injuries related to activity.
- Irregular or absent menstrual periods.

Disordered eating can include any combination of anorexia, bulimia, and/or excessive exercise.[19] It can lead to malnutrition, which obviously has a negative impact on the ability of the female to perform athletically. In addition, chronic fatigue, compromise of the immune system, and often depression have been associated with disordered eating. Certainly disordered eating can lead to serious illness and even death.[19]

Amenorrhea is the absence of the menstrual cycle for more than 6 months. Normal hormonal cycles stop when body weight is too low. Normal estrogen levels are essential for bones to use calcium. A decrease in estrogen levels also interferes with the activity of bone-producing cells, which eventually causes the bones to become weak and increases the likelihood of stress fracture.[19]

Osteoporosis includes not only bone loss but also new bone formation. Fractures can occur in the hip, spine, foot, or other sites without any visible evidence.

The effects of female athletic triad can be reversed by returning to normal exercise and eating patterns that allow for return of normal menstrual periods thus preventing further bone loss.[23]

## Contraceptives

Female athletes have been known to take extra oral contraceptive pills to delay menstruation during competition. This practice is not recommended because the pills should be taken no more than 21 days, followed by a 7-day break. Side effects range from nausea, vomiting, fluid retention, and amenorrhea to the extreme effects of hypertension and double vision. Some oral contraceptives make women hypersensitive to the sun. Any use of oral contraceptives related to physical performance should be under the express direction and control of a physician. However, oral contraceptive use is acceptable for females with no medical problems who have coitus at least twice a week. New low-dose preparations, containing less than 50 mg of estrogen, add negligible risks for the healthy woman.[17]

## Exercise During Pregnancy

During pregnancy, athletes exhibit high levels of muscle tonicity. Women who suffer from a chronic disability after childbirth usually have a record of little or no physical exercise in the decade immediately preceding pregnancy.[4] Generally, competition may be engaged in well into the third month of pregnancy unless bleeding or cramps are present and can frequently be continued until the seventh month if no handicapping or physiological complications arise. Such activity may make pregnancy, childbirth, and postparturition less stressful. Many athletes do not continue beyond the third month because of a drop in their performance that can result from a number of reasons, some related to their pregnancy, others perhaps psychological. It is during the first 3 months of pregnancy that the dangers of disturbing the pregnancy are greatest. After that period there is less danger to the mother and fetus because the pregnancy is stabilized. There is no indication that mild to moderate exercise during pregnancy is harmful to fetal growth and development or causes reduced fetal mass, increased perinatal or neonatal mortality, or physical or mental retardation.[4] It has been found, however, that extreme exercise may lower birth weight.

Many athletes compete during pregnancy with no ill effects. Most physicians, although advocating moderate activity during this period, believe that especially vigorous performance, particularly in activities in which there may be severe body contact or heavy jarring or falls, should be avoided.

## SEXUALLY TRANSMITTED INFECTIONS (STIs)

Sexually transmitted infections (STIs) are of major concern in sports because many athletes are at an age during which they are more sexually active than they will be at any other time in their lives. While it is true that STIs do not occur with participation in sport activities, because of the personal relationships that exist between coaches, fitness professionals, health care providers, and athletes, some understanding of how these infections can affect an individual athlete is warranted. Sexually transmitted infections are infectious diseases that can be contracted through sexual contact. Any of the STIs can potentially be transmitted through sexual contact (including vaginal and anal intercourse and oral-genital contact) with an infected partner who may or may not show any signs or symptoms. STIs may be caused by bacteria or viruses. Bacterial infections such as gonorrhea, syphilis, and chlamydia may be cured with antibiotics in the majority of cases. Serious health problems are prevented if these infections are diagnosed and treated early. Viral infections such as herpes, genital warts, and HIV are much more difficult to treat, and in some cases no cure exists.

STIs do not go away by themselves, and in many cases, relatively quick, painless treatments are available. No one is immune to STIs. Everyone who is sexually active can get or transmit an STI. The current trend is to emphasize prevention through "safer sex" practices and treatment of STIs rather than focus on the ethics of sexual behavior. Most important, some of these diseases have the potential to cause serious, long-term health problems, even death.

Table 23-3 discusses the common STIs, their symptoms, treatment, and potential effects.

## SUMMARY

- Most common skin infections in athletes are caused by viruses, bacteria, and fungi. Viral infections include herpes simplex (e.g., the cold sore) and herpes zoster. The two most common types of bacterial infections are streptococcus and staphylococcus. Ringworm, or tinea, is the fungus infection commonly attacking all areas of the body; tinea pedis (athlete's foot) is the most common.

**TABLE 23-3** Sexually Transmitted Infections

| STI | Signs | Care | Possible Problems |
|---|---|---|---|
| Chlamydia | About 75% of infected people have no symptoms. However, there may be a mild mucuslike discharge from the genitals or stinging when urinating. Also, there may be pain in the testicles (men) or abdomen (women). | Infected persons and their sexual partners must be tested and treated with antibiotics. | Painful infections of the reproductive organs, which may lead to infertility in both men and women. |
| Genital herpes | Sores around genitals or anus, often with small, painful blisters. Some people have no symptoms but are still infected and contagious. | Infected persons should avoid intimate sexual contact while sores persist. Acyclovir capsules or ointment may be helpful but will not cure herpes. | May contribute to cervical cancer and be transmitted to infants during childbirth. |
| Crab lice | Visible, blood-sucking lice in pubic hair. Causes itching. Eggs (nits) attached to hair shafts. | Treatments to kill lice. Recent sexual partners, clothing, and bed linen should be treated. | None. |
| Genital warts | Usually painless growths around the genitals or anus occur about 1–3 months after contact. In rare cases, growths may itch, burn, or bleed, or may not appear for years. | Chemical treatment, liquid nitrogen, laser beam, or surgery. May return after treatment. | May obstruct the urethra or complicate vaginal delivery in childbirth; may be connected to cervical cancer. |
| Trichomoniasis | Among women, symptoms may include a vaginal discharge, discomfort during sexual intercourse, abdominal pain, pain when urinating, and itching in the genital area. Most men have no symptoms, but some men may experience a penile discharge, painful urinating, or a "tingly" feeling in the penis. | Infected persons and their partners are treated with antibiotics. | If untreated, may lead to bladder and urethral infections in men and women. |
| Gonorrhea | Men may have a creamy puslike penile discharge and pain when urinating, or they may have no symptoms. Women may have vaginal discharge and pain when urinating, but often have no symptoms. | Infected persons and their sexual partners must be tested and treated with antibiotics. | If untreated, can cause arthritis, dermatitis, heart problems, and reproductive problems in both men and women. Can be transmitted to infants at birth, causing blindness. |
| Syphilis | Painless ulcer (chancre) at point of contact, usually penile shaft, around vaginal opening, or anus. Secondary stage may include rash or swollen lymph nodes. | Infected persons and their sexual partners must be tested and treated with antibiotics. | If untreated, may affect brain or heart, or even be fatal. Pregnant women can transmit to unborn infants. |
| AIDS (Acquired immunodeficiency syndrome) | Increased susceptibility to common infections and unusual cancers. Most people infected with the virus may show no symptoms for many years but are still contagious. | No current proven treatment. Avoid sexual contact or practice safe sex. | Full-blown AIDS almost always is fatal. Outlook for carriers of the virus is uncertain. |

For more information on HIV/AIDS, see Chapter 8.

- The common cold, sinusitis, sore throat, hay fever, and asthma are respiratory tract illnesses that can adversely affect the athlete. Asthma can be chronic (e.g., bronchial) or induced by physical activity. Care of the athlete who is having an acute asthmatic attack requires an understanding of the early symptoms and signs and responding accordingly.

- A number of conditions of the digestive system, such as diarrhea, vomiting, constipation, and gastroenteritis, commonly affect the athletic population.

- Anemia is a problem for some athletes. Iron-deficiency anemia is a condition found most often in women. In an athlete with iron-deficiency anemia, the red blood cells are either too small or too large and hemoglobin is decreased. The athlete with sickle-cell anemia may have an adverse reaction at high altitudes at which the sickle-shaped red blood cell is unable to transport oxygen adequately.

- Diabetes mellitus is a complex hereditary or developmental disease. Decreased effectiveness of insulin or an insufficient amount of insulin is responsible for most cases of diabetes. The diabetic athlete must carefully monitor his or her energy output to ensure a balance of food intake and the burning of sugars via insulin. If this balance is not maintained, diabetic coma or insulin shock may result.

- Epilepsy is defined as "a recurrent paroxysmal disorder of cerebral function characterized by sudden, brief attacks of altered consciousness, motor activity, sensory phenomena, or inappropriate behavior." A coach must recognize that an athlete is going into a seizure and be able to provide immediate care.

- The athlete with high blood pressure may have to be carefully monitored by the physician. Hypertension may require the avoidance of heavy resistive activities.

- Because communicable viral diseases such as German measles, mumps, and infectious mononucleosis can infect many athletes on a team, early recognition is necessary. When such a disease is suspected, the athlete should be isolated from other athletes and immediately referred to a physician for diagnosis.

- Sexually transmitted infections have their highest incidence among younger, sexually active persons. Because most athletes are in this high-risk age group, coaches should be concerned about the spread of these diseases. Suggestions to avoid these infections are safe sex, which involves the use of a condom or the elimination of multiple partners, and complete abstinence from sexual intercourse.

- The highly active female may have menstrual irregularities, including dysmenorrhea, amenorrhea, or oligomenorrhea. Female athletic triad is a combination of amenorrhea, disordered eating, and osteoporosis.

- Many female athletes compete during pregnancy with no ill effects. There is no indication that mild to moderate exercise during pregnancy is harmful to fetal development.

- The sexually transmitted infections with the highest incidence among the young athletic population are chlamydia, genital herpes, trichomoniasis, genital warts, crab lice, gonorrhea, and syphilis.

---

### *Solutions to Critical Thinking* Exercises

**23-1** Tinea pedis causes severe itching underneath and between the toes and on the sole of the foot. A red, white, or grayish scaling appearance may also be present. Scratching can cause infection. Generally this condition can be prevented by wearing clean, dry socks and making certain that the feet and toes are dry following bathing.

**23-2** It appears that the athlete is exhibiting signs and symptoms associated with the flu. In general the flu is caused by a viral infection, and thus the illness must simply be allowed to run its course while dealing with it symptomatically.

**23-3** The female athletic triad includes some form of eating disorder, amenorrhea, and osteoporosis. The eating disorder causes amenorrhea, in which menstruation stops, thus reducing the production of estrogen, which ultimately causes a loss of calcium from the bone.

## REVIEW QUESTIONS AND CLASS ACTIVITIES

1. Describe the organisms underlying the common skin infections seen in athletes. Name a disease caused by each one.
2. Invite a dermatologist or other professional to speak to the class about skin conditions, skin disease, and their care. He or she may wish to discuss specific conditions that pose a serious threat to the athlete's health and to others.
3. Describe the anemias that most often affect the athlete. How should each be managed?
4. What are the most common conditions related to the digestive system?
5. What is diabetes mellitus? What is the difference between diabetic coma and insulin shock? How is each managed?
6. What is epilepsy? What should be done for the athlete during a seizure? After it?
7. What is hypertension and how should it be addressed in athletics?
8. In a sports setting, what is the indication that an athlete has a contagious disease?
9. Discuss menstrual irregularities that occur in highly active athletes. Why do they occur? How should they be managed? How do they relate to reproduction? What is the female athletic triad and how can it be prevented?

## REFERENCES

1. Adams BB: 2002. Dermatologic disorders of the athlete, *Sports medicine* 32(5):309–321.
2. Barnes, DE, editor: 2004. *Action plan for diabetes*, Champaign, IL, Human Kinetics, pp. 1–11; 139–141.
3. Bender, M, 2007. 4 reasons your allergies are worse than ever, *Shape* 26(9):142.
4. Brown W: 2002. The benefits of physical activity during pregnancy, *Journal of science and medicine in sport* 5(1):37–45.
5. Brukner P, Khan K: 2002. Gastrointestinal symptoms during exercise. In Brukner, P, editor: *Clinical sports medicine*, 2nd rev. ed, Sydney, McGraw-Hill.
6. Brukner P, Khan K, McCrory P: 2002. The athlete with epilepsy. In Brukner, P, editor: *Clinical sports medicine*, 2nd rev. ed, Sydney, McGraw-Hill.
7. Chintanadilok J, Lowenthal DT: 2002. Exercise in treating hypertension: tailoring therapies for active patients, *Physician and sportsmedicine* 30(3):11–14; 16; 19–20; 23; 50.
8. Colberg SR, Swain DP: 2000. Exercise and diabetes control: a winning combination, *Physician and sportsmedicine* 28(4):63.
9. Dougherty, TM: 2003. Sports dermatology: what certified athletic trainers and therapists need to know, *Athletic therapy today* 8(3): 46–48.
10. Eichner R: 2002. Anemia pointers for diagnosis and treatment, *Physician and sportsmedicine* 30(10):29.
11. Eichner, R: 2007. Sports medicine pearls and pitfalls—sickle cell trait and athletes: three clinical concerns, *Current sports medicine reports* 6(3):134.
12. Eichner, R: 2008. Asthma in athletes: scope, risks, mimics, trends, *Current sports medicine reports* 7(3):118.
13. Eichner R: 2002. Athletes and viral infections, *Sports medicine digest* 24(3):34–35.
14. Fallon, K: 2006. Athletes with gastrointestinal disorders. In Burke, L, editor: *Clinical sports nutrition*, 3rd ed, Sydney, McGraw-Hill.
15. Fountain, NB, May, AC: 2003. Epilepsy and athletics, *Clinics in sports medicine* 22(3):605–616.
16. Goss J, Langley S: 2001. Detecting the female athlete triad: the coach's role, *Coaches' report* 7(3): 31–33; 35.
17. Harmon KG: 2002. Evaluating and treating exercise-related menstrual irregularities, *Physician and sportsmedicine* 30(3):29–30; 33–35.
18. Johnson, R: 2004. Herpes gladiatorum and other skin diseases, *Clinics in sports medicine* 23(3):473–484.
19. Kawaguchi, J: 2008. Redefining the female athlete triad, *Athletic therapy today* 13(1):11.
20. Keles, N: 2002. Testing allergic rhinitis in the athlete, *Rhinology* 40(4):211–214.
21. Leaver-Dunn D, Robinson JB, Laubenthal J: 2000. Assessment of respiratory conditions in athletes, *Athletic therapy today* 5(6): 14–19.
22. Loucks, A: 2006. Menstrual disorders in athletes, *Current sports medicine reports* 5(6):273.
23. MacKnight JM: 1999. Hypertension in athletes and active patients: tailoring treatment to the patient, *Physician and sportsmedicine* 27(4): 35.
24. McCormick, I: 2004. Understanding the female athlete triad: components of the triad not only affect female athletes, but also fitness enthusiasts, *IDEA personal trainer* 15(5):28–33.
25. McCulloch JM, Kloth LC: 2002. *Wound healing: alternatives in management*, 3rd ed, Philadelphia, FA Davis.

26. Mylonakis, E, Dickinson, BP, Rich, JD: 2003. Influenza vaccination for athletes: facts and controversies, *American journal of medicine & sports* 5(1):67–71.

27. O'Kane JW: 2002. Coping with upper respiratory infections, *Physician and sportsmedicine* 39(9):49–50.

28. Page, C, Diehl, J: 2007. Upper respiratory tract infections in athletes, *Clinics in sports medicine* 26(3):345.

29. Pescatello, LS, Franklin, BA, Fagard, R: 2004. American College of Sports Medicine position stand: Exercise and hypertension, *Medicine and science in sports and exercise* 36(3):533–553.

30. Pleacher, M, Dexter, W: 2007. Cutaneous fungal and viral infections in athletes, *Clinics in sports medicine* 26(3):397.

31. Putukian, M, O'Connor, F, Stricker, P: 2008. Mononucleosis and athletic participation: an evidence-based subject review, *Clinical journal of sport medicine* 18(4):309.

32. Ram, F: 2002. Does regular exercise help in the treatment and management of bronchial asthma?, MacAuley, D, editor: *Evidence-based sports medicine*, London, BMJ Books, pp. 165–180.

33. Rogers, S: 2008. Practical approach to preventing CA-MRSA infections in the athletic setting, *Athletic therapy today* 13(4):37.

34. Rundell, KW: 2004. Overuse of asthma medication in athletics?, *Medicine and science in sports and exercise* 36(6):925.

35. Rush S: 2002. Sports dermatology, *ACSM's health & fitness journal* 6(4):24–26.

36. Saladin, K: 2006. *Anatomy and physiology: the unity of form and function*, New York, McGraw-Hill.

37. Schnirring L: 1999. New drugs should help fight influenza this winter, *Physician and sportsmedicine* 27(12):15.

38. Taylor, P: 2005. A menace in the locker room: MRSA, a strain of antibiotic-resistant staphylococcus once confined to hospitals, is striking athletes at an alarming rate with dire consequences, *Sports illustrated* 102(9):50–53.

39. Turbeville, S, Cowan, L: 2006. Infectious disease outbreaks in competitive sports: a review of the literature, *American journal of sports medicine* 34(11):1860–1865.

40. Vantu RV: 1998. Epilepsy and athletics, *Clinical Sports Medicine* 17(1):61.

41. Vinci DM: 2002. Athletes and Type I diabetes mellitus, *Athletic therapy today* 7(6):48–49.

42. Vossen, DP, McArel, H, Vossen, JV: 2005. Physical activity and the common cold in undergraduate university students: implications for health professionals, *Physical & health education journal*: 70(3):43.

43. Weaver J, Denegar CR, Hertel J: 2000. Exercise-induced asthma, *Athletic therapy today* 5(3):38.

## ANNOTATED BIBLIOGRAPHY

Beers M: 2006. editor: *The Merck manual of medical information: home edition*, New York, Merck & Co.

*This textbook is one of the classical medicine references available to the health care professional. It covers most medical conditions.*

Cuppett, M, Walsh, K: 2005. *General medical conditions in the athlete*, St. Louis, Elsevier Mosby.

*Provides a comprehensive discussion of general medical conditions and associated pathologies in the athletic population.*

Hamann B: 2006. *Diseases: identification, prevention, and control*, New York, McGraw-Hill.

*An excellent reference guide for the health professional on the most common human diseases.*

Rundell, KW: 2002. *Exercise-induced asthma: pathophysiology and treatment*, Champaign, IL, Human Kinetics.

*This reference book presents current research and information on exercise-induced asthma, especially as it affects athletes and others who are physically active.*

*Tabor's cyclopedic medical dictionary:* 2005. Philadelphia, FA Davis.

*Despite the dictionary format, this volume contains a wealth of valuable information on various health conditions.*

## WEB SITES

American Academy of Dermatology: www.aad.org/

*The American Academy of Dermatology is committed to advancing the science of promoting a lifetime of healthier skin, hair, and nails.*

Asthma and Allergy Foundation of America (AAFA): www.aafa.org/

*Asthma and Allergy Foundation of America (AAFA) is dedicated to helping people with asthma and allergic diseases through education and support for research.*

American Board of Obstetrics and Gynecology: www.abog.org/

American Gastroenterological Association: www.gastro.org/

*Includes information for physicians and the public about digestive disease symptoms, treatments, and research.*

American Diabetes Association: www.diabetes.org/

*This site offers the latest information on diabetes and living with the disease.*

American Epilepsy Society: www.aesnet.org/

*The American Epilepsy Society promotes research and education for professionals dedicated to the prevention, treatment, and cure of epilepsy.*

Hypertension Network: BloodPressure.com: www.bloodpressure.com/

*Information for the consumer on hypertension (high blood pressure).*

Sexually Transmitted Infections: Index: www.plannedparenthood.org/library/STI/STI-facts.html

# Substance Abuse

*When you finish this chapter you will be able to:*

- Discuss the issue of substance abuse in the athletic and physically active population.
- Identify the signs of substance abuse.
- Describe the effects of performance-enhancing drugs commonly used by athletes.
- Discuss the negative effects of alcohol and tobacco on an athlete's health.
- Identify the primary recreational drugs and their effects.
- Briefly discuss drug testing programs to identify the substance abuser.

The use, by athletes, of nutritional supplements to improve performance was discussed in Chapter 5. This chapter focuses on the abuse of a variety of substances, particularly drugs and medications, as ergogenic aids and the negative impact they can potentially have on the health of the athlete.

Certainly, concern about the number of athletes engaging in substance abuse is increasing (Focus Box 24-1).[27] Some athletes use performance-enhancing drugs in an attempt to improve performance, whereas others use drugs as a recreational pursuit. The use of performance-enhancing drugs among Olympic athletes and the widespread use of street drugs by high school, collegiate, and professional athletes has been much written about and discussed.[31] **Clearly, substance abuse has no place in the athletic population.**[1,17,27]

## PERFORMANCE-ENHANCING DRUGS

In sports medicine, the administration of a drug that is designed to improve the competitor's performance is known as **doping**. Doping has been defined as "the administration or use of substances in any form alien to the body or of physiological substances in abnormal amounts and with abnormal methods by healthy persons with the exclusive aim of attaining an artificial and unfair increase in performance in sports."[11]

**doping**
The administration of a drug that is designed to improve the competitor's performance.

### Stimulants

The intention of the athlete when he or she ingests a stimulant may be to increase alertness, to reduce fatigue, or in some instances, to increase

24-1   *Focus Box*

**Identifying the Substance Abuser**

The following are signs of drug abuse:

1. Sudden personality changes
2. Severe mood swings
3. Changing peer groups
4. Decreased interest in extracurricular and leisure activities
5. Worsening grades
6. Disregard for household chores and curfews
7. Feeling of depression most of the time
8. Breakdown in personal hygiene habits
9. Increased sleep and decreased eating
10. Clothes and skin smell of alcohol or marijuana
11. Sudden weight loss
12. Lying, cheating, stealing, etc.
13. Arrests for drunk driving or for possessing illegal substances
14. Truancies from school
15. Frequent job changes or loss
16. Defensiveness at the mention of drugs or alcohol
17. Increased isolation (spends time in room)
18. Family relationship deteriorates
19. Drug paraphernalia (needles, empty bottles, etc.) found
20. Others make observations about negative behavior
21. Signs of intoxication
22. Constantly misses appointments
23. Falls asleep in class or at work
24. Has financial problems
25. Misses assignments or deadlines
26. Diminished productivity

competitiveness; use can produce hostility. Some athletes respond to stimulants with a loss of judgment that may lead to personal injury or injury to others.[1]

### Amphetamines

Amphetamines, caffeine, and cocaine are the stimulant drugs most commonly used in sports.[17] (Cocaine is discussed in the section on recreational drug abuse.) Amphetamines present an extremely difficult problem in sports because they are commonly found in cold remedies, nasal and ophthalmic decongestants, and most asthma preparations.

Amphetamines are extremely powerful and dangerous drugs. They may be injected, inhaled, or taken as tablets. Amphetamines are among the most abused of the drugs used for enhancing sports performance.

In ordinary doses, amphetamines can produce an increased sense of well-being and heightened mental activity—until fatigue sets in (from lack of sleep), accompanied by nervousness, insomnia, and anorexia. In high doses, amphetamines reduce mental activity and impair performance of complicated motor skills. The athlete's behavior may become irrational. The chronic user may get hung up, or in other words, become stuck, in a repetitive behavioral sequence. This behavior may last for hours, becoming increasingly more irrational. The long-term, or even short-term, use of amphetamines can lead to amphetamine psychosis, manifested by auditory and visual hallucinations and paranoid delusions. Physiologically, high doses of amphetamines can cause abnormal pupillary dilation, increased blood pressure, and hyperthermia.

Athletes believe that amphetamines improve sports performance by promoting quickness and endurance, delaying fatigue, and increasing confidence, thereby causing increased aggressiveness. Studies indicate that there is no improvement in performance, but there is an increased risk of injury, exhaustion, and circulation collapse.

### Caffeine

Caffeine is found in coffee, tea, cocoa, and cola and is readily absorbed into the body[25] (Table 24-1). It is a central nervous system stimulant and diuretic and also stimulates gastric secretion. One cup of coffee can contain from 100 to 150 mg of caffeine. In moderation, caffeine results in wakefulness and mental alertness.[32] In larger amounts and in individuals who ingest caffeine daily, it raises blood pressure and decreases, then increases, the heart rate. It affects coordination, sleep, mood, behavior, and thinking processes. In terms of exercise and sports performance, caffeine is controversial.[25] Like amphetamines, caffeine can affect some athletes by acting as an ergogenic aid during prolonged exercise. A habitual user of caffeine who suddenly stops may experience withdrawal, including headache, drowsiness, lethargy, rhinorrhea, irritability, nervousness, depression, and loss of interest in work.[25] Caffeine also acts as a diuretic when hydration is important.[32]

**24-1 *Critical Thinking***
Exercise

A women's lacrosse player is concerned that she has been chosen for a random drug test later that afternoon. She met her boyfriend for lunch and drank a large cup of espresso. She is worried that she will test positive for a performance enhancing drug.

? What should she be told to reduce her anxiety about the drug test?

**TABLE 24-1** Examples of Caffeine-Containing Products

| Product | Dose |
| --- | --- |
| Coffee (1 cup) | 100 mg |
| Diet Coke (12 oz) | 45.6 mg |
| Diet Pepsi (12 oz) | 36.0 mg |
| No-Doz (1) | 100.0 mg |
| Anacin (1) | 32.0 mg |
| Excedrin (1) | 65.0 mg |
| Midol (1) | 32.4 mg |

## Narcotic Analgesic Drugs

Narcotic analgesic drugs are derived directly or indirectly from opium. Morphine and codeine (methylmorphine) are examples of substances made from opium. Narcotic analgesics are used for the management of moderate to severe pain. They have been banned by the NCAA because of the high risk of physical and psychological dependency and because of many other problems stemming from their use. Slight-to-moderate pain can be effectively dealt with by drugs other than narcotics.[1]

## Beta Blockers

In sports, beta blockers have been used by athletes who require steadiness, whose signs of nervousness must be in control while engaging in sports such as target shooting, sailing, archery, fencing, ski jumping, and luge. Beta blockers relax the blood vessels. This relaxation, in turn, slows heart rate and decreases cardiac output. Therapeutically, beta blockers are used for a variety of cardiac diseases and for treating hypertension.[17]

## Diuretics

Diuretics are used for a variety of cardiovascular and respiratory conditions (e.g., hypertension) in which elimination of fluids from tissues is necessary. Sports participants have misused diuretics mainly in two ways: to reduce body weight quickly or to decrease a drug's concentration in the urine (increasing its excretion to avoid the detection of drug misuse). In both cases, there are ethical and health grounds for banning certain classes of diuretics from use during competition.

## Anabolic Steroids, Human Growth Hormone, and Androstenedione

Three substances related to increasing muscle build, strength, power, and growth are anabolic steroids, human growth hormone (HGH), and androstenedione.[18]

### Anabolic Steroids

*Anabolic steroids are different from corticosteroids which have anti-inflammatory capabilities.*

Androgenic hormones are products of the male testes. Of these hormones, testosterone is the principal one; it possesses the ability to function androgenically (to stimulate male characteristics) and anabolically (through improved protein assimilation, increase muscle mass and weight, general growth, bone maturation, and virility).[28] When prescribed by a physician to improve certain physiological conditions, these drugs have value. In 1984, the American College of Sports Medicine (ACSM) reported that anabolic androgenic steroids taken with an adequate diet could contribute to an increase in body weight and, with a heavy resistance program, to a significant gain in strength. However, in sports, anabolic steroids constitute a major threat to the health of the athlete[23] (Focus Box 24-2). Anabolic steroids present an ethical dilemma for the sports world. It is estimated that more than a million young male

*Focus Box*

**Examples of Deleterious Effects of Anabolic Steroids**

■ *Teens*—premature closure of long bones, acne, hirsutism, voice deepening, enlarged mammary glands (gynecomastia) of the male

■ *Men*—male-pattern baldness, acne, voice deepening, mood swings, aggressive behavior, decreased high-density lipoprotein, increased cholesterol, reduction in size of testicles, reduced testosterone production, changes in libido

■ *Women*—female-pattern baldness, acne, voice deepening (irreversible), increased facial hair, enlarged clitoris (irreversible), increased libido, menstrual irregularities, increased aggression, decreased body fat, increased appetite, decreased breast size

■ *Abuse*—may lead to liver tumors and cancer, heart disease, and hypertension

and female athletes are taking them, with most being purchased through the black market. It is estimated that 6.5 percent of male and 1.4 percent of female high school students take or have taken anabolic steroids.[34] Also an estimated 2 to 20 percent of male intercollegiate athletes take anabolic steroids.[33]

If these drugs are given to the prepubertal boy, a most certain hazard is a decrease in his ultimate height because of the cessation of long bone growth. Acne, hirsutism, a deepening of the voice in the prepubescent boy, and in some cases, a swelling of the breasts, called *gynecomastia*, are among other androgen effects.[10] The ingestion of steroids by females can result in **hirsutism** (excessive hair growth or the presence of hair in unusual places) and in a deepening of the voice because of vocal cord alteration. When the dosage is halted, the hirsutism may cease, but the change in the vocal cords is irreversible.[10] As the duration and dosage increase, the possibility of producing androgen effects also increases. Because self-administered overdosage seems to be the pattern of those who use steroids, the preceding statement is most significant. Abuse of these drugs may also lead to cancer of the liver and prostate glands and to heart disease.[8]

Anabolic steroids are most abused in sports that involve strength.[10] Power lifting, the throwing events in track and field, and American football are some of the sports in which the use of anabolic steroids is a serious problem.[15] Because female athletes are developing the attitude of "win at all costs," their abuse of anabolic steroids is also becoming a major health concern.

### Human Growth Hormone

Human growth hormone (HGH) is a hormone produced by the pituitary gland. It is released into circulation in a pulsating manner. This release can vary with a person's age and developmental period. A lack of HGH

*24-2 Critical Thinking*
Exercise

A high school football player has been taking anabolic steroids to get stronger and faster.

? What are the potential negative side effects of using anabolic steroids?

**hirsutism (her** soot ism)
Excessive hair growth and/or the presence of hair in unusual places.

can result in dwarfism. In the past, HGH was in limited supply because it was extracted from cadavers. Now, however, it can be made synthetically and is more available.[22]

Experiments indicate that HGH can increase muscle mass, skin thickness, connective tissues in muscle, and organ weight and can produce lax muscles and ligaments during rapid growth phases. It also increases body length and weight and decreases body fat percentage.[22]

The use of HGH by athletes throughout the world is on the increase because it is more difficult to detect in urine than anabolic steroids are.[29] There is currently a lack of concrete information about the effects of HGH on the athlete who does not have a growth problem. It is known that an overabundance of HGH in the body can lead to premature closure of long-bone growth sites or, conversely, can cause acromegaly, a condition that produces elongation and enlargement of bones of the extremities and thickening of bones and soft tissues of the face.[22] Also associated with acromegaly is diabetes mellitus, cardiovascular disease, goiter, menstrual disorders, decreased sexual desire, and impotence. *It may decrease the life span by up to 20 years.* Like anabolic steroids, HGH presents a serious problem for the sports world. At this time there is no proof that an increase of HGH combined with weight training contributes to strength and muscle hypertrophy.[29]

### Androstenedione

Androstenedione is a relatively weak androgen that is produced primarily in the testes.[13] It has been used in humans to produce transient increases in testosterone in males and particularly in females primarily for the purpose of enhancing athletic performance.[13] To date there is no scientific evidence or research to support the efficacy or safety of using this ergogenic aid.[13] In 2004 the FDA banned its sale, and it is currently illegal to buy or sell androstenedione.

### Blood Reinjection (Blood Doping, Blood Packing, and Blood Boosting)

Not only is the use of blood reinjection in competition unethical, but when conducted by nonmedical personnel, it could prove dangerous.

Endurance, acclimatization, and altitude make increased metabolic demands on the body, which responds by increasing blood volume and red blood cells to meet the increased aerobic demands.[9]

Recently researchers have replicated these physiological responses by removing 900 ml of blood, storing it, and reinfusing it after 6 weeks. The reason for waiting at least 6 weeks before reinfusion is it takes that long for the athlete's body to reestablish a normal hemoglobin and red blood cell concentration. Using this method, endurance performance has been significantly improved. From the standpoint of scientific research, such experimentation has merit and is of interest. However, not only is use of such methods in competition unethical, but when conducted by nonmedical personnel, it could prove to be dangerous, especially when a matched donor is used.[9]

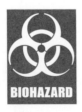

BIOHAZARD

There are serious risks with transfusing blood and related blood products. The risks include allergic reactions, kidney damage (if the wrong type of blood is used), fever, jaundice, the possibility of transmitting infectious diseases (viral hepatitis or HIV), or blood overload, resulting in circulatory and metabolic shock.

## RECREATIONAL DRUG ABUSE

Just as it has become a part of the general world, recreational drug use has become a part of the world of sports.[7] Reasons for using these substances may include desire to experiment, to temporarily escape from problems, or to just be part of a group (peer pressure). For some, recreational drug use leads to abuse and dependence. There are two general aspects of dependence: psychological and physical. *Psychological dependence* is the drive to repeat the ingestion of a drug to produce pleasure or to avoid discomfort. *Physical dependence* is the state of drug adaptation that manifests itself as the development of tolerance and, when the drug is removed, causes a withdrawal syndrome. *Tolerance* of a drug is the need to increase the dosage to create the effect that was obtained previously by smaller amounts. The *withdrawal syndrome* consists of an unpleasant physiological reaction when the drug is abruptly stopped. Some drugs that are abused by the athlete overlap with those thought to enhance performance. Examples include amphetamines and cocaine. Tobacco (nicotine), alcohol, cocaine, marijuana, crystal methamphetamine, ecstasy, and ADHD medications are the most abused recreational drugs. Athletes have also been known to abuse barbiturates, nonbarbiturate sedatives, psychotomimetic drugs, or different inhalants.[27]

### Tobacco

A number of current problems are related to tobacco and sports. They can be divided into two headings: cigarette smoking and the use of smokeless tobacco.

#### Cigarette Smoking

On the basis of various investigations into the relationship between smoking and performance, the following conclusions can be drawn:[2,11]

- Individuals vary in sensitivity to tobacco, and relatively high sensitivity may seriously affect performance. Because more than one-third of men studied indicate tobacco sensitivity, it may be wise to prohibit smoking by athletes.

- Tobacco smoke has been associated with as many as 4,700 different chemicals, many of which are toxic.

- As few as ten inhalations of cigarette smoke cause an average maximum decrease in airway conductance of 50 percent. This decrease occurs as well in nonsmokers who inhale secondhand smoke.

- Smoking reduces the oxygen-carrying capacity of the blood. A smoker's blood carries five to ten times more carbon monoxide than normal; thus the red blood cells are prevented from picking up sufficient oxygen to meet the demands of the body's tissues. The carbon monoxide also tends to make arterial walls more permeable to fatty substances, a factor in atherosclerosis.

- Smoking aggravates and accelerates the heart muscle cells through overstimulation of the sympathetic nervous system.
- Total lung capacity and maximum breathing capacity are significantly decreased in heavy smokers; this is important to the athlete because both changes impair the capacity to take in oxygen and make it readily available for body use.
- Smoking decreases pulmonary diffusing capacity.
- After smoking, an accelerated thrombolic tendency is evidenced.
- **Smoking is a carcinogenic factor in lung cancer and is a contributing factor to heart disease.**

The addictive chemical of tobacco is nicotine, which is one of the most toxic drugs. When ingested, nicotine causes blood pressure elevation, increased bowel activity, and an antidiuretic action. Moderate tolerance and physical dependence occur. It also has been noted that passive inhalation of cigarette smoke can reduce maximum aerobic power and endurance capacity.

### Use of Smokeless Tobacco

It is estimated that 36 percent of athletes use smokeless tobacco, which comes in three forms: loose-leaf, moist or dry powder (snuff), and compressed.[5] The tobacco is placed between the cheek and the gum, where it is sucked and chewed. Aesthetically, this is an unsavory habit during which an athlete is continually spitting into a container. Besides the unpleasant appearance, **the use of smokeless tobacco poses an extremely serious health risk.** Smokeless tobacco causes bad breath, stained teeth, tooth sensitivity to heat and cold, cavities, gum recession, tooth bone loss, leukoplakia, aggressive oral and throat cancer, and periodontal destruction (with tooth loss).[6] The major substance ingested is nitrosonornicotine, which is the drug responsible for this habit's addictiveness. This chemical makes smokeless tobacco a more addictive habit than smoking is. Smokeless tobacco increases heart rate but does not affect reaction time, movement time, or total response time among athletes or nonathletes.

Coaches, fitness professionals, health care providers, and professional athletes themselves must avoid the use of smokeless tobacco to present a positive role model.[5,6]

### Alcohol

Alcohol is the number one abused drug in the United States.[26] Alcohol is absorbed directly into the bloodstream through the small intestine. It accumulates in the blood because alcohol absorption is faster than its oxidation. It acts as a central nervous system depressant, producing

Alcohol consumption, at any time or in any amount, does not improve mental or physical abilities and should be avoided by athletes.

sedation and tranquility.[14] Characteristically, alcohol consumption, at any time and in any amount, does not improve mental or physical abilities, and athletes should completely avoid it.[14] Alcohol consumption on a large scale can lead to a moderate degree of tolerance. Alcohol has no place in sports participation.

## Cocaine

Cocaine, sometimes called "coke," "snow," "toot," "happy dust," and "white girl," is a powerful central nervous system stimulant and a local anesthetic and vasoconstrictor. Besides being a banned performance enhancer, cocaine is one of the most abused recreational drugs. It can be inhaled, smoked, or injected (intravenously, subcutaneously, or intramuscularly).[30]

In high doses cocaine, which is found in the leaves of the coca bush, causes a sense of excitement and euphoria. On occasion it also produces hallucinations. When applied locally to the skin, cocaine acts as an anesthetic; however, when taken into the body through inhalation, snorting, or injection, it acts on the central nervous system.[30]

### Crack

Crack, a highly purified form of cocaine, is smoked and is known to produce a virtually instantaneous high. Habitual use of cocaine does not lead to physical tolerance or dependence but does cause psychological dependence and addiction.[30] When cocaine is used recreationally, the athlete feels alert, self-satisfied, and powerful. Heavy usage can produce paranoid delusions and violent behavior. Overuse can lead to overstimulation of the sympathetic nervous system and can cause tachycardia, hypertension, extra heartbeats, coronary vasoconstriction, strokes, pulmonary edema, aortic rupture, and sudden death.

## Marijuana

Marijuana is another one of the most abused drugs in Western society. It is more commonly called "grass," "weed," "pot," "dope," or "hemp." The marijuana cigarette is called a "joint," "j," "number," "reefer," or "root." Marijuana is not a harmless drug. The components of marijuana smoke are similar to those of tobacco smoke and the same cellular changes are observed in the user.[4]

Continued use leads to respiratory diseases such as asthma and bronchitis and to a decrease in vital capacity of 15 to 40 percent (certainly detrimental to physical performance). Among other deleterious effects are lowered sperm counts and testosterone levels. Evidence of interference with the functioning of the immune system and cellular metabolism has also been found. The most consistent sign of this interference is an increase in pulse rate, which averages close to 20 percent higher during exercise and is a definite factor in limiting performance. Some decrease in leg, hand, and finger strength has been found at higher dosages. Like tobacco, marijuana must be considered carcinogenic.[4]

Psychological effects such as a diminution of self-awareness and judgment, a slowdown of thinking, and a shorter attention span appear early in the use of the drug. Postmortem examinations of habitual users reveal not only cerebral atrophy but alterations of anatomical structures, which suggest irreversible brain damage. Marijuana also contains unique substances (cannabinoids) that are stored, in much the same manner as are fat cells, throughout the body and in the brain tissues for weeks and even months. These stored quantities result in a cumulative deleterious effect on the habitual user.

A drug such as marijuana has no place in sports. Claims for its use are unsubstantiated, and the harmful effects, both immediate and long-term, are too significant to permit indulgence at any time.[4]

## Crystal Methamphetamine

This drug is used by individuals of all ages and is increasingly gaining in popularity as a club drug. It is a colorless, odorless, and highly addictive synthetic stimulant. Crystal methamphetamine resembles small fragments of glass or shiny blue-white "rocks" of various sizes. Like powdered methamphetamine, it is abused because of the long-lasting euphoric effects it produces. But it has a higher purity level and may produce even longer-lasting and more intense physiological effects than the powdered form of the drug. It may either be smoked using glass pipes similar to pipes used to smoke crack cocaine or it may be injected. A user who smokes or injects the drug immediately experiences an intense sensation followed by a high that may last 12 hours or more.[12]

Crystal methamphetamine use is associated with numerous serious physical problems, which may include rapid heart rate, increased blood pressure, and damage to the small blood vessels in the brain that can lead to stroke. Overdoses can cause increased temperature, convulsions, and death. People who use crystal methamphetamine may have episodes of paranoia, anxiety, violent behavior, confusion, and insomnia. The drug can produce psychotic symptoms that persist for months or years after an individual has stopped using the drug.[12]

## Ecstasy

Considered the most commonly used designer drug, ecstasy is a close derivative of methamphetamine and can be described as a hallucinogenic stimulant. Designer drugs are illicit variations of other drugs. Ecstasy is most often found in tablet, capsule, or powder form and is usually consumed orally, although it can also be injected. Ecstasy can cause euphoria and feelings of well-being, enhanced mental or emotional clarity, anxiety, and paranoia. Heavier doses can cause hallucinations, sensations of lightness and floating, depression, paranoid thinking, and violent, irrational behavior. Physical reactions can include loss of appetite, nausea, vomiting, blurred vision, increased heart rate and blood pressure, muscle tension, faintness, chills, sweating, tremors, insomnia, convulsions, and loss of control over voluntary body movements. Some reactions have been reported to persist up to 14 days after taking ecstasy.[24]

## ADHD Medications

The abuse of medications commonly used for treating attention deficit and hyperactivity disorder (ADHD) is a relatively new phenomenon, but one that has become a major cause for concern, especially in the college population. These medications usually are amphetamines such as Ritalin, Adderall, and Dexedrine. They are stimulants but they also decrease an individual's distractibility and facilitate concentration and focus. Reasons for abusing or misusing stimulant medication include improving attention, partying, reducing hyperactivity, and improving grades. Some individuals illegally or illicitly obtain the medications for their own use or for sale. Common signs and symptoms include shakiness, rapid speech or movements, difficulty sitting still, difficulty concentrating, lack of appetite, sleep disturbance, and irritability.

## DRUG-TESTING PROGRAMS

Professional sports leagues, the NCAA, and the United States Antidoping Agency (USADA) have clearly established "banned substance" lists and drug-testing programs in response to problems created by drug use among athletes at those levels.[19] The National Federation of State High School Associations (NFHS) does not currently have a list of banned substances or specific policies on drug testing. They have left the choice of whether to drug test athletes up to individual schools. However, they have provided guidelines for those schools wishing to institute a drug-testing program.[20]

Testing high school athletes for drugs has been occurring since the mid-1970s, when efforts to reduce drug use increased.[16] Drug testing among high school athletes has been done infrequently and with varying degrees of success. However, court decisions in 1995 removed some hurdles for drug testing of high school athletes. Drug testing can be done for a variety of different drugs. It appears that high school drug-testing programs most commonly screen athletes for amphetamines, marijuana, cocaine, opiates, and phencyclidine (PCP). These standard drug-testing packages leave out several commonly used substances such as alcohol, tobacco, and steroids.[16]

## SUMMARY

- Substance abuse involves the use of performance-enhancing drugs and the widespread use of recreational drugs, or street drugs. It is important to be knowledgeable about substance abuse in the athletic population and to be able to recognize signs that an athlete is engaging in substance abuse. Substance abuse has no place in the athletic population.

- The use of performance-enhancing drugs (ergogenic aids) by athletes must be discouraged because of potential health risks and to ensure equal competition. Among the more common ergogenic aids used by athletes are stimulants, beta blockers, narcotic analgesics, diuretics, anabolic steroids, human growth hormone, and blood doping.

- Recreational drug abuse among athletes is of major concern. It can lead to serious psychological and physical health problems.

- The most prevalent substances that are abused are tobacco, alcohol, cocaine, marijuana, crystal methamphetamine, ecstasy, and ADHD medications.

- Drug testing of athletes for the purpose of identifying individuals who may have some problems with drug abuse is done routinely by the NCAA and the USADA. The major goals of drug testing are to protect the health of athletes and to help ensure that competition is fair and equitable. Most professional teams and colleges and universities have initiated drug-testing programs for their athletes. Unfortunately, drug testing is rarely done at the high school level because of cost constraints.

---

*Solutions to Critical Thinking* Exercises

**24-1** The athlete should be informed that her drug test is designed to screen for recreational drugs rather than for performance-enhancing drugs, and so this should not be a problem, Additionally, even if the test was screening for performance-enhancing drugs, it is highly unlikely that one cup of espresso would contain enough caffeine for her to test positive.

**24-2** The visible signs of steroid abuse include male pattern baldness, acne, voice deepening, mood swings, aggressive behavior, gynecomastia,

reduction in the size of a testicle, and changes in libido.

**24-3** Point out the potential long-term effects of using smokeless tobacco, which include bad breath, stained teeth, tooth sensitivity to heat and cold, cavities (with tooth loss), gum recession, periodontal destruction, and oral and throat cancer. Also try to suggest a substitute for the tobacco, such as gum or sunflower seeds, so that the athlete's habitual need to chew on something and spit while playing baseball is satisfied.

## REVIEW QUESTIONS AND CLASS ACTIVITIES

1. How do stimulants enhance an athlete's performance?
2. What are the purposes of narcotic analgesic drugs in sports? How do they affect performance?
3. What type of athlete would use beta blockers? Why are they used?
4. Describe why athletes use anabolic steroids, diuretics, and growth hormone. What are their physiological effects on the athlete?
5. Describe blood doping in sports. Why is it used? What are its dangers?
6. Contrast psychological and physical dependence, tolerance, and withdrawal syndromes.
7. List the dangers of smokeless tobacco. List the effects of nicotine on the body.
8. Why is cocaine use a danger to the athlete?
9. Select a recreational drug to research. What are the physiological responses to it, and what dangers does it pose to the athlete?
10. How can an athlete who is abusing drugs be identified? Describe behavioral identification as well as drug testing.
11. Debate the issue of drug testing in athletics.

## REFERENCES

1. Avois, L, Robinson, N: 2006. Central nervous system stimulants and sport practice, *British journal of sports medicine* 40(1):16–20.

2. Bellenir, K: 2004. Smoking concerns sourcebook: basic consumer health information about nicotine addiction and smoking cessation, featuring facts about the health effects of tobacco use, Detroit, Omnigraphics.

3. Browne, A, Lachance, V, Pipe A: 1999. The ethics of blood testing as an element of doping control in sport, *Medicine & science in sports & exercise* 31(4):497.

4. Campos, DR, Yonamine, M, de Moraes Moreau, RL: 2003. Marijuana as doping in sports, *Sports medicine* 33(6):395–399.

5. Chiamulera, C, Leone, R: 2007. Smokeless tobacco use in sports: 'legal doping'? *Addiction* 102(12): 1847.

6. Cooper, J, Ellison, J, Walsh M: 2003. Spit (smokeless)-tobacco use by baseball players entering the professional ranks, *Journal of athletic training* 38(2):126.

7. De Rose, E. 2008. Doping in athletes—an update, *Clinics in sports medicine* 27(1):107.

8. Earnest, CP: 2001. Dietary androgen 'supplements': separating substance from hype, *Physician and sportsmedicine* 29(5):63.

9. Eichner, R: 2007. Blood doping, *Sports medicine* 37(4):389.

10. Graham, M, Davies, B: 2008. Anabolic steroid use, *Sports medicine* 38(6):505.

11. Green, GA, Uryasz, FD, Petr, TA, Bray, CD: 2001. NCAA study of substance use and abuse habits of college student-athletes, *Clinical journal of sport medicine* 11(1): 51–56.

12. Iritani, B, Hallfors, D: 2007. Crystal methamphetamine use among young adults in the USA. *Addiction* 102(7):1102.

13. Kersey, RD: 2001. What athletic trainers and therapists should know about androstenedione, *Athletic therapy today* 6(1):59.

14. Kinney, J: 2005. Loosening the grip: A handbook of alcohol information, New York, McGraw-Hill.

15. Koziris L: 2000. Anabolic-androgenic steroid abuse, *Physician and sportsmedicine* 28(12):67.

16. Lassiter, D, Deere, R, Hey W: 2000. Overview of drug testing in secondary school athletics, *K.A.H.P.E.R.D. journal* 36(2):10–13.

17. Lumpkin, A, Stoll, SK, Beller, JM: 2003. Ergogenic aids for sport performance. In Lumpkin, A, editor: *Sport ethics: applications for fair play*, 3rd ed, Boston, McGraw-Hill, pp. 207–225.

18. Matheson, GO: 2005. Steroids in sports: are drugs the only ones being used?, *Physician and sportsmedicine* 33(5):6.

19. Mazur AF: 2001. Substance abuse and NCAA drug testing: are we being fair?, *NCAA sports sciences education newsletter*.

20. National Collegiate Athletic Association: 2007. *NCAA drug testing: education programs*, Indianapolis, NCAA.

21. O'Connor, M: 2004. Promoting a responsible approach to alcohol in sport (abstract), *Journal of science and medicine in sport* 7(4 Supplement):88.

22. O'Mathuna, D: 2006. Human growth hormone for improved strength and increased muscle mass in athletes, *Alternative medicine alert* 9(9):97–101.

23. Powers M: 2002. The safety and efficacy of anabolic steroid precursors: what is the scientific evidence?, *Journal of athletic training* 37(3):300.

24. Puente, C, González, J: 2008. Sensation seeking, attitudes toward drug use, and actual use among adolescents: testing a model for alcohol and ecstacy use, *Substance use & misuse* 43(11): 1618.

25. Reid, TR: 2005. Caffeine, *National geographic* 207(1). p. 2–33.

26. Steinbach, P: 2003. Team spirits: student-athletes are apt to abuse alcohol, prompting one researcher to ponder why, *Athletic business* 27(12):26; 28; 30.

27. Stewart, B, Smith, A: 2008. Drug use in sport: implications for public policy, *Journal of sport & social issues* 32(3): 278.

28. Stilger VG et al: 2000. Androstenedione and anabolic-androgenic steroids: what you need to know, *Athletic therapy today* 5(1):56.

29. Trulock SC: 2000. Drug use in athletics: abuse of the human growth hormone in amateur athletes, *Sports Medicine Update*, 14(4):18.

30. Williams, J, Pacula, R: 2006. College students' use of cocaine, *Substance use & misuse* 41(4):489.

31. Wilson W, editor: 2001. Doping in elite sport: the politics of drugs in the Olympic movement, Champaign, IL, Human Kinetics.

32. Woolf, K, Bidwell, W: 2008. The effect of caffeine as an ergogenic aid in anaerobic exercise, *International journal of sport nutrition & exercise metabolism* 18(4):412.

33. Yesalis CE, editor: 2000. *Anabolic steroids in sport and exercise*, 2nd ed. Champaign, IL, Human Kinetics.

34. Yesalis, CE, Bahrke, MS: 2005. Anabolic-androgenic steroids: incidence of use and health implications, *President's council on physical fitness and sports research digest* 5(5): 1–8.

## ANNOTATED BIBLIOGRAPHY

Williams M: 1997. *The ergogenics edge: pushing the limits of sports performance*, Champaign, IL, Human Kinetics.

   *This text for athletes, coaches, and personal trainers provides the most recent information on a wide variety of ergogenics and analyzes their positive and negative effects on sports performance factors.*

Wilson W, editor: 2001. *Doping in elite sport: the politics of drugs in the Olympic movement*, Champaign, IL, Human Kinetics.

   *This book examines the issues related to elite athletes' use of banned substances and explores the critical issues surrounding efforts to control doping.*

Yesalis CE, editor: 2000. *Anabolic steroids in sport and exercise*, 2nd ed. Champaign, IL, Human Kinetics.

   *This book attempts to answer questions and provide information on the use and abuse of anabolic steroids in sports.*

## WEB SITES

NCAA Drug Testing Program
   www.ncaa.org/wps/
   ncaa?ContentID=282
   *Provides an updated list of banned drugs and drug testing information.*

www.usantidoping.org/
   *This organization is dedicated to eliminating the practice of doping in sport.*

www.olympic-usa.org/
   *Contains information about drug testing from the USOC.*

www.wada-ama.org/en/
   prohibitedlist.ch2
   *A comprehensive list of all medicines (over 5,000) showing which are prohibited or permitted in international sport.*

Substance Abuse and Mental Health Service Administration:
   www.samhsa.gov/

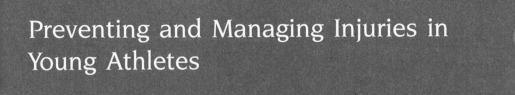

# Preventing and Managing Injuries in Young Athletes

*When you finish this chapter you will be able to:*

- Explain why young athletes are more susceptible to injuries than adults.
- Identify where, how, and to whom youth sports injuries are occurring in the United States.
- Discuss matching of young athletes as a criterion for determining competitive levels.
- Understand that young athletes can safely engage in a strength-training program.
- Discuss the psychological considerations relative to young athletes competing in sport activities.
- Identify different organizations that have established certification programs for coaches of youth sports.
- Discuss recognition and management of the types of injuries that are likely to occur in the young athlete.
- Explain what parents and coaches can do to help prevent or minimize injuries in the young athlete.

Under the best of circumstances, sports programs for young participants promote responsible social behaviors, greater academic success, confidence in physical abilities, an appreciation of personal health and fitness, and the development of strong social bonds. Sports, when specifically planned for, can provide a venue for learning positive ethical behaviors.[24,32]

Sports can promote
- responsible social behaviors
- greater academic success
- confidence in physical abilities
- appreciation of health and fitness
- positive ethical behaviors

## CULTURAL TRENDS

In recent years there has been a significant increase in the participation of young children, particularly females, in both organized and informal sports, as well as recreational activities (Figure 25-1). It has been estimated that approximately 75 percent of U.S. households with school-age children have at least one child who plays organized sports.[22] Unfortunately, along with this growth in sports participation, comes an increase in sports- and recreation-related injuries. Certainly, the risk of physical injury is inherent in sports participation. Young athletes are more susceptible to these injuries because they are continuously gaining motor and cognitive skills throughout the growth process.[17]

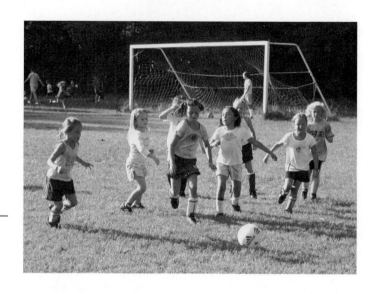

**Figure 25-1**

Unsupervised play is
generally more dangerous
than organized sports
activities.

Many parents and health
professionals question the
value of sports for the
immature child.

Parents and professionals in the areas of education, psychology, and medicine have long questioned whether vigorous physical training and competition are advisable for the immature child.[17] Increasingly, children, and particularly females, are engaging in intense programs of training that may require many hours of daily commitment extending over many years. Swimmers may practice 2 hours, two times a day, covering 6,000 to 10,000 meters each session; gymnasts may practice 3 to 5 hours per day; and runners may cover as many as 70 miles each week.

Forty-six million young
people between the ages of
five and seventeen engage in
sports.

The number of young people between 5 and 17 years of age in the United States engaging in youth sports is estimated at more than 46 million. The National Youth Sports Safety Foundation estimates that between 20 and 30 million U.S. children are in organized out-of-school sports with another 25 million participating in competitive school sports (Table 25-1).[24]

## Where Are Injuries Occurring? The Facts*[23]

- More than 30 million children participate in sports each year in the United States.
- Nearly three-quarters of U.S. households with school-age children have at least one child who plays organized sports.
- Each year, more than 3.5 million children ages 14 years and under receive medical treatment for sports injuries.
- Each year, approximately 715,000 sports and recreation injuries occur in school settings alone.
- Collision and contact sports are associated with higher rates of injury; however, injuries from individual sports tend to be more severe.

*Modified from National SAFE KIDS Campaign, *Childhood sports injuries and their prevention: a guide for parents with ideas for kids.* NIH Pub. 06-4821, 2006.[23]

**TABLE 25-1** Estimated Number of Young People Ages 5–17 Enrolled in Specific Categories of Youth Sports[3]

| Activities | Estimated number of participants |
|---|---|
| Agency-sponsored sports (Little League baseball, Pop Warner football) | 22 million |
| Club sports (Fee-based services such as gymnastics, ice skating, and swimming) | 2.4 million |
| Recreational sports programs (Everyone Plays, sponsored by recreational departments) | 14.5 million |
| Intramural sports (in middle, junior, senior high schools) | 0.5 million |
| Interscholastic sports (in middle, junior, senior high schools) | 7.5 million |

- Most organized sports-related injuries (62 percent) occur during practice rather than games; however, approximately 33 percent of parents often do not take the same safety precautions during their child's practice as they would for a game.

- The highest rates of sports injury for boys are ice hockey, rugby, and soccer. Soccer, basketball and gymnastics seem to incur the highest rates of injury in girls.[1]

- A recent survey found that among athletes ages 5 to 14 years, 15 percent of basketball players, 28 percent of football players, 22 percent of soccer players, 25 percent of baseball players, and 12 percent of softball players have been injured while playing their respective sports.

- In 2004, nearly 391,800 children ages 5 to 14 years were treated in hospital emergency rooms for either football or basketball-related injuries.

- Children ages 5 to 14 years are at a higher risk of winter sports injuries; each year, approximately 49,000 injuries are sustained among this age group involving skiing, snowboarding, or sledding.

- The most common types of sport-related injuries in children are sprains (mostly ankle), muscle strains, bone or growth plate injuries, repetitive motion injuries, and heat-related illness.

- Approximately two out of five traumatic brain injuries among children are associated with participation in sports and recreational activities. Brain injury is the leading cause of sports-related death to children.

- Children who do not wear or use protective equipment are at greater risk of sustaining sports-related injuries. Inappropriate or unavailable equipment are reasons for children's not wearing protective gear.

Proven Interventions

- Children should have access to and consistently use the appropriate gear necessary for each respective sport.
- Organized sports through schools, community clubs, and recreation areas that are properly maintained assist in preventing injuries to children.
- Coaches should be trained in first aid and CPR and should have a plan for responding to emergencies. Coaches should be well versed in the proper use of equipment and should enforce rules on equipment use.
- Sports programs with adults on staff who are Certified Athletic Trainers are ideal because such trainers can help prevent or provide immediate care for athletic injuries.

## PHYSICAL MATURITY ASSESSMENT IN MATCHING ATHLETES

Children are at greater risk than adults for sports and recreational injuries because they are unable to assess the risks involved and have less coordination, slower reaction times, and less accuracy (Figure 25-2). Children ages 5 to 14 account for nearly 40 percent of all sports-related injuries treated in hospital emergency departments. The rate and severity of sports-related injuries increase with a child's age. Among children ages 5 to 9, sports-related injuries occur more frequently among girls than boys. However, during puberty, ages 10 to 14, boys are injured more frequently and more severely than girls. Among children ages 5 to 14, boys account for nearly 75 percent of all sports-related injuries. In addition, boys are more likely than girls to suffer from multiple injuries.[23]

**Figure 25-2**

The risk of injury is inherent in both recreational and organized youth sport activities.

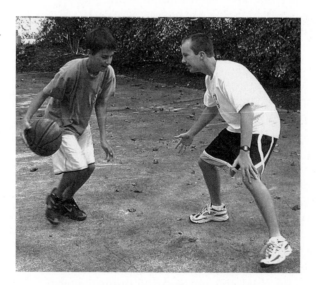

**TABLE 25-2** Tanner Stages of Maturity

| | |
|---|---|
| Males | Stage 1. No evidence of pubic hair. |
| | Stage 2. Slightly pigmented hair laterally at the base of the penis, usually straight. |
| | Stage 3. Hair becomes darker, coarser, begins to curl and spreads over the pubes. |
| | Stage 4. Hair is adult in type but does not extend onto thighs. |
| | Stage 5. Hair extends onto the thighs and frequently up the linea alba. |
| Females | Stage 1. No evidence of pubic hair. |
| | Stage 2. Long, slightly pigmented, downy hair along the edges of the labia. |
| | Stage 3. Darker, coarser, slightly curled hair spread sparsely over the mons pubis. |
| | Stage 4. Adult type of hair but it does not extend onto thighs. |
| | Stage 5. Adult distribution including spread along the medial aspects of the thighs. |

However, the risk of sports injury is associated more with a child's stage of development than age or body size. A less developed child competing against a more mature child of the same age and weight is at a disadvantage and may be at greater risk for injury. **Therefore all youth sports participants should be matched by physical maturation, weight, size, and skill level.**

Maturity assessment should be part of the preparticipation physical examination as a means of protecting the young physically developing athlete. The most commonly used method for estimating physical maturity is Tanner's Stages of Maturity, indicating development of secondary sexual characteristics.[27] The Tanner approach evaluates pubic hair and genitalia development in boys and pubic hair and breast development in girls (Table 25-2). Other indicators that may be noted are facial and axillary hair. Stage one indicates that puberty is not evident, and stage five indicates full development. The crucial stage in terms of collision and high-intensity noncontact sports is stage three, in which there is the fastest bone growth. In this stage, the growth plates are two to five times weaker than the joint capsule and tendon attachments. Tanner's staging emphasizes that young athletes in grades 7 to 12 must be matched by maturity, not age.[27]

The American Academy of Pediatrics indicates that there is no physical reason to separate preadolescent girls and boys by gender in recreational or competitive sports activities. Separation of genders should occur in collision-type sports once boys have attained greater muscle mass in proportion to their body weight.[2]

There is no need to separate preadolescent girls and boys in competitive sports.

## PHYSICAL CONDITIONING AND TRAINING

**Guidelines and training philosophies developed for and used by adults should not be imposed on youngsters who are anatomically, physiologically, or psychologically less mature.** In conditioning programs, young athletes should focus on developing muscular strength and endurance, cardiovascular fitness, and flexibility[6] (see Chapter 4). Young athletes should work with fitness professionals, coaches, and/or athletic trainers, if available, year-round, to ensure they maintain their conditioning with appropriate exercises and nutrition. In addition, young athletes should engage in appropriate conditioning programs for a minimum of six weeks before the start of daily practice.[12] A minimum of a 15-minute warm-up period before any game or practice, and an appropriate cool-down period afterward, is recommended. Young athletes should also warm up for five minutes during any prolonged breaks in activity (including half time, between periods, etc.). Young athletes should routinely stretch properly before and after workouts of any kind. Workouts and practices should be limited to no more than two hours, since injuries are more likely to occur when the athlete becomes fatigued.[10]

Strength training refers to a systematic program of exercises designed to increase an individual's ability to exert or resist force[10] (Figure 25-3). Contrary to the traditional belief that strength training is dangerous for children, the American College of Sports Medicine (ACSM), the American Orthopedic Society for Sports Medicine, and the American Academy of

**Figure 25-3**

Several professional organizations have recommended strength training for young athletes in properly designed and supervised programs.

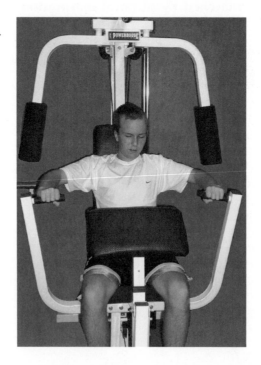

**TABLE 25-3** Recommendations for Strength Training Programs from the American Academy of Pediatrics*[2]

1. Strength training programs for preadolescents and adolescents can be safe and effective if proper resistance training techniques and safety precautions are followed.
2. Preadolescents and adolescents should avoid competitive weight-lifting, power lifting, body building, and maximal lifts until they reach physical and skeletal maturity.
3. In recommending or evaluating strength training programs for children and adolescents, the following issues should be considered:
   a. Before beginning a formal strength training program, a physician should perform a medical evaluation. If indicated, a referral may be made to a sports medicine physician who is familiar with various strength training methods as well as risks and benefits in preadolescents and adolescents.
   b. Aerobic conditions should be coupled with resistance training if general health benefits are the goal.
   c. Strength training programs should include a warm-up and cool-down component.
   d. Specific strength training exercises should be learned initially with no load (resistance). Once the exercise skill has been mastered, incremental loads can be added.
   e. Progressive resistance exercise requires successful completion of 8 to 15 repetitions in good form before increasing weight or resistance.
   f. A general strengthening program should address all major muscle groups and exercise through the complete range of motion.
   g. Any sign of injury or illness from strength training should be evaluated before continuing the exercise in question.

*Modified from the American Academy of Pediatrics Committee on Sports Medicine and Fitness: Strength Training by Children and Adolescents, *Pediatrics* 107(6):1470–1472, 2001.[2]

Pediatrics maintain that for young athletes who have the emotional maturity to accept and follow directions, strength training can be a safe and effective activity, provided that the program is properly designed and competently supervised[1,2,3] (Table 25-3). Even some seven- and eight-year-old boys and girls have benefited from strength training. There is no reason why younger children could not participate in strength-related activities, such as push-ups and sit-ups, if they can safely perform the exercises and follow instructions.[3] In general, if children are ready for participation in organized sports or activities—such as Little League baseball, soccer, or gymnastics—then they are ready for some type of strength training.[10] It must be emphasized, however, that strength training is a form of physical conditioning distinct from the competitive sports of competitive weightlifting and power-lifting.[3] It has been suggested that in young athletes strength training may also decrease the incidence of some sports injuries by increasing the strength of tendons, ligaments, and bone.[11]

**25-1 Critical Thinking**
Exercise

A parent of a 10-year-old boy asks the coach of a youth football team if it is all right to have his son begin strength training with weights.

? How should the coach respond to this?

Sports should allow boys and
girls to develop positive self-
esteem.

## PSYCHOLOGICAL AND LEARNING CONCERNS

Of even more concern than the physical aspects of sports are the psychological stresses that may be placed on children by overzealous parents, coaches, and fitness professionals.[13] Children must not be considered to be miniature adults. Although children can mimic adult skills, they often cannot understand sports concepts such as playing fair unless specifically taught.

Children usually are eager to please adults, making them vulnerable to coercion and manipulation. A positive approach should be used by giving children frequent encouragement with positive reinforcements followed by corrective[14] feedback. With this method the young athlete has the opportunity to develop a sense of self-worth and positive self-esteem.[8]

Not all children are equal in ability. Some children respond well to competition, others respond poorly, as usually demonstrated by their level of performance. A child must be shown that there are benefits in experiencing a loss and that trying to the best of his or her ability is the most important factor in competition. Parents and coaches must realize that children are not good at making performance corrections unless instructions are given instantly at the time of the situation. In other words, half-time performance suggestions given a half-hour later may have little effect on the child.[8]

**Enjoyment of an activity, rather than winning at all costs, should be the focus of a child's training, conditioning, and competition** (Figure 25-4).[33] Too often parents who were fine athletes or who wanted to be great athletes coerce their young children to the point of anxiety and a dislike for the sport.[16]

**Figure 25-4**

It is critical that the young athlete makes enjoying the activity the focus rather than concentrating on training competition and winning.

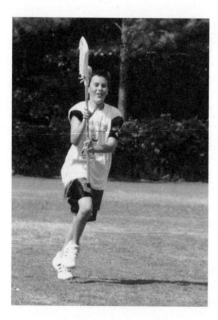

There are many differences between free-flowing play and organized sports. Organized sports, fortunately or unfortunately, carry the obligatory win or lose connotations of competition and also involve adults who coach and train the youngster, as well as adults who interpret and enforce the rules that govern competition. The adverse effect of adult influences upon the young athlete is but one potential negative psychological aspect of youth sport participation.[30]

Participation in organized sport can be taken to an extreme. Intensive participation can be described in terms of frequency and/or intensity.[33] Examples of intensive participation include the ice skater or gymnast who trains daily for hours and competes all year round for years on end. Other examples include the multisport athlete who trains and competes on a daily basis all year round. This intensive participation places significant physical demands on the body, demands that may result in serious overuse or stress-failure injury. Just as the young body grows to accept greater physical demands, so does the young mind. Intensive participation places many demands on the youngster, some of which may be unrealistic. As this relates to intense competition, research demonstrates that a child's cognitive ability to develop a mature understanding of the competition process does not occur until the age of 12. It is not until between the ages of 10 and 12 years of age that children develop the capacity to comprehend more than just one other viewpoint. Finally, after the age of 12 years the youngster can readily adopt a team perspective.

Psychological issues may also enter the picture when rehabilitating youth sport participants involved in intense competition and training. Risk factors for psychological complications in the injured child include stress in the family, high-achieving siblings, over- or underinvolved parent(s), a paradoxical lack of leisure in athletic activity, self-esteem that is reliant on athletic prowess, and a narrow range of interests beyond athletics.

## COACHING QUALIFICATIONS

No federal laws require coaching education at any level of competition.[5] Currently, the way to become trained as a coach in the United States is to complete a university degree program, a National Body of Sports certification program, and/or a youth sports coaching education program.[24] Until 1996 no coaching standards had been developed.[20] The National Association for Sport and Physical Education (NASPE) has developed the National Standards for Athletic Coaches. The standards are not intended to be a certification program or the basis of a single national assessment for all coaches. The standards are put forth to help organizations and agencies who currently certify coaches, provide coach education/training, evaluate select coaches, or design programs to meet the needs of prospective and practicing coaches.[20] The United States Olympic Committee (USOC) has mandated that all coaches participating under the governance of USOC receive certification in the safety training course developed by the American Red Cross/USOC.[31]

Recognition and
Management of Specific
Injuries and Conditions

Youth sport coaches must be
certified and educated in
• techniques of coaching
• supervising conditioning
• sport safety
• first aid
• child development
• CPR

10 percent of youth in
organized sports sustain an
injury.

Often coaches of youth sports have little or no background in providing safe and positive sports experiences. It is estimated that 2.5 million volunteer coaches lack formal preparation.[7] Every youth sport coach should be certified and dedicated to the highest ideals of coaching.[25] One organization that promotes such ideals is the National Youth Sports Coaches Association (NYSCA).[20] Currently the NYSCA has a membership of more than 143,000 that serves more than 2 million boys and girls in the United States. This association offers three levels of certification consisting of the fundamentals of coaching, first aid and safety, and common sports injuries; it also offers instruction in the psychological aspects of losing and in discipline. All youth sport coaches must also have a good understanding of normal child development—physical, emotional, and psychological.[4]

Other nationally recognized coaching certification programs include the American Sport Education Program (ASEP) and the Program for Athletic Coaches Education (PACE). Coaching certification programs are also available through individual National Sport Governing Bodies (NGBs) such as the United States Soccer Federation (USSF).[20]

## COMMON INJURIES IN THE YOUNG ATHLETE

Children are susceptible to many of the same sport injuries that the physically mature athlete is, including joint sprains, muscle and tendon strains, and skeletal fractures.[27]

Many pediatric physicians are concerned about these repeated microtraumas that can occur to the young athlete over time. Such small traumas can compound and produce chronic and, in some cases, degenerative conditions within the immature musculoskeletal system.[6]

### Growth Plate Fractures

The bones of young athletes and adults share many of the same risks for injury. However, a young athlete's bones are also subject to an injury called a growth plate fracture. The growth plate (physis) is an area of developing tissue near the ends of long bones, between the shaft of the bone (the diaphysis) and the end of the bone (the epiphysis). The long bones of the body do not grow from the center outward but grow instead at each end of the bone around the growth plate.[15] The growth plate regulates and determines the length and shape of the mature bone and is the last portion of the bone to harden (ossify), thus leaving it vulnerable to fracture. Fractures can result either from a single traumatic event, such as a fall, or from chronic stress and overuse. Most growth plate fractures occur in the radius of the forearm, the tibia and fibula in the lower leg, and the fingers.[15]

About one-third of all growth plate injuries occur in competitive sports, such as football, basketball, or gymnastics, while about 20 percent occur with participation in recreational activities, such as biking, sledding, skiing, or skateboarding. Females between the ages of 11 and 12 and 14-year-old males are most likely to experience this injury, although all children who are still growing are at risk. Males are twice as likely to have growth plate fractures as females.[15]

If a fracture of any bone is suspected the young athlete should be immediately referred to a physician for x-ray to determine the type of fracture. If a fracture of the growth plate has occurred, the severity of the injury is determined depending on the degree of damage to the growth plate itself. Treatment may range from immobilization in a cast to surgery for repair and internal fixation.

Growth plate fractures must be carefully monitored to ensure proper long-term results. In some cases, the injury prevents the bone from getting longer. In other cases, the fracture actually stimulates growth so that the injured bone is longer than the uninjured bone. Complicated fractures need to be followed until the young athlete reaches skeletal maturity.

## Apophysitis

The apophysis is a specialized area of cartilage within the growth plate. At certain locations throughout the body, a large tendon inserts into the bone at the apophysis. The apophysis is very susceptible to injury because it is developing cartilage and not mature bone. The repetitive stresses of running, jumping, and other actions produce an inflammation or irritation of the apophysis at these tendon insertions. Apophysitis is inflammation of an apophysis. The most common sites for apophysitis are at the insertion of the patellar tendon on the tibial tubercle in the knee and at the insertion of the Achilles tendon on the calcaneous at the heel. Osgood-Schlatters disease is an apophysitis of the tibial tubercle in the knee and Sever's disease is an apophysitis of the calcaneous.[19] They usually result from repetitive actions rather than from a specific episode, though sometimes an injury will first bring attention to the problem. The symptoms of these conditions usually begin between 8 and 15 years of age. The pain that occurs is primarily related to activities and does not typically awaken the adolescent at night. In these conditions, the tenderness is well localized, and there are no other significant abnormalities of the knee, ankle, or other surrounding parts.

Diagnosis is usually made from information from the history and physical examination. A physician may order radiographs (x-rays) to confirm the diagnosis or to exclude other problems. It is most important to understand that these are not serious conditions. They do not affect the joints themselves, so they do not lead to anything serious such as arthritis, though they can take up to several years to resolve. Most treatment is directed toward reducing the symptoms.

## Avulsion Fractures

In a growing child, it is clear that the muscles must grow and adapt to the increasing length of the skeletal bones. It appears that a change in muscle length results from changes within the muscle belly itself and/or an increase in tendon length. When changes in muscle length do not match changes in long bone growth, stresses occurring in the muscle predispose the young athlete to injury. Injuries range from varying degrees of muscle strain to situations where the bony attachment of the muscle fails before the muscle is damaged. An avulsion fracture as defined previously is one in which a piece of bone is fractured and pulled away from the rest of the bone at the site of tendon or ligament attachment. The most common sites for these avulsion injuries in the young athlete include the anterior superior and inferior iliac spines in the ilium, the ischial spine, and the fifth metatarsal in the foot. As forces across the joints of the lower extremity due to running, jumping, and kicking exceed most forces across the upper extremity, avulsion fractures of the lower extremity outnumber avulsion fractures of the upper extremity. Stresses across the shoulder and elbow of the young throwing athlete, however, are sufficient to result in avulsion of the medial humeral epicondyle and proximal humerus.

### Spondylolysis

Spondylolysis is a defect or fracture in the bony structures of the spine that occurs most often in young athletes.[29] Physical forces encountered by youngsters involved in physical activities play a significant role in the development of spondylolysis. Activities that involve repetitive loading, especially with the lumbar spine in extension/hyperextension, such as ballet, gymnastics, diving, football, weight lifting, and wrestling, have been implicated in spondylolysis. Spondylolysis originates in children between the ages of 5 and 10 years and most frequently occurs at the fifth lumbar vertebra, with the fourth lumbar vertebra being involved second most frequently. Many youngsters with spondylolysis remain asymptomatic for long periods of time and are often not diagnosed until later in their skeletal development. X-rays are required to visualize the fracture.[29]

Spondylolisthesis is a condition in which a vertebra slips anterior to the vertebra immediately below it. Spondylolisthesis most frequently takes place between the fifth lumbar and first sacral vertebrae, although the condition can occur at more than one spinal segment.

Treatment of spondylolysis and spondylolisthesis centers on healing the bony defect and decreasing the patient's symptoms. Treatment depends upon the physician's personal preference and ranges from relative rest without a brace to 23 hours of bracing each day. When bracing is used, the brace is typically a rigid custom-fit lumbar spinal orthosis designed to keep the youngster out of extension. In addition to activity modification, hamstring stretching is an integral part of the treatment program.[29]

## SPORTS INJURY PREVENTION

One of the primary goals of every parent, coach, and administrator involved with youth sports should be to do everything possible to minimize the chances of injury to the young athlete. While it is certainly true that injuries are inherent with participation in sport activities, it is also true that many sports injuries can be prevented by paying attention to some common-sense guidelines such as ensuring proper physical and psychological conditioning, using appropriate safety equipment, creating a safe playing environment, providing adequate adult supervision, and enforcing safety rules in any sports program.

Parents and coaches should ensure that each athlete receives a pre-participation physical exam, either from the family physician or from a team physician. The physical should consist of a general exam, which includes checks on height, weight, pulse, respiration, blood pressure, eye, ear, nose, chest, and abdomen. It should also include an orthopedic exam that focuses on joint flexibility, joint range of motion, muscle strength, and a history of past bone and joint injuries[18] (see Chapter 2).

As stressed earlier in this chapter, young athletes should be encouraged to focus on developing muscular strength and endurance, cardiovascular fitness, and flexibility. The young athletes who consistently work on conditioning and training are not only likely to enhance their performance but also to reduce the likelihood of injury because they are more fit (see Chapter 4).

The young athlete should be educated about, and pay attention to, sound nutritional practices, which include eating a balanced diet from the basic food groups. A young athlete's diet should be high in carbohydrates while also including essential proteins and fats (see Chapter 5).

Young athletes must be acclimatized to practicing or playing in hot, humid, sunny environments. Practices and games should be held early in the morning or late in the afternoon if at all possible. Coaches and parents can minimize the chances of the young athlete having a heat-related problem by making certain that the athlete is appropriately hydrated. Fluid breaks should be offered at consistent intervals, and young athletes should be strongly encouraged to consume sufficient fluids to help prevent dehydration (see Chapter 10).

Athletes should use appropriate, properly fitted protective equipment. This equipment should be constantly checked to ensure that it is in good condition. Defective equipment should be replaced or repaired immediately if any problems are noted. Appropriate protective equipment should be worn in all practices as well as during competitions (see Chapter 6).

Coaches and parents should also take responsibility for making certain that schools at the junior high, middle school, or high school levels establish and implement specific plans, guidelines, and policies for dealing with injuries to the young athletes competing at that institution. Table 25-4 recommends safety plans, guidelines, and policies that schools should establish for the injured athletes.

Parents and coaches should do everything possible to create a safe playing environment. They must ensure adequate adult supervision, make sure playing conditions (e.g., field surfacing, maintenance) are safe and develop and enforce safety rules that help reduce the number and severity of sports and recreational injuries. Table 25-5 provides injury prevention guidelines for specific sports.[28]

Youth athletes must practice good hygiene and other health habits.

**TABLE 25-4** Plans, Policies, and Guidelines for Managing Injuries in School
Athletic Programs*

**25-4 Critical Thinking**
Exercise

A new high school has opened,
and the new athletic director
has been directed by the school
board to develop a written
policies and procedures plan for
dealing with the injured athlete.

? What issues should be
addressed and included in this
document?

- Have a preestablished emergency plan.
- Provide a full time on-site certified athletic trainer.
- Identify a team physician/consulting physician.
- Develop an injury protection manual describing how injuries are handled
  and who is responsible for overseeing injury management.
- Provide preparticipation physical evaluations for all athletes annually.
- Compile emergency medical authorization cards that give parental
  permission for emergency medical care if required.
- Establish specific inclement weather protocols/guidelines (i.e., lightning
  storms and extreme heat).
- Require coaches to participate in ongoing education in coaching techniques,
  CPR, and first aid.
- Establish a protocol for "return to participation following injury" decisions.
- Develop a field/facility maintenance plan.
- Develop policies on purchase, fitting, and maintenance of athletic
  equipment.
- Provide a supervised year-round conditioning program for ALL student
  athletes.

*Modified from "Safety Items Parents Should Look for in a High School Athletic
Program," National Athletic Trainers' Association, Secondary School Athletic Trainers'
Committee, 1999.

**TABLE 25-5** Sport-Specific Guidelines for Injury Prevention*

| | |
|---|---|
| Baseball/ Softball | • Most injuries in baseball and softball involve the throwing arm and shoulder, but these injuries usually emerge gradually. Young athletes should not abuse the throwing arm by overusing it.<br>• Players should incorporate conditioning and stretching exercises for the shoulder into their overall program.<br>• It is to the player's advantage to warm up and cool down the throwing arm properly to minimize the risk of injuries.<br>• Condition all shoulder muscles, emphasizing muscles in the back of the shoulder that are required to stop the pitching motion. Muscles in the front of the arm are naturally stronger—shoulder injuries can result from weaker muscles in the back. |
| Basketball | • Players should focus on conditioning exercises for the total body, including upper and lower extremities.<br>• Players should focus on good warm-up and stretching prior to any ballistic movements.<br>• Footwear should fit properly to minimize the risk of ankle- and foot-related injuries.<br>• Replace footwear when the shock absorption is no longer adequate. |
| Football | • Intentional spearing of opponents should be discouraged.<br>• Blocking below the waist should be minimized during practice.<br>• Block and tackle with the head up to reduce the risk of neck injuries. |

*Modified from "Minimizing the Risks of Injury in High School Athletics" National Athletic Trainers Association, Dallas TX,
2002.

**TABLE 25-5** (Continued)

| | |
|---|---|
| Football (cont'd) | • In addition to total strengthening and conditioning, football-specific conditioning exercises should strengthen the neck to allow players to keep their heads firmly erect while making contact during blocks or tackles. |
| | • Make sure the practice and playing areas are safe. Look for holes, broken glass, and other hazards on and around the practice field, game field, and blocking sleds. |
| | • Ample fluid replacement should be available at all times. |
| Soccer | • Players should be encouraged to wear appropriate shin guards during practice and play. |
| | • Provide fluids on the sidelines throughout practice and games. Although soccer requires non-stop play with no time-outs, athletes should be encouraged to come to the sidelines or touch line where they can replenish fluids without penalty. |
| | • Warm up for approximately 15 minutes, beginning for half that time without a ball. Warm-up exercises should include light jogging and stretching. Without these warm-ups, the explosive action of shooting can result in strained muscles. |
| | • Adhere to the rules of the game when tackling. |
| | • Although soccer does not provide time-outs, injuries should be evaluated immediately to ensure the athlete is not worsening the injury. |
| Track and Field | • Stretching is key to minimizing the risk of injury in every event. |
| | • Conditioning programs should concentrate on muscular strength, muscular endurance, and flexibility. Individual event training should be emphasized. |
| | • All athletes involved in running events should work to maintain year-round cardiovascular endurance. |
| | • Before and after each event, athletes should warm up and cool down, stretch, and hydrate with fluids. |
| | • Special attention should be paid to the nutritional needs of the endurance athlete. |
| Volleyball | • An overall strength base with emphasis on leg, back, and posterior shoulder (rotator cuff) strengthening during the preseason is vital. |
| | • Proper equipment should include volleyball-specific shoes and knee pads for shock absorption. |
| | • A proper warm-up and stretching program should emphasize the shoulder, low back, and legs. Do not start spiking before warming up and stretching the shoulder. After stretching, start throwing a volleyball easily, gradually increasing intensity until the muscles are warm. |
| | • Advanced drills and conditioning, such as plyometrics or jump training, should not be conducted unless the athlete has been tested and can demonstrate balance, flexibility, and strength. |
| | • Ample fluid replacement should be available at all times. |
| Wrestling | • Depleting food and fluid to make a particular weight class may be detrimental to the health and safety of the athlete. Body composition and weight loss should be closely monitored. |
| | • Wrestlers should be encouraged to wear protective headgear that provides ear protection. |
| | • Wrestlers should be encouraged to wear protective knee pads. |
| | • To reduce the risk of skin diseases, wrestlers should shower before and after workouts; wash their workout clothes daily; dry their skin adequately; clean mats daily; avoid wearing street shoes on wrestling mats or wrestling shoes off the mats; wipe headgear down with alcohol pads after each use; and conduct daily total body skin inspections. |
| | • Wrestlers with open wounds, broken skin, or diseases of the skin should be discouraged from participating until the skin is healed or the wrestler has been cleared to participate by a licensed physician. If allowed to wrestle, the athlete should have the affected skin covered to prevent cross-contamination. |
| | • Proper strength and conditioning regimes should be encouraged. |

## Athletic Injury Management Checklist

Following is a checklist of things that might potentially result in youth sports injuries.

☐ Inadequate preparticipation exams.
☐ Improper, poorly fitted, or lack of protective equipment.
☐ Grouping teams by age instead of size.
☐ Hazardous playing fields and other environmental hazards.
☐ Training errors.
☐ Undue fatigue or overtraining.
☐ Lack of coaching education.
☐ Insufficient or incorrect instruction.
☐ Failure to do proper warm-up stretching and cooldown.
☐ Allowing the athlete to play when injured.
☐ Delayed or insufficient medical care.
☐ Poor nutrition.
☐ Poor health habits.

## SUMMARY

- The extent to which young athletes train and compete must be carefully monitored to avoid physical and emotional injuries.

- The estimated number of young people engaging in some sport in the United States is 30 million.

- A major concern to some parents and health care professionals is the stress placed on the young body from intense sports competition and training.

- All youth sport participants should be matched by physical maturation, weight, size, skill level, and experience.

- Young athletes can positively respond to some type of conditioning exercises, if the exercises are properly supervised and conducted.

- Activities such as falling, jumping, landing on straight legs, repeated hard throwing motions, running very long distances, and lifting heavy weights may produce injuries to the immature musculoskeletal system.

- Children are not miniature adults; coaching must be based on their emotional and cognitive level.

- Separation of genders in sport activities needs to occur only when boys have attained greater muscle mass in proportion to their body weight.

- Enjoyment of an activity, rather than winning at all costs, must be stressed to children as the most important factor in sports participation.

- An overzealous coach can cause the young athlete great emotional stress.
- Coaches participating in youth sports must be trained in techniques and skills, safety and injury prevention, first aid, and growth and development.
- Coaches should be certified.
- Each year more than 775,000 young athletes under 15 years of age are treated for sports-related injuries.
- Young athletes are prone to the same injuries that the mature athlete is, but they must also contend with injuries to their skeletal growth centers.
- Injuries to young athletes can be avoided through proper conditioning and supervision, proper matching, use of proper equipment, and appropriate rules of competition.
- Young athletes must be encouraged to practice good health habits.

---

*Solutions to Critical Thinking* Exercises

---

**25-1** Strength training is safe and effective for this 10-year-old as long as (1) the program is properly designed and competently supervised, and (2) the boy has the emotional maturity to accept and follow directions. If this boy is ready to participate in organized sports, he is ready for some type of strength training.

**25-2** Based on the symptoms, it is likely this girl has a fracture. Call the rescue squad and do not move her until the injury has been immobilized. Of greatest concern in a young girl of this age is that she has fracture of the physis or growth plate.

**25-3** It is likely the young gymnast has a spondylolysis. This condition typically occurs from repeated forced hyperextensions of the low back. Make certain that this girl is evaluated by her family physician before she is allowed to resume practice or competition.

**25-4** Some of the more important issues that should be addressed in the policies and procedures plan include having an emergency action plan; providing preparticipation physical evaluations for all athletes; compiling emergency medical authorization cards that give parental permission for emergency medical care; establishing inclement weather guidelines; developing a field/facility maintenance plan; employing a certified athletic trainer and identifying a team physician; requiring coaches to be certified in CPR and first aid; developing policies on purchase and maintenance of protective equipment; and providing a supervised year-round conditioning program.

## REVIEW QUESTIONS AND CLASS ACTIVITIES

1. Why are young athletes more susceptible to injuries than adults?
2. Discuss where, how, and to whom youth sports injuries are occurring in the United States.
3. What criteria should be used for matching young athletes in terms of their competitive levels?

4. Describe Tanner's Stages of Maturity and explain how this scale is applied to matching athletes.

5. Under what circumstances is it all right for young athletes to engage in a strength training program?

6. What are some of the psychological considerations relative to young athletes' competing in organized sport activities?

7. Identify different organizations that have established certification programs for coaches of youth sports.

8. Discuss recognition and management of the types of injuries that are likely to occur in the young athlete.

9. What can parents and coaches do to help prevent or minimize injuries in the young athlete?

## REFERENCES

1. American Academy of Orthopedic Surgeons, P.O. Box 1998, Des Plaines, IL 60017.

2. American Academy of Pediatrics Committee on Sports Medicine and Fitness: 2001. Strength training by children and adolescents, *Pediatrics* 107(6):1470–1472.

3. American College of Sports Medicine http://www.acsm.org/health/currentcomments/YSTRNGTH.pdf

4. Bach, G: 2003. What coaches should know: certification programs lay a foundation for volunteer coaches to work effectively with youngsters in organized sports, *Athletic business* 27(11):70–72; 74; 76.

5. Barfield, WR, Kirkendall, DT, McBryde Jr., AM: 2003. Who can coach our youth in sports?, *ACSM's health & fitness journal* 7(5):10–15.

6. Benjamine, HJ, Glow, KM: 2003. Strength training for children and adolescents. What can physicians recommend?, *Physician and sportsmedicine* 31(9):19–26.

7. Carnegie Corporation of New York, 437 Madison Ave, New York, NY 10022.

8. Cherubini, JM, Hamstra, KL, Swanik, CB: 2002. Athletic injury and parental pressure in youth sports, *Athletic therapy today*, 7(6): 36–41.

9. Duri ZA: 2002. The immature athlete, *Clinics in sports medicine* 21(3): 461–482.

10. Faigenbaum AD, Micheli LJ: 1998. Youth resistance training, *Sports medicine bulletin* 32(2):28.

11. Faigenbaum, AD, Schram, J: 2004. Can resistance training reduce injuries in youth sports?, *Strength and conditioning journal* 26(3):16–21.

12. Faigenbaum AD: 2001. Preseason conditioning for high school athletes, *Strength and conditioning journal* 23(1):70–72.

13. Hamstra KL: 2002. Athletic injury and parental pressure in youth sports, *Athletic therapy today* 7(6): 36–41.

14. Holt, N, Tamminen, K, Black, D: 2008. Parental involvement in competitive youth sport settings, *Psychology of sport & exercise* 9(5):663.

15. Hunt TN: 2003. Epiphyseal-plate fracture in an adolescent athlete, *Athletic therapy today* 8(1):34–36.

16. Kanters, M, Bocarro, J: 2008. Supported or pressured? An examination of agreement among parents and children on parent's role in youth sports, *Journal of sport behavior* 31(1):64.

17. Koester MC: 2002. Adolescent and youth sports medicine: a "growing" concern, *Athletic therapy today* 7(6):6–12.

18. Koester MC: 2000. Youth sports: a pediatrician's perspective on coaching and injury prevention, *Journal of athletic training* 35(4): 466–470.

19. Mitchell, D: 2008. Sever's disease: what does the literature really tell us? *American Academy of Podiatric Sports Medicine newsletter* 3:7.

20. National Association for Sports and Physical Education (NASPE), 1900 Association Dr., Reston, VA 22091.

21. National Electronic Injury Surveillance System, US Consumer Product Safety Commission, National Injury Information Clearinghouse, 1998.

22. National Safe Kids Campaign: Injury facts: Sports Injuries, http://www.safekids.org/

23. National SAFE KIDS Campaign: 2006. Childhood sports injuries and their prevention: a guide for parents with ideas for kids, NIH Pub. 06-4821.

24. National Youth Sports Safety Foundation, 333 Longwood Ave, Suite 202, Boston, MA 02115.

25. Perkins, D: 2007. Coaches: making youth sports a positive experience. *Coaching update* 22(2):4–5; 24–25.

26. Pfeiffer RP: 2002. Pediatric sports injuries, *Athletic therapy today* 7(6):5.

27. Prentice B: 2009. *Arnheim's Principles of athletic training*, 13th ed. New York, McGraw-Hill.

28. Shimon JM: 2002. Youth sport injury prevention: prevention is key, *Strategies* 15(5):27–30.

29. Standaert CJ: 2002. Spondylolysis in the adolescent athlete, *Clinical journal of sport medicine* 12(2): 119–122.

30. Torres, C, Hager, P: 2007. De-emphasizing competition in organized youth sport: misdirected reforms and misled children, *Journal of the philosophy of sport* 34(2):194.

31. United States Olympic Committee (USOC), National Governing Bodies of Sports, One Olympic Plaza, Colorado Springs, CO 80909.

32. Wells, M, Arthur-Banning, S, Paisley, K: 2008. Good (youth) sports: using benefits-based programming to increase sportsmanship, *Journal of park & recreation administration* 26(1):1.

33. Whisenant, W, Jordan, J: 2008. Fairness and enjoyment in school sponsored youth sports. *International review for the sociology of sport* 43(1):91.

## ANNOTATED BIBLIOGRAPHY

American Academy of Pediatrics: 1991. *Sports medicine: health care for young athletes*, Elk Grove Village, IL, American Academy of Pediatrics.

*A comprehensive guide to training, conditioning, and injury care of the young athlete.*

Appenzeller H: 2000. *Youth sports and the law: a guide to legal issues*, Chapel Hill, NC, Carolina Academic Press.

*Studies various court cases to understand the legal principles involved in sport participation. The objective of the book is to provide better and safer sporting experiences for today's children.*

*Athletic Therapy Today* 7(6):2002. Special edition on pediatric sports injury.

Birrer R, Griesmer B, Cataletto M: 2002. *Pediatric sports medicine for primary care*, Baltimore, Lippincott, Williams & Wilkins.

*Provides useful information on the management of sports-related injuries, discusses the preparticipation physical examination, the athlete's growth and maturation, nutrition, the psycho-social aspects of sports participation, and common medical problems.*

*Coaching youth sports*, Bimonthly journal.

*Features excellent information and advice for individuals who are youth sport coaches.*

Crisfield P, Carm S: 2001. *The young athlete's handbook*, Champaign, IL, Human Kinetics.

*Discusses how to manage training; develop techniques and skills; and maintain a healthy balance between sports, school, friends, and family.*

Kraemer, WJ, Fleck, SJ: 2005. *Strength training for young athletes*, 2nd ed.; Champaign, IL, Human Kinetics.

*Provides answers as the authoritative guide to strength development for 7- to 18-year-old athletes. Presents the latest facts on the effects of strength training on growth, development, and performance and makes recommendations relative to starting age, choice of exercises, frequency of training, rate of progression, and philosophical aspects of program design.*

Lair C, Murdoch S: 2002. *Feeding the young athlete: Sports nutrition made easy for players and parents*, Seattle, Moon Smile Press.

*Provides detailed discussion of nutritional practices for serious and committed student athletes.*

Litt, A, editor: 2004. *Fuel for young athletes*, Champaign, IL, Human Kinetics.

*Provides guidelines for meeting the essential nutritional needs of adolescent athletes to set the stage for good health and optimal performance throughout their sport careers.*

Metzl J, Shookhoff C: 2002. *The young athlete: A sports doctor's complete guide for parents*, New York, Little Brown and Company.

*Explores how to be a good sports parent, hallmarks of good coaching, nutrition and nutritional supplements, and keeping values and perspective intact (including topics such as preventing sports from taking over the family's life, good sportsmanship, and ethics).*

**WEB SITES**

National Youth Sports Safety Foundation:
www.nyssf.org

American Academy of Pediatrics:
www.aap.org

National Association for Sport and Physical Education:
www.aahperd.org

KidsHealth:
www.kidshealth.org

National Safe Kids Campaign:
www.safekids.org

National Youth Sport Coaches Association
www.nays.org/coaches/

Parents Alliance for Youth Sports
http://paysonline.nays.org/

Academy for Youth Sports Administrators
www.nays.org/IntMain.cfm?Page=28&Cat=18

National Alliance for Youth Sports
www.nays.org/

Tips for Soccer Moms and Dads
www.calstatela.edu/faculty/dfrankl/soccer/soccer01.htm
www.nays.org/academy/

Youth Sports Network
www.myteam.com/

The Institute for the Study of Youth Sports
http://ed-web3.educ.msu.edu/ysi/

North American Youth Sports Institute
www.naysi.com/

# Employment Settings for the Athletic Trainer

Opportunities for employment as an athletic trainer have changed dramatically during recent years. Athletic trainers no longer work only in athletic training clinics at the college, university, or secondary school level. The employment opportunities for athletic trainers are more diverse than ever. A discussion of the various employment settings follows.

## Clinics and Hospitals

Today, more than 40 percent of certified athletic trainers are employed in clinics and hospitals—more than in any other employment setting. The role of the athletic trainer varies from one clinic to the next. Athletic trainers may be employed in an outpatient ambulatory rehabilitation clinic working in general patient care, as health, wellness, or performance enhancement specialists, or as clinic administrators. Their job may also involve ergonomic assessment, working hardening, CPR training, or occasionally overseeing drug testing programs. They may also be employed by a hospital but work in a clinic. Other clinical athletic trainers see patients during the morning hours in the clinic. In the afternoons, athletic trainers' services are contracted out to local high schools or small colleges for practice, game, or single-event coverage. For the most part, private clinics have well-equipped facilities in which to work. In many sports medicine clinics, the athletic trainer may be responsible for formulating a plan to market or promote athletic training services offered by that clinic throughout the local community.

### Physician Extenders

Some athletic trainers work in clinics that are owned by physicians. While virtually all athletic trainers work under the direction of a physician, those employed as a physician extender actually work in the physician's office where patients of all ages and backgrounds are being treated. The educational preparation for athletic trainers allows them to function in a variety of domains, including injury prevention, evaluation, management and rehabilitation, health education, nutrition, training and conditioning, organizing preparticipation physicals, and maintaining essential documentation. While the contact with only the physically active population may not be as great as in other employment settings, the physician extender can expect regular hours, little weekend or evening responsibilities, opportunity for growth, and in general, better pay. All of these factors collectively make physician extender positions attractive for the athletic trainer. Potentially many new jobs could be created as physicians become more and more aware of the value that an athletic trainer, functioning as a physician extender, can provide to their medical practice.

## Industrial/Occupational Settings

It is becoming relatively common for industries to employ athletic trainers to oversee fitness and injury rehabilitation programs for their employees. The athletic trainer working in an industrial or occupational setting must have a sound understanding of the principles and concepts of workplace ergonomics, including inspecting, measuring, and observing dimensions of the work space, as well as specific tasks that are performed at the workstation. Once a problem has been identified, the athletic trainer must be able to implement proper adjustments to workplace ergonomics to reduce or minimize possible risks for injury. In addition to these responsibilities, athletic trainers may be assigned to conduct wellness programs and provide education and individual counseling. It is likely that many job opportunities will exist for the athletic trainer in corporate/industrial settings in the next few years.

## Corporate Settings

Opportunities are expanding for athletic trainers to use their educational background as preparation for working in business, sales, or marketing of products that other athletic trainers may use. Athletic trainers might also be employed by a company to administer health, wellness, and fitness programs, or perhaps to provide some patient care to their employees.

## Colleges or Universities

At the college or university level, clinical positions for athletic trainers vary considerably from institution to institution. In smaller institutions, the athletic trainer may be a half-time teacher in physical education and half-time athletic trainer. In some cases, if the athletic trainer is a physical therapist rather than a teacher, he or she may spend part of the time in the school health center and part of the time in athletic training. Increasingly at the college level, athletic training services are being offered to members of the general student body who participate in intramural and club sports. In most colleges and universities, the athletic trainer is full-time, does not teach, works in the department of athletics, and is paid by the institution.

Some athletic trainers working at colleges and universities are employed as faculty members. These individuals may or may not be assigned clinical responsibilities. In addition to faculty responsibilities it is most likely that these faculty members also serve as program directors and/or as researchers.

## Secondary Schools

It would be ideal to have certified athletic trainers serve every secondary school and middle school in the United States. Many of the physical problems that occur later from improperly managed sports injuries could be avoided initially if proper care from an athletic trainer had been provided. If a secondary school or middle school hires an athletic trainer, it is very often in a faculty–athletic trainer capacity. This individual is usually employed as a teacher in one of the school's classroom disciplines and performs athletic training duties on a part-time or extracurricular basis. Thus, student athletic trainers who hope to find a position in a secondary school setting should be encouraged to seek teacher certification. In this instance compensation usually is on the basis of released time from teaching, a stipend as a coach, or both. Salaries for the secondary school athletic trainer are continuing to improve. Another means of obtaining secondary school athletic training coverage is using a certified graduate student from a nearby college or university. The graduate student receives a graduate assistantship with a stipend paid by the secondary school or community college. In this situation both the graduate student and the school benefit. However, this practice may prevent a school from employing a certified athletic trainer on a full-time basis.

### School Districts

Some school districts have found it effective to employ a centrally placed certified athletic trainer. In this case the athletic trainer, who may be full- or part-time, fills a nonteaching position that serves a number of schools. The advantage is savings; the disadvantage is that one individual cannot provide the level of service usually required by a typical school.

## Professional Sports

Although positions for athletic trainers working at the professional level are limited, opportunities to work in this setting continue to expand. Virtually every professional team, regardless of the sport, employs at least one and occasionally as many as four certified athletic trainers. Athletic trainers work with both male and female professional teams including football, basketball, baseball, hockey, soccer, lacrosse, softball, golf, and tennis. They are also employed in professional rodeo, auto racing (NASCAR), and wrestling. The athletic trainer for professional sports teams usually performs specific team athletic training duties for six to eight months out of the year; the other four to six months are spent in off-season conditioning and individual rehabilitation. The athletic trainer working with a professional team is involved with only one sport and is paid according to contract, much like a player. Playoff and championship money may add to the yearly income.

## Amateur/Recreational/Youth Sport

Athletic trainers are working at all levels of amateur sport. The United States Olympic Committee employs athletic trainers and interns at three training centers. Every national governing body (NGB) for each of the Olympic sports employs either a single athletic trainer or a group of trainers to work with the national teams and developmental programs for younger athletes. Some municipal or community-based recreational programs either employ athletic trainers full time or as independent contractors to cover their programs. The Amateur Athletic Union (AAU) also employs athletic trainers to cover their tournaments.

## Performing Arts

A relatively new and expanding employment opportunity exists in the performing arts and entertainment industry. Athletic trainers can be found working with dance companies and theater performance groups. They are employed by Disney and the large casinos. Some touring bands even employ athletic trainers to work with their performers and road crew who sustain injuries while traveling.

## The Military/Law Enforcement/Government

The United States military, particularly the Navy, the Marines, and the Army, have demonstrated increased emphasis on injury prevention and health care for the troops. Treatment centers are being developed that closely resemble and, to a great extent, function as athletic training clinics. The centers are staffed by sports medicine physicians, orthopedists, athletic trainers, physical therapists, and support staff. Injured personnel are seen as soon as possible by an athletic trainer, who evaluates an injury, makes decisions on appropriate referral, and begins an immediate rehabilitation program. There are currently over 100 athletic trainers in the military either as active duty or reserve personnel. Occasionally some contract positions are available as well. It is likely that the role of the athletic trainer in the military will increase substantially over the next several years.

Opportunities are also increasing for athletic trainers to become involved with local, state, and federal law enforcement groups or agencies. Athletic trainers are working with police and firefighters as well as with agencies such as the FBI and ATF.

Other athletic trainers are employed by government agencies such as the United States Senate, NASA, and the Pentagon.

## Health and Fitness Clubs

It is likely that a significant number of job opportunities for athletic trainers will exist in health and fitness clubs. Some clubs may offer patient care but it is more likely that the athletic trainer will be a performance enhancement specialist or instructor. These clubs may be chains, franchises, or independent.

# Requirements for Certification as an Athletic Trainer

An athletic trainer who is certified by the Board of Certification (BOC) is a highly qualified paramedical professional educated and experienced in dealing with the injuries that occur with participation in sports. Candidates for certification are required to have an extensive background of both formal academic preparation and supervised practical experience in a clinical setting, according to JRC-AT guidelines. The guidelines listed in Focus Box A-1 have been established by the Board of Certification.

## THE CERTIFICATION EXAMINATION

Once the requirements have been fulfilled, applicants are eligible to sit for the certification examination. The certification examination is computer based and consists of three sections: a written portion, a practical portion, and a written-simulation portion. The examination tests for knowledge and skill in six major domains: (1) athletic injury prevention and risk management; (2) recognition, evaluation, and assessment of injuries; (3) immediate care of injuries and illnesses; (4) rehabilitation and reconditioning of athletic injuries; (5) health care organization and administration; and (6) professional development and responsibility. Successful performance on the certification exam leads to certification as an athletic trainer (ATC).

---

**A-1** ⟩ **Focus Box**

**Board of Certification Requirements for Certification as an Athletic Trainer**

Purpose of certification

The Board of Certification (BOC) was incorporated in 1989 to provide a certification program for entry-level athletic trainers and recertification standards for certified athletic trainers. The purpose of this entry-level certification program is to establish standards for entry into the profession of athletic training. Additionally, the BOC has established the continuing education requirements that a certified athletic trainer must satisfy to maintain current status as a BOC-certified athletic trainer.

The Process

Annually, the Board of Certification reviews the requirements for certification eligibility and standards for continuing education. Additionally, the Board reviews and revises the certification examination in accordance with the test specifications of the BOC Role Delineation Study that is reviewed and revised every five years.

---

A-1 ⟩ **Focus Box (continued)**

The Board of Certification uses a criterion-referenced passing point for the anchor form of the examination. Each new examination version is equated to the anchor version to ensure that candidates are not rewarded or penalized for taking different versions of the examination.

Procedures for certification

**Requirements for Candidacy for the BOC Certification Examination**

1. Candidates must successfully complete an entry-level athletic training program accredited by the Committee for Accreditation of Athletic Training Education (CAATE).

2. Proof of graduation (an official transcript) at the baccalaureate level from an accredited college or university located in the United States of America. Graduates of foreign universities may petition for a substitution of this degree requirement. Such a request will be evaluated at the candidate's expense by an independent consultant selected by the BOC.

    Students who have begun their last semester or quarter of college are permitted to apply to take the certification examination prior to graduation provided all academic and clinical requirements of the section used for candidacy have been satisfied. A candidate will be permitted to take the examination on the date closest to his or her date of graduation.

3. Endorsement of the examination application by the CAATE Accredited Program Director.

4. Proof of current certification in CPR (Note: CPR certification must be current at the time of initial application and at any subsequent exam retake registration.)

## CONTINUING EDUCATION REQUIREMENTS

To ensure ongoing professional growth and involvement by the certified athletic trainer, the BOC has established requirements for continuing education.[1] To maintain certification, all certified athletic trainers must document a minimum of 75 CEUs* attained during each 3-year recertification term. CEUs may be awarded for attending symposiums, seminars, workshops, or conferences; serving as a speaker, panelist, or certification exam model examiner; participating in the USOC program; authoring a research article in a professional journal; completing an NATA journal quiz; completing postgraduate course work; and obtaining CPR, first aid, or EMT certification. All certified athletic trainers must also demonstrate proof of CPR certification at least once during the 3-year term.

REFERENCES
1. Board of Certification
   http://www.bocatc.org/

*1 ceu = 1 contact hour

# Glossary

**abduction**   A movement of a body part away from the midline of the body

**accident**   An act that occurs by chance or without intention

**accommodating resistance**   Form of isokinetic exercises in which speed is an element

**acute injury**   An injury with sudden onset and short duration

**ad libitum**   In the amount desired

**adduction**   A movement of a body part toward the midline of the body

**afferent nerve fibers**   Nerve fibers that carry messages toward the brain

**agonist muscles**   Muscles directly engaged in contraction as related to muscles that relax at the same time

**ambulation**   Move or walk from place to place

**ameboid action**   A leukocyte moving through a capillary wall through the process of diapedisis

**amenorrhea**   Absence or suppression of menstruation

**amnesia**   Loss of memory

**analgesia**   Pain inhibition

**anaphylaxis**   An immediate transient allergic reaction resulting in swelling of tissues and dilation of capillaries

**anemia**   Lack of iron

**anesthesia**   Partial or complete loss of sensation

**angioedema**   A well-defined area of swelling occurring as a result of an allergic response

**anomaly**   Deviation from the norm

**anorexia**   Lack or loss of appetite; aversion to food

**anorexia nervosa**   Eating disorder characterized by a distorted body image

**anoxia**   Lack of oxygen

**antagonist muscles**   Muscles that counteract the action of the agonist muscles

**anterior**   Before or in front of

**anterior cruciate ligament**   Stops external rotation

**anteroposterior**   Refers to the position of front to back

**anxiety**   A feeling of uncertainty or apprehension

**apophysis**   A bone outgrowth to which muscles attach

**arrhythmical movement**   Irregular movement

**arthroscopic examination**   Viewing the inside of a joint via the arthroscope, which utilizes a small camera lens

**articulation**   A joint

**assumption of risk**   The individual, through expressed or implied agreement, assumes some risk or danger will be involved in a particular undertaking

**asymmetries (body)**   A lack of symmetry of sides of the body

**ATC**   An athletic trainer certified by the Board of Certification

**atrophic necrosis**   Death of an area due to lack of circulation

**atrophy**   Wasting away of tissue or of an organ; diminution of the size of a body part

**automatism**   Automatic behavior before consciousness or full awareness has been achieved following a brain concussion

**avascular necrosis**   Death of tissue resulting from a lack of blood supply

**avulsion**   A tearing away

**axial loading**   A blow to the top of the athlete's head while in flexion

**axilla**   Armpit

**ballistic stretching**   Older stretching technique that uses repetitive bouncing motions

**bandage**   A strip of cloth or other material used to hold a dressing in place

**bilateral**   Pertaining to both sides

**biomechanics**   Branch of study that applies the laws of mechanics to living organisms and biological tissues

**bipedal**   Having two feet or moving on two feet

**body composition**   Percent body fat plus lean body weight

**boil (furuncle)**   A staph infection originating in a hair follicle

**bowlegged**   Bending outward of the lower joint

**bradykinin**   Peptide chemical that causes pain in an injured area

**bulimia**   Binge-purge eating disorder

**bursae**   Pieces of synovial membrane that contain a small amount of fluid

**bursitis**   Inflammation of a bursa, especially those bursae located between bony prominences and a muscle or tendon, such as those of the shoulder or knee

**calcific tendinitis**   Deposition of calcium in a chronically inflamed tendon, especially the tendons of the shoulder

**calisthenic**   Exercise involving free movement without the aid of equipment

**callus**   New bone formation over a fracture

**calorie (large)**   Amount of heat required to raise 1 kg of water 1° C; term used to express the fuel or energy value of food or the heat output of the organism; the amount of heat required to heat 1 lb of water to 4° F

**catastrophic injury**   A permanent injury to the spinal cord that leaves the athlete quadriplegic or paraplegic

**cauterization**   A purposeful destruction of tissue

**cerebrovascular accident**   Stroke

**chondromalacia**   A degeneration of a joint's articular surface, leading to softening

**chronic injury**   An injury with long onset and long duration

**circuit training**   Exercise stations that consist of various combinations of weight training, flexibility, calisthenics, and aerobic exercises

**circumduct**   Act of moving a limb such as the arm or hip in a circular motion

**clavus durum**   Hard corn

**clavus molle**   Soft corn

**clonic muscle cramp**   Involuntary muscle contraction marked by alternate contraction and relaxation in rapid succession

**closed fracture**   Fracture that does not penetrate superficial tissue

**collagenous tissue**   The white fibrous substance composing connective tissue

**collision sport**   Sport in which athletes use their bodies to deter or punish opponents

**commission (legal liability)**   Performing an act outside of an individual's legal jurisdiction

**communicable disease**   A disease that may be transmitted directly or indirectly from one individual to another

**concentric (positive) contraction**   The muscle shortens while contracting against resistance

**conduction**   Heating by direct contact with a hot medium

**conjunctivae**   Mucous membrane that lines the eyes

**contact sport**   Athletes make physical contact, but not with the intent to produce bodily injury

**contrecoup brain injury**   After head is struck, brain continues to move within the skull and becomes injured opposite the force

**convection**   Heating indirectly through another medium, such as air or liquid

**conversion**   Heating by other forms of energy (e.g., electricity)

**convulsions**   Paroxysms of involuntary muscular contractions and relaxations

**core temperature**   Internal, or deep body, temperature monitored by cells in the hypothalamus, as opposed to shell, or peripheral, temperature, which is registered by the layer of insulation provided by the skin, subcutaneous tissues, and superficial portions of the muscle masses

**corticosteroid**   A steroid produced by the adrenal cortex

**coryza**   Profuse nasal discharge

**counterirritant**   An agent that produces a mild inflammation and in turn acts as an analgesic when applied locally to the skin (e.g., liniment)

**crepitus**   A crackling feel or sound

**cryokinetics**   Cold application combined with exercise

**cryotherapy**   Cold therapy

**cubital fossa**   Triangular area on the anterior aspect of the forearm directly opposite the elbow joint (the bend of the elbow)

**cutaneous**   Of or pertaining to the skin

**cyanosis**   Slightly bluish, grayish, slatelike, or dark purple discoloration of the skin due to a reduced amount of blood hemoglobin

**debride**   Removal of dirt and dead tissue from a wound

**deconditioning**   A state in which the athlete's body loses its competitive fitness

**degeneration**   Deterioration of tissue

**dermatome**   A segmental skin area innervated by various spinal cord segments

**diapedisis**   Passage of blood cells by ameboid action through the intact capillary wall

**diaphragm**   A musculomembranous wall separating the abdomen from the thoracic cavity

**diarthrodial joint**   Ball and socket joint

**diastolic blood pressure**   The residual pressure when the heart is between beats

**diplopia**   Seeing double

**dislocation**   A bone is forced out and stays out until surgically or manually replaced or reduced

**distal**   Farthest away from a point of reference

**doping**   The administration of a drug that is designed to improve the competitor's performance

**dorsiflexion**   Bending toward the dorsum or rear, opposite of plantar flexion

**dorsum**   The back of a body part

**dressing**   A material, such as gauze, applied to a wound

**duration**   Length of time that an athlete works during a bout of exercise

**duty of care** An individual who has the responsibility of caring for an injury

**dysmenorrhea** Painful or difficult menstruation

**dyspepsia** Imperfect digestion

**dyspnea** Difficulty in breathing

**eccentric (negative) contraction** The muscle lengthens while contracting against resistance

**ecchymosis** Black and blue skin discoloration due to hemorrhage

**ectopic** Located in a place different from normal

**ectopic bone formation** Bone formation occurring in an abnormal place

**edema** Swelling as a result of the collection of fluid in connective tissue

**electrolyte** Solution that is a conductor of electricity

**electrotherapy** Treating disease by electrical devices

**embolus** Fat or plaque that migrates through the vascular system

**encephalon** The brain

**endurance** The ability of the body to undergo prolonged activity

**entrapment** Organ becomes compressed by nearby tissue

**epidemiological approach** The study of sports injuries involving the relationship of as many injury factors as possible

**epilepsy** Recurrent paroxysmal disorder characterized by sudden attacks of altered consciousness, motor activity, and sensory perception

**epiphysis** The cartilagenous growth region of a bone

**epistaxis** Nosebleed

**etiology** Pertaining to the cause of a condition

**eversion of the foot** To turn the foot outward

**exostoses** Benign bony outgrowths that protrude from the surface of a bone and are usually capped by cartilage; callus formations

**extraoral mouth guard** A protective device that fits outside the mouth

**extravasation** Escape of a fluid from its vessels into the surrounding tissues

**exudates** Accumulation of a fluid in an area

**fascia** Fibrous membrane that covers, supports, and separates muscles

**fasciitis** Fascia inflammation

**fibrinogen** A protein present in blood plasma that is converted into a fibrin clot

**fibroblast** Any cell component from which fibers are developed

**fibrocartilage** A type of cartilage in which the matrix contains thick bundles of collagenous fibers (e.g., intervertebral disks)

**fibrosis** Development of excessive fibrous connective tissue; fibroid degeneration

**flash-to-bang method** Provides an estimation of how far away lightning is occurring

**folliculitis** Inflammation of hair follicles

**foot pronation** Combined foot movements of eversion and abduction

**foot supination** Combined foot movements of inversion and abduction

**frequency** Number of times per week that an athlete exercises

**genitourinary** Pertaining to the reproductive and urinary organs

**genu recurvatus** Hyperextension at the knee joint

**genu valgum** Knock knees

**genu varum** Bow legs

**glycogen supercompensation** High carbohydrate diet

**good samaritan law** Provides limited protection to someone who voluntarily chooses to provide first aid

**hemarthrosis** Blood in a joint cavity

**hematoma** Blood tumor

**hematuria** Blood in the urine

**hemoglobin** Molecules that carry oxygen in the blood

**hemoglobinuria** Hemoglobin in the urine

**hemophilia** A hereditary blood disease in which coagulation is greatly prolonged

**hemorrhage** Discharge of blood

**hemothorax** Bloody fluid in the pleural cavity

**hirsutism** Excessive hair growth and/or the presence of hair in unusual places

**homeostasis** Maintenance of a steady state in the body's internal environment

**hyperemia** An unusual amount of blood in a body part

**hyperextension** Extreme stretching out of a body part

**hyperflexibility** Flexibility beyond a joint's normal range

**hyperhidrosis** Excessive sweating; excessive foot perspiration

**hypermobility** Mobility of a joint that is extreme

**hypertension** High blood pressure; abnormally high tension

**hyperthermia** Increased body temperature

**hypertonic** Having a higher osmotic pressure than a compared solution

**hypertrophy** Enlargement of a part caused by an increase in the size of its cells

**hyperventilation** Abnormally deep breathing that is prolonged, causing a depletion of carbon dioxide, a fall in blood pressure, and fainting

**hypoallergenic**  Low allergy producing

**hypothermia**  Decreased body temperature

**hypoxia**  Lack of an adequate amount of oxygen

**idiopathic**  Of unknown cause

**iliotibal band friction syndrome**  Runner's knee

**impetigo**  A bacterial strep infection

**injury**  An act that damages or hurts

**innervation**  Nerve stimulation of a muscle

**integument**  A covering or skin

**intensity**  Increasing the work-load

**interosseous membrane**  Connective tissue membrane between bones

**interval training**  Alternating periods of work with active recovery

**intervertebral**  Between two vertebrae

**intramuscular bleeding**  Bleeding within a muscle

**intraoral mouth guard**  A protective device that fits within the mouth and covers the teeth

**intravenous**  Substances administered to a patient via a vein

**inversion of the foot**  To turn the foot inward. Inner border of the foot lifts

**ions**  Electrically charged atoms

**ipsilateral**  Situated on the same side

**ischemia**  Local anemia

**isokinetic exercise**  Resistance is given at a fixed velocity of movement with accommodating resistance

**isokinetic muscle resistance**  Accommodating and variable resistance

**isometric exercise**  Contracts the muscle statically without changing its length

**isometric muscle contraction**  Muscle contracts statically without a change in its length

**isosceles triangle**  Triangle with two sides equal in length

**isotonic exercise**  Form of exercise that shortens and lengthens the muscle through a complete range of motion

**isotonic muscle contraction**  Shortens and lengthens the muscle through a complete range of motion

**joint**  Point at which two bones join together

**joint capsule**  Saclike structure that encloses the ends of bones in a diarthrodial joint

**keloid**  An overgrowth of collagenous scar tissue at the site of a wound of the skin

**keratolytic**  Pertaining to loosening the horny layer of skin

**knock knee**  Bending inward of the lower joint

**kyphosis**  Exaggeration of the normal thoracic spine

**labile**  Unsteady; not fixed; easily changed

**lactase deficiency**  Difficulty digesting dairy products

**lateral**  Pertaining to point of reference away from the midline of the body

**liability**  Legal responsibility for the harm one causes to another person

**lordosis**  Abnormal lumbar vertebral convexity

**luxation**  Total dislocation

**lysis**  Breakdown

**macerated skin**  Skin softened by soaking

**malaise**  Discomfort and uneasiness caused by an illness

**malfeasance or an act of commission**  Where an individual commits an act that is not legally theirs to perform

**managed care**  Costs of health care are monitored closely by insurance carriers

**margination**  Accumulation of leukocytes on blood vessel walls at the site of injury during early stages of inflammation

**mechanoreceptors**  Located in muscles, tendons, ligaments, and joints; provide information on position of a joint

**medial**  Pertaining to point of reference closest to the midline of the body

**medical insurance**  A contract between the insurance company and policy holder

**menarche**  Onset of menses

**meninges**  Any one of the three membranes that enclose the brain and the spinal cord, comprising the dura mater, the pia mater, and the arachnoid

**menorrhagia**  Abnormally heavy or long menstrual periods

**metabolites**  Products left after metabolism has taken place

**metatarsalgia**  Pain in the metatarsal

**metatarsophalangeal joint**  Joint at which the phalanges meet the metatarsal bones

**microtrauma**  Small musculoskeletal traumas that are accumulative

**misfeasance**  When an individual improperly does something he or she has the legal right to do

**mononucleosis (infectious)**  A disease, usually of young adults, causing fever, sore throat, and lymph gland swelling

**muscle**  Tissue that when stimulated contracts and produces motion

**muscle contracture**  Abnormal shortening of muscle tissue in which there is a great deal of resistance to passive stretch

**muscle cramps**  Involuntary muscle contractions

**muscle guarding** Muscle contraction in response to pain

**muscular endurance** The ability to perform repetitive muscular contractions against some resistance

**muscular strength** The maximum force that can be applied by a muscle during a single maximum contraction

**musculoskeletal** Pertaining to muscles and the skeleton

**myoglobin** A respiratory pigment in muscle tissue that is an oxygen carrier

**myositis** Inflammation of muscle

**myositis ossificans** Calcium deposits that result from repeated trauma

**myotatic reflex** Stretch reflex

**necrosis** Death of tissue

**negative resistance** Slow eccentric muscle contraction against resistance with muscle lengthening

**negligence** The failure to use ordinary or reasonable care

**nerve entrapment** A nerve that is compressed between bone or soft tissue

**neuritis** Chronic nerve irritation

**neuroma** Enlargement of a nerve

**NOCSAE** National Operating Committee on Standards for Athletic Equipment

**noncontact sport** Athletes are not involved in any physical contact

**nonfeasance or an act of omission** Where an individual fails to perform a legal duty

**nystagmus** A constant involuntary back and forth, up and down, or rotary movement of the eyeball

**occlusion** Alignment of the teeth; malocclusion means that the upper and lower teeth do not line up

**omission (legal)** Person fails to perform a legal duty

**open fracture** Overlying skin has been lacerated by protruding bone fragments

**orthosis** Used in sports as an appliance or apparatus to support, align, prevent, or correct deformities or to improve function of a movable body part

**orthotic** A custom-designed insert that can be placed in the shoe and worn to correct a variety of biomechanical abnormalities that can potentially lead to injury

**osteoarthritis** A wearing down of hyaline cartilage

**osteoblasts** Bone-forming cells

**osteochondral** Refers to relationship of bone and cartilage

**osteochondritis** Inflammation of bone and cartilage

**osteochondritis dissecans** Fragment of cartilage and underlying bone is detached from the articular surface

**osteochondrosis** A disease state of a bone and its articular cartilage

**osteoclasts** Cells that absorb and remove osseous tissue

**osteoporosis** A decrease in bone density

**palpate** To use the hands or fingers to examine

**palpation** Feeling an injury with the fingers

**papule** Pimple

**paraplegia** Paralysis of lower portion of the body and of both legs

**paresthesia** Abnormal sensation such as numbness, prickling, and tingling

**patellar tendinitis** Jumper's knee

**pathology** Study of the nature and cause of disease

**pediatrician** A specialist in the treatment of children's diseases

**periodization** Varying training techniques during different seasons

**periosteum** The fibrous covering of a bone

**peristalis** A progressive, wavelike movement that occurs in the alimentary canal

**pes planus** Flat feet

**phagocytosis** Process of ingesting microorganisms, other cells, or foreign particles, commonly by monocytes, or white blood cells

**phalanges** Bones of the fingers and toes

**phalanx** Any one of the bones of the fingers and toes

**photophobia** An intense intolerance of light

**plantarflexion** The forepart of the foot is depressed relative to the ankle

**plica** A fold of tissue within the body

**plyometric exercise** Uses a quick eccentric stretch of the muscle to facilitate a concentric contraction

**pneumothorax** A collapse of a lung due to air in the pleural cavity

**point tenderness** Pain is produced when the site of injury is palpated

**polymers** Natural or synthetic substances formed by the combination of two or more molecules of the same substance

**positive resistance** Slow concentric muscle contraction against resistance with muscle shortening

**posterior** Toward the rear or back

**posterior cruciate ligament** A ligament that stops internal rotation

**posttraumatic amnesia** Inability of athlete to recall events since injury

**power** Ability to accelerate a load, depending on the level of strength and velocity of a muscle contraction

**primary assessment** Initial first aid evaluation

**prophylactic** Pertaining to prevention, preservation, or protection

**prophylaxis** Guarding against injury or disease

**proprioceptive neuromuscular facilitation (PNF)** Stretching techniques that involve combinations of alternating contractions and stretches

**proprioceptors** Organs within the body that provide the athlete with an awareness of where the body is in space (kinesthesis)

**prostaglandin** Acidic lipids widely distributed in the body; in musculoskeletal conditions it is concerned with vasodilation; it has a histaminelike effect; it is inhibited by aspirin

**prothrombin** Interacts with calcium to produce thrombin

**proximal** Nearest to the point of reference

**psychogenic** Of psychic origin; that which originates in the mind

**psychophysiological** Involving the mind and the body

**psychosomatic** Showing effects of mind-body relationship; physical disorder caused or influenced by the mind (i.e., by the emotions)

**quadriplegia** Paralysis affecting all four limbs

**referred pain** Pain that is felt at a point of the body other than its actual origin

**regeneration** Repair, regrowth, or restoration of a part such as tissue

**residual** That which remains; often used to describe a permanent condition resulting from injury or disease (e.g., a limp or a paralysis)

**resorption** Act of removal by absorption

**retrograde amnesia** Memory loss for events occurring immediately before trauma

**revascularize** Restoration of blood circulation to an injured area

**rhinitis** Inflammation of the nasal mucus lining

**RICE** Rest, ice, compression, and elevation

**rotation** Turning around an axis in an angular motion

**SAID principle** Specific adaptations to imposed demands

**Scheuermann's disease (osteochondrosis)** A degeneration of the vertebral epiphyseal endplates

**sciatica** Inflammatory condition of the sciatic nerve; commonly associated with peripheral nerve root compression

**sclera** White outer coating of the eye

**scoliosis** A lateral deviation curve of the spine

**secondary assessment** Follow up; a more detailed examination

**seizure** Sudden attack

**shin splints** Medial tibial stress syndrome; anterior lower leg pain

**sign** Objective evidence of an abnormal situation within the body

**sling psychrometer** Instrument for establishing the wet-bulb, globe temperature index

**spasm** A sudden, involuntary muscle contraction

**spica** A figure-eight, with one of the two loops being larger

**spondylolisthesis** Forward slipping of a vertebral body, usually a lumbar vertebra

**spondylolysis** A degeneration of the vertebrae and a defect in the pars intermedia of the articular processes of the vertebrae

**sprain** Injury to a ligament that connects bone to bone

**staleness** Deterioration in the usual standard of performance

**standard of reasonable care** Assumes that an individual is a person of reasonable and ordinary prudence

**staphylococcus** A genus of micrococci, some of which are pathogenic, causing pus and tissue destruction

**static stretching** Passively stretching an antagonist muscle by placing it in a maximal stretch position and holding it there

**statute of limitation** A specific length of time to sue for damages from negligence

**strain** A stretch tear, or rip in the muscle or its tendon

**strength** Ability of a muscular contraction to exert force to move an object (dynamic) or to perform work against a fixed object (static)

**streptococcus** Oval bacteria that appear in a chain

**stress** The positive and negative forces that can disrupt the body's equilibrium

**stress fracture** Spot of irritation on the bone

**stressor** Anything that affects the body's physiological or psychological condition

**stroke volume** The heart's capacity to pump blood

**subcutaneous** Beneath the skin

**subluxation** A bone is forced out but goes back into place

**subthreshold** Below the point at which a physiological effect begins to be produced

**symptom** Subjective evidence of an abnormal situation within the body

**syndrome** Group of typical symptoms or conditions that

characterize an injury, a deficiency, or a disease

**synergy** To work in cooperation with

**synovia** A transparent lubricating fluid found in joints, bursae, and tendons

**synovitis** Inflammation of a synovial membrane

**synthesis** Buildup

**systolic blood pressure** The pressure caused by the heart's pumping

**tendinitis** Inflammation of the tendon

**tendon** Tough band of connective tissue that attaches muscle to bone

**tennis leg** Strain of the gastrocnemius muscle

**tenosynovitis** Inflammation of a tendon and its synovial sheath

**tetanus toxoid** Tetanus toxin modified to produce active immunity against *Clostridium tetani*

**thrombi** Plural of thrombus

**thromboplastin** Substance within the body's tissues that accelerates blood clotting

**thrombus** Blood clot that blocks small blood vessels or a cavity of the heart

**time-loss injuries** Injuries that require the player to suspend activity within a day of an injury's onset

**tinea** Ringworm; skin fungus disease

**tonic muscle cramp** Continuous muscle contraction that is long in duration

**tonic muscle spasm** Rigid muscle contraction that lasts over a period of time

**tonus (muscle)** Residual state of muscle contraction

**torque** A twisting force produced by contraction of the medial femoral muscles that tends to rotate the thigh medially

**torsional** Rotating or twisting of a body part

**tort** Legal wrong committed against another

**training effect** Stroke volume increases while heart rate is reduced at a given exercise load

**transitory paralysis** Temporary inability to move

**traumatic** Pertaining to the course of an injury or wound

**traumatic arthritis** Arthritis stemming from repeated joint injury

**traumatic asphyxia** Result of a violent blow to, or compression of, the rib cage, causing cessation of breathing

**trigger point** Area of tenderness in a tight band of muscle

**urticaria** Sudden vascular reaction of skin resulting in weals or papules and itching

**valgus** Bent outward

**variable resistance** Resistance is varied throughout the range of motion

**varus** Bent inward

**vasoconstriction** Decrease in the diameter of a blood vessel

**vasodilation** Increase in the diameter of a blood vessel

**vasospasm** Blood vessel spasm

**venule** Tiny vein fed by a capillary

**verruca** Virus causing a wart

**viscera** Internal organs

**viscus (organs)** Any internal organ enclosed within a cavity

**volar** Referring to the palm or the sole

**water ad libitum** Unlimited access to water

**xerostomia** Having a dry mouth

**xiphoid process** Smallest of three parts of the sternum

# Credits

## Chapter 2

**Focus Box 2-5,** from *NCAA Sports Medicine Handbook 2000–2001;* **Figs. 2-1, 2-2,** Used with permission from *The Physician and Sports Medicine;* **Fig. 2-3,** Courtesy: D. Bailey, California State University at Long Beach.

## Chapter 3

**Fig. 3-2,** Courtesy: The University of North Carolina at Chapel Hill.

## Chapter 4

**Figs. 4-2A&B, 4-50,** From Prentice, WE: *Arnheim's Principles of Athletic Training,* ed. 13, New York, NY: McGraw-Hill, 2009; **Fig. 4-21,** Courtesy of Cybex; **Figs. 4-35 through 4-38, Figs. 4-44 through 4-45,** From Prentice, WE: *Rehabilitation techniques for sports medicine and athletic training,* ed. 4, New York, NY: McGraw-Hill, 2004; **Fig. 4-48,** Courtesy of Biodex.

## Chapter 5

**Fig. 5-2,** from Prentice, WE: *Get Fit Stay Fit,* ed. 5, New York, NY: McGraw-Hill, 2009; **Fig. 5-3,** U.S. Department of Agriculture, Center for Nutrition Policy and Promotion, April 2005, CNPP-16.

## Chapter 6

**Figs. 6-1, C&D, 6-3, 6-4B, 6-6, 6-8, 6-9, 6-11 through 6-14, 6-16 B, 6-17 A-C, 6-19, 6-20, 6-22,** Courtesy Sports Authority (www.sportsauthority.com); **Figs. 6-15 through 6-16A,** From Nicholas, JA, Hershman, EB: *The lower extremity and spine in sports medicine,* ed. 2, St. Louis: Mosby, 1993; **Fig. 6-17D,** Courtesy TKO; **Figs. 6-27, 6-29A-D,** Courtesy, Mueller Sports Medicine; **Figs. 6-29E,** From Prentice, WE:

*Arnheim's Principles of Athletic Training,* ed. 13, New York, NY: McGraw-Hill, 2009.

## Chapter 7

**Fig. 7-19,** Courtesy, Neann, Victoria, Australia.

## Chapter 8

**Focus Box 8-1,** From Payne, WA, Hahn, DB: *Understanding Your Health,* ed. 9, New York, NY: McGraw-Hill, 2007; **Fig. 8-5A,** © Tierbild Okapia/Photo Researchers, Inc.; **Fig. 8-5B&C,** Dr. P Marazzi/Photo Researchers, Inc.; **Fig. 8-5D,** © NMSB/Custom Medical Stock Photo, Inc.

## Chapter 9

**Table 9-2,** Modified from Berkow, R: *The Merck manual of diagnosis and therapy,* ed. 14, Rahway; **Fig. 9-1,** Courtesy National Weather Center; **9-2,** Courtesy Borreal Laboratory, Tonawonda, NY; **Fig. 9-4,** Courtesy Nova Lynx, Green Valley, CA.

## Chapter 10

**Figure 10-1,** From Prentice, WE: *Arnheim's Principles of Athletic Training,* ed. 13, New York, NY: McGraw-Hill, 2009.

## Chapter 13

**Figs. 13-1 – 13-3, 13-5,** Saladin, KS: *Anatomy and Physiology,* ed. 3, Dubuque, IA: McGraw-Hill 2004; **Fig. 13-7,** Courtesy Chris Bartlett, Central Davidson High School, Lexington, NC; **Fig. 13-10,** Courtesy Zimmer, Inc.; **Fig. 13-12,** From McKinley, M & O'Loughlin, V: *Human Anatomy,* ed. 1, New York: McGraw-Hill Higher Education, 2006.

## Chapter 14

**Fig. 14-1,** From Van De Graaf, K: *Human Anatomy,* ed. 6, Dubuque, IA: McGraw-Hill Higher Education, 2002; **Figs. 14-3, 14-7** From Prentice, WE: *Arnheim's Principles of Athletic Training,* ed. 13, New York, NY: McGraw-Hill, 2009; **Fig. 14-8,** Courtesy Arun Shanghag; **Figs. 14-4 through 14-5,** From Thompson, CW and Floyd, RT: *Manual of Structural Kinesiology,* ed. 15, Dubuque, IA: McGraw-Hill 2004; **Fig. 14-17,** Courtesy Myfootshop.com; **Fig. 14-18,** From Habif, TP: *Clinical dermatology,* ed. 3, St. Louis: Mosby, 1996.

## Chapter 15

**Figs. 15-2 through 15-3,** From Saladin, KS: *Anatomy and Physiology,* ed. 3, Dubuque, IA: McGraw-Hill 2004; **Fig. 15-7,** Courtesy Cramer Products, Garder, KS; **Figs. 15-8, 15-14C, 15-19,** From Prentice, WE: *Arnheim's Principles of Athletic Training,* ed. 13, New York, NY: McGraw-Hill, 2009; **Fig. 15-17,** Courtesy, Cramer Products, Gardner, KS; **Fig. 15-18,** From Williams, JPG: *Color Atlas of Injury in Sport,* ed. 2, Chicago, IL: Yearbook Medical Publishers, 1990.

## Chapter 16

**Figs. 16-1, 16-3, 16-16, 16-17,** From Saladin, KS: *Anatomy and Physiology,* ed. 3, Dubuque, IA: McGraw-Hill 2004; **Fig. 16-18,** From Van De Graaff, K: *Human anatomy,* ed. 6, Dubuque, IA: McGraw-Hill Higher Education, 2002; **Fig. 16-22,** Cramer Products, Garder, KS.

## Chapter 17

**Figs. 17-1 through 17-5,** From Saladin, KS: *Anatomy and Physiology,* ed. 3,

Dubuque, IA: McGraw-Hill, 2004; **Figs. 17-6 through 17-7, 17-9B,** From Prentice, WE: *Arnheim's Principles of Athletic Training,* ed. 13, New York, NY: McGraw-Hill, 2009; **Fig. 17-8,** Courtesy Ken Bartlett, California State University at Long Beach; **Fig. 17-10,** From Williams, JPG: *Color Atlas of Injury in Sport,* ed. 2, Chicago, IL: Yearbook Medical Publishers, 1990; **Fig. 17-16,** Courtesy BRACE International, Phoenix, AZ; **Fig. 17-19,** Courtesy Robert Barclay and Renee Reavis Shingles, Central Michigan University; **Fig. 17-20,** Courtesy Scott Barker, California State University—Chico.

## Chapter 18

**Figs. 18-2 through 18-4, 18-20,** From Saladin, KS: *Anatomy and Physiology,* ed. 3, Dubuque, IA: McGraw-Hill 2004; **Fig. 18-5,** From Nicholas, JA and Hershman, EB: *The upper extremity in sports medicine,* ed. 2, St. Louis: Mosby; **Figs. 18-6, 18-16A, 18-19,** From Prentice, WE: *Arnheim's Principles of Athletic Training,* ed. 13, New York, NY: McGraw-Hill, 2009; **Fig. 18-18,** Art by Don O'Conner.

## Chapter 19

**Figs. 19-1 through 19-2, 19-10 through 19-11, 19-13 through 19-15,** From Saladin, KS: *Anatomy and Physiology,* ed. 3, Dubuque, IA: McGraw-Hill 2004; **Fig. 19-19 through 19-22A, 19-24,** From Nicholas, JA and Hershman, EB: *The upper extremity in sports medicine,* ed. 2, St. Louis: Mosby; **Fig. 19-6B,** Gallaspy, J: *Sights and Symptoms of Athletic Injury,* ed. 1, New York; McGraw-Hill, 1996; **Figs. 19-8, 19-16 through 19-17,19-23,** From

Prentice, WE: *Arnheim's Principles of Athletic Training,* ed. 13, New York, NY: McGraw-Hill, 2009; **Fig. 19-12,** From Booher, JM and Thibodeau, GA: *Athletic Training Injury Assessment,* ed. 4, Dubuque, IA: McGraw-Hill, 2000.

## Chapter 20

**Fig. 20-1,** From Van De Graaf, K: *Human Anatomy,* ed. 6, Dubuque, IA: McGraw-Hill Higher Education, 2002; **Figs. 20-2, through 20-6, 20-8,** From Saladin, KS: *Anatomy and Physiology,* ed. 3, Dubuque, IA: McGraw-Hill 2004; **Figs. 20-7, 20-17, 20-18A,** From McKinley, M & O'Loughlin, V: *Human Anatomy,* ed. 1, New York: McGraw-Hill Higher Education, 2006; **Fig. 20-9,** From Seeley, RR, Stephens, TD, Tate, P: *Anatomy & physiology,* ed. 7, New York, NY: McGraw-Hill 2006; **Fig. 20-10,** Art by Donald O'Connor; **Fig. 20-20B,** From Williams, JPG: *Color Atlas of Injury in Sport,* ed. 2, Chicago, IL: Yearbook Medical Publishers, 1990.

## Chapter 21

**Fig. 21-2, 21-4 through 21-5,** From Saladin, KS: *Anatomy and Physiology,* ed. 3, Dubuque, IA: McGraw-Hill 2004; **Fig. 21-3,** From Seeley, RR, Stephens, TD, Tate, P: *Anatomy & physiology,* ed. 7, New York, NY: McGraw-Hill 2006; **Fig. 21-9, 21-13A,** From McKinley, M & O'Loughlin, V: *Human Anatomy,* ed. 1, New York: McGraw-Hill Higher Education, 2006; **Fig. 21-12 A,** Modified from Carola R, Harley JP, Noback, CR: *Human Anatomy,* ed. 1, New York, NY: McGraw-Hill, 1992; **Fig. 21-13B,** modified from Saladin, KS: *Anatomy and Physiology,* ed. 3, Dubuque, IA: McGraw-Hill 2004.

## Chapter 22

**Fig. 22-1, 22-12, 22-14,** From Saladin, KS: *Anatomy and Physiology,* ed. 3, Dubuque, IA: McGraw-Hill, 2004; **Fig. 22-3,** from Prentice, WE: *Rehabilitation techniques for sports medicine and athletic training,* ed. 4, Dubuque, IA: McGraw-Hill 2004; **Fig. 22-4 through 22-7B, 22-15,** From Prentice, WE: *Arnheim's Principles of Athletic Training,* ed. 13, New York, NY: McGraw-Hill, 2009; **Fig. 22-8,** From National Safety Council, *First Aid: Taking Action,* ed. 1, New York: McGraw-Hill Higher Education, 2007; **Fig. 22-9,** From McKinley, M & O'Loughlin, V: *Human Anatomy,* ed. 1, New York: McGraw-Hill Higher Education, 2006; **Fig. 22-10A-C,** From Seeley, RR, Stephens, TD, and Tate, P: *Anatomy and physiology,* ed. 8, New York: McGraw-Hill Higher Education, 2008; **Fig. 22-10D, 22-13,** From Williams, JPG: *Color Atlas of Injury in Sport,* ed. 2, Chicago, IL: Yearbook Medical Publishers, 1990; **Fig. 22-11,** Photo Courtesy of the contributor, Wikipedia user Rls.

## Chapter 23

**Table 23-3,** Modified from American College Health Association: Making sex safer, Baltimore: American College Health Association, 1990; **Fig. 23-2, 23-3 A&B, 23-5,** From Habif, TP: *Clinical dermatology,* ed. 3, St. Louis: Mosby, 1996; **Fig. 23-4,** Courtesy of MetroWest CleanGear Group; **Fig. 23-3,** From Stewart WP, Danito, JL, Madden, S: *Dermatology: diagnosis and treatment of cutaneous disorders,* ed. 4, St. Louis: The CV Mosby Co., 1978; **Fig. 23-4,** From Prentice, WE: *Arnheim's Principles of Athletic Training,* ed. 13, New York, NY: McGraw-Hill, 2009.

# Index